BEHAVIOR CHANGE CONTRACT

My behavior change: _____

1. Three important short-term benefits I've discovered from my research about my behavior change are:
   1. _____
   2. _____
   3. _____

2. My SMART goal for this behavior change is:
   _____
   _____
   _____

3. Keeping my current stage of behavior change in mind, these short-term goals and rewards will make my SMART goal more attainable:

Short-term goal	Target date	Reward
_____	_____	_____
Short-term goal	Target date	Reward
_____	_____	_____
Short-term goal	Target date	Reward

4. Barriers I anticipate to making this behavior change are:
   1. _____
   2. _____
   3. _____

   The strategies I will use to overcome these barriers are:
   1. _____
   2. _____
   3. _____

5. Resources I will use to help me change this behavior include:
   a friend, partner, or relative: _____
   a school-based resource:_____
   a health-care resource: _____
   a community-based resource: _____
   a book or reputable website: _____

6. When I achieve the long-term behavior change described above, my reward will be:
   _____   _____
   Reward   Target date

7. I intend to make the behavior change described above. I will use the strategies and rewards above to achieve the goals that will contribute to a healthy behavior change.

Signed: _____

CHOOSING HEALTH'S
STUDENT ADVISORY BOARD

96 Student Story Contributors   **1750** Student Class Testers!   **175** Student Advisory Board Members

We would like to thank the following students at: University of California at Berkeley, Stanford University, East Carolina University, Central Piedmont Community College, East Mecklenburg High School, The University of Texas at Austin, New York University, University of Pennsylvania, University of Texas at San Antonio, Clemson University, University of Massachusetts at Amherst, University of Windsor, The University of Alabama at Birmingham, University of Florida, University of Central Florida, Franklin W. Olin College of Engineering, University of Ottawa, University of Michigan, Palm Beach State College, Vanderbilt University, San Francisco State University, University of California at Davis, California Polytechnic State University San Luis Obispo, and Georgia Southern University for their help in developing the text and media for *Choosing Health*.

Warren Adderley	Joshua Cole	Amanda Jane Holland	Michelle McGovern	Christopher Sorianao
Stephany Aguilar	Michael Cooper	Caleb Hopkins	Katherine McGrath	Bryon Spencer
Anuella Alexander	Joan Craig	Allison Huberlie	Courtney A. Meier	Demauria Arielle Squires
Raquel Alleyne	Lorriane Crook	Curt Hughes	Madonna Messana	Jessica Stark
Samantha Alridge-Taylor	Molly Crowther	Amanda Humphrey	Chris Morris	Brandon J. Staton
Miroslava Alvarado	Logan Cuddington	Holly Christine Ipock	Cody Morris	Corinne Steiner
Erika Amaya	Viege Delva	Seresa'u Ivey	Christy Nance	Tara Sterling
Yeani Anthony	Sarah Dobbs	Molly Jack	Seeta Nath	Lamin Subaneh
Elizabeth Ann Arline	Carrie Grey Downing	Douglas Jackson	Elizabeth Negrete	Lee Tavasso
Janine Armstrong	Emily Ehlers	Stefani M. Janvier	Linda Nguyen	David Theologou
Syed Azfar	Aaron Evans	Sara Jaramillo	Nidya Ortiz	Catina T. Thrasher
Paige Baratta	Taeilor Evans	Caitlin Jensen	Brittney Nicole Partridge	Bradford Threlkeld
Abbey Barber	Corey Fletcher	Ahmed Kabore	Joseph Patterson	Greg Toner
Stephen Barbieri	Joshua Fletcher	Bryson Keen	Daleine Paulinis	Michael Torres
Shelby Barry	Betty S. Foh	D'Jillisser Kelly	Eboni Peoples	Ashley Traywick
Tabitha B. Bednarczyk	Akoye O. Gamory	Reza Kermani	Bruce Pittman	Christian Tripp
Ombria Bell	David Garcia	Angela Maria Korleski	Brianna Pomatico	Sandra A. Trybus
Antonio Bellocchio	Javier Garcia	Danuel Laan	Raven A. Pritchett	Daniel Udo
Addison Benson	Marvin Gary	Steven Le	Jasmine Raeford	Melissa Updyke
Karen Anne Bernatavitz	Natashia George	Chloe Anne Lebatard	Christopher Rahim	Luis Urrea
Kenneth Bethea Jr.	Nick Geraine	Stephanie Jane Leibfried	Camille Reynolds	Ana von Son
Tarmeshia Bivins	Andrew Gines	Terri Lewis	Yessica Rivas	Briana Verdugo
Paulette Blanc	Danielle Goldman	Munir Limant	Ally Rodgers	Christine Vo
Steven Briones	Danielle Gonzalez	Michael Lopez	Krystal Rodriguez	Jerri Ashley Waller
Allen Brooks	Nancy Greene	Claudia-Regina Lopez-Ferrer	Rebecca L. Rooks	Annie Wang
Mark Brooks	Morgan P. Grissom	Hilary Louis	Rachel Rozier	Brian Watson
Ryan Burnside	Katherine Guzman	Courtney Lugo	Diana Salazar	Lydia Wearden
Melissa Ann Byrum	Rachel Halverson	Lauraine Lynch	Julius Scott	Freddie Weinberg
Cara Elizabeth Carr	Derek V. Hampton Jr.	Stephen Malone	Emmanuel Seide	Laura White
Jessica Lynne Carr	Jasmine Harris	Samantha Mandel	Alexandra Rose Seidman	Kaitlin Emily Wiggins
Jaketa Cash	Monique Heath	Margot Markman	Freeman Senecharles	Shana Wilkins
Brendan Chan	Lauren Heather Helms	Ashley Marie Mason	Jessica Seracino	Kristina Nicole Williamson
Amelia Carolyn Chappell	Danon Elora Hirsch	Brittany Rae Massey	John Michael Sheahan	Charles H. Wilson
Jephthe Louis Charles	Ted Hoffman	Whitney Allison McCall	Evan Skinner	Katherine D. Wilson
Jessica Cocke	Martin Hogarty	Jonathan McClure	Annie Snodgrass	Ceili R. Wonilowicz

THE TEXT THAT SPEAKS
THE LANGUAGE
OF TODAY'S
STUDENTS

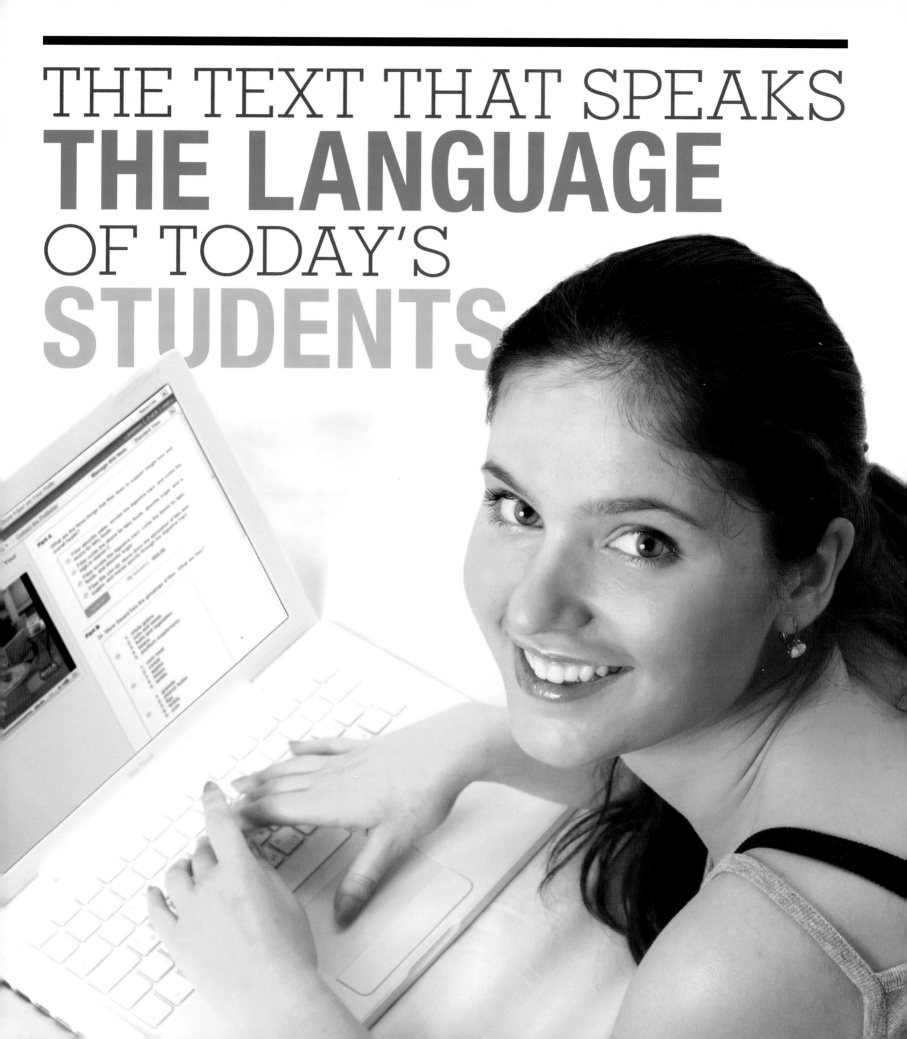

HELP YOUR STUDENTS
CHOOSE HEALTH

Help your students put better choices into practice

NEW! Choose This, Not That

boxes highlight good vs. bad choices students make about common health issues. Each box promotes the healthy choice and explains why the poor choice is problematic.

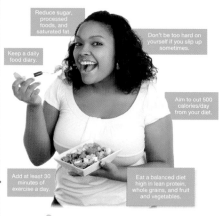
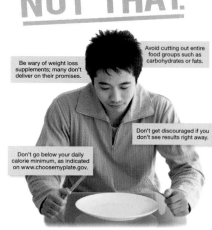
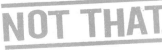

When you want to lose some **weight**, you can reach your goal healthfully, or set yourself up for frustration. To drop pounds in a healthy way:

CHOOSE THIS.

Reduce sugar, processed foods, and saturated fat.

Keep a daily food diary.

Don't be too hard on yourself if you slip up sometimes.

Aim to cut 500 calories/day from your diet.

Add at least 30 minutes of exercise a day.

Eat a balanced diet high in lean protein, whole grains, and fruit and vegetables.

NOT THAT.

Be wary of weight loss supplements; many don't deliver on their promises.

Avoid cutting out entire food groups such as carbohydrates or fats.

Don't get discouraged if you don't see results right away.

Don't go below your daily calorie minimum, as indicated on www.choosemyplate.gov.

Choose This:
A Pound or Two Each Week
When you want to lose weight, you want the pounds gone NOW. But a slower, steadier pace will be more manageable and bring longer-lasting results.

Not That:
Crash Diet
Trendy diets may sound like a path to getting skinny fast, but they are often not balanced and will leave you feeling depleted. They also don't help keep weight off later.

- **Androstenedione.** A steroid precursor that is thought to enhance athletic performance and boost testosterone, androstenedione has been linked to many high-profile controversies among professional athletes. Androstenedione is illegal for sale or use in the United States, and its side effects include breast development and impotence in men, abnormal periods and facial hair in women, and liver disease and blood clots.

- **Ephedra.** Typically used to boost energy and promote weight loss, ephedra has such serious adverse effects that the U.S. Food and Drug Administration has banned its sale. Research has not shown ephedra to be effective in boosting energy or athletic performance, and its side effects include high blood pressure, irregular heartbeat, stroke, gastrointestinal distress, and psychological problems.[43]

Change Yourself, Change Your World

Improved fitness is as much a public health goal as it is a personal one. Some of the factors that contribute to one's level of fitness reflect individual choice—whether to drive or cycle, watch TV or go outside, spend time online or spend time at the gym. But the communities in which we live also play a key role. Getting fit starts with you, but

through the choices you make, you also have the potential to help improve the lives of others.

Personal Choices

In the busy life of a student, scheduling regular exercise may seem daunting. But if you set goals, find activities you enjoy, and periodically reassess your progress, you'll be able to stay motivated, have fun, and enjoy the benefits of fitness.

Set Realistic Goals

One of the most important aspects of a fitness program is working at an intensity and rate that makes sense for you as you are. It is important to realistically assess your current fitness level in order to set fitness goals that are appropriate. Fitness goals can be based on a specific activity-related improvement you want to make, such as cycling 40% farther than you currently can; a health-related goal you may have, such as reducing your blood pressure; or a social or lifestyle desire, like preparing for a backpacking trip with your friends. Make sure your goals are easily measurable, so you can clearly tell when you've met one. If you don't make a particular goal you have set, don't get discouraged. Take that chance to reevaluate your goal and possibly break it down into smaller sub-goals.

> Take this self-assessment for a quick idea of how fit you are:
> www.nhs.uk/Tools/Pages/Fitness.aspx.

NEW! Change Yourself, Change Your World

sections at the end of each chapter give students solid, specific advice about how they can improve their own behaviors, help friends or family members, and advocate for changes in their environments to promote health for everyone.

NEW! Choosing to Change Worksheets

replace the former Behavior Change Workshops and help students implement behavior change for topics in every chapter of the book. The first step asks students to determine their stage of change, and the remainder of the worksheet walks them through their change.

Choosing to Change Worksheet

To complete this worksheet online, visit MasteringHealth™

You have acquired extensive information from this chapter about stressors and how to manage them. You had the opportunity to make observations about whether or not your perceptions of negative events in your life may be contributing to making you feel distressed by completing the **Negative Event Scale for University Students** Self-Assessment on page 58.

Directions: Fill in your stage of change in Step 1 and complete the remaining steps with your stage of change in mind.

Step 1: *Your Stage of Behavior Change.* Please check one of the following statements that best describes your readiness to change your perception of stressors.

_____ I do not intend to change my perception of stressors in the next six months. (Precontemplation)

_____ I might change my perception of stressors in the next six months. (Contemplation)

_____ I am prepared to change my perception of stressors in the next month. (Preparation)

_____ I have been changing my perception of stressors for less than six months. (Action)

_____ I have been changing my perception of stressors for more than six months. (Maintenance)

Engage Students...

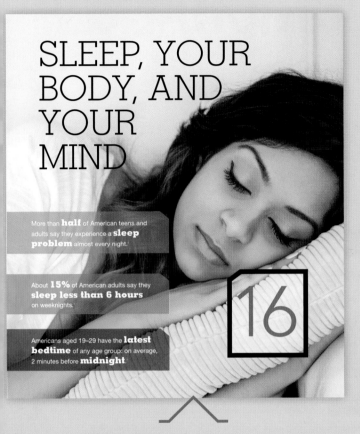

SLEEP, YOUR BODY, AND YOUR MIND

More than **half** of American teens and adults say they experience a **sleep problem** almost every night.

About **15%** of American adults say they **sleep less than 6 hours** on weeknights.

Americans aged 19–29 have the **latest bedtime** of any age group: on average, 2 minutes before **midnight**.

16

NEW! Chapter 16: Sleep, Your Body, and Your Mind

engages students in one of their favorite topics: sleep! Chapters 16 & 17 are available electronically via the Pearson eText in MasteringHealth™.

Student Stories

in every chapter of the book demonstrate that even college-aged students have to deal with health concerns.

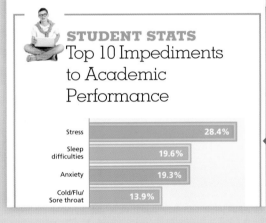

Sleep Deprived

STUDENT STORY

"HI, I'M JASMINE. I'm a freshman and I'm a child development major. Each night, I'm very lucky if I get four hours of sleep. I'm just a night owl. I like staying up at night. My father's the exact same way. It's like 3 o'clock in the morning and we'll still be up watching the food channel. Around exam time, I find myself awake at 7:30 in the morning, still up—knowing that I have a test at 9:30. Why, I don't know.

I don't think I'm doing my best right now because when I drag myself to class, I'm half asleep. I do need to change and get better rest so that I can do better in school. I don't think I've gotten 8 hours of sleep since 19, so that's six years of not getting a full night's sleep.

STUDENT STATS
Top 10 Impediments to Academic Performance

Stress	28.4%
Sleep difficulties	19.6%
Anxiety	19.3%
Cold/Flu/ Sore throat	13.9%

Student Stats

throughout the book present up-to-date national statistics and research on key health topics that apply to today's college population.

...and help them think critically

Media and... Boxes

disuss how today's media—everything from TV commercials to phone apps—affect our actions and feelings concerning a variety of health topics.

media and HEALTH

Evaluating Health Information in the Media

Is the health information you just researched on the Internet accurate? Can you trust your favorite actor's television advertisement for a weight-loss product? Was last week's episode of *The Dr. Oz Show* based on any kind of medical reality? How can you make sense of the endless stream of media headlines trumpeting health studies that sometimes contradict one another?

The term *media* can mean a variety of things. We use it here to include books, newspapers, magazines, television, advertisements, Internet/websites, and even mobile apps.

Whenever you encounter information from the media, critically assess it. Is someone trying to sell you something? Are there other ways to solve problems like being overweight without resorting to pills? Do you realize that many of the images of celebrities you see in magazines have been digitally altered to make them look more attractive than they really are?

When you come across an article about the results of the latest health-related study, consider: Was the study conducted by an unbiased source, or was it carried out by an individual or organization with

by many credible, nonprofit, noncommercial sites, but it is sometimes used by commercial entities as well.

- What is the purpose of the site? Is it to inform and educate, or is it to sell you something? If it is to sell you something, be aware that the information presented is more likely to be biased.
- Does the site tell you where the information it presents is coming from? If so, is the content based on scientific evidence, or was it written by someone hired by the site to produce marketing information? Sites that are able to provide citations and links to scientific studies and journals are more likely to be credible than sites lacking these references.
- Does the site specify when its content was last updated? Health information can sometimes change quickly, so you want to seek out information that is as current as possible.
- Does the site list a reputable professional accreditation? Many reputable health sites, for example, are accredited by the Health on the Net Foundation, and bear an insignia reading "HON."

Other features that help students go deeper:

- **NEW! CRITICAL-THINKING QUESTIONS** appear in each Diversity & Health and Media and... box.
- **GET CRITICAL** features at the end of each chapter ask students to analyze a hot topic from the news and think deeply about it.

MAKE THE CONNECTION BETWEEN
LECTURE & BEHAVIOR CHANGE

MasteringHealth™

Mastering is the most effective and widely used online homework, tutorial, and assessment system for the sciences. It delivers self-paced tutorials that focus on your course objectives, provides individualized coaching, and responds to each student's progress.

For Students

Proven, assignable, and automatically graded health activities reinforce course learning outcomes.

51 *ABC News* Videos

with assessment and feedback, help health come to life and show how it's related to the real world.

Health Coaching Activities

Coaching activities guide students through key health and fitness concepts with interactive mini-lessons that provide hints and feedback.

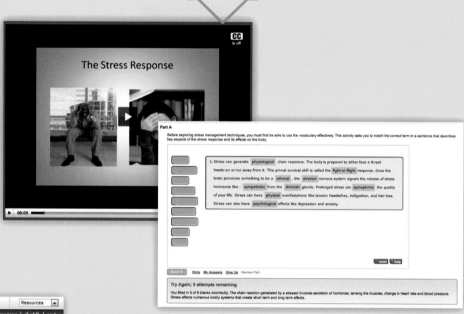

NutriTools Build-A-Meal Activities

These unique activities allow students to combine and experiment with different food options and learn firsthand how to build healthier meals.

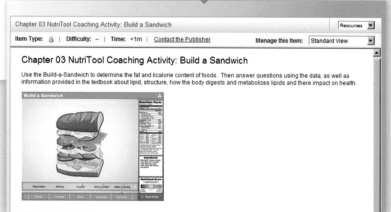

Other automatically graded health and fitness activities include:

- Behavior Change Video Activities
- Reading Quizzes
- Chapter MP3s
- Student Story Videos

Students Want to Practice on Their Own?

MasteringHealth™ also provides students with the tools to study effectively and practice on their own time at their own pace.

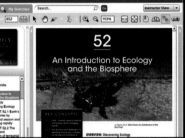

Study Area

Students can access the Study Area for use on their own or in a study group.

eText

The Pearson eText gives students access to the text whenever and wherever they can access the Internet. The eText can be viewed on PCs, Macs, and tablets, including iPad and Android. New for the Second Edition of *Choosing Health* are two additional electronic chapters covering sleep (Chapter 16) and environmental health (Chapter 17), available only through the eText.

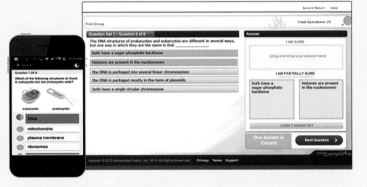

NEW! Dynamic Study Modules

enable students to study effectively on their own in an adaptive format. Students receive an initial set of questions with a unique answer format asking them to indicate their confidence level. Once completed, reviews include explanations using materials taken directly from the text. These modules can be accessed on smartphones, tablets, and computers.

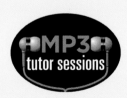

MP3 tutor sessions

with rapid review explain the big picture concepts for each chapter and can be downloaded to student smartphones, tablets, and computers.

All Self-Assessments

are available under the Study Area in an interactive PDF format.

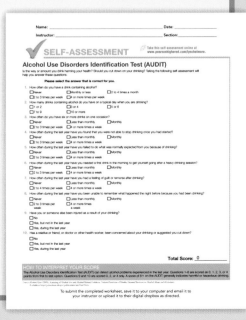

The Study Area also includes:

A Cumulative Test, RSS Feeds, Audio Case Studies, *ABC News* Videos, and book-specific activities.

EASY TO GET STARTED, USE, AND MAKE YOUR OWN

MasteringHealth™

For Instructors

MasteringHealth™ helps instructors maximize class time with easy-to-assign, customizable, and automatically graded assessments that motivate students to learn outside of the class and arrive prepared for lecture.

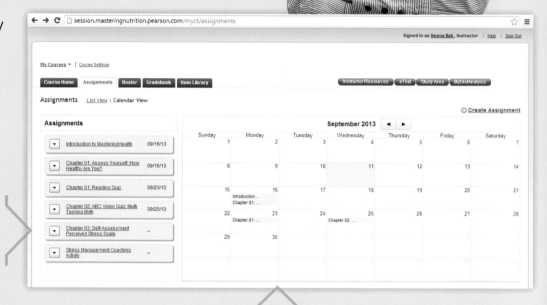

Customize Publisher-provided Problems or Quickly Add Your Own

MasteringHealth™ makes it easy to edit any questions or answers, import your own questions, and quickly add images or links to further enhance the student experience.

Calendar Feature for Instructors and Students

The Course Home default page now features a Calendar View displaying upcoming assignments and due dates.

- Instructors can schedule assignments by dragging and dropping the assignment onto a date in the calendar.

- The calendar view lets students see at-a-glance when an assignment is due, and resembles a syllabus.

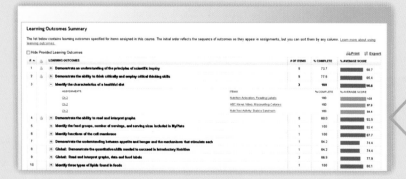

Learning Outcomes

Tagged to book content and tied to Bloom's Taxonomy, Learning Outcomes are designed to let Mastering do the work in tracking student performance against your learning outcomes. Mastering offers a data-supported measure to quantify students' learning gains and to share those results quickly and easily:

- Add your own or use the publisher-provided learning outcomes.
- View class performance against the specified learning outcomes.
- Export results to a spreadsheet.

Now that students come more prepared to class with MasteringHealth™, # Flip Your Classroom

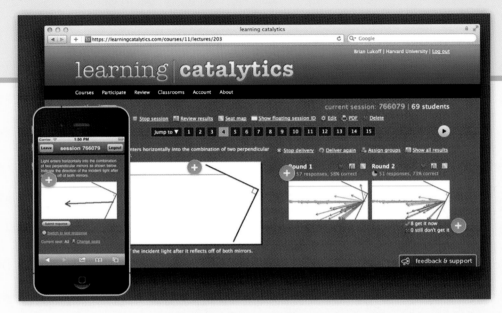

NEW! Learning Catalytics™

Learning Catalytics™ allows students to use their smartphones, tablets, or laptops to respond to questions in class. With Learning Catalytics™ you can:

Use a wide variety of question types to engage students:

multiple choice, word clouds, sketch a graph, annotate art, highlight a passage, compute a numeric answer, and more.

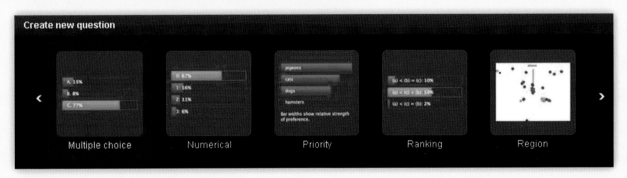

Use multiple question types to get into the minds of students

and understand what they do or don't know and adjust lectures accordingly.

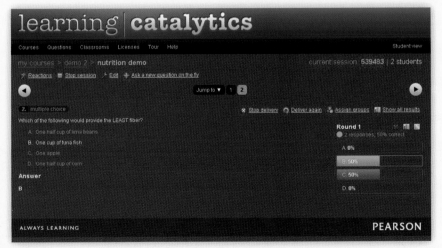

- Access rich analytics to understand student performance.
- Add your own questions to make Learning Catalytics™ fit your course exactly.
- Assess and improve students' critical-thinking skills, and so much more.

Learning Catalytics™ is included with the purchase of MasteringHealth™.

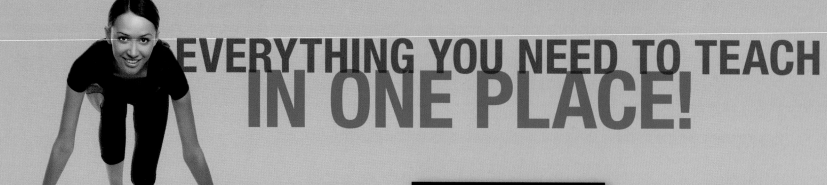

EVERYTHING YOU NEED TO TEACH IN ONE PLACE!

Teaching Toolkit DVD for *Choosing Health*

The Teaching Toolkit DVD replaces the former printed Teaching Toolbox by providing everything you need to prep for your course and deliver a dynamic lecture in one convenient place. Included on three discs are these valuable resources:

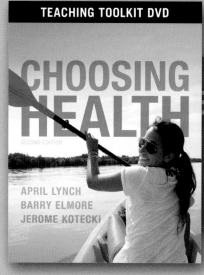 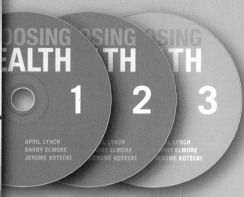

Disc 1 — Robust media assets for each chapter

- 51 *ABC News* Lecture Launcher videos
- PowerPoint® Lecture Outlines
- PowerPoint Abbreviated Lecture Outlines
- PowerPoint clicker questions and Jeopardy-style quiz show questions
- Files for all illustrations and tables and selected photos from the text
- Transparency Masters

Disc 2 — Comprehensive Test Bank

- Test Bank in Word and RTF formats
- Computerized Test Bank, which includes all the questions from the Test Bank in a format that allows you to easily and intuitively build exams and quizzes.

Disc 3 — Additional innovative supplements for instructors and students

For Instructors:
- *Instructor's Resource Support Manual*
- Introduction to MasteringHealth™
- Introductory video for Learning Catalytics™
- *Great Ideas: Active Ways to Teach Health & Wellness*
- *Teaching with Student Learning Outcomes*
- *Teaching with Web 2.0*

For Students:
- *Take Charge of Your Health! Worksheets*
- *Behavior Change Log Book and Wellness Journal*
- *Eat Right! Healthy Eating in College and Beyond*
- *Live Right! Beating Stress in College and Beyond*
- *Food Composition Table*

User's Quick Guide for *Choosing Health*

This easy-to-use printed supplement accompanies the Teaching Toolkit and offers easy instructions for both experienced and new faculty members to get started with the rich Toolkit content, how to access assignments within MasteringHealth™, and how to flip the classroom with Learning Catalytics™.

CHOOSING HEALTH

SECOND EDITION

April Lynch

Barry Elmore, M.A.
Formerly of East Carolina University

Jerome Kotecki, HSD
Ball State University

With contributions by
Laura Bonazzoli
Karen Vail-Smith, M.S., M.P.A.
East Carolina University

PEARSON

Boston   Columbus   Indianapolis   New York   San Francisco   Upper Saddle River
Amsterdam   Cape Town   Dubai   London   Madrid   Milan   Munich   Paris   Montréal   Toronto
Delhi   Mexico City   São Paulo   Sydney   Hong Kong   Seoul   Singapore   Taipei   Tokyo

Executive Editor: *Sandra Lindelof*
Director of Development: *Barbara Yien*
Senior Project Development Editor: *Marie Beaugureau*
Editorial Assistant: *Tu-Anh Dang-Tran*
Art Development Editor: *Kelly Murphy*
Associate Content Producer: *Julia Akpan*
Project Manager, Instructor Media: *Kyle Doctor*
Text Permissions Project Manager: *Alison Bruckner*
Text Permissions Specialist: *Creative Compliance*
Managing Editor: *Michael Early*
Production Project Manager: *Lori Newman*
Program Manager: *Susan Malloy*
Production Management: *S4Carlisle Publishing Services*

Compositor: *S4Carlisle Publishing Services*
Design Manager: *Marilyn Perry*
Interior and Cover Designer: *Tandem Creative Inc.*
Illustrators: *Precision Graphics*
Photo Permissions Management: *PreMediaGlobal*
Photo Researcher: *PreMediaGlobal, Tandem Creative Inc.*
Manager of Image Resources: *Maya Melenchuck*
Executive Marketing Manager: *Neena Bali*
Director of Marketing: *Christy Lesko*
Senior Procurement Specialist: *Stacey Weinberger*
Cover and Text Printer: *Courier, Kendallville*

Cover Photo Credit: *Getty Images/Roberto Westbrook*

Credits and acknowledgments for materials borrowed from other sources and reproduced, with permission, in this textbook appear on the appropriate page within the text or on p. CR-1.

Library of Congress Cataloging-in-Publication Data
Lynch, April.
    Choosing health/April Lynch, Barry Elmore, and Jerome Kotecki.—Second edition.
        pages cm
    Includes index.
    ISBN-13: 978-0-321-92965-5
    ISBN-10: 0-321-92965-9
    1. Health—Popular works.   I. Elmore, Barry.   II. Kotecki, Jerome Edward.   III. Title.
    RA776.5.L96   2015
    613—dc23   2013025088

ISBN 10: 0-321-92965-9; ISBN 13: 978-0-321-92965-5 (Student Edition)
ISBN 10: 0-321-96314-8; ISBN 13: 978-0-321-96314-7 (Instructor's Review Copy)
ISBN 10: 0-321-96312-1; ISBN 13: 978-0-321-96312-3 (Books a la Carte Edition)

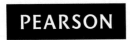

www.pearsonhighered.com

1 2 3 4 5 6 7 8 9 10—CRK—18 17 16 15 14

" *This book is dedicated to my husband, Colin, daughter, Ava, and son, Van. In the ever-changing love and laughter project that is our family, I'm inspired to reach for better choices, every single day.*"

—April Lynch

" *To Rick, Billie, Sudie, my colleagues at ECU, and my students. Without you this book would not have been possible.*"

—Barry Elmore

" *This book is dedicated to my friends and family for their continued support and love. They allowed me the time and energy to focus my passion and write this book.*"

–Jerome Kotecki

About the Authors

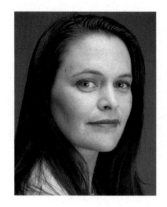

April Lynch

April Lynch is an award-winning author and journalist who specializes in health, the medical and biological sciences, and human genetics. During her tenure with the *San Jose Mercury News,* the leading newspaper of Silicon Valley, she served as the Science and Health editor, focusing the paper's coverage on personal health and scientific developments in the field of disease prevention. She has also worked as a writer and editor for the *San Francisco Chronicle.* April has written numerous articles on personal health, medical and scientific advances, consumer issues such as health insurance, and the ways that scientific breakthroughs are redefining our understanding of health. She has been a frequent contributor to leading university textbooks covering applied biology, nutrition, and environmental health and science. Along with *Choosing Health*, April has co-authored *Health: Making Choices for Life*, an innovative personal health textbook for users who desire a more detailed, in-depth book for students majoring in health-related subjects. Together with a leading genetic counselor, April is also the co-author of *The Genome Book,* a hands-on guide to using genetic information in personal health decisions. Her work has won numerous awards from organizations such as the Society of Professional Journalists, the California Newspaper Publishers Association, and the Associated Press. Her current interests include a focus on how people receive and interact with health information online as well as how complex scientific and medical information is best shared compellingly and effectively in digital media. She lives in the San Francisco Bay Area with her husband and children.

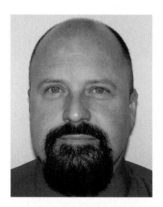

Barry Elmore, M.A.

Formerly of East Carolina University

Barry Elmore is a former faculty member at East Carolina University in the College of Health and Human Performance. He obtained a B.S. from Mount Olive College and an M.A. in Health Education at East Carolina University, where he was a merit scholar. Barry has extensive experience in the field of community health, with particular focus on sexually transmitted infections. He served as the Executive Director of the Pitt County AIDS Service Organization, the third largest AIDS service organization in North Carolina, before beginning his teaching career and worked as a health educator in the nonprofit sector for nearly 20 years. He is a member of the American Public Health Association (APHA), the Society for Public Health Education (SOPHE), and the North Carolina Association for Research in Education (NCARE). Barry has been recognized for outstanding teaching by East Carolina University.

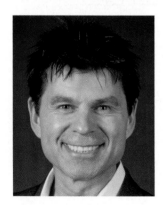

Jerome Kotecki, HSD

Ball State University

Jerome E. Kotecki is a professor of Health Science in the Department of Physiology and Health Science at Ball State University. Dr. Kotecki earned his doctorate in health education and his master's degree in exercise science from Indiana University. He has published more than 40 scientific research papers on the prevention, arrest, and reversal of the most common chronic diseases facing Americans today. Jerome has authored or co-authored multiple textbooks on the importance of healthy lifestyle habits to enhance the multidimensional components of human health and prevent cardiovascular disease, diabetes, cancer, and other chronic conditions. Jerome has extensive experience in health promotion, with particular focus on physical activity and health. An experienced teacher and researcher, he is devoted to helping students adopt and maintain healthy lifestyles. Jerome has been recognized for his contributions to the scholarship of teaching and learning by his department, college, and university. He is an avid fitness participant and enjoys cycling, resistance training, running, mountain biking, hiking, swimming, and yoga.

About the Contributors

Laura Bonazzoli

Laura Bonazzoli has been writing and editing in the health sciences for over 20 years. Her early work in human anatomy and physiology, chemistry, and other core sciences laid the foundation for writing projects in nursing, pathology, nutrition, complementary and alternative medicine, and personal health. Her commitment as a writer is to help her readers appreciate the power of small choices to improve their health and the health of their communities. In her free time, Laura and her daughter enjoy exploring the gardens, byways, and beaches of mid-coast Maine.

Karen Vail-Smith, M.S., M.P.A.

East Carolina University

Karen Vail-Smith received a B.S. from The University of North Carolina at Chapel Hill and an M.S. and an M.P.A. from East Carolina University. She has been a faculty member in East Carolina University's Department of Health Education and Promotion for 22 years. She specializes in personal health and human sexuality. She has received numerous teaching awards, including the prestigious UNC Board of Governor's Distinguished Professor for Teaching award. She has published more than 25 articles in health professional journals.

Brief Contents

1 Health in the 21st Century 1

2 Psychological Health 23

3 Stress Management 48

4 Nutrition and You 70

5 Physical Activity for Fitness & Health 99

6 Body Image, Body Weight 125

7 Drug Use and Abuse 152

8 Alcohol and Tobacco Use and Abuse 174

9 Social Relationships and Communication 202

10 Sexuality, Contraception, and Reproductive Choices 222

11 Preventing Infectious Diseases & Sexually Transmitted Infections 257

12 Diabetes, Cardiovascular Disease, and Cancer 284

13 Consumer Health 320

14 Personal Safety and Injury Prevention 342

15 Aging Well 364

Additional Electronic Chapters
Access these chapters online through MasteringHealth™

16 Sleep, Your Body, and Your Mind 388

17 Your Environment, Your Health 408

Contents

Preface xxiii

Acknowledgments xxviii

Chapter 1
Health in the 21st Century 1

What Is Health? 2
  Health Versus Disease 2
  Health Versus Wellness 3
  Dimensions of Health and Wellness 3

Current Health Challenges 4
  Health Across America 4
  Health on America's Campuses 6
  Health Around the World 7

Determinants of Health 8
  Biology and Genetics 8
  Individual Behaviors 9
  Social Determinants 9
  Physical Determinants 10
  Health Services 10
  Policy-Making 12

Achieving Successful Behavior Change 12
  Factors That Influence Behavior Change 12
  Models of Behavior Change 13

Change Yourself, Change Your World 14
  Personal Choices 15
  Campus Advocacy 17

Choosing to Change Worksheet 19

Chapter Summary 20

Get Connected 21

Test Your Knowledge 21

Get Critical 22

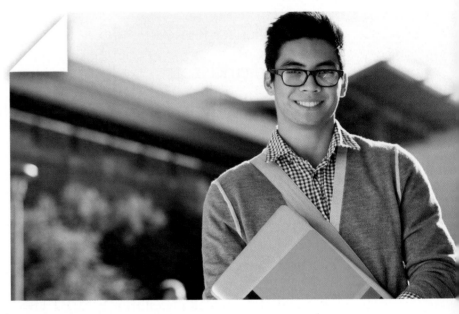

Chapter 2
Psychological Health 23

What Is Psychological Health? 24
  Components of Psychological Health 24
  Facets of Psychological Health 24
  The Role of Emotional Intelligence 25
  The Value of Optimism 25

Factors Affecting Psychological Health 26
  Maslow's Hierarchy of Needs 26
  Family History 27
  Social Support 27
  The Role of Spiritual Health 27

Common Psychological Challenges 29
  Shyness 29
  Loneliness 29
  Anger 29

Mental Disorders in the United States: An Overview 30

Mood Disorders 31
  Depressive Disorders 31
  Bipolar Disorder 34

Anxiety Disorders 34
    Generalized Anxiety Disorder (GAD) 34
    Panic Attacks and Panic Disorder 35
    Social Anxiety Disorder 35
    Phobias 35
    Obsessive-Compulsive Disorder (OCD) 35
    Post-Traumatic Stress Disorder (PTSD) 36
    Treating Anxiety Disorders 36

Other Disorders 37
    Attention Disorders 37
    Schizophrenia 37

Self-Injury and Suicide 38
    Self-Injury 38
    Suicide 38

Getting Help for a Psychological Problem 39
    Options on Campus 39
    Clinical Options 39

Change Yourself, Change Your World 41
    Personal Choices 41
    Helping a Friend 42
    Campus Advocacy 42

Choosing to Change Worksheet 43
Chapter Summary 45
Get Connected 46
Test Your Knowledge 46
Get Critical 47

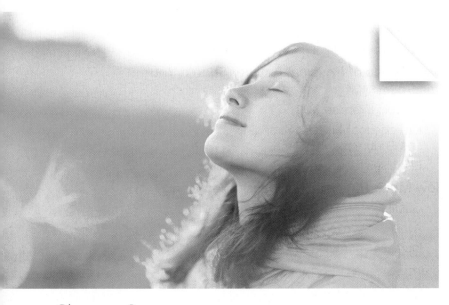

Chapter 3
Stress Management 48

What Is Stress? 49
The Body's Stress Response 49
    Alarm Phase: The Fight-or-Flight Response 50
    Resistance Phase 51
    Exhaustion Phase and Allostatic Overload 52

Health Effects of Chronic Stress 52
    Effects on the Cardiovascular System 52
    Effects on the Digestive System 52
    Effects on Weight 53
    Effects on the Immune System 54
    Effects on Sleep 54
    Effects on Relationships 54
    Effects on Mood, Mind, and Mental Health 54

What Influences Our Stress Response? 55
    The Role of Personality Types 55
    The Role of Personality Traits 56

Common Causes of Stress 56
    Financial Stressors 56
    Daily Hassles 56
    Academic Pressure 56
    Job-Related Stressors 56
    Social Stressors 56
    Major Life Events 57
    Environmental Stressors 57
    Internal Stressors 59

Getting Help for Managing Stress 59
Change Yourself, Change Your World 59
    Personal Choices 59
    Helping a Friend 65
    Campus Advocacy 65

Choosing to Change Worksheet 66
Chapter Summary 68
Get Connected 68
Test Your Knowledge 68
Get Critical 69

Chapter 4
Nutrition and You 70

What Are Nutrients? 71
    Energy and Calories 71
    Carbohydrates 72
    Fats 74
    Proteins 77
    Vitamins 77
    Minerals 78
    Water 80
    What About Dietary Supplements? 81

Other Healthful Substances in Foods 83
    Phytochemicals 83
    Antioxidants 83
    Probiotics and Prebiotics 84

Tools to Help You Eat Right 85
    Learn About the Dietary Reference Intakes (DRIs) 85
    Read Food Labels 85
    Follow the *Dietary Guidelines for Americans* 87
    Log Onto MyPlate 87

How Do Nutrition Guidelines Vary for Different Groups? 90

Is Our Food Supply Safe? 90
    Foodborne Illness 90
    Food Allergies and Intolerances 91
    Food Residues 92
    Genetically Modified Foods 92

Change Yourself, Change Your World 92
    Personal Choices 93
    Campus Advocacy 95

Choosing to Change Worksheet 96
Chapter Summary 97
Get Connected 97
Test Your Knowledge 98
Get Critical 98

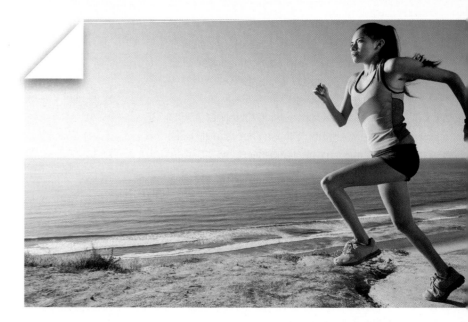

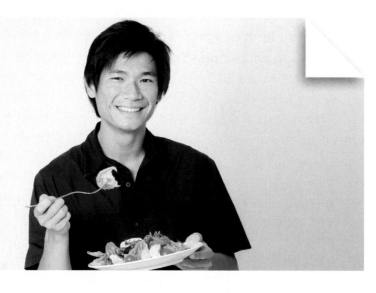

    Reduced Risk of Some Cancers 102
    Increased Immune Function 102
    Stronger Bones 102
    Reduced Risk of Injury 103
    Healthful Weight Management 103
    Benefits to Psychological Health, Stress Management, and Sleep 103

Principles of Fitness Training 103
    Overload 103
    Specificity 104
    Reversibility 104
    Individuality 104

What Types of Physical Activity Should You Consider? 104
    Aerobic Exercise 105
    Exercise for Muscular Strength and Endurance 106
    Exercises for Improving Flexibility 110

How Much Physical Activity Do You Need? 111
    Guidelines for Health Maintenance 111
    Avoid Sustained Sitting 111
    Increase Your Level of Activity 111

Exercise Safe, Exercise Smart 115
    Get Medical Clearance 115
    Warm Up and Cool Down 115
    Get Training 115
    Wear Suitable Clothes 115
    Eat Right 116
    Stay Hydrated 116
    Prepare for Hot or Cold Weather 116
    Start Slow and Watch Out for Red Flags 118

Chapter 5
Physical Activity for Fitness & Health 99

What Is Physical Fitness? 100
    Cardiorespiratory Fitness 100
    Muscular Strength 101
    Muscular Endurance 101
    Flexibility 101
    Body Composition 101

What Are the Benefits of Physical Activity? 102
    Stronger Heart and Lungs 102
    Management and Prevention of Type 2 Diabetes 102

Care for Injuries 118
Be Wary of Performance-Enhancing Drugs 118
Change Yourself, Change Your World 120
Personal Choices 120
Campus Advocacy 121
Choosing to Change Worksheet 122
Chapter Summary 123
Get Connected 123
Test Your Knowledge 124
Get Critical 124

Change Yourself, Change Your World 136
Personal Choices 136
Helping a Friend 144
Campus Advocacy 144
Body Image and Eating Disorders 144
Body Image Disorders 144
Eating Disorders 144
Other Unhealthful Eating Behaviors 146
Getting Help for a Body Image or Eating Disorder 147
Personal Choices: Develop a More Positive Body Image 147
Choosing to Change Worksheet 148
Chapter Summary 149
Get Connected 150
Test Your Knowledge 150
Get Critical 151

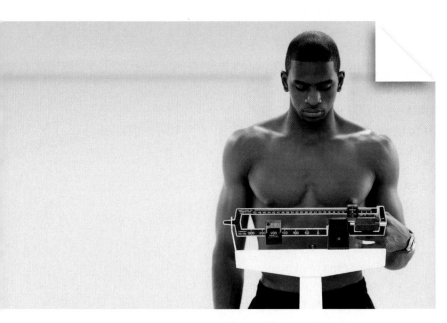

Chapter 6
Body Image, Body Weight 125

Body Image and Body Weight 126
Many Factors Influence Body Image 127
Defining a Healthful Body Weight 127
Alarming Trends in Body Weight 130
Weight Trends in the United States 130
Weight Trends Around the World 130
Weight Trends on Campus 131
Risks and Costs of Obesity 131
Health Risks 131
Financial Burden of Obesity 133
Factors That Contribute to Weight Gain 133
Biology and Genetics 133
Individual Behaviors 134
Social Factors 136
Physical Factors 136
Public Policy 136

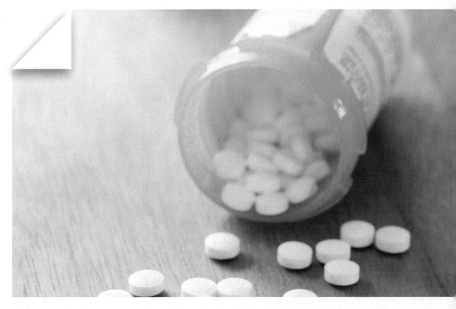

Chapter 7
Drug Use and Abuse 152

An Overview of Addiction 153
What Is Addiction? 153
What Are Some Behavioral Addictions? 154
Patterns of Drug Use 155
How the Body Responds to Drugs 156
Drug Misuse and Abuse 156
Initial Effects on the Brain 156
Effects of Chronic Use 156
How Drugs Leave the Body 157
Commonly Abused Drugs 157
Prescription and Over-the-Counter Medications 157
Marijuana 158

Stimulants 160
Hallucinogens 162
"Club Drugs" 163
Inhalants 164
Depressants 164
Heroin 165

Prevention Strategies: Do They Work? 165
Getting Help for a Drug Problem 167
Campus and Community-Based Options 167
Clinical Options 167
Change Yourself, Change Your World 168
Personal Choices 168
Helping a Friend 169
Campus Advocacy 169

Choosing to Change Worksheet 170
Chapter Summary 172
Get Connected 172
Test Your Knowledge 172
Get Critical 173

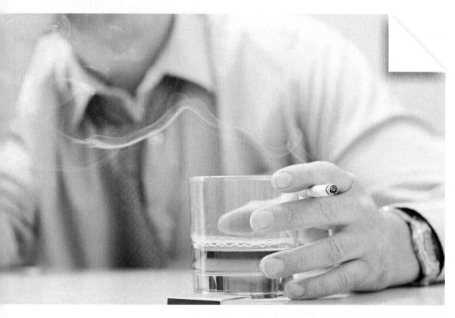

Chapter 8
Alcohol and Tobacco Use and Abuse 174

Alcohol Use in the United States 175
Alcohol Use and Binge Drinking on Campus 175
The Makeup of Alcohol 177
How the Body Absorbs and Metabolizes Alcohol 178
Blood Alcohol Concentration 179
Intoxication 180
The Effects of Alcohol on the Body 180
Immediate Effects of Alcohol on the Body 180

Long-Term Effects of Alcohol on the Body 182
Alcohol and Pregnancy 183
The Effects of Alcohol on Behavior 183
Drinking and Driving 183
Alcohol and Sexual Activity 184
Alcohol and Other Problems 184
Alcohol Abuse 184
Alcoholism 184
Getting Help for a Drinking Problem 185
Change Yourself, Change Your World 186
Personal Choices 187
Helping a Friend 187
Campus Advocacy 187
Smoking in the United States 187
Smoking on Campus 187
What's in a Cigarette? 189
Effects of Smoking on Health 191
Short-Term Health Effects 191
Long-Term Health Effects 192
Smoking and Pregnancy 192
Secondhand Smoke 193
Other Forms of Tobacco 194
Cigars 194
Clove Cigarettes 194
Bidis 194
Smokeless ("Spit") Tobacco 195
Electronic Cigarettes 195
Getting Help to Quit Smoking 195
Treatment Options 196
Dealing with Relapse 196
Change Yourself, Change Your World 196
Personal Choices 197
Campus Advocacy 197

Choosing to Change Worksheet 199
Chapter Summary 200
Get Connected 200
Test Your Knowledge 201
Get Critical 201

Chapter 9
Social Relationships and Communication 202

Communication in Relationships 203
Communicating Feelings 203
Being a Good Listener 204
Resolving Conflicts 205
Gender Roles and Communication 205

Developing Relationships 205

    Self-Perception 205

    Early Relationships 206

    Gender Roles 207

Friendships 207

    Maintaining Old Friendships 208

Intimate Relationships 208

    Sternberg's Triangular Theory of Love 208

    What Causes Attraction? 210

    Dating 210

    Same-Sex Relationships 211

    Healthy Relationships 211

    Dysfunctional Relationships 211

    When Relationships End 213

Committed Relationships 213

    Cohabitation 213

    Marriage 213

    Domestic Partnerships 215

    Staying Single 215

Starting a Family 216

    Choosing Children 216

    Stepfamilies 216

    Single Parenthood 217

    Characteristics of Happy Families 217

Change Yourself, Change Your World 217

    Personal Choices 217

    Campus Advocacy 218

Choosing to Change Worksheet 219

Chapter Summary 220

Get Connected 220

Test Your Knowledge 221

Get Critical 221

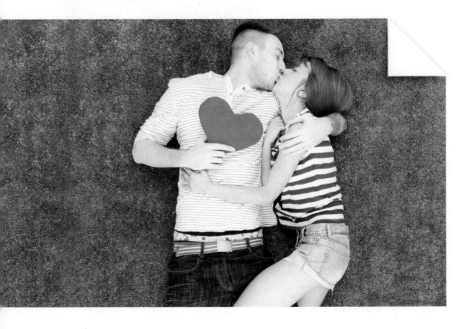

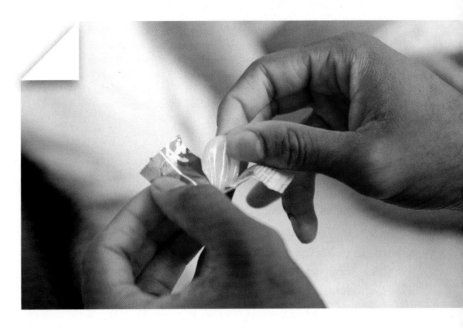

Chapter 10

Sexuality, Contraception, and Reproductive Choices 222

Sexual Anatomy and Health 223

    Female Sexual Anatomy 223

    Common Sexual Health Problems in Females 225

    Male Sexual Anatomy 225

    Common Sexual Health Problems in Males 227

The Menstrual Cycle 227

    Phases of the Menstrual Cycle 227

    Disorders Associated with the Menstrual Cycle 228

The Sexual Response Cycle 229

    Sexual Dysfunctions 230

Sexual Behavior 231

    Abstinence and Celibacy 231

    Non-Intercourse Sexual Activity 231

    Sexual Intercourse 232

    Communicating About Sex 232

Sexual Orientation and Gender Identity 232

    Heterosexuality 232

    Homosexuality 233

    Bisexuality 235

    Transgenderism and Transsexuality 236

Conception and Contraception 236

    Conception 236

    Contraceptive Options 237

    Which Method Is the Best? 243

Abortion 244

    Methods of Abortion 245

Physical and Psychological Complications
of Abortion 246
Legal Status of Abortion 246

Pregnancy and Childbirth 246
Pregnancy 246
Childbirth 250

Infertility 252
Causes of Infertility 252
Options for Infertile Couples 252

Change Yourself, Change Your World 253
Personal Choices 253
Campus Advocacy 253

Choosing to Change Worksheet 254
Chapter Summary 255
Get Connected 255
Test Your Knowledge 256
Get Critical 256

Protozoan Infections 270
Parasitic Worm Infections 271

Sexually Transmitted Infections 271
Risk Factors for STIs 271
HIV and AIDS 272
Hepatitis B 273
Genital Herpes 273
Human Papillomavirus 274
Chlamydia 275
Gonorrhea 277
Pelvic Inflammatory Disease 277
Syphilis 277
Pubic Lice and Scabies 278
Trichomoniasis 278

Change Yourself, Change Your World 279
Personal Choices 279
Campus Advocacy 279

Choosing to Change Worksheet 280
Chapter Summary 281
Get Connected 282
Test Your Knowledge 282
Get Critical 283

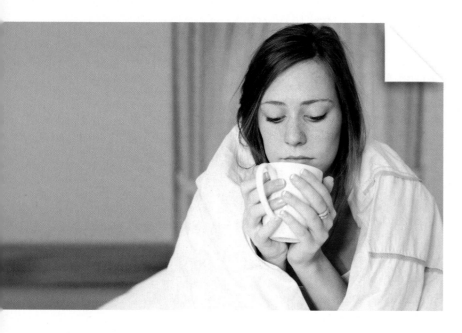

Chapter 11
Preventing Infectious Diseases & Sexually Transmitted Infections 257

How Are Infections Spread? 258

Protecting Against Infections 260
The Body's First Line of Defense 260
The Body's Immune Response 260
Immunization 262
Immune Disorders 263

Infectious Diseases 264
Viral Infections 264
Bacterial Infections 266
Fungal Infections 270

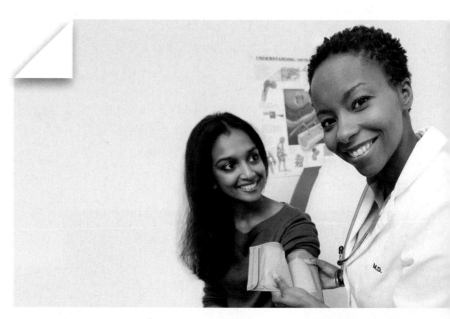

Chapter 12
Diabetes, Cardiovascular Disease, and Cancer 284

Overview of Chronic Diseases 285
Scope of the Problem 285
Influence of Four Key Behaviors 286

Diabetes 286
Types of Diabetes 286

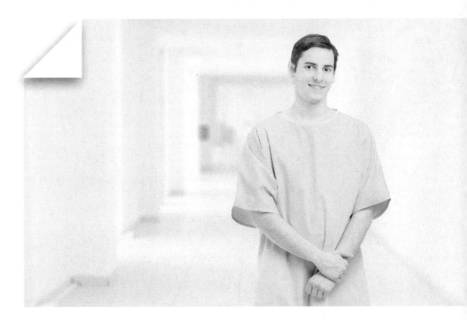

Detecting Diabetes 289

Long-Term Effects of Diabetes 289

Risk Factors for Type 2 Diabetes 289

Clinical Management of Diabetes 290

Cardiovascular Disease 291

The Healthy Cardiovascular System 292

Atherosclerosis 293

Hypertension (High Blood Pressure) 294

Coronary Heart Disease 295

Congestive Heart Failure 298

Stroke 298

Other Forms of Cardiovascular Disease 299

Risk Factors for Cardiovascular Disease 299

Cardiometabolic Risk 301

Cancer 303

What Is Cancer? 303

Risk Factors for Cancer 304

Detecting Cancer 306

Types of Cancer 306

Common Cancers in Men and Women 307

Common Cancers in Men 309

Common Cancers in Women 309

Treating Cancer 311

Change Yourself, Change Your World 311

Personal Choices 312

Supporting a Friend with a Chronic Disease 314

Campus Advocacy 315

Choosing to Change Worksheet 316

Chapter Summary 317

Get Connected 318

Test Your Knowledge 318

Get Critical 319

Chapter 13

Consumer Health 320

Choosing Self-Care 321

Practicing Prevention 321

Finding Accurate Health Information 322

Options for Self-Care 323

When to See a Doctor 324

Checkups and Preventive Care 324

Health Problems Beyond Self-Care 326

Conventional Medicine 327

Where to Find Conventional Health Care 327

Choosing a Provider 328

Being a Smart Patient 328

Handling Prescription Medications Properly 329

Complementary and Alternative Medicine (CAM) 329

Evaluating Complementary and Alternative Therapies 330

Paying for Health Care 332

Discount Programs 332

Health Insurance 332

Health Savings Accounts and Flexible Spending Accounts 333

Students and Health Insurance 335

What Happens When I Graduate? 335

"Personalized Medicine" and the Future of Consumer Health 336

A Short Course in Genetics and Genomics 336

Uses of Genomic Information 337

Ethical, Social, and Legal Implications of Genomic Advances 338

Change Yourself, Change Your World 338

Personal Choices 338

Campus Advocacy 338

Choosing to Change Worksheet 339

Chapter Summary 340

Get Connected 340

Test Your Knowledge 341

Get Critical 341

Chapter 14

Personal Safety and Injury Prevention 342

Overview of Unintentional Injuries 343

Motor Vehicle Accidents 343

What Factors Increase the Risk for Motor Vehicle Accidents? 344

How Can You Reduce Your Risk for Motor Vehicle Accidents? 345

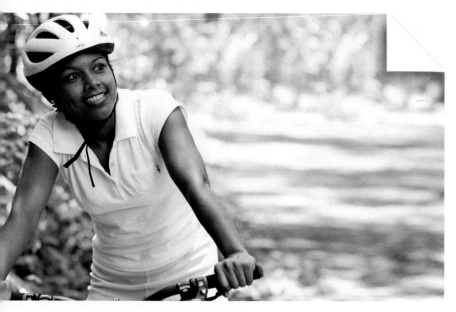

Choosing to Change Worksheet 361

Chapter Summary 362

Get Connected 362

Test Your Knowledge 363

Get Critical 363

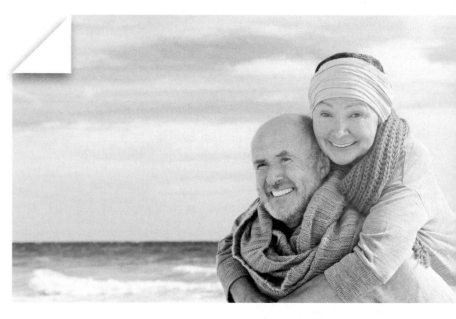

Other Traffic Injuries 346

    Accidents Involving Pedestrians and Cyclists 347

    Safety Tips for Pedestrians and Cyclists 347

Residential, Occupational, and Recreational Injuries 347

    Unintentional Poisoning 347

    Choking and Suffocation 347

    Drowning and Other Water Injuries 348

    Fire Injuries 349

    Work-Related Injuries 350

Overview of Intentional Injuries and Violence 351

Violence Within Communities 352

    Assault 352

    Murder 353

    School and Campus Violence 353

    Hate Crimes 355

    Terrorism 355

Violence Within Relationships 355

    Intimate Partner Violence 355

    Stalking and Cyberstalking 356

    Addressing Violence Within Relationships 357

Sexual Violence 357

    Risk Factors for Sexual Violence 357

    Sexual Harassment 357

    Rape 358

    Effects of Sexual Violence 359

Change Yourself, Change Your World 359

    Personal Choices 359

    Helping a Friend 360

    Campus Advocacy 360

Chapter 15

Aging Well 364

Aging in the United States 365

    Trends in Health and Health Care 366

    Life Expectancy 366

    Gender and Longevity 366

What Happens As You Age? 367

    Physical Changes 367

    Psychosocial Changes 370

What Contributes to Successful Aging? 372

    Physical Activity 372

    Good Nutrition 373

    Weight Management 374

    Avoiding Tobacco 374

    Mental Exercise 375

    Stress Management 375

Understanding Death and Dying 375

    What Is Death? 376

    How Do We Develop Our Concepts of
    Death and Dying? 376

Planning for the End of Life 377

    Complete Advance Directives 377

    Consider Organ Donation 377

    Write a Will 378

Research Your Options for End-of-Life Care 378
Clarify Your Beliefs and Values 378
After a Death 379
Autopsy 379
Care of the Body 379
Planning a Service 379
Experiencing Grief 380
Change Yourself, Change Your World 380
Personal Choices 380
Supporting a Loved One Who Is Dying 381
Supporting a Loved One Who Is Grieving 382
Campus Advocacy 383
Choosing to Change Worksheet 384
Chapter Summary 385
Get Connected 386
Test Your Knowledge 386
Get Critical 387

Why Is Ample Sleep Important? 393
Health Effects 393
Effects on Academic Performance 394
Risk for Traumatic Injury 394
What Factors Influence Sleep? 395
Biology and Genetics 395
Individual Behaviors 396
Factors in the Environment 396
Sleep Disorders 397
Insomnia 397
Snoring 397
Sleep Apnea 397
Narcolepsy 398
Parasomnias 399
Getting Help for a Sleep Disorder 400
Campus and Community Support 400
Clinical Diagnosis and Treatment 400
Complementary and Alternative Therapies 400
Change Yourself, Change Your World 401
Personal Choices 401
Campus Advocacy 403
Choosing to Change Worksheet 404
Chapter Summary 406
Get Connected 406
Test Your Knowledge 407
Get Critical 407

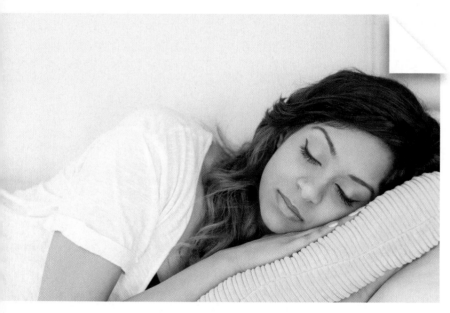

Additional Electronic Chapters

Access these chapters online through MasteringHealth™

Chapter 16
Sleep, Your Body, and Your Mind 388

What Is Sleep? 389
Regions and Rhythms of Sleep 389
Stages of Sleep 390
Cycles of Sleep 391
Sleep: How Much Is Enough? 392
Research on Short and Long Sleep 392
Short Sleep: The American Way? 393

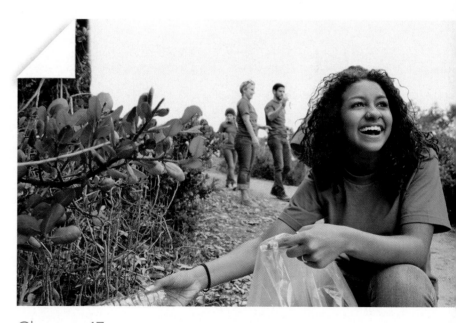

Chapter 17
Your Environment, Your Health 408

Overview of Environmental Health 409
Defining Your Environment 410

Environmental Health Is a Global Issue 410

The Evolution of Environmental Health 410

Toward Sustainability 411

Overpopulation and Globalization 411

Factors Contributing to Population Growth 411

Effects of Overpopulation 412

Reversing Population Growth 412

Air Pollution 413

Common Air Pollutants 413

Environmental Phenomena Associated with Air Pollution 414

What Can Be Done to Reduce Air Pollution and Climate Change? 417

Water Pollution 419

Types of Pollutants Found in Water 419

Is Bottled Water Worth It? 421

What Can You Do to Reduce Water Pollution? 422

Land Pollution 422

Municipal Waste and Its Management 422

Hazardous Waste and Its Management 423

What Can You Do to Manage Household Hazardous Waste? 424

Pollution at Home 426

Pollutants in Foods and Beverages 426

Pollutants in Indoor Air 427

Health Effects of Pollutants at Home 427

Noise Pollution 429

Radiation 431

Types and Health Effects of Radiation 431

What Can You Do to Reduce Your Exposure to Radiation? 431

Change Yourself, Change Your World 432

Personal Choices 432

Campus Advocacy 433

Choosing to Change Worksheet 434

Chapter Summary 435

Get Connected 436

Test Your Knowledge 436

Get Critical 437

Test Your Knowledge Answers AN-1

Credits CR-1

Glossary GL-1

References RF-1

Index I-1

Feature Boxes

STUDENT STORIES

Corey: Proud of My Scars   4

Jasmine: Sleep Deprived   14

Javier: Dealing with Depression   33

Kristina: A Friend's Suicide   38

David: Balancing School and Family   52

Jessica: Handling School Stress   59

Peter: Fixing a Poor Diet   84

Nidya: Why I'm Vegetarian   89

Sean: Cardiorespiratory Fitness   104

Molly: Adapting Exercise to My Needs   121

Josh: Losing Weight   136

Viege: Eating Disorders   147

Andrea: Tainted Drugs   160

Ana: Coping with Addiction   167

Courtney: Negative Effects from Drinking   183

Addison: Quitting Cold Turkey   197

Brittany and Sandy: Good Friends   207

Jonathan and Yeani: How to Be a Healthy Couple   210

Betty: Deciding to Get on the Pill   236

Abbey: Talking Honestly About Sex   245

Jessica: How I Avoid Infections   262

Gabe: Unprotected Sex   279

Michael: A Family History of Diabetes   291

Amanda: Surviving Cancer   307

Holly: Living Without Health Insurance   328

Anuella: Waiting for Health Coverage   335

Caleb: Car Accident   347

Jenny: Abusive Relationship   356

Stephen: Handling Aging   371

Michelle: Grieving   380

Remy: Sleep Apnea   398

Rachel: Setting a Sleep Schedule   403

Toby: Car vs. Campus Shuttle   419

Camille: Recycling Cell Phones   424

media and ...

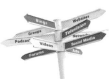

Media and Health: Evaluating Health Information in the Media   11

Media and Fitness: Do Fitness Apps Work?   117

Media and Body Image: Beauty in the Age of Photoshop: Seeing Shouldn't Be Believing   128

Media and Alcohol and Tobacco Use: How Entertainment and Ads Drive Drinking and Smoking   190

Media and Sexuality: Is Porn a Problem?   234

Media and Violence: Does the Media Encourage Violent Crime—or the Fear of Violent Crime?   354

Media and Aging: Do High-Tech Games Boost the Brain?   375

CHOOSE THIS. NOT THAT.

Stress: Exercise vs. Alcohol   64

Hunger: A Healthful Lunch vs. A High-Fat Lunch   82

Fitness: Slow and Steady vs. Fast and Furious   119

Weight Loss: A Pound or Two Each Week vs. Crash Diet   142

Conflict: A Fair Fight vs. Full-On "Fight Club"   206

Motor Vehicle Accidents: Attentive and Defensive Driving vs. Distracted, Impaired, or Aggressive Driving   346

Dietary Guidelines: A Blueprint for Better Nutrition   88
Are "Study Drugs" Smart—and Safe?   159
Peer Pressure: Resisting the Pitch   188
Social Media, Communication, and Cyber-Bullies   209
Emerging Infectious Diseases   269

Helping Someone in a CVD Emergency   297
What the Affordable Care Act Means for You   334
10 Tips for Campus Safety   360
Starting Right for a Restful Night   402

SELF-ASSESSMENT

How Healthy Is Your Current Lifestyle?   18
Anxiety Assessment   36
Negative Event Scale for University Students   58
Do You Eat Well?   94
Determining Your Maximum Heart Rate and Target Heart
   Rate Range   106
Assessing Your Weight-Related Health Risks   130
Could I Have an Eating Disorder?   146
Should You Seek Drug Treatment?   168
Alcohol Use Disorders Identification Test (AUDIT)   186
Is My Relationship Healthy?   211

Are You and Your Partner Ready for Sex?   235
Are You at Risk for an STI?   271
Are You at Risk for Type 2 Diabetes?   290
What's Your Risk for a Heart Attack?   302
Am I at Risk for Cancer?   305
How Proactive Are You About Preventive Health
   Care?   338
Are You an Aggressive Driver?   345
Are You Comfortable with Death?   377
Are You Getting Enough Sleep?   403
Is Loud Music Damaging Your Hearing?   431

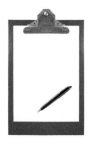

Choosing to Change Worksheet

Behavior Change Contract   19
Improving Psychological Health   43
Adopting Stress Management Techniques   66
Improving Diet   96
Improving Overall Fitness   122
Changing Body Weight and Improving Body Image   148
Reducing or Eliminating Drug Use   170
Quitting or Cutting Back on Drinking or Tobacco
   Use   199

Building Healthy Relationships   219
Practicing Safer Sex   254
Reducing STI Risk   280
Reducing the Risk of Chronic Disease   316
Taking Part in Preventive Care   339
Improving Driving   361
Aging Well   384
Increasing the Quantity or Quality of Sleep   404
Improving Environmental Health   434

Practical Strategies

Building Optimism   26
Questions to Ask Before Starting an Antidepressant   34
Spotting Destructive Thoughts   41
Building Self-Esteem   42
Recognizing the Signs of Stress Overload   55
Coping with Financial Stress   57

Exercising for Stress Management   62
Choosing Complex Carbohydrates   74
Choosing Healthful Fats   76
Eating Right While on the Run   95
Safe Weight Lifting   110
Cutting Calories, Not Nutrition   140

Warning Signs of Addiction   154

How to Protect Yourself from Risky Alcohol-Related
   Behavior   184

Quitting Smoking   198

Tips for Maintaining a Strong Relationship   212

Communicating Effectively About Sex and Birth
   Control   244

Protecting Yourself Against Infectious Diseases   270

Reducing Your Risk of STIs   274

Healthy Food Choices   314

Tips for Affordable Health Care   336

Preventing RSI When Working on a Computer   351

Coping with Grief   382

Reducing Your Energy Consumption   418

Reducing Pollution at Home   429

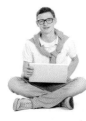

STUDENT STATS

Common Health Problems Reported by College
   Students   7

Psychological Health on Campus   30

Top 10 Impediments to Academic Performance   54

Top Supplements Used by Students   81

Overweight, Obesity, and Dieting on Campus   132

Drug Use Among Young Adults   156

Alcohol Use on Campus   177

Smoking on Campus   189

Students and Relationships   215

Sex and the College Student   240

STIs in People Aged 15–24   278

CAM Use Among College Students   330

Top Five Causes of Death in the United States
   Among People Aged 15–24   344

Sleepless on Campus   393

How Many College Students Think Green?   411

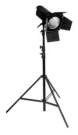

SPOTLIGHT

Science Discovers Stress   51

Feeding Your Bones   80

Core Concerns: Why You Should Strengthen
   Your Core   107

Can Alcohol Have Health Benefits?   182

Celibacy: The New Sexual Revolution?   233

Hand Washing and Hand Sanitizers   260

MRSA   268

Testicular Self-Exam   310

Breast Awareness and Self-Exam   312

Should You Get Vaccinated?   326

Exercise: The Life Preserver   374

Naps: Helpful or Harmful?   392

MYTH OR FACT?

Can Stress Give You an Ulcer?   53

Does Stretching Prevent Injury?   116

Can Coffee Cure a Hangover?   181

Should Boys Be Circumcised for Health Reasons?   226

Do Vaccines Cause Autism?   263

Do Hybrid Cars Merit Their Hype?   420

Does Using a Cell Phone Fry Your Brain?   432

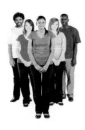

DIVERSITY & HEALTH

Health Disparities Among Different Racial and Ethnic
   Groups   6

Mental Health Through the Lenses of Ethnicity and
   Sexuality   32

Stress Through the Lenses of Gender, Age, and
   Geography   60

Vegetarian Diets   91

Men, Women, and Building Muscle   101

Safe Exercise for Special Populations   120

Overweight, Obesity, Ancestry, and the
   "Thrifty Gene"   135

Drug Use Through the Lenses of Sex, Race, Age, and Geography   155

Alcohol Use Through the Lenses of Sex, Race/Ethnicity, Age, Education, and Geography   176

Tobacco Use Through the Lenses of Sex, Race/Ethnicity, Age, Education, and Geography   191

Same-Sex Marriage: The State of Our Current Debate   214

Rates of STIs for Different Sexes, Ages, Races, and Sexual Orientations   276

Socioeconomic, Racial, and Ethnic Disparities in Chronic Disease   288

Gender Differences in Risk for Heart Disease   300

Injuries and Violence: Special Concerns for Young Men   353

Aging in the Blue Zones   373

Sleep Through the Lenses of Sex and Ethnicity   395

Working for Environmental Justice   425

CONSUMER CORNER

Choosing a Therapist Who's Right for You   40

Drinking Calories: What's in Your Bottle?   81

Organic, Local, All Natural, and Fair Trade: What to Choose?   93

Choosing Athletic Shoes   118

Are "Light" Cigarettes Safer to Use?   194

Using an Over-the-Counter Medication Safely   324

How to Choose a Bike Helmet   348

Should You Try OTC Sleep Aids?   401

What's in That Bottle?   422

Preface

When it comes to your health, what will you choose? You might think that question pertains to something in your future, such as who your next doctor should be, or how you can avoid illness down the road.

But the truth is you will also answer that question several times today, in ways both large and small. Did you get enough sleep last night? What will you have for lunch? Will you really hit the gym this afternoon, or just think about it? Are you waiting until the last minute to begin that paper due next week, or are you planning ahead so that you don't get overwhelmed?

In an era filled with medical innovations and high-tech health care, it's easy to overlook the fact that much of your health still rests in your hands. We all have to live with some factors we can't immediately control, such as our genetics or the physical environment that surrounds us. But beyond these fixed elements, your decisions and lifestyle habits count for a lot. This book is called *Choosing Health* to underscore that your actions and behavior *matter*. You can consciously make decisions now that greatly reduce your chances of developing health problems later. The health you choose is an essential part of creating the life you want, both on campus now and in the years ahead.

Key Features of this Text

We wrote this book to help you make the best possible health choices, using the most recent and scientifically accurate information available. Other textbooks provide plenty of health information but offer little guidance for actively improving your health. *Choosing Health*, Second Edition, makes health information more relevant to you with unique features such as these:

- **New! Electronic Chapter 16: Sleep, Your Body, and Your Mind** (available in the eText through MasteringHealth™) covers the most up-to-date research on sleep, its effects on health, and how to get your best night's rest. Also available as an electronic chapter is Chapter 17: Your Environment, Your Health.

- **New! Choose This, Not That** boxes highlight good vs. bad choices students make about common health issues. Each box promotes the healthy choice and explains why the poor choice is problematic.

- **New! Media and...** boxes discuss how today's media—everything from TV commercials to phone apps—affect our actions and feelings concerning a variety of health topics.

- **New! Choosing to Change Worksheets** (also available online through MasteringHealth™) in every chapter replace the former Behavior Change Workshops and help you target a behavior you want to change, determine your stage of behavior change based on the transtheoretical model of behavior change, think through the steps necessary to make a positive change, and put yourself on a path to success.

- **New! Change Yourself, Change Your World** sections at the end of each chapter show you how to implement the health information you've just learned. Each section offers advice on personal choices, helping a friend, and campus advocacy.

- **New! Critical-Thinking Questions** prompt you to think deeply and appear in each Diversity & Health and Media and... box.

- **Student Stories** appear throughout the text, and videos of real college students telling health-related stories stream on our course management platform, MasteringHealth™. New for the second edition, QR codes next to select Student Stories in the text link directly to that student's video. These stories reveal how students have dealt with health challenges and may inspire you to make changes in your own life.

- **Health Online** links throughout the book guide you to relevant health-related quizzes, tools, websites, videos, and podcasts. These links can also be found on MasteringHealth™, where they will be updated as needed.

- **Self-Assessments** (also available online through MasteringHealth™) enable you to evaluate your current health behaviors and identify areas you may wish to work on.

- **A magazine-style design** makes the book fun to read!

- **The lively, engaging writing** is informative, scientifically reliable, and authoritative.

- **Student Stats** throughout the book show you how health issues affect the college student population. Colorful graphs display statistics compiled by national surveys of college students.

- **Practical Strategies** boxes replace the previous Practical Strategies for Health and Practical Strategies for Change boxes. They provide concrete tips you can use to develop and maintain healthful behaviors.

- **Consumer Corner** boxes examine consumer-related issues such as using over-the-counter medications safely, choosing athletic shoes, and deciding whether or not to purchase organic produce.

- **Diversity & Health** boxes highlight how health issues can affect certain populations disproportionately, depending on sex, racial/ethnic background, socioeconomic class, and other factors.

- **Myth or Fact?** boxes provide scientific evidence supporting or refuting common health-related claims.

- **Special Feature** boxes highlight hot topics in health, including subjects like what the Affordable Care Act means for you; social networking, communication, and cyber-bullying; and emerging infectious diseases.
- **Get Critical** features at the end of each chapter ask you to think deeply about a health story from the news.

New in the Second Edition

The entire text has been reviewed and updated for the most current research, data, and statistics. In addition, the organization of many chapters has been updated to promote readability and clarity. The addition of **Choose This, Not That** boxes, **Change Yourself, Change Your World** sections, and **Choosing to Change Worksheets** enhance an already robust behavior change emphasis throughout the text. The addition of the **Media and...** boxes addresses instructor requests for more information about the effects of traditional and new media on health, and the new **Critical-Thinking Questions** included in the Diversity & Health and Media and... boxes encourage students to use their higher thinking skills. Above and beyond these improvements, each chapter has undergone specific changes.

Chapter 1:

- Additional information provided about how we as a society have come to our current definition of health.
- Revised and updated the information about the differences between health and wellness.
- Revised and updated the information about predisposing factors and enabling factors.
- New explanation of illness vs. disease added and new discussion of the ever-changing balance between the dimensions of wellness added.
- More information about health disparities added.
- Changed the Get Critical to one about Beyonce's "Move Your Body" video.

Chapter 2:

- Added information about the Ryff Scales of Psychological Well-Being.
- Revised information about Maslow's hierarchy of needs pyramid.
- Removed information about shyness and bad mood.
- Added more information about the benefits of spirituality and added information on Acceptance and Commitment Therapy (ACT).
- Added a section on campus options for help with mental issues.
- New Student Story: Javier: Dealing with Depression.

Chapter 3:

- Added a Choose This, Not That box on handling stress.
- Added information about the roles of personality types and personality traits on the stress response.
- Moved the Special Feature on getting enough sleep and the section on effects of stress on sleep to the new sleep chapter.
- Removed the Consumer Corner on stress and video games.
- Added a section about the effect of stress on weight.
- Replaced the Self-Assessment covering college students and stress.

- Completely updated and revised the Diversity & Health box.
- New Student Stories: David: Balancing School and Family, and Jessica: Handling School Stress

Chapter 4:

- Added a Choose This, Not That on healthful eating.
- Updated USDA MyPyramid to MyPlate.
- Created new Figure 4.3 showing the differences between AMDRs and DRIs.
- Moved information about dietary supplements into this chapter (from the consumer health chapter).
- Added information about glycemic index.
- Added a section about vitamin deficiencies and toxicities.
- Expanded Consumer Corner box to include not only a discussion of organic foods but also organics, "all natural," local, and fair trade.
- Added a section on food label claims.
- New Student Story: Nidya: Why I'm Vegetarian.

Chapter 5:

- Added QR codes that link directly to videos showing the exercises depicted in Figures 5.2 and 5.3.
- Added a Choose This, Not That box on how to begin a fitness program.
- Added a Media and... box on fitness apps.
- Added a Diversity & Health box on men, women, and building muscle mass.
- Removed the Consumer Corner box on low- or no-cost exercise equipment, removed the Self-Assessment about whether you should see a doctor before beginning an exercise program. Moved the content of the Practical Strategies for Health box on red flags during exercise into the body of the chapter.
- Changed the Get Critical to one covering Lance Armstrong's recent admission of performance-enhancing drug use.
- New Student Story: Molly: Adapting Exercise to My Needs.

Chapter 6:

- Added a Choose This, Not That box on weight-loss techniques.
- Removed the Diversity & Health box about eating disorders in men.
- Added information about the "thrifty gene theory" of weight gain.
- Added information about body image disorders.
- Added Figure 6.6 on health effects of anorexia and increased eating disorders content.
- Removed the table on body composition analysis methods.
- New Student Story: Viege: Eating Disorders
- New Get Critical on fashion-designer Karl Lagerfeld's comments about the singer Adele's weight.

Chapter 7:

- Added information about addiction in general and behavioral addictions.
- Added sections on how drugs affect the brain and how drugs leave the body
- Removed the Special Feature on other addictive behaviors and converted the previous Consumer Corner into a new Special Feature on study drugs.

- New Student Story: Ana: Coping with Addiction
- New Get Critical on the Adderall-related death of college student Richard Fee.

Chapter 8:
- Added a Media and... box on the media's effects on alcohol and tobacco use.
- Added a Special Feature box on resisting peer pressure.
- New Self-Assessment: Alcohol Use Disorders Identification Test (AUDIT).
- Moved drunk driving content to this chapter from the personal safety chapter.
- Updated information about smoking on campus and why some students smoke.
- Added a section on electronic cigarettes.
- Removed the Practical Strategies for Change box on beating relapse.
- New Student Story: Courtney: Negative Effects from Drinking.
- New Get Critical on the proposal to add graphic images to tobacco packaging.

Chapter 9:
- Added a Choose This, Not That on dealing with conflict.
- Added a Diversity & Health box on the state of same-sex marriage legalization.
- Changed the Special Feature that was on Facebook to a new Special Feature about social media, communication, and cyber-bullies.
- Added definitions of the terms homonegative and LGBTQI.
- Removed the Diversity & Health box on gender roles and communication.
- Updated the single parenthood section.
- New Get Critical on the American Academy of Pediatrics supporting gay marriage.

Chapter 10:
- Added a Media and... box on whether porn is a problem and updated and expanded content on porn.
- Added information on the Kinsey Scale of sexual orientation.
- Added more practical information about choosing the contraceptive that is right for you in the "Which Method Is Best?" section.
- Expanded the Practical Strategies box on talking about sex to include also talking about contraception.
- Added Table 10.2, arguments in opposition and support of abortion rights.
- Removed content on toxic shock syndrome.
- New Get Critical on NBA-star Jason Collins coming out as gay.

Chapter 11:
- Added new Figure 11.1 on the chain of infection and discussion of the chain of infection.
- Increased information on trichomoniasis.
- Reduced information on parasitic worm infections.
- New Get Critical on George Clooney, malaria, and the availablity of malaria drugs in the developing world.

Chapter 12:
- Added Figure 12.2, long-term complications of diabetes; Figure 12.7, warning signs of heart attack in men vs. women; Figure 12.9, cardiometabolic risk, and Figure 12.11, signs of skin cancer.
- Added Self-Assessments "Am I At Risk for Diabetes?," What's Your Risk for Heart Attack?," and "Am I At Risk for Cancer?" Removed the Self-Assessment "Are You At Risk for Chronic Disease?"
- Expanded the Practical Strategies box on healthy foods for chronic disease prevention.
- Added a section about cardiometabolic risk (CMR).
- Updated screening recommendations for cancer.
- Updated information about breast self-awareness and breast self-exams.
- Expanded the Diversity & Health box to not just cover racial disparities but also socioeconomic and ethnic disparities.
- Moved information about lowering risk for cancer from a Practical Strategies for Health box into the text discussion of each type of cancer.
- New Student Story: Michael: A Family History of Diabetes.
- New Get Critical on the pink ribbon campaign.

Chapter 13:
- Updated information on the Affordable Care Act.
- Added a new section on handling prescription medications properly.
- Updated the section on paying for health care.
- Moved information about dietary supplements into the nutrition chapter.
- Updated all health screenings information.
- Changed the Student Stats to one about CAM use among college students.
- Removed the Diversity & Health box on the uninsured.
- New Get Critical on genetic sequencing.

Chapter 14:
- Added a Choose This, Not That on safe driving.
- Added a Media and... box on whether viewing violence promotes violent behavior or the fear of violence.
- Updated the choking section and added photos showing back blows and abdominal thrusts.
- Moved drunk driving information to the alcohol chapter.
- Removed some information on car safety features.
- Removed the Practical Strategies for Health box on preparing for a home emergency.
- Removed information about falls, weather-related injuries, gangs, and child abuse.
- New Get Critical about hazing.

Chapter 15:
- Added a Media and... box on high-tech brain games and aging.
- Expanded the Diversity & Health box to cover aging in Blue Zones.
- Added a section on andropause.
- Reduced the "End of Life" section.

- Reduced information on osteoporosis, arthritis, and Alzheimer's disease.
- Removed the Consumer Corner on alternative medications for menopause.
- New Student Story: Stephen: Handling Aging.
- New Get Critical on physician-aid-in-dying.

Chapter 16:
- This chapter is entirely new and covers the latest research about sleep, sleep's effects on health, and how to get your best night's rest. This chapter is electronic and available through MasteringHealth™.

Chapter 17:
- This chapter has been moved from the printed text and has become electronic; it is available through MasteringHealth™.
- Added a Myth or Fact? box on hybrid cars.
- Added information about the evolution of the field of environmental health.
- Added sections about the effects of overpopulation and reversing population growth.
- Expanded sections on what can be done to reduce various types of pollution.
- Updated information about pollution drifting across the Pacific Ocean from China and affecting western states.
- Updated information about the effects of climate change on health.

Student Supplements

The student supplements for this textbook include:

- **MasteringHealth™ (www.masteringhealthandnutrition.com)** Mastering is the most effective and widely used online homework, tutorial, and assessment system for the sciences. It delivers self-paced tutorials that focus on course objectives, provides individualized coaching, and responds to your progress. Through MasteringHealth™, access:
  - Health Coaching Activities that guide you through key health and fitness concepts with interactive mini-lessons that provide hints and feedback.
  - NutriTools Build-A-Meal Activities, which allow you to combine and experiment with different food options and learn firsthand how to build healthier meals.
  - Dynamic Study Modules that enable you to study effectively on your own in an adaptive format. You receive an initial set of questions with a unique answer format asking you to indicate your confidence level. Once completed, reviews include explanations using materials taken directly from the text. These modules can be accessed on smartphones, tablets, and computers.

MasteringHealth™ also contains a complete set of student videos; health-related *ABC News* videos; online behavior change tools; interactive versions of the in-text Choosing to Change Worksheets and Self-Assessments; practice tests and additional self-assessments; links to updated websites, videos, and podcasts; and a rich suite of additional study tools, including MP3 audio files, mobile tips you can access on your smartphone, audio case studies, an online glossary, and flashcards.

- **Mobile Tips!** Now you can access health tips covering everything from stress management to fitness wherever you go, via your smartphone. A set of four different tip "cards" per chapter are available. Access them by navigating to **http://chmobile.pearsoncmg.com** on any mobile device. Or go straight to each chapter's cards by scanning the QR code provided at the end of the chapter.
- **A YouTube channel (www.youtube.com/ch00singhealth)** features selected student videos as well as videos from around the web.
- ***The Behavior Change Log Book and Wellness Journal*** is a booklet you can use to track your daily exercise and nutritional intake and create a long-term nutrition and fitness prescription plan.
- **A Digital 5-Step Pedometer** measures steps, distance (miles), activity time, and calories.
- **MyDietAnalysis (www.pearsonhighered.com/mydietanalysis)** is an online tool powered by ESHA Research, Inc., that features a database of nearly 20,000 foods and multiple reports. It allows you to track your diet and physical activity, receive analyses of what nutrients you may be lacking, and generate and submit reports electronically.
- ***Eat Right! Healthy Eating in College and Beyond*** is a guidebook that provides practical tips, shopper's guides, and recipes so that you can start putting healthy principles into action. Topics include healthy eating in the cafeteria, dorm room, and fast food restaurants; eating on a budget; weight-management tips; vegetarian alternatives; and guidelines on alcohol and health.
- ***Live Right! Beating Stress in College and Beyond*** is a guidebook that provides useful strategies for coping with a variety of life's challenges, during college and beyond. Topics include sleep, managing finances, time management, coping with academic pressure, relationships, and being a smart consumer.
- ***Take Charge of Your Health! Worksheets*** is a collection of 50 self-assessment exercises that you can fill out to assess your health and wellness. Worksheets are available as a gummed pad and can be packaged at no additional charge with the main text.

Instructor Supplements

This textbook comes with a comprehensive set of supplemental resources to assist instructors with classroom preparation and presentation.

- **MasteringHealth™ (www.masteringhealthandnutrition.com)** MasteringHealth™ helps instructors maximize class time with easy-to-assign, customizable, and automatically graded assessments that motivate students to learn outside of the class and arrive prepared for lecture. Through MasteringHealth™, access:
  - Publisher-provided problems with easy-to-edit questions and answers. It is also easy to import your own questions or quickly add images or links to further enhance the student experience.
  - Learning Outcomes that are tied to Bloom's Taxonomy and are designed to let Mastering do the work in tracking student performance against your learning outcomes. Mastering offers a data-supported measure to quantify students' learning gains and to share those results quickly and easily.
  - Learning Catalytics that let you use a wide variety of question types to engage students and understand what they do or don't know.

MasteringHealth™ also has a new Calendar View displaying up-coming assignments and due dates and allows instructors to easily schedule assignments.

- **The Teaching Toolkit DVD** replaces the former printed Teaching Toolbox and provides everything you need to prep for your course and deliver a dynamic lecture in one convenient place. It includes 51 *ABC News* Lecture Launcher videos, PowerPoint® Lecture Outlines and abbreviated Lecture Outlines, PowerPoint® clicker questions and *Jeopardy*-style quiz show questions, files for all illustrations and tables and selected photos from the text, Transparency Masters, the Test Bank in Word and RTF formats, the Computerized Test Bank, the Instructor's Resource Support Manual, Introduction to MasteringHealth™, Introductory video for Learning Catalytics, *Great Ideas! Active Ways to Teach Health and Wellness*, *Teaching with Student Learning Outcomes*, *Teaching with Web 2.0*, *Take Charge of Your Health! Worksheets*, *Behavior Change Log Book and Wellness Journal*, *Eat Right! Healthy Eating in College and Beyond*, and *Live Right! Beating Stress in College and Beyond*.

Electronic Editions

Choosing Health, Second Edition, is available in two electronic versions:

- **The Pearson eText available through MasteringHealth™** gives students access to the text whenever and wherever they can access the Internet. The eText pages look exactly like the printed text and include powerful interactive and customization functions. Students can create notes, highlight text, create bookmarks, zoom in and out, click hyperlinked words and phrases to view definitions, and search quickly and easily for specific content. Instructors can add notes to guide students, upload documents, and customize presentations using Whiteboard mode. The eText also contains the electronic chapters, Chapter 16: Sleep, Your Body, and Your Mind, and Chapter 17: Your Environment, Your Health. Contact your local Pearson sales representative for more information.

- **CourseSmart eTextbooks** are an exciting new choice for students looking to save money. As an alternative to purchasing the print textbook, students can subscribe to the same content online and save 40% off the suggested list price of the print text. Access the CourseSmart eText at **www.coursesmart.com.**

We are a team of health educators and communicators whose work reflects our deeply held belief that discussions of health are always a dialogue in progress. We hope this book will help you make changes toward better health. We also hope you'll let us know how those changes are going, and how we can make *Choosing Health* even more useful. Go to MasteringHealth™, and share your stories with us!

April Lynch
Barry Elmore
Jerome Kotecki

Acknowledgments

Authoring a new textbook can feel like a solitary job during countless hours alone researching topics or drafting chapters. But in reality, we as authors were supported not only by each other, but by an amazing team of editors, publishing professionals, content contributors, supplement authors, and reviewers.

Collectively, the authors would like to thank everyone at Pearson for their support and belief in our vision and our book, and call out a few of the key players for special thanks. First off, this book would not be possible without the support of Vice President, Editorial Director, Frank Ruggirello, who was always there to provide backing and funds for the project and to be our advocate to the highest reaches of the organization. Another lifeline for the book is Executive Editor Sandra Lindelof, who believed in our team from the start, provided creative and enthusiastic guidance for the book as a whole, and really fosters our student-centric approach to teaching health. This book would not be what it is today without the razor-sharp, insightful, and deeply knowledgeable edits, feedback, and management of Director of Development Barbara Yien. Senior Project Development Editor Marie Beaugureau stepped in and supplied even more editorial vision, direction, coordination, and management—her continuous contact with the team and good cheer in the face of tight schedules kept us all happy and on-track. Art Development Editor Kelly Murphy helped visualize the new Choose This, Not That feature, with great results. We'd also like to thank Editorial Assistant Tu-Anh Dang-Tran; Project Manager, Instructor Media Kyle Doctor; and Associate Content Producer Julia Akpan who, together, commissioned and managed the supplements and robust and innovative interactive media for the book. Megan Power and Lori Newman, Project Managers, expertly handled the production aspects of the book, from coordinating the design to making sure manuscript was being sent to the correct places to double-checking all aspects of page proofs. We must also thank everyone at S4Carlisle Publishing Services, especially Senior Project Editor Mary Tindle, for their wonderful work on the production and composition of the book—no matter how tight the schedule, they were always able to turn out the next round of page proofs. Senior Procurement Specialist Stacey Weinberger researched all types of paper and printing methods for us, to help us produce the most beautiful printing of the book possible. And speaking of beautiful, a million thanks to Yvo Riezebos, who designed the modern, engaging, and lively cover and interior for the book. Carolyn Arcabascio and Marta Johnson at PreMedia Global provided invaluable expertise in the researching and coordinating of hundreds of photos for the book, and Maya Melenchuk offered valuable help overseeing the photo program. A huge thanks goes out to Neena Bali, Executive Marketing Manager, who has worked tirelessly to get the message of *Choosing Health* out to instructors across the country.

We would also like to thank our contributors, all of whom truly left their stamps on the book and whom we can't thank enough for their time and expertise. Without Laura Bonazzoli, this book would not have been made. Her creativity, attention to detail, and passion for explaining complex health issues show throughout the entire text. Karen Vail-Smith at East Carolina University was invaluable at creating and vetting the content this text is based on.

The creation of the instructor and student supplements for *Choosing Health,* Second Edition, could not have been completed without the excellent work of our supplement authors. The Test Bank was created by Judy Kaufman, Monroe Community College, and Natalie Stickney, Georgia Perimeter College. The PowerPoint Lecture Outlines and Jeopardy-style quiz shows were written by Sloane Burke Winkelman, California State University, Northridge. Nicole George-O'Brien authored the Instructor Resource and Support Manual. Many thanks to all of them.

And, finally, we'd like to thank all the reviewers who spent their time reading and commenting on our chapters—we listened to each and every one of your comments and are extremely grateful for your feedback. A full list of reviewers begins on the next page.

From April Lynch

I have countless people to thank, beginning with those who helped with the heavy lifting of turning ideas into a new way to teach the subject of health, and of putting words to page. This project would have never gotten off the ground without the deep knowledge, health expertise, teaching wisdom, and killer sense of humor held by co-author Barry Elmore. It wouldn't have stayed off the ground without the invaluable contributions of co-author Jerome Kotecki and contributor Laura Bonazzoli, who brought a new level of expertise and polish to our team. I'll always be grateful to long-time colleague and fellow writer Julie Sevrens Lyons. Julie's prose has a deft, highly approachable touch, and this book is far the stronger for her contribution. For particular guidance on the topic of human and clinical genetics, I'm indebted to Vickie Venne, M.S., C.G.C., an excellent genetic counselor, advisor, and friend. And for some occasional real-world perspective, student-style, there's no one I'd turn to before my niece Emma Lynch Marini, whose insights and help on this book have always been smart, funny, and spot-on. Maybe, Emma, you just might use this book when you reach college!

From Barry Elmore

I have so many people to thank for their hard work and contributions to this book. Thanks to Matt Cox, for his help with the initial research. Thank you to all of the people at Pearson who worked so diligently on this book. I'd like to offer my sincere appreciation to Karen Vail-Smith, Dr. Sloane Burke, Sandra Walz, Julie Sevrens Lyons, Mary Jane Niles, and Laura Bonazzoli for their varied and invaluable contributions. It took a talented team of many players to bring this book to press, and I'd like to thank everyone who was a part of the effort.

From Jerome Kotecki

First, I am privileged to have had the opportunity to work with the extremely gifted team of April Lynch, Barry Elmore, and Pearson Education. Second, I am deeply grateful to those who continue to teach me on a daily basis: my students. The way in which they embrace learning—by being intellectually curious and inquisitive—provides a feedback loop that helps keep me focused on my own research and on investigating the latest findings in health research to expand my perspicacity as a professor. Third, I am fortunate to work with administrators who maintain that a well-written textbook based on expert knowledge reflects an important faculty contribution when it comes to the scholarship of teaching and learning. I appreciate the support of Dr. Michael Maggiotto, Dean of the College of Sciences and Humanities, Dr. Terry King, Provost and Vice President for Academic Affairs, and Dr. Jo Ann Gora, President, of Ball State University. Finally, I wish to extend my gratitude to my mentors. Thank you to Dr. James Stewart, my undergraduate advisor, for having faith in my abilities and encouraging me to stretch myself intellectually; and to Dr. Budd Stalnaker, Dr. John Seffrin, Dr. Mohammad Torabi, and Dr. Morgan Pigg, my graduate advisors, for your expertise and high standards and for guiding me on a path of enlightenment during my years at Indiana University and beyond.

SECOND EDITION REVIEWERS

Ni Bueno
Cerritos College

Lisa Shanti N. Chaudhari
Northern Arizona University

Max Faquir
Palm Beach State College

Autumn Hamilton
Minnesota State University

Kim Heffernan
University of Maryland

Annette Carrington Johnson
North Carolina Central University

Cheryl A. Kerns-Campbell
Grossmont College

Ayanna Lyles
California University of Pennsylvania

Debbie Lynch
Rose State College

Donna McGill-Cameron
Woodland Community College

Grace Pokorny
Long Beach City College

Andrea S. Salis
Queensborough Community College—CUNY

Terese A. Sheridan
University of Nebraska—Kearney

Kelly Fisher Shobe
Georgia Perimeter College

Amanda Tapler
Elon University

Iva Toler
Prince George's Community College

Ladona Tornabene
University of Minnesota, Duluth

Cody Trefethen
Palomar College

Gayle Truitt-Bean
Clarion University of Pennsylvania

MasteringHealth REVIEWERS

Steve Hartman
Citrus College

Kris Jankovitz
California Polytechnic State University, San Luis Obispo

Ayanna Lyles
California University of Pennsylvania

Karla Rues
Ozarks Technical and Community College

Debra Smith
Ohio University

FIRST EDITION REVIEWERS

Katherine Lewis Allen
Northern Arizona University

Elizabeth Barrington
San Diego Mesa College

Linda Beatty
McLennen Community College

R. Cruz Begay
Northern Arizona University

Robin Benton
Salem State College

James Brenner
West Chester University

Liz Brown
Rose State College

Jocelyn Buck
Wake Technical Community College

Ni Bueno
Cerritos College

Sloane Burke
East Carolina University

Angela Burroughs
North Carolina Central University

Annette Carrington
North Carolina Central University

Dusty Childress
Ozarks Technical Community College

Fay Cook
Lock Haven University of Pennsylvania

Jane Curth
Georgia Perimeter College

Dan Czech
Georgia Southern University

Asad Dalia
University of Cincinnati

Brent Damron
Bakersfield College

Kathleen Dayton
Montgomery College, Rockville

Jennifer Dearden
Morehead State

Jacqueline Dove
Baylor University

Maureen Edwards
Montgomery College

Paul Finnicum
Arkansas State University

Ari Fisher
Louisiana State University

Kelly Fisher Shobe
Georgia Perimeter College

Autumn Hamilton
Minnesota State University

Chris Harman
California University of Pennsylvania

Valarie L. Hilson
Arkansas State University

Yvonne Hilton
Lincoln University

Kathy Hixon
Northeastern State University

Angela D. Holley
Georgia Perimeter College

Jane House
Wake Technical Community College

Guoyuan Huang
University of Southern Indiana

Hollie Huckabee
Arkansas State University

Emogene Johnson-Vaughn
Norfolk State University

Aaron Junta
Shasta College

Patricia Kearney
Bridgewater College

Bill Kernan
William Patterson University

Brian Kipp
Grand Valley State University

John Kowalczyk
University of Minnesota, Duluth

Gary Ladd
Southwestern Illinois College

Ellen Larson
Northern Arizona University

Ayanna Lyles
California University of Pennsylvania

Debbie Lynch
Rose State College

Bridget Melton
Georgia Southern University

Roseann Poole
Tallahassee Community College

Mary Jo Preti
MiraCosta College

Elizabeth Ridings
Montgomery College

Albert Simon
Jackson State University

Becky Slonaker
McLennen Community College

Carol Smith
Elon University

Deborah Stone
Louisiana State University

Nancy Storey
Georgia Perimeter College

Cody Trefethen
Palomar College

Sandra Walz
West Chester University

Lesley Wasilko
Montgomery College

Linda White
Metropolitan State College

Sharon Woodard
Wake Forest University

PERSONAL HEALTH FORUM AND FOCUS GROUP PARTICIPANTS

Kim Archer
Stephen F. Austin State

Brian Barthel
Utah Valley University

Laura Blitzer
Long Island University

Dan Czech
Georgia Southern University

Jennifer Dearden
Morehead State University

Joel Dering
Cameron University

Joyce Fetro
Southern Illinois University

Paul Finnicum
Arkansas State University

Teresa Hardman
Moorehead University

Emogene Johnson-Vaughn
Norfolk State University

Andrew Kanu
Virginia State University

Patricia Marcum
University of Southern Indiana

Bridget Melton
Georgia Southern University

Maria Okeke
Florida A&M University

Dana Sherman
Ozarks Technical Community College

CLASS TESTERS

Fran Babich
Butte College

Elizabeth Bailey
Elon University

Stephanie Bennett
University of Southern Indiana

Tina Cummings
Bakersfield College

Dan Czech
Georgia Southern University

Kathy Deresinski
Triton College

Melody Durrenberger
Georgia Perimeter College

Max Faquir
Palm Beach State College

Renee Fenwick-Frimming
University of Southern Indiana

Kendra Guilford
University of Alabama, Tuscaloosa

Essam Hamido
Tennessee State University

Chris Harman
California University of Pennsylvania

Guoyuan Huang
University of Southern Indiana

Hollie Huckabee
Arkansas State University

Emogene Johnson-Vaughn
Norfolk State University

Tim Jones
Tennessee State University

Walt Justice
Southwestern College

September Kirby
South Dakota State University

Ayanna Lyles
California University of Pennsylvania

Bridget Melton
Georgia Southern University

Susan Milstein
Montgomery College

Kim Queri
Rose State College

Lesley Rennis
Borough of Manhattan Community College

Bernard Smolen
Prince George's Community College

Resa Walch
Elon University

Sharon Woodard
Wake Forest University

INTERVIEWEES

Duro Agbede
Southwestern College

Mike Basile
Borough of Manhattan Community College

Philip Belcastro
Borough of Manhattan Community College

Rebecca Brey
Ball State University

Elaine Bryan
Georgia Perimeter College

Ni Bueno
Cerritos College

Laura Burger-Simm
Grossmont College

Lynda Butler-Storsved
Elon University

Michael Calhoun
Elon University

Cheryl Campbell
Grossmont College

Doug Casey
Georgia Perimeter College

Steve Chandler
Florida A&M University

Kim Clark
California State University, San Bernardino

Mary Conway
Sierra College

Marianne Crocker
Ozarks Technical Community College

Paula Dahl
Bakersfield College

Brent Damron
Bakersfield College

James Deboy
Lincoln University

Eva Doyle
Baylor University

Melanie Durkin
Southwestern College

Maureen Edwards
Montgomery College

Kelly Falcone
Palomar College

Paul Finnicum
Arkansas State University

Barb Francis
Metropolitan State College

Valerie Goodwin
Southwestern College

Michelle Harcrow
University of Alabama, Tuscaloosa

Chris Harrison
Montgomery College

Bryan Hedrick
Elon University

Casie Higginbotham
Middle Tennessee State University

Valerie Hilson
Arkansas State University

Yvonne Hilton
Lincoln University

Kris Jankovitz
California Polytechnic State University, San Luis Obispo

Carol Jensen
Metropolitan State College

David Jolly
North Carolina Central University

Shannon Josey
Middle Tennessee State University

Beth Kelley
Grossmont College

Jerome Kotecki
Ball State University

Aaron Krac
Queensborough Community College

Randy Maday
Butte College

Rick Madson
Palm Beach State College

Vance Manakas
Moorpark College

Patricia Marcum
University of Southern Indiana

Mitch Mathias
Arkansas State University

Connie Mettille
Winona State University

Gavin O'Connor
Ozarks Technical Community College

Maria Okeke
Florida A&M University

Kevin Petti
San Diego Miramar College

Rod Porter
San Diego Miramar College

Regina Prodoehl
James Madison University

Elizabeth Ridings
Montgomery College

Karla Rues
Ozarks Technical Community College

Todd Sabato
James Madison University

Dana Sherman
Ozarks Technical Community College

Agneta Sibrava
Arkansas State University

Jeff Slepski
Mt. San Jacinto College

Nancy Storey
Georgia Perimeter College

Debra Sutton
James Madison University

Amanda Tapler
Elon University

Karen Thomas
Montgomery College

Silvea Thomas
Kingsborough Community College

Iva Toler
Prince George's Community College

Tim Wallstrom
Riverside Community College

Lesley Wasilko
Montgomery College

Patti Waterman
Palomar College

Linda White
Metropolitan State College

Susanne Wood
Tallahassee Community College

LaShawn Wordlaw-Stinson
North Carolina Central University

Bonnie Young
Georgia Perimeter College

Thank You to Our Student Advisory Board

The *Choosing Health* Student Advisory Board consists of students who submit stories, videos, questions, or feedback to us about *Choosing Health*. Many of them are thanked on the Student Advisory Board page at the beginning of the book.

HEALTH IN THE 21ST CENTURY

The current **life expectancy** at birth in the United States is **78.7 years**.[i]

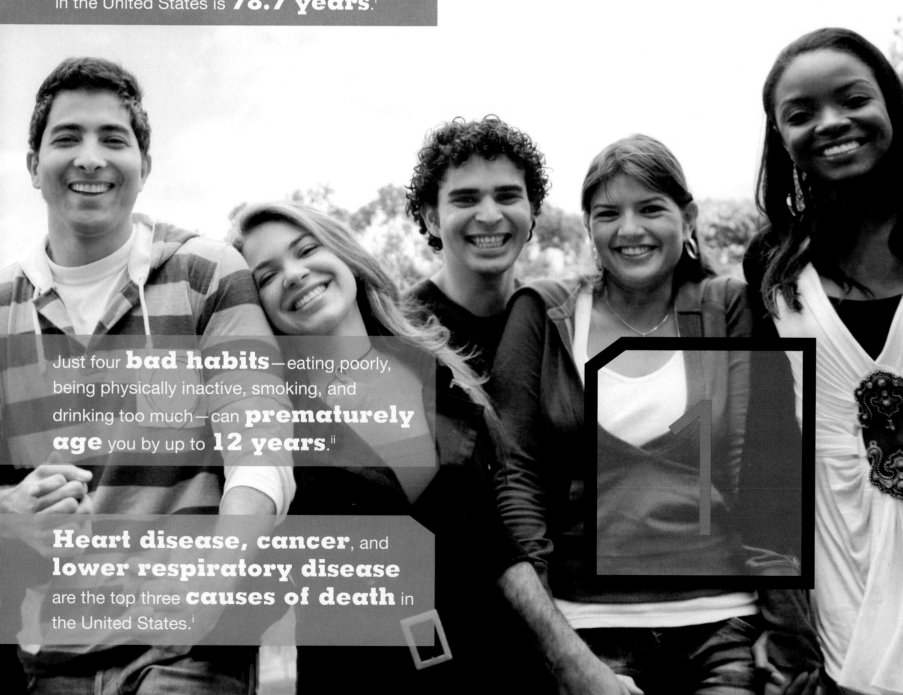

Just four **bad habits**—eating poorly, being physically inactive, smoking, and drinking too much—can **prematurely age** you by up to **12 years**.[ii]

Heart disease, cancer, and **lower respiratory disease** are the top three **causes of death** in the United States.[i]

Learning Objectives

DISCUSS the evolution of our current understanding of health and wellness.

IDENTIFY and describe the multiple dimensions of health.

COMPARE health challenges across America and around the world.

IDENTIFY four lifestyle choices that profoundly influence health.

PROVIDE examples of the six categories of determinants of health.

DESCRIBE three models of behavior change.

LIST seven steps for creating an effective behavior-change contract.

Have you ever noticed that, when you're ill, stressed, or sleep deprived, you're more likely to doubt yourself, argue with your roommate, and feel overwhelmed by even simple tasks? But when you're bursting with strength and stamina, you feel calm and confident. Even daunting challenges—like hiking a grueling trail or solving a calculus proof—can seem like fun.

Intuitively, you know health matters. But do your choices each day—what to eat, how much to sleep, whether to exercise, smoke, or abuse alcohol—really make health a priority? A theme of this textbook is that these so-called *lifestyle choices* can have a profound influence on your health. That's because, over many years, the cumulative effects of lifestyle choices can greatly increase or decrease your risk for disease and early death. If health matters, then your choices matter, too.

This textbook provides the facts you need to begin evaluating your current lifestyle choices. But information is just a first step. Each chapter concludes by identifying a variety of practical strategies to improve your own health, as well as ways to get involved in promoting a more healthful environment on campus. With this support, you can start making healthy changes for yourself and your world.

What Is Health?

If health matters, then it's worth taking a moment to explore what the term means. Let's begin by considering how the concept of health has evolved from a narrow focus on freedom from disease to a broad focus on wellness in multiple dimensions of life.

Health Versus Disease

For many centuries, the term *health* was generally understood to mean the absence of disease. Disease itself was recognized, fundamentally, as an imbalance, whether in temperature (hot versus cold), elements (fire, air, earth, and water), or *humors* (body fluids, including black and yellow bile, phlegm, and blood). As science and technology advanced in the 19th and 20th centuries, our understanding of the nature of this imbalance shifted. Physicians came to recognize that, in a state of health, the body has a variety of regulatory mechanisms that enable it to maintain stable internal conditions. The healthy body continually maintains this internal stability even as external factors—environmental temperature, food and water intake, and so forth—change. **Disease** therefore came to be understood as an alteration in body structure or biochemistry that is significant enough to cause the body's regulatory mechanisms to fail. This failure is often temporary—as when we experience congestion for several days before throwing off a cold. But in many cases, the body is unlikely to be able to return to a balanced state without medical care.

With this understanding of disease, you can probably appreciate that the traditional definition of health as "the absence of disease" is problematic for several reasons. People can and do experience **illness,** a subjective state in which a person feels unwell, whether or not true disease is present. Should we describe such a person as healthy? Conversely, people can experience themselves as entirely well despite having a serious disease. For example, certain types of cancer can go unrecognized until they are in a very advanced stage because they produce no obvious symptoms. Moreover, some people who have a diagnosed disease live highly productive lives and do not perceive themselves as unwell. Are they healthy?

In 1948, the newly formed World Health Organization (WHO)—the global health unit of the United Nations—published a radical new definition of **health** as "a state of complete physical, mental,

disease An alteration in body structure or biochemistry that is significant enough to cause the body's regulatory mechanisms to fail. Symptoms may or may not be present.

illness A subjective state in which a person feels unwell. Disease may or may not be present.

health More than merely the absence of disease, a state of well-being that encompasses physical, social, psychological, and other dimensions and is a resource for everyday life.

Premature
death Disability Symptoms Signs Awareness Education Growth High-level
wellness

|
Neutral point
(no discernible illness or wellness)

FIGURE 1.1 The Illness–Wellness Continuum. Your general direction on the continuum matters more than your specific point on it at any given time.

Source: Adapted from "Illness - Wellness Continuum" from *Wellness Workbook: How to Achieve Enduring Health and Vitality,* 3rd Edition, by John W. Travis, MD and Regina Sara Ryan. Copyright © 1981, 1988, 2004 by John W. Travis. Adapted and reprinted with permission.

and social well-being, and not merely the absence of disease or infirmity."[1] This holistic view was praised for acknowledging that, in a healthy person, many different dimensions of life work together harmoniously. However, the WHO definition's insistence upon "complete" physical well-being led to charges that it excluded people who are positive, fulfilled, and even vibrant despite having a disability or disease. This concern led to the introduction of a broader concept of health we now know as wellness.

> **wellness** An active process through which people become aware of, and make choices toward, a more successful existence.

Health Versus Wellness

Although the term wellness can be traced back to the 17th century, its first modern use was by Halbert L. Dunn, M.D., in a 1959 article in the *American Journal of Public Health.* Influenced by the WHO definition of health, Dunn argued that health-care providers should stop focusing so narrowly on disease, and begin studying the factors that support good health. He proposed thinking about disease and health as a "graduated scale" with death at one extremity and "peak wellness" at the other. He defined "peak wellness" as "performance at full potential in accordance with an individual's age and makeup."[2]

Dunn's work directly influenced that of John W. Travis, M.D., who founded the first "wellness center" in the United States in 1975. Travis developed a model of wellness he called the *illness–wellness continuum,* which has two extremes: premature death at one end and high-level wellness on the other **(Figure 1.1)**. At any given moment, most of us fall somewhere in between these extremes, shifting between states of feeling sick, "neutral," and vibrantly healthy. Your general direction on the continuum (either toward high-level wellness or toward premature death) matters more than your place on it at any given time. You may have a cold, for instance, and not feel particularly well—but if you are taking care of yourself and have a positive attitude, your general direction will be toward greater wellness. Moreover, people who have a chronic disease or disability and even people who are dying can experience high-level wellness, if they feel they are learning, growing, and contributing creatively to their world.

Today, the National Wellness Institute defines **wellness** as "an active process through which people become aware of, and make choices toward, a more successful existence."[3] People who have a high level of wellness make decisions that promote health in multiple areas of their lives.

Dimensions of Health and Wellness

Recall that the WHO definition of health identifies three dimensions—physical, mental, and social—all of which are working harmoniously. Though some researchers accept these three dimensions as adequate, others have identified more or different dimensions appropriate for the

populations they serve. In this textbook, we acknowledge the following seven dimensions of health and wellness: physical, intellectual, psychological, spiritual, social, environmental, and occupational **(Figure 1.2)**.

Physical Health

Physical health focuses on the body: how well it functions, and how well you care for it. Optimal physical health includes being physically active, eating nutritiously, getting enough sleep, making responsible decisions about sex, drinking, and drugs, and taking steps to avoid injuries and infectious diseases.

Intellectual Health

Intellectual health is marked by a willingness to take on new intellectual challenges, an openness to new ideas and skills, a capacity to think critically, and a sense of humor and curiosity. People who have a high level of intellectual health not only recognize problems quickly, but also seek and create solutions.

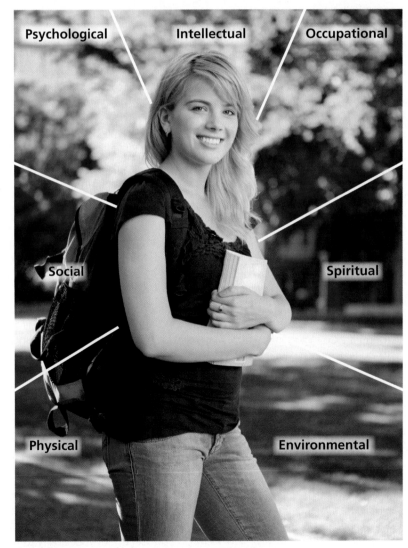

Psychological Intellectual Occupational

Social Spiritual

Physical Environmental

FIGURE 1.2 Dimensions of Health and Wellness. More than just the absence of disease, health and wellness encompass multiple dimensions of life.

Proud of My Scars

"HI, I'M COREY. I'm 19 and I'm a sophomore park and rec management major. I was born with a skeletal condition where the left side of my body is bigger than the right side. The doctors had to even out my legs so that I could walk flat-footed and wouldn't have back problems later in life. I've had a total of three surgeries, which left me with some scars. I also have a scar from my belly button all the way to the side of my rib cage. Growing up, I was always self-conscious, especially during the summer when everybody was out at the beach in swimsuits, and all these guys had six-pack abs. I knew I'd never be able to have abs like that because I have this scar running straight through my abdominal muscle.

Now, though, I've realized that my scars are a great conversation starter. People will see me and ask 'Oh, cool scar, how'd you get it?' I've learned over the years that everybody has a fail point and mine just happens to be physical. I've just learned to live with it. Those scars are what make me 'me.' I also have friends who don't really care what I look like or whether I'm the strongest or best-looking guy in the world. My friends are there whether I'm having surgeries or I'm on top of the world."

1. Where do you think Corey falls on the wellness continuum?

2. Assess how Corey is doing in at least three different dimensions of wellness.

STUDENT STORY

Psychological Health

Psychological health is a broad category encompassing autonomy, self-acceptance, and the ability to respond appropriately to our environment. It also includes the ability to maintain nurturing relationships and to pursue meaningful goals. Finally, people who are psychologically healthy sense that they are continually growing as individuals.

Spiritual Health

Spiritual health is influenced by the beliefs and values we hold and the ways in which we express them—for instance, in humanitarian activities, religious practices, or efforts on behalf of nature and the environment. Spiritual health contributes to a sense of place and purpose in life, and can be a source of support when we face challenges.

Social Health

Social health describes the quality of our interactions and relationships with others. How satisfying are your relationships with your family, your friends, and others in your life? How do you feel about your ability to fulfill social roles, whether as a friend, roommate, or community volunteer? Good social health is also characterized by an ability to provide support to others and receive it in return.

Environmental Health

Environmental health describes the quality of our home, work, school, and social environments—as well as the health of our planet. Air quality, availability of clean water and nutritious food, crime rates, weather, pollution, and exposure to chemicals are just a few of the variables that factor into environmental health.

Occupational Health

Occupational health describes the quality of your relationship to your work. Rather than a paying job, your "work" may consist of your studies, an athletic endeavor, or an artistic pursuit—whatever you consider your primary occupation. Challenges to occupational health include stress, lack of fulfillment in the work, poor relationships with colleagues, inadequate compensation, and sudden unemployment.

Current Health Challenges

In the past century, dramatic technological advances have enabled people worldwide to enjoy longer, healthier lives. Advances in public health, such as municipal water purification, sanitation, and food service inspection, have decreased the prevalence of disease. At the same time, new diagnostic techniques such as MRI scans and DNA testing, as well as vaccines, medications, and new types of surgery have helped us to find and treat disease earlier and more successfully. Despite such progress, many health challenges remain.

Health Across America

By one very basic measure of health—how long the average person born in the United States can expect to live—we are in far better shape than our predecessors. The current **life expectancy** at birth in the United States is a record 78.7 years—more than 15 years longer than it was in 1940.[4] The causes of *mortality* (the term used in public health for deaths within a population) have also changed dramatically over the years. In 1900, the leading causes of mortality were infectious diseases such as pneumonia, influenza, and tuberculosis.[5] Today, the leading causes in the United States are chronic diseases (see **Table 1.1**).

≫ **Want to know your life expectancy?** Try an online longevity calculator like the ones at www.northwesternmutual.com/learning-center/the-longevity-game.aspx **and** www.livingto100.com.

TABLE 1.1 **Top Five Causes of Death in the United States**

	Cause of Death
All ages	1. Heart disease 2. Cancer 3. Chronic lower respiratory disease 4. Stroke 5. Accidents/unintentional injuries
15–24 years old	1. Accidents/unintentional injuries 2. Suicide 3. Assault/homicide 4. Cancer 5. Heart disease

Source: Data from *Deaths: Preliminary Data for 2011*, by D. L. Hoyert and J. Xu, 2012, *National Vital Statistics Reports, 61* (6), pp. 29–30.

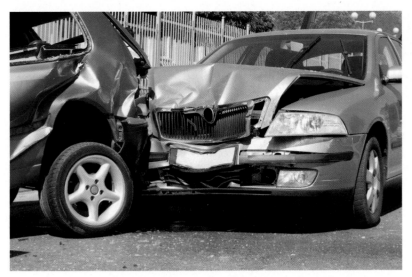

Accidents are the leading cause of death among people aged 15–24 in the United States.

America's Health Challenges

In 2011, just two chronic diseases—heart disease and cancer—were responsible for almost half of all deaths (46.6%) in the United States.[4] Almost 1 out of every 2 adults has at least one chronic disease.[6] These statistics are all the more shocking when you realize that chronic diseases are among the most preventable of all health problems in the United States.[6] That's why one of the world's oldest and largest public health agencies—the U.S. Centers for Disease Control and Prevention (CDC)—is sponsoring a national initiative to reduce our rate of chronic disease. As part of this initiative, the CDC has identified four common behaviors that are responsible for most of the suffering and early death related to chronic diseases. They are **(Figure 1.3)**:[6]

- Lack of physical activity
- Poor nutrition
- Tobacco use
- Excessive alcohol consumption

Are Americans paying attention, and if so, are we changing our behaviors? Recent national health surveys reveal the following trends among U.S. adults:

- Less than half (48%) meet the 2008 *Physical Activity Guidelines*.[7]
- More than 33% are overweight and another 35.9% are obese.[8]
- 22% of males and 17% of females smoke.[8]
- More than 23% admitted to binge drinking within the last year.[8]

As these statistics suggest, it's time for Americans to make healthful lifestyle choices a priority.

Organizations That Promote America's Health

The U.S. Department of Health and Human Services (HHS) is the U.S. government's principal agency for protecting the health of all Americans and providing essential human services, especially for those who are least able to help themselves.[9] Its primary division is the U.S. Public Health Service (PHS), which is directed by the Office of the Surgeon

> **life expectancy** The average number of years a person may expect to live.
>
> **Healthy People initiative** A federal initiative to facilitate broad, positive health changes in large segments of the U.S. population every 10 years.

General. The PHS includes a dozen operating divisions that work together to promote and protect the health of Americans. Among these is the CDC, as well as the following:[9]

- The *Food and Drug Administration (FDA)* is responsible for assuring the safety, efficacy, and security of medications, medical devices, the food supply, cosmetics, and products that emit radiation.
- The *National Institutes of Health (NIH)* is the primary center for medical research in the United States.
- The *Substance Abuse and Mental Health Services Administration* is an agency whose mission is to reduce the impact of substance abuse and mental illness on America's communities.

The Healthy People Initiative

In 1979, HHS launched the **Healthy People initiative** with a report of the Surgeon General on health promotion and disease prevention efforts in the United States. This laid the groundwork for the publication in 1980 of *Healthy People 1990*, a set of 10-year objectives for improving the health of all Americans. Every decade since, HHS has updated *Healthy People* to include both new objectives and a report of the progress made over the previous decade. Called both a "road map and a compass for better health," the most recent effort, *Healthy People 2020*, was released in December 2010.[10]

Healthy People 2020 poses two main questions:[10]

- What makes some people healthy and others unhealthy?
- How can we create a society in which everyone has a chance to live long, healthy lives?

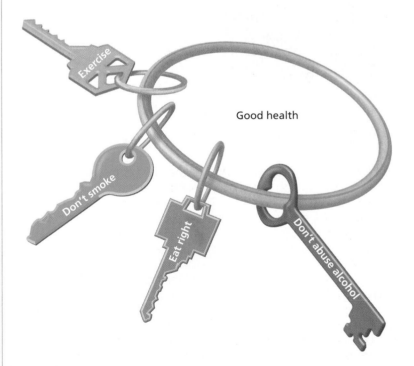

FIGURE 1.3 Four Keys to Good Health. These four behaviors can significantly reduce your risk of chronic disease and early death.

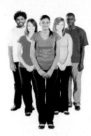

Health Disparities Among Different Racial and Ethnic Groups

Whether the causes are socioeconomic, biological, cultural, or still not well understood, health disparities exist among different racial and ethnic populations. For example:

- Hispanics are more likely to live in an area with poor air quality than any other ethnic group, and are more likely to suffer from asthma. They have the highest adolescent birth rate, and are less likely to receive prenatal care early in pregnancy. Hispanic children have the highest rates of obesity, and are less likely to receive all recommended childhood vaccinations.[1]

- African Americans experience the same leading causes of death as the general population, but tend to experience these diseases and injuries more often and die of them at younger ages and higher rates than other

groups. These differences start in infancy, when African American babies experience a higher infant mortality rate—more than twice that of Caucasians, Hispanics, or Asian Americans. African American adults have the highest homicide rate, for example: 23.1 per 100,000 versus 2.7 per 100,000 for Caucasians. They also have the highest rates of obesity and hypertension of any ethnic group, and the highest death rate from heart disease, stroke, and cancer.[1]

- Asians and Asian Americans, overall, tend to have a life expectancy longer than that of the general population. Their rates of chronic disease tend to be lower, as do their rates of substance abuse, fatal motor vehicle accidents, homicides, and suicides. For example, the rate of drug-induced deaths among Asian Americans is just 2 per 100,000, compared with over 15 per 100,000 for Caucasians.[1]

- Native Americans experience lower than average rates of some of the more common health concerns in the United States, such as heart disease or cancer. But they also tend to have a shorter life expectancy than the general population, due to high rates of smoking, alcohol abuse, fatal motor vehicle accidents, drug-induced deaths, and suicide.[1] Diabetes and its complications is an especially important concern—Native Americans as a group have the highest rate of diabetes.[2]

- Caucasians share many health risks with Native Americans, including high rates of alcohol abuse, fatal motor vehicle accidents, drug-induced deaths, and suicide.[1] In addition, Caucasian women have the highest incidence of any kind of cancer.[3, 4]

Critical-Thinking Questions

1. According to the United States Census Bureau, in 2010, the median income for African American families was $39,988, whereas the median income for Asian American families was $68,780. Relate this income disparity to the health disparities identified above.

2. In 2012, a report from the American Cancer Society announced that cancer had surpassed heart disease as the leading cause of death among Hispanics, but not other ethnic groups. Use the following link to access an online article summarizing this report, and list at least three factors that the American Cancer Society identifies as contributing to this trend: www.cancer.org/cancer/news/news/report-cancer-now-leading-cause-of-death-among-hispanic-americans.

References: **1.** "CDC Health Disparities and Inequalities Report—United States, 2011," by the Centers for Disease Control and Prevention, January 14, 2011, *Morbidity and Mortality Weekly Report,* vol. 60 (Supplement). Available at http://www.cdc.gov/mmwr/pdf/other/su6001.pdf. **2.** "National Diabetes Fact Sheet, 2011," by the Centers for Disease Control and Prevention, 2011. Atlanta, GA: Centers for Disease Control and Prevention, U.S. Department of Health and Human Services. http://www.cdc.gov/diabetes/pubs/pdf/ndfs_2011.pdf. **3.** "Breast Cancer Rates by Race and Ethnicity," by the Centers for Disease Control and Prevention, November 14, 2012, retrieved from http://www.cdc.gov/cancer/breast/statistics/race.htm. **4.** "Cancer Rates by Race and Ethnicity," by the Centers for Disease Control and Prevention, May 2, 2012, retrieved from http://www.cdc.gov/cancer/dcpc/data/race.htm.

In exploring these questions, *Healthy People 2020* emphasizes an *ecological approach* to health, one that considers the relationship between an individual's health and the many factors that influence it—from biology and lifestyle choices to level of education, access to health-care services, and even the foods available in the individual's neighborhood. Later in this chapter, we'll discuss these influences in more detail.

One of the primary goals of the Healthy People initiative is to achieve *health equity*—the attainment of the highest level of health for all people.[10] This requires the elimination of **health disparities**—differences in the rate and burden of disease and the access to and quality of health care among various population groups. These include groups based on race or ethnicity, religion, socioeconomic status, sex, age, mental health, disability, sexual orientation or gender identity, geographic location, or other characteristics historically linked to discrimination or exclusion.[10] For example, gays and lesbians experience certain health disparities—including a lower quality of health

care—associated with the discrimination they experience. The nearby **Diversity & Health** box identifies key health disparities specific to race and ethnicity, and we'll examine the role of poverty and other disparities as we continue in this chapter.

>> **For more information on** *Healthy People 2020*, **visit** www.healthypeople.gov.

health disparities Gaps in the rate and burden of disease and the access to and quality of health care among various population groups.

Health on America's Campuses

Centers of higher learning, as microcosms of our larger society, have come to recognize that promoting students' health helps the institution meet its goal of providing the best education possible. Stress, sleep deprivation, poor nutrition, depression, anxiety, alcohol and tobacco use, and sexually transmitted infections are just a few of the health issues that can affect academic performance and achievement.

> *The behaviors that increase the risk of developing chronic diseases—including unhealthy eating habits and a lack of physical activity—are common among college students."*

Campus Health Challenges

The **Student Stats** box lists common health issues reported by college students in a recent nationwide study.[11] The same study reported that more than 60% of students describe their health as either "very good" or "excellent."

Among Americans aged 15–24, the leading causes of death are accidents, suicide, and homicide (see Table 1.1). These sudden, traumatic deaths lead mortality in this age group because younger people do not experience the same high rates of chronic diseases (such as heart disease and cancer) that increase mortality among the adult population as a whole. However, the behaviors that increase the risk of developing chronic diseases—including unhealthy eating habits and a lack of physical activity—are common among college students. Although 62% of students report being at a healthy weight, 21% are overweight and 11% are obese.[11] Furthermore, although 46.5% of college students meet national recommendations for physical activity (moderate exercise for at least 30 minutes at least 5 days per week or vigorous exercise for at least 20 minutes at least 3 days per week), over half do not.[11]

Interestingly, research has shown that students tend to vastly overestimate how many of their peers are regularly using alcohol, tobacco, or other drugs.[11] For example:

- Students believe that 92.9% of their peers consumed alcohol during a given 30-day period. The actual percentage was 62.0%.
- Students believe that 79.7% of their peers had smoked cigarettes during a given 30-day period. The actual percentage was 13.2%.
- Students believe that 80.1% of their peers had smoked marijuana during a given 30-day period. The actual percentage was 15.3%.
- Students believe that 74.8% of their peers used illicit drugs (excluding marijuana) during a given 30-day period. The actual percentage was 12.7%.

The lesson here: When it comes to drugs and alcohol, it's simply not true that "everyone is doing it."

The Healthy Campus Initiative

In conjunction with the Healthy People initiative, the American College Health Association publishes an initiative called **Healthy Campus** for use in student settings. Colleges and universities participating in this program can choose to focus on improving health topics most relevant to them, such as:

- Reducing stress and depression
- Decreasing student abuse of alcohol and drugs

Healthy Campus An offshoot of the Healthy People initiative, specifically geared toward college students.

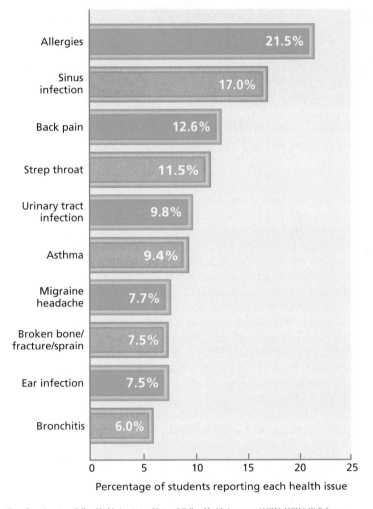

STUDENT STATS
Common Health Problems Reported by College Students

Percentage of students reporting each health issue

Health Issue	Percentage
Allergies	21.5%
Sinus infection	17.0%
Back pain	12.6%
Strep throat	11.5%
Urinary tract infection	9.8%
Asthma	9.4%
Migraine headache	7.7%
Broken bone/fracture/sprain	7.5%
Ear infection	7.5%
Bronchitis	6.0%

Data from *American College Health Association National College Health Assessment (ACHA-NCHA II) Reference Group Executive Summary, Fall 2012,* by the American College Health Association, 2013, retrieved from http://www.acha-ncha.org.

- Improving opportunities for daily physical activity on campus
- Improving sexual health among students

>> **A full list of student objectives for** *Healthy Campus 2020* **is available at** www.acha.org/HealthyCampus/student-obj.cfm.

Health Around the World

In our increasingly mobile and connected world, where a country experiencing a dangerous infectious disease is just a plane ride away, global health has become a top concern.

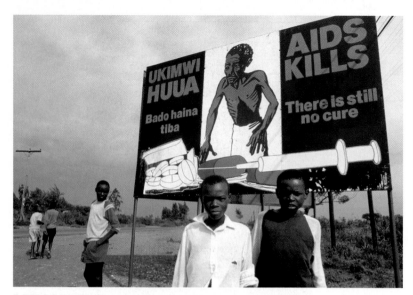

HIV/AIDS continues to be a serious concern worldwide, especially in sub-Saharan Africa.

Some countries with lower levels of economic development and less stable political systems continue to experience high rates of infectious diseases that have largely been eradicated in other parts of the world. For example, parts of Africa, Asia, and South America continue to grapple with cholera, an infectious disease transmitted via contaminated water, and malaria, which is transmitted by mosquitoes. Although the rate of new infections from the human immunodeficiency virus (HIV) dropped by 50% between 2010 and 2012, the United Nations Programme on HIV/AIDS reports that, at the end of 2011, 34 million people were living with HIV. The most heavily affected regions of the world are sub-Saharan Africa, the Caribbean, Eastern Europe, and Central Asia.[12]

Some infections are now resisting conventional treatment with antimicrobial drugs. A wide range of disease-causing microorganisms—including the bacteria that cause tuberculosis, the viruses that cause influenza, and the parasites that cause malaria—are becoming resistant to the antimicrobial agents used for treatment.[13] People infected with resistant strains of microorganisms are more likely to have longer hospital stays and to die as a result of the infection.[13] This is a concern not only in developing nations, but across the globe.

>> For more information on infectious diseases around the world, visit the World Health Organization website at www.who.int/topics/infectious_diseases/en.

Nutritional diseases are also still a concern in developing nations: In 2012, 870 million people in the world remained chronically undernourished. Nearly 98% of these hungry people live in the developing world.[14] Deficiency of certain vitamins and minerals causes a variety of diseases rarely seen in the United States and Europe, such as night blindness, which develops when vitamin A is deficient, and a form of mental retardation called cretinism, which is due to iodine deficiency. Malnutrition also increases an individual's susceptibility to infection, as well as the risk that infection will result in death.

To address these global disparities, a number of privately funded international health organizations have joined with public efforts carried out by international agencies such as the WHO. These groups are currently funding immunizations, mosquito nets, water filters, vitamin drops, and the addition of iodine to salt. These efforts are improving global health.

Whereas global rates of HIV and certain other infectious diseases have begun to stabilize or decline, rates of chronic diseases such as heart disease and type 2 diabetes are rising worldwide. That's because obesity—a risk factor for chronic diseases—is increasing. Two trends contribute to the rising prevalence of "globesity": A greater percentage of the world's population now has access to high-fat, high-sugar processed foods. At the same time, more people have access to motorized transportation, labor-saving devices, and sedentary forms of entertainment. These trends have contributed to an alarming statistic: The WHO estimates that in developing nations 115 million people now suffer from obesity-related disease.[15]

Determinants of Health

Earlier we noted that *Healthy People 2020* takes an ecological approach to health—one that considers the relationship of individual human beings to their environment. In this view, individuals share responsibility for the state of their health with a range of social, economic, and environmental factors. The WHO, as well as the CDC and other agencies of the HHS, refers to these factors as **determinants of health.** Any steps taken to improve health—both for individuals and for populations—are likely to be more successful when they target multiple determinants of health.[16]

>> To watch a video explaining and providing examples of how determinants influence an individual's health, go to www.healthypeople.gov/2020/about/DOHAbout.aspx.

Determinants of health fall into six broad categories, all of which overlap to a greater or lesser extent. Let's take a closer look.

Biology and Genetics

Biological and genetic determinants influence your health but are beyond your control. The following are the most significant determinants in this category:

- **Age.** Incomplete growth and development make children more susceptible to certain health problems, such as infectious diseases. At the other end of the age spectrum, the physical and cognitive effects of aging increase an older adult's vulnerability to poor health.[16]

- **Sex.** The genes you inherited at conception determined your sex—that is, the anatomical and physiological features that differentiate males from females. Sex has a powerful role on health, with biological differences between men and women resulting in many different health outcomes. Women tend to live about four years longer than men, for example, but have higher rates of arthritis and osteoporosis (low bone density). Men are more likely to develop hypertension (high blood pressure) and heart disease, to abuse alcohol, and to die in a motor vehicle accident, by homicide, by suicide, from a drug overdose, or from heart disease.[17]

- **Genetics.** In addition to your sex, many other aspects of your genetic inheritance influence your health. Most obviously, these include the presence or absence of genetic conditions such as color blindness or hemophilia (a failure of

determinants of health The range of personal, social, economic, and environmental factors that influence health status.

blood clotting). You may also have inherited from one or both parents a particular gene or genes that increases your susceptibility to a disease. For instance, women who carry the BRCA1 or BRCA2 gene have an increased risk for breast and ovarian cancer.

- **Race/Ethnicity.** Certain population groups have an increased or decreased risk for certain diseases when compared with the general population. (See the **Diversity & Health** box on page 6.) Awareness of these differences can prompt you to make better lifestyle choices, and can prompt your physician to provide more targeted care. For example, because African Americans have higher rates of hypertension, informed doctors may encourage more frequent blood pressure screenings for their African American patients at an earlier age.

- **Health history.** Some conditions that you experienced in the past may still be influencing your health today. For instance, have you ever had chickenpox? If so, you're at increased risk for a disorder called shingles, which is characterized by a painful, itchy rash that forms blisters. After a person recovers from chickenpox, the virus remains in the body, and can become active decades later as shingles. Similarly, many sexually transmitted infections can reduce your fertility or cause other health problems. Past injuries can also permanently affect health.

- **Family history.** You—and your children—are at increased risk for developing some of the same diseases that members of your family have experienced. This is true not only for recognized genetic diseases, but also for many chronic diseases such as hypertension and type 2 diabetes, and even for some psychological disorders such as depression. It's important to know your family health history so that you and your health-care provider can take steps to reduce any risks.

 Create and print out your own family health history tree using the interactive tool *My Family Health Portrait* **from the U.S. Surgeon General at** https://familyhistory.hhs.gov/fhh-web/home.action.

Individual Behaviors

Although you can't turn back the clock on aging or select different genes, other health determinants—such as your individual lifestyle choices—are very much within your ability to control.

We noted earlier that the CDC has identified four behavioral decisions with a profound ability to influence your health. These are: (1) the level of physical activity you engage in, (2) the type of diet you eat, (3) your choice about whether or not to smoke, and (4) how much alcohol you consume. Making healthful choices in these four key areas can greatly decrease your risk of developing chronic disease later in life. On the other hand, poor choices in these areas can prematurely age you by up to 12 years![18]

Other lifestyle choices that play a significant role in promoting health include: managing your stress level, getting enough sleep, refraining from illicit drug use, developing supportive relationships with others, making responsible sexual health decisions, and taking basic steps to ensure your personal safety, such as wearing a seat belt. These behaviors are discussed later in this text.

Social Determinants

Individual behaviors are undeniably important in determining health, but the ecological approach also recognizes the influence of a variety of social

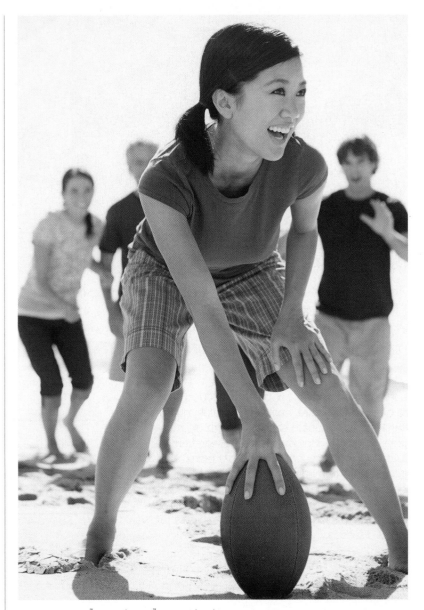

Regular physical activity is a key component of staying healthy.

status syndrome The disparity in health status and rates of premature mortality between the impoverished and the affluent within any given society.

conditions that you can work to improve, but can't fully control. Social determinants are the economic and societal conditions in which people live. They include, for example, interpersonal and community relationships, discrimination, poverty, educational and job opportunities, transportation, and public safety.[16]

Research over the past two decades has increasingly acknowledged the significant influence of social determinants on health. For example, a family may understand the value of regular physical activity, but live in a high-crime area where they're afraid to go out walking, and can't afford the cost of membership in a fitness club. If you're getting the sense that poverty is a fundamental social determinant of health, you're right: Rates of both disease and premature death are dramatically higher among the poor than among the rich.[19] Called the **status syndrome,** this disparity in health and mortality has been observed not only in developing nations, but also in Europe and the United States. The status syndrome has traditionally

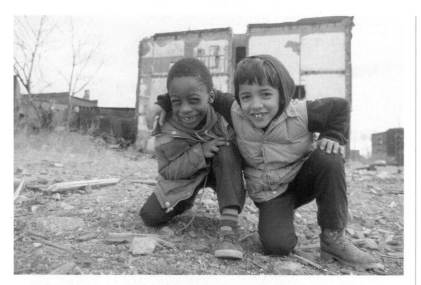

These boys live in a poor area of South Bronx, NY. Living in a neighborhood that lacks access to resources increases their risk for a variety of health problems.

been attributed to a poor person's reduced access to quality health care, health information, nutritious foods, safe, adequate shelter, and opportunities for physical activity. However, some researchers believe that it occurs because, in people who are poor, two fundamental human needs go unmet: These are the needs for autonomy and for full social participation. These unmet needs dramatically increase stress, causing physiological changes that can lead to a variety of diseases.[19]

Physical Determinants

Physical determinants are physical conditions in the environment. Examples include:[16]

- Aspects of the natural environment, such as plants and climate
- Aspects of the so-called *built environment*, which includes all buildings, spaces, and products that are made or modified by people
- Presence or absence of toxic substances and other physical hazards

For example, heat waves, extreme cold, floods, wildfires, and other natural hazards are aspects of the physical environment that threaten health, whereas a nearby park, community swimming pool, and farmers' market support health.

Health Services

Health services include availability of quality health care as well as access to that care. Health literacy is also included in health services.

Access to Health Services

In countries with a national health service, health insurance status does not usually affect access to quality care. In the United States, health insurance status directly affects access to health services. People with inadequate health insurance are less likely to have a regular doctor or

place of care. They are also less likely to receive preventive care, and more likely to delay medical treatment. Many uninsured wait until a condition has advanced to a crisis stage before visiting a local hospital emergency room—a habit that greatly increases the level of care required as well as the cost of that care.

Supporting the understanding that access to quality care is a key determinant of health, studies have found that while higher-income Americans have enjoyed a wide range of health gains, these improvements have not been shared equally by lower-income Americans.[17] In part to address this disparity, in 2010 the U.S. Congress passed into law a set of comprehensive new health-care reforms. Called the Affordable Care Act, the legislation aims to substantially reduce the number of Americans who do not have health insurance.[20] Among other measures, it supports the creation of affordable insurance exchanges where consumers without access to health insurance from an employer can find an affordable plan that meets their needs. They may also be eligible for tax credits and other financial assistance to help them pay for coverage.

>> **For updates on the Affordable Care Act, visit** www.healthcare.gov.

Health Literacy

In the 21st century, quality health care increasingly depends upon **health literacy,** the ability to evaluate and understand health information and to make informed choices for your own care. It includes the ability to read, understand, and follow instructions in medical brochures and prescription drug labels; the ability to listen to health-care providers, ask good questions, and analyze the information you receive; and the ability to navigate an often-confusing and complex health-care system.[21] Increasingly, health literacy also requires a degree of computer literacy and media awareness.

Another goal of this text is to increase your health literacy by providing you with strategies to critically evaluate all the health

health literacy The ability to evaluate and understand health information and to make informed choices for your health care.

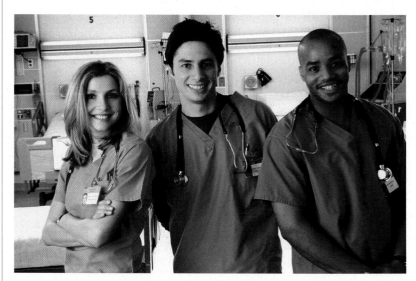

Can you trust medical information from doctors (real or fictional) on TV?

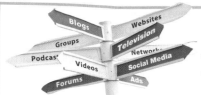

media and HEALTH

Evaluating Health Information in the Media

Is the health information you just researched on the Internet accurate? Can you trust your favorite actor's television advertisement for a weight-loss product? Was last week's episode of *The Dr. Oz Show* based on any kind of medical reality? How can you make sense of the endless stream of media headlines trumpeting health studies that sometimes contradict one another?

The term *media* can mean a variety of things. We use it here to include books, newspapers, magazines, television, advertisements, Internet/websites, and even mobile apps.

Whenever you encounter information from the media, critically assess it. Is someone trying to sell you something? Are there other ways to solve problems like being overweight without resorting to pills? Do you realize that many of the images of celebrities you see in magazines have been digitally altered to make them look more attractive than they really are?

When you come across an article about the results of the latest health-related study, consider: Was the study conducted by an unbiased source, or was it carried out by an individual or organization with a vested interest in the outcome? Have the results been replicated by other researchers? Was the sample size of the study large or small? Was the study conducted over a short or long period of time? Is the study only showing what may be a coincidental *correlation* between two things, or is it truly showing that one variable is the direct result of another variable?

The Internet deserves special attention in discussions of health in the media, as it is increasingly where people turn for information. When you're evaluating health information online, ask yourself the following questions to determine whether or not the information is credible:

- Is the sponsor of the site identified? Is it a commercial, nonprofit, academic, or government site? In general, sites with URLs ending in ".gov" (signifying a U.S. government site) or ".edu" (signifying an educational institution) are more likely to provide credible information than those that end in ".com." Note that the domain ".org" is used by many credible, nonprofit, noncommercial sites, but it is sometimes used by commercial entities as well.

- What is the purpose of the site? Is it to inform and educate, or is it to sell you something? If it is to sell you something, be aware that the information presented is more likely to be biased.

- Does the site tell you where the information it presents is coming from? If so, is the content based on scientific evidence, or was it written by someone hired by the site to produce marketing information? Sites that are able to provide citations and links to scientific studies and journals are more likely to be credible than sites lacking these references.

- Does the site specify when its content was last updated? Health information can sometimes change quickly, so you want to seek out information that is as current as possible.

- Does the site list a reputable professional accreditation? Many reputable health sites, for example, are accredited by the Health on the Net Foundation, and bear an insignia reading "HON."

Throughout this text, the **Get Connected** feature at the end of each chapter lists health-related websites where you can obtain reliable health information. Still, keep in mind that information on the Internet is never a substitute for consulting a health-care professional. Do not rely solely on online information to make important decisions about your health! Make an appointment with your doctor and don't be afraid to ask questions to be certain that you are receiving the most accurate information about any health issue you may be facing.

Critical-Thinking Questions

1. How often do you encounter an advertisement for prepackaged snack foods or meals? In contrast, how often have you encountered an advertisement for fresh fruits and vegetables? Does this alter your eating habits at all?

2. How often have you seen an advertisement promoting prescription drugs—for everything from weight loss to social anxiety? Does this affect the way you think about prescription drugs or your guess as to how many people take prescription drugs? Do you think seeing advertisements makes you more or less likely to take prescription drugs, or do ads have no effect?

3. How regularly are you exposed to images of seemingly perfect celebrities? How does this affect your feelings about your own body and your self-esteem?

Sleep Deprived

"HI, I'M JASMINE. I'm a freshman and I'm a child development major. Each night, I'm very lucky if I get four hours of sleep. I'm just a night owl. I like staying up at night. My father's the exact same way. It's like 3 o'clock in the morning and we'll still be up watching the food channel. Around exam time, I find myself awake at 7:30 in the morning, still up— knowing that I have a test at 9:30. Why, I don't know.

I don't think I'm doing my best right now because when I drag myself to class, I'm half asleep. I do need to change and get better rest so that I can do better in school. I don't think I've gotten 8 hours of sleep since I was 13. I'm 19, so that's six years of not getting a full night's sleep. That takes a toll on your body and your mind."

1. What stage of the *transtheoretical model of behavior change* would you guess that Jasmine is in?

2. Apply the health belief model to Jasmine's situation. What is the perceived threat? What is the perceived benefit to changing her behavior? What are the perceived barriers she may face?

3. Look at Jasmine's situation through an ecological model approach. What factors in her environment are reinforcing her late-night behavior? What factors are going against it?

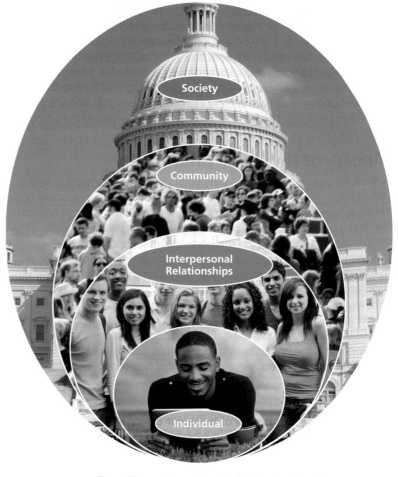

FIGURE 1.5 An Ecological Model of Behavior Change. Like ecological approaches to health itself, ecological models of behavior change acknowledge the influence of many factors at different levels, from individual to societal. They also emphasize the effectiveness of coordinated interventions at multiple levels.

development of a variety of **ecological models** of behavior change, in which the creation of a supportive environment is acknowledged to be as important to achieving change as is an individual's acquisition of health information and development of new skills.

Ecological models emphasize these principles:[26]

- Multiple levels of factors—from individual behavior to family values, community support, and public policy—influence health behaviors **(Figure 1.5)**.

- Influences at different levels interact to promote or impede change.

- For successful behavior change, interventions at multiple levels are most effective.

For example, an individual's motivation to lose weight might interact positively with a physician's advice to exercise, an employer's financial incentive for logging time at the company gym, and a city's construction of a new bike path. On the other hand, personal motivation is less effective when environments and policies make it difficult to choose healthful behaviors.

This means that, if you want to make lasting change, you shouldn't try to go it alone. You're more likely to succeed if you reach out for support from your health-care provider, your campus health services,

> **ecological model** Any of a variety of behavior-change models that acknowledge the creation of a supportive environment as being equally important to achieving change as an individual's acquisition of health information and development of new skills.

and other resources in your community. In the next section, we talk more about recruiting support for your change. And if the resources you need don't currently exist—advocate for them! Every chapter of this text concludes with ideas on campus advocacy for health-related change.

Even with support, making healthful behavior change is still tough, so it helps to follow a systematic plan. The plan provided ahead uses an ecological framework to help you make effective and lasting behavior change.

Change Yourself, Change Your World

By enrolling in a personal health course and reading this text, you've already taken the initial step toward achieving better health and wellness. Throughout this book you'll find **Self-Assessments** that will help you assess your current health status, as well as **Choosing to Change**

Worksheets that guide you on how to set appropriate goals and implement plans for behavior change. Each Choosing to Change Worksheet will prompt you to list your level of readiness for change—also known as your stage of behavior change—based on the transtheoretical model you read about earlier in this chapter. The Worksheets will then walk you through behavior-change techniques appropriate for your stage of change, promoting a greater chance of success. To find electronic versions of the Self-Assessments and Choosing to Change Worksheets, online practice quizzes and activities, videos of real health students talking about their health issues, *ABC News* videos about current health news, and more, visit **MasteringHealth** at **www.mastering healthandnutrition.com**.

This chapter's **Self-Assessment** on page 18 is a general self-survey evaluating your current health behaviors. Complete the survey, then read the instructions for interpreting your score. Now, is there a particular area of health you'd like to turn around? Once you've identified the health behavior you most want to change . . . how do you begin? Let's look at the personal choices that help people succeed in making behavior change.

Personal Choices

Changing your targeted behavior will require more than a quick decision to "just do it." Effective change is a process and starts with information, a SMART goal, and a practical plan. You also need to identify and tackle your barriers, recruit support, promise yourself some rewards—and commit. Let's consider these seven steps one at a time.

Step 1. Get Informed

You've identified a goal—"Get fit!"—but how much do you really know about the behavior you want to change? For instance, what are the components of fitness, what are the benefits, how is it achieved, and how is it measured? If you're going to set a fitness goal and create a plan for reaching it, you need to be able to answer these questions. So your first step is to do some homework. The information in this text, together with the **Get Connected** links at the end of each chapter, are good resources for researching your health concerns. You can also find information at your campus health services center, from your health-care provider, and from reputable professional journals. Answering specific questions will, among other things, help you identify a more effective behavior-change goal; that is, a SMART goal.

---

shaping A behavior-change technique based on breaking broad goals into more manageable steps.

Step 2. Set a SMART Goal

If you don't know precisely where you're going, how will you know when you've arrived? Experts in business, health care, and personal development agree that goals are more likely to be achieved when you put them in writing following the acronym SMART. SMART stands for the five qualities of an effective goal:[27]

- **Specific.** When writing your goal, include specific details. For example, "I'm going to try to lose weight" is not a SMART goal. How much weight do you want to lose? Or if precise numbers don't motivate you, specify how you want to look or feel: "I want my new jeans to feel comfortable, not tight."

- **Measurable.** Include objective criteria for evaluating your success. What data would make it clear to anyone that you have succeeded? For instance, "By the end of this semester . . . I'll have lost 10 pounds . . . I'll be meditating for at least 20 minutes a day . . . I'll have paid off my credit card debt . . ."

- **Attainable.** Does the research you did earlier convince you that you can achieve your goal? If not, you probably won't. So make

sure your goal isn't unreasonable. For instance, for most people who are overweight, it's sensible to aim to lose about ½–1 pound of body weight per week; however, 3 pounds a week is not attainable without putting your health at risk.

- **Relevant.** Don't borrow somebody else's health goal! Make sure that the goal you've written feels right for you. For instance, let's say you can't even climb a flight of stairs without feeling winded. You've been looking for some inspiration to get moving when a friend invites you to join him in training for a local marathon. Your friend has been running cross-country since middle school. The goal is relevant for him, but it's not SMART for you.

- **Time based.** A SMART goal has a time frame. For instance: "For the next six months, each time I weigh myself—on the 15th and the 30th of each month—I'll have lost at least one pound. In five months' time, by December 30th, I'll have lost 10 pounds."

The National Institutes of Health also advises that your goal be *forgiving*.[28] That is, it should allow for the occasional intervention of unforeseen events. A goal of walking for 30 minutes a day, 5 days a week, is forgiving. A goal of walking for 30 minutes a day, every day, is not.

Step 3. Make a Plan

A SMART goal is like a guiding vision, but to make it happen, you need an action plan, and that means you need to break down your goal into day-to-day actions that will enable you to achieve it. In doing this, it helps to use a technique called **shaping;** that is, breaking a big goal into a series of smaller, measurable steps. If you'd like to eventually run a 10K, for instance, set yourself a goal of a shorter distance at first, and then gradually increase your distance a little each week.

When shaping, it can be helpful to ask yourself questions like: who, what, when, where, why, how, and how long? Here is an example:

- On Sunday morning, I'll weigh myself and write down my weight.

- Monday to Friday, I'll skip the regular sodas and have diet soda, skim milk, or water, and I'll have an apple instead of fries with my sandwich.

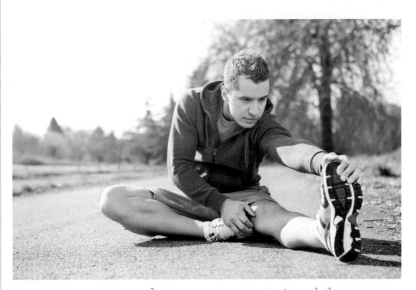

Set a goal that is relevant and attainable and you're more likely to reach it.

- Also, after my last class on M/W/F, I'll walk to the fitness center. I'll do at least 10 minutes on the stationary bike and 10 minutes on the stair-climber. On Saturday morning, I'll take the drop-in yoga class.
- On Sunday morning, I'll weigh myself again. If I've lost one pound or more, I'll continue with my plan for another week. And I'll call my best friend to celebrate! If I haven't, I'll increase my exercise next week to 15 minutes per machine.

Step 4. Identify Barriers and How You'll Overcome Them

Barriers are factors that stand in the way of successful change. Barriers can emerge from any of the multiple levels of influence on human behavior, including psychological factors, the social and physical environment, and access to health services.

One of the most important psychological barriers to change is a quality known as low self-efficacy. Psychologist Albert Bandura of Stanford University was the first to recognize the importance of self-efficacy in behavior change. In a 1977 paper, he described **self-efficacy** as the conviction that you can successfully execute the behavior required to make the change you desire.[29] Bandura explained that your expectations of personal efficacy determine whether you'll initiate a behavior change process, how much effort you'll expend, and how long you'll sustain it in the face of obstacles.[29] If you believe in your ability to get in better shape, for example, you'll keep exercising, even if a few workouts leave you tired or sore. This persistence will further reinforce your sense of efficacy. In contrast, if you have low self-efficacy, you may give up quickly and, as a result, you're likely to retain your self-defeating expectations.

Your sense of self-efficacy is closely tied to your **locus of control,** a concept first developed by psychologist Julian B. Rotter in 1954.[30] If you have an *internal* locus of control, you are more likely to believe that you are the master of your own destiny. When a barrier presents itself, you'll look for ways to overcome it. If you have an *external* locus of control, you are more likely to believe that events are out of your hands—that there's little you can do to overcome barriers.

What barriers might exist in your social environment? Let's say you want to lose weight, but your roommate is constantly baking the most delectable treats—and asking you to try them. You might overcome this barrier by telling your roommate about your weight-loss plan, and inviting him or her to create some low-calorie meals and snacks. Self-advocacy is an essential—though sometimes uncomfortable—skill to practice in demonstrating self-efficacy.

Aspects of your physical environment can act as barriers, too. But with some ingenuity, you can often find ways to overcome them. For example, if you struggle with binge eating, make sure you go through your apartment or dorm room and get rid of any junk foods.

We discussed earlier the significant disparity in access to quality health services in the United States. This is a barrier to change for millions of Americans. Fortunately, as a college student, you may have access to low-cost health services and programs.

People with a high level of self-efficacy and an internal locus of control may be able to overcome most barriers to behavior change. You can increase your own sense of self-efficacy by turning to clearly defined techniques that help change behavior in positive ways specific to your health concerns. Throughout this book, we offer **Practical Strategies** boxes to help you do just that.

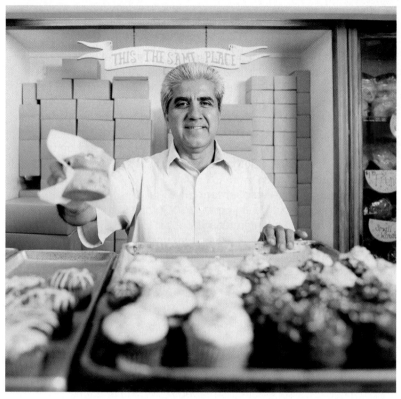

Factors in your environment can be barriers to behavior change.

Step 5. Recruit Some Support

According to the ecological models of behavior change, your plan for change will be more likely to succeed if you have different levels of support. Start with your family members and friends. With whom do you feel comfortable sharing your plans for change? Give your support group members specific instructions about how they can help, and when your motivation wanes, call on them to cheer you on. If family members and friends can't provide the consistent support you need, consider joining a campus or community self-help group.

A subtle form of social support comes through **modeling,** learning behaviors by watching others who have already made successful change. If you'd like to eat less junk food, for example, observe the habits of a health-conscious friend who has already scoped out the options for healthy eating on campus. A rarely acknowledged benefit of modeling is that it lets you imagine yourself engaging in the same healthful behavior—in a sense, you *rehearse* it. Frequent rehearsal through modeling helps you become more familiar and comfortable with the actions required for the behavior change.

Step 6. Promise Yourself Rewards

Rewards keep you motivated to sustain change. For example, you might promise yourself new clothing after you've reached a target weight goal. However, rewards don't have to be material objects. For instance, the natural "high" people often feel after physical exercise can be its own positive reinforcement.

End-goal rewards are important, but it's also important to reward yourself for small steps along

self-efficacy The conviction that you can successfully execute the behavior required to make the change you desire.

locus of control A person's belief about where the center of power lies in his or her life; it can be external or internal.

modeling A behavior-change technique based on watching and learning from others.

the way. For instance, if you enroll in an aerobics class that meets Tuesdays and Thursdays, you might promise yourself that, in the weeks that you attend both sessions, you'll reward yourself with an act of "self-kindness," such as a call to a loved one.[28]

Step 7. Commit in Writing

Many people find it helps to write out and sign their name at the bottom of a behavior-change contract—indicating that they've made a pact with themselves that they intend to keep. So if you're ready to take the plunge, turn to the **Choosing to Change Worksheet** on page 19 for a form you can use. Notice that the steps in this contract follow those just discussed.

Make copies of your behavior-change contract, and place them anywhere you want support.

Believe It!

Once you have your contract, it's time to make it happen. When barriers arise—and they will—don't give in to discouragement. Try to fill your mind with positive **self-talk:** thoughts that affirm your ability to change and acknowledge the help available to you from your environment. At all costs, avoid negative self-talk—the inner chatter that says you can't do this, or you don't have the time or money, or it's not important anyway.

Another tip for maintaining your belief in yourself is to engage in **self-monitoring;** that is, to observe and record aspects of your behavior-change process, such as how many servings of fruits and vegetables you eat each day, or how many hours of sleep you get each night. This solid evidence of improvement can boost your confidence when it starts to slip. Your record can also show you when it's time to shift your change plan into higher gear.[28]

Cope With Relapse

When people attempt to change a long-term behavior, a lapse—a temporary "slip" back to the previous behavior—is highly likely. For instance, a person trying to quit smoking who takes a drag on a friend's cigarette is experiencing a lapse. Unfortunately, a **relapse,** a complete return to the previous pattern of behavior, is also common.[31] For example, according to the American Cancer Society, a majority of the people who successfully quit smoking have tried to quit—and relapsed—several times before.[32]

Preventing a relapse is easy if you can prevent a lapse in the first place! Two strategies for preventing lapses include the following:

- **Control cues.** With **cue control,** you learn to change the stimuli that provoke your unwanted behavior. For example, you may learn from your self-monitoring records that you're more likely to overeat while you're watching television, or whenever your mom leaves her latest batch of homemade cookies on the kitchen counter, or when you're around a certain friend. You might then try to change the behavior by:[28]
  - Separating the behavior from the cue (don't eat while watching television)
  - Taking action to avoid or eliminate the cue (ask your mom to put her cookies in a closed container out of sight)

- Changing the environment or other circumstances surrounding the cue (plan to meet your friend in a nonfood setting)
- **Find a substitute.** For cue control to work, you have to have the capacity to change the stimulus. Fortunately, there's a technique called **counter-conditioning,** in which you learn to substitute a healthful or neutral behavior for the unwanted behavior when it's triggered by a cue beyond your control. One of the simplest examples is the urge to have something in their mouths that strikes most smokers repeatedly in the first few weeks after they quit. With counter-conditioning, the person replaces cigarette smoking with chewing on something, whether gum, licorice, or even a toothpick. Peer pressure commonly triggers lapses, but countering can be surprisingly effective in overcoming it. Write out and memorize one or more short, assertive statements such as, "No thanks, I've had enough." Then, in situations in which you'd usually give in, substitute your assertion.

Campus Advocacy

When a barrier to change exists in your social or physical environment, or results from poor health services or policy-making, your best chance for change might just be in **advocacy;** that is, working independently or with others to directly improve aspects of your world. You may think of advocacy as lobbying to legislators, and while that's one form, there are many others available to you in your role as a college student. These include the following:

- Get better informed about the issue, especially what's happening on campus and within your community.
- Use your social networking pages to heighten awareness of the issue among your contacts.
- Meet with campus faculty or staff members to share your suggestions on the issue.
- Write about the issue for campus news services.
- Speak about the issue at campus gatherings.
- Organize a letter-writing campaign to your dean of students or other decision-makers.
- Organize a student demonstration related to the issue.
- Join a campus organization already working on the issue.
- Found an organization of your own.

Concluding every chapter of this book, you'll find suggestions for campus advocacy specific to the topics addressed in that chapter, from fitness to discrimination to climate change. These suggestions may or may not be appropriate for your campus. Still, we hope they'll provide you with examples of strategies that have worked for others, and some inspiration for advocacy of your own.

---

self-talk A person's internal dialogue.

self-monitoring A behavior-change technique in which the individual observes and records aspects of his or her behavior-change process.

relapse A return to the previous state or pattern of behavior.

cue control A behavior-change technique in which the individual learns to change the stimuli that provoked the lapse.

counter-conditioning A behavior-change technique in which the individual learns to substitute a healthful or neutral behavior for an unwanted behavior triggered by a cue beyond his or her control.

advocacy Working independently or with others to directly improve aspects of the social or physical environment, or to change policies or legislation.

>> **Watch videos of real students discussing their health at** MasteringHealth™

SELF-ASSESSMENT
How Healthy Is Your Current Lifestyle?

Complete one section at a time by circling the number under the answer that best describes your behavior. Then add the numbers you circled to get your score.

Smoking

	Almost Always	Sometimes	Almost Never

If you are currently a nonsmoker, enter a score of 10 for this section and go to the next section on Alcohol and Drugs.

	Almost Always	Sometimes	Almost Never
1. I avoid smoking cigarettes.	2	1	0
2. I smoke only low-tar and -nicotine cigarettes or I smoke a pipe.	2	1	0

Smoking Score _____

Alcohol and Drugs

	Almost Always	Sometimes	Almost Never
1. I avoid drinking alcoholic beverages or I drink no more than 1 (for women) or 2 (for men) drinks a day.	4	1	0
2. I avoid using alcohol or other drugs (especially illegal drugs) as a way of handling situations or problems.	2	1	0
3. I am careful not to drink alcohol when taking certain medicines (for example, medicine for sleeping, pain, colds, and allergies) or when pregnant.	2	1	0
4. I read and follow the label directions when using prescribed and over-the-counter drugs.	2	1	0

Alcohol and Drugs Score _____

Eating Habits

	Almost Always	Sometimes	Almost Never
1. I eat a variety of foods each day, such as fruits and vegetables, whole-grain breads and cereals, lean meats, low-fat dairy products, beans and legumes, and nuts and seeds.	4	1	0
2. I limit the amount of fat, saturated fat, *trans* fat, and cholesterol I eat (including fat on meats, eggs, butter, cream, shortenings, and organ meats such as liver).	2	1	0
3. I limit the amount of salt I eat by cooking with only small amounts, not adding salt at the table, and avoiding salty snacks.	2	1	0
4. I avoid eating too much sugar (especially frequent snacks of sticky candy or soft drinks).	2	1	0

Eating Habits Score _____

Exercise/Fitness

	Almost Always	Sometimes	Almost Never
1. I do vigorous exercises for 30 minutes a day at least 5 times a week (examples include jogging, swimming, brisk walking, or bicycling).	4	2	0
2. I do exercises that enhance my muscle tone for 15–30 minutes at least 3 times a week (examples include using weight machines or free weights, yoga, or calisthenics).	3	1	0
3. I use part of my leisure time participating in individual, family, or team activities that increase my level of fitness (such as gardening, dancing, bowling, golf, or baseball).	3	1	0

Exercise/Fitness Score _____

Stress Control

	Almost Always	Sometimes	Almost Never
1. I have a job, go to school, or do other work that I enjoy.	2	1	0
2. I find it easy to relax and express my feelings freely.	2	1	0
3. I recognize early, and prepare for, events or situations likely to be stressful for me.	2	1	0
4. I have close friends or others with whom I can talk about personal matters and call on for help.	2	1	0
5. I participate in group activities (such as religious worship and community organizations) and/or have hobbies that I enjoy.	2	1	0

Stress Control Score _____

Safety/Health

	Almost Always	Sometimes	Almost Never
1. I wear a seat belt while riding in a car.	2	1	0
2. I avoid driving while under the influence of alcohol and other drugs, or riding with someone else who is under the influence.	2	1	0
3. I obey traffic rules and avoid distractions like texting and talking on the phone when driving.	2	1	0
4. I am careful when using potentially harmful products or substances (such as household cleaners, poisons, and electrical devices).	2	1	0
5. I get at least 7 hours of sleep a night.	2	1	0

Safety/Health Score _____

HOW TO INTERPRET YOUR SCORE

Examine your score for each section and refer to the key below.

Scores of 9 and 10
Excellent. Your answers show that you are aware of the importance of this area to your health. More important, you are putting your knowledge to work for you by practicing good health habits.

Scores of 6 to 8
Good. Your health practices in this area are good, but there is room for improvement. Look again at the items you answered with a "Sometimes" or "Almost Never." What changes can you make to improve your score? Even a small change can help.

Scores of 3 to 5
At Risk. Your health risks are showing. Do you want to know why it is important for you to change these behaviors? Perhaps you need help in deciding how to make the changes you desire. In either case, help is available. You can start by contacting your health-care provider or a registered dietitian.

Scores of 0 to 2
Seriously at Risk. Obviously, you were concerned enough about your health to take this test. But your answers show that you may be taking serious risks with your health. You can easily get the information and help you need to reduce your health risks and have a healthier lifestyle if you wish. Are you ready to take the next step?

To complete this Self-Assessment online, visit MasteringHealth™

Source: "Healthstyle: A Self-Test" adapted by Linda Bobroff, Ph.D from U.S. Department of Health and Human Services, DHHS Publication Number (PHS) 81-50155. Department of Family, Youth and Community Services, University of Florida. Used by permission of the University of Florida, Institute of Food and Agricultural Services.

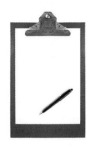

Choosing to Change Worksheet

To complete this worksheet online, visit MasteringHealth™

The Choosing to Change Worksheets guide you on how to implement your behavior-change plans based on the stages of change identified by the transtheoretical model.

Stages of Behavior Change:

Precontemplation: I do not intend to make a change in the next six months.

Contemplation: I might make a change in the next six months.

Preparation: I am prepared to make a change in the next month.

Action: I have been making a change for less than six months.

Maintenance: I have been maintaining a change for more than six months.

After you have completed the Self-Assessment in this chapter, consider what stage of change you are in for each of the categories listed. Remember, it is common to be at various stages of change for different behaviors. Then, select one behavior in which you are at either the contemplation or preparation stage that you would like to target for change over the next few months. Next, fill out the Behavior-Change Contract below. Make sure you sign it, and either display it where you'll see it often, or discuss it with your health instructor as part of your work toward your long-term goal.

Behavior-Change Contract

My behavior change: _____

1. Three important short-term benefits I've discovered from my research about my behavior change are:

1. _____

2. _____

3. _____

2. My SMART goal for this behavior change is:

_____

_____

_____

3. Keeping my current stage of behavior change in mind, these short-term goals and rewards will make my SMART goal more attainable:

Short-term goal	Target date	Reward
Short-term goal	Target date	Reward
Short-term goal	Target date	Reward

4. Barriers I anticipate to making this behavior change are:

1. _____

2. _____

3. _____

The strategies I will use to overcome these barriers are:

1. _____
2. _____
3. _____

5. Resources I will use to help me change this behavior include:

- a friend, partner, or relative: _____
- a school-based resource: _____
- a health-care resource: _____
- a community-based resource: _____
- a book or reputable website: _____

6. When I achieve the long-term behavior change described above, my reward will be:

_____   _____
Reward   Target date

7. I intend to make the behavior change described above. I will use the strategies and rewards above to achieve the goals that will contribute to a healthy behavior change.

Signed: _____

Chapter Summary

MasteringHealth™

Build your knowledge—and health!—in the Study Area of **MasteringHealth**™ with a variety of study tools.
www.masteringhealthandnutrition.com
(or www.pearsonmastering.com)

- *Disease* occurs when the body is unable to compensate for some sort of alteration in its structure or its function. The body's natural regulatory mechanisms fail, and the person may begin to experience symptoms of this failure, such as pain or weakness.
- *Health* is more than merely the absence of disease. In a healthy person, many different dimensions of life work together harmoniously.
- *Wellness* is defined by the National Wellness Institute as an active process through which people become aware of, and make choices toward, a more successful existence.
- Seven dimensions of health and wellness include physical, intellectual, psychological, spiritual, social, environmental, and occupational.
- Although life expectancy in the United States is a record 78.7 years, many health challenges remain. For example, just two chronic diseases—heart disease and cancer—are responsible for almost half of all deaths in the United States, and almost half of American adults have at least one chronic disease.
- The four common behaviors responsible for most of the suffering and early death related to chronic disease in the United States are lack of physical activity, poor nutrition, tobacco use, and excessive alcohol consumption.

- The U.S. Department of Health and Human Services (HHS) is the U.S. government's principal agency for protecting the health of all Americans. Its primary division is the U.S. Public Health Service, and one of its leading agencies is the Centers for Disease Control and Prevention (CDC).
- The HHS Healthy People initiative takes an ecological approach to health that considers the relationship between an individual's health and the many factors that influence it. One of the key goals of Healthy People is to eliminate health disparities, differences in the rate and burden of disease and the access to and quality of health care among various population groups.
- Among Americans aged 15–24, the leading causes of death are accidents, suicide, and homicide. Stress, depression, anxiety, alcohol and tobacco use, and sexual health are all common health concerns faced by college students.
- An alarming global health problem is infection, especially the growth of drug-resistant strains of infectious microbes. Although malnutrition is overwhelmingly a concern of developing nations, obesity-related diseases are common concerns throughout the world.
- Determinants of health are a broad range of biological, economic, and other factors that influence health. The six broad categories of determinants of health are biology and genetics, individual behaviors, social

determinants, physical determinants, health services—including access to quality health care and health literacy—and policy-making.

- *Predisposing, enabling,* and *reinforcing factors* can all influence our success in making and maintaining health-related behavior change.

- The *transtheoretical model of behavior change* proposes six stages, from precontemplation, contemplation, and preparation, to action, maintenance, and termination, that a person progresses through before achieving sustained behavior change.

- The *health belief model* identifies four factors as instrumental in predicting health-related behavior change, including perceptions of threat, severity, and benefit, and cues to action.

- Ecological models of behavior change acknowledge that the creation of a supportive environment is as important to achieving change as an individual's acquisition of health information and development of new skills.

- After identifying a health-related behavior you want to change, seven steps for implementing that change include: becoming informed, setting a SMART goal, breaking down your goal into a sequential action plan, identifying barriers to change and how you'll overcome them, recruiting support, promising yourself rewards, and committing in writing.

- As you put your plan into action, identify thoughts constituting negative self-talk and replace them with affirmations and other examples of positive self-talk. Use self-monitoring to see your real progress and move closer to your goal.

- Prevent relapse by taking inventory of the full ecological spectrum of factors that might trigger a lapse, and then identifying strategies for coping, including cue control and counter-conditioning.

- Advocacy can be effective when a barrier to change exists in your social or physical environment, or results from poor health services or policy-making.

GET CONNECTED

>> Visit the following websites for further information about the topics in this chapter:

- Centers for Disease Control and Prevention
  www.cdc.gov
- Go Ask Alice (answers to health questions, sponsored by Columbia University)
  http://goaskalice.columbia.edu
- U.S. Department of Health and Human Services' healthfinder.gov
  http://healthfinder.gov
- U.S. Department of Health and Human Services' *Healthy People 2020*
  www.healthypeople.gov
- Medline Plus
  www.nlm.nih.gov/medlineplus
- Mayo Clinic
  www.mayoclinic.com

MOBILE TIPS!

Scan this QR code with your mobile device to access additional health tips. Or, via your mobile device, go to **http://chmobile.pearsoncmg .com** and navigate to Chapter 1.

- World Health Organization
  www.who.int/en
- Media Literacy Project
  www.medialiteracyproject.org

Website links are subject to change. To access updated web links, please visit MasteringHealth™

TEST YOUR KNOWLEDGE

1. An appreciation of the capacity of people with a disability or chronic disease to make choices toward a more successful existence contributed to
   a. the concept of disease as a state of imbalance.
   b. the 1948 WHO definition of health.
   c. the development of the concept of wellness.
   d. the recognition of the importance of self-efficacy in behavior change.

2. Which dimension of health is characterized by the quality of your interactions and relationships with other people?
   a. intellectual health
   b. psychological health
   c. spiritual health
   d. social health

3. Which of the following statements about current health challenges is true?
   a. Obesity is the top cause of mortality throughout the world.
   b. Infections due to drug-resistant microbes are an increasing health concern throughout the world.
   c. The rate of new infections from the human immunodeficiency virus (HIV) increased by 20% between 2010 and 2012.
   d. Nearly 10% of chronically undernourished people live in the wealthiest countries of the world.

4. The CDC recognizes several behaviors as responsible for much of the suffering and early death related to chronic disease. These are
   a. lack of physical activity, overeating, and tobacco use.
   b. lack of physical activity, poor nutrition, tobacco use, and excessive alcohol consumption.
   c. failing to meet current physical activity guidelines, overeating, tobacco use, and alcohol consumption.
   d. poor nutrition, tobacco use, and alcohol consumption.

5. Health literacy is an example of which type of health determinant?
   a. individual behaviors
   b. social determinants
   c. health services
   d. policy-making

6. In the transtheoretical model of behavior change, which stage indicates the period during which a person has modified the behavior in an observable way?
   a. precontemplation
   b. contemplation
   c. preparation
   d. action

7. Which of the following is a principle of the ecological models of behavior change?
   a. The individual's belief that making a change will reduce a threat to his or her health is the primary factor in behavior change.
   b. Interventions at multiple levels—from individual to society—are most effective in making health-related behavior change.
   c. The individual must be able to admit the potential environmental consequences of changing a behavior.
   d. All of these answers describe principles of the ecological models of behavior change.

8. You're determined to get fit, and have begun to walk from your apartment to campus daily. The fact that you live in a warm, sunny climate is an example of
   a. a predisposing factor for behavior change.
   b. an enabling factor for behavior change.
   c. a reinforcing factor for behavior change.
   d. none of these answers.

9. Damian's strength-training program hits a snag when he pulls a muscle in his thigh. After a course of physical therapy, he resumes his program, modifying it as prescribed. Damian's behavior demonstrates
   a. self-efficacy.
   b. a strong external locus of control.
   c. cue control.
   d. counter-conditioning.

10. Relapse is
   a. less likely when the person views the lapse as due to external circumstances.
   b. almost always due to circumstances beyond the person's individual control.
   c. a temporary "slip" back to the previous behavior.
   d. uncommon.

Get Critical

What happened

In the spring of 2011, Grammy award–winning singer Beyoncé released a music video for kids entitled, "Move Your Body!" Wearing a simple T-shirt, short shorts, and high heels, Beyoncé bursts into a school cafeteria and gets the kids dancing. The video was created to support First Lady Michelle Obama's "Let's Move!" campaign to fight childhood obesity.

Although the film has many supporters, who've praised Beyoncé for increasing awareness of childhood obesity as well as showcasing the fun of physical activity, critics charge that videos such as "Move Your Body" can cause obese kids and teens to feel ashamed of their bodies and drive them toward fad dieting. Experts also point out that weight is not an isolated factor, and simply watching a fun video is unlikely to have any effect whatsoever on children's health.

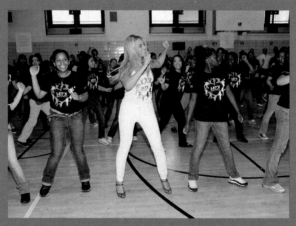

Beyoncé visits a school in New York, NY, to support the "Move Your Body!" video and "Let's Move!" campaign.

What do you think?

- What's your opinion of celebrity efforts such as Beyoncé's "Move Your Body" video? Are you in favor of such efforts or do you find them offensive?

- One of the kids shown throughout the video is an obviously overweight boy who is dancing just as enthusiastically—and as skillfully—as all the other kids. In addition, most of the video's dance moves are simple, such as stepping from side to side or "shimmying" in place. Given this, what do you think of the charge that viewing the video could cause obese kids to feel ashamed?

- Review the three principles of the ecological models of behavior change. Discuss these principles in view of the critique of the "Move Your Body" video that "weight is not an isolated factor."

Watch the "Move Your Body" video here: www.youtube.com/watch?v=mYP4MgxDV2U.

PSYCHOLOGICAL HEALTH

About 50% of college students report having felt **overwhelming anxiety** at some time within the past year.[i]

During the **college years** (late adolescence/young adulthood) the first symptoms of **panic disorder, bipolar disorder**, and **obsessive-compulsive disorder** may begin to appear.[ii]

More than 1 in 10 college students report being recently diagnosed or treated for **depression**.[i]

The **second** leading cause of death among 15- to 24-year-olds is **suicide**.[iii]

Learning Objectives

IDENTIFY two components and six facets of psychological health.

DISCUSS a variety of factors that influence psychological health.

DESCRIBE common psychological challenges and ways to address them.

COMPARE the prevalence of mental disorders in the United States and other countries.

DISCUSS the characteristics, possible causes, and treatment of mood disorders.

DIFFERENTIATE five common types of anxiety disorder.

IDENTIFY the characteristic symptoms of attention disorders and schizophrenia.

LIST the warning signs of suicide and describe suicide prevention methods.

DESCRIBE the different options for treatment of mental disorders.

IDENTIFY strategies for improving your psychological health and for helping a friend.

Look at a brochure advertising any college in the country, and you'll find photos

of happy students enjoying their studies and having fun. But as you know, real life for college students is more complicated than such images suggest. When worry, anger, or loneliness arises, good psychological health can help you maintain your balance and resolve the challenge effectively.

So what does it mean to have "good" psychological health? How do you develop it? We discuss these questions ahead.

What Is Psychological Health?

The field of psychology emerged in the late 19th century, when German and American scientists began conducting experiments to try to discover a physical basis for mental disorders. At the same time, the Austrian neurologist Sigmund Freud began exploring the role of past traumas in prompting unconscious conflicts that lead to mental disorders. But decades passed before researchers began to study the question of what constitutes psychological health. Here, we explore a few of the key concepts such work has revealed.

Components of Psychological Health

At its most basic, **psychological health** can be defined as the dimension of health and wellness that encompasses both mental and emotional components. **Mental health** can be described as the "thinking" component of psychological health. The term describes your ability to perceive reality accurately and respond to its challenges rationally and effectively. **Emotional health** refers to the "feeling" component of psychological health. It describes how you react emotionally to the ups and downs of life. People with good emotional health are able to "roll with the punches," keeping less happy times in perspective.

Mental and emotional health affect other dimensions of health. Your physical health, for example—your breathing, heart rate, and immune response—is influenced by your thoughts and emotions. So is your social health: An upbeat mood can draw others to you, whereas stormy emotions can cause others to disengage.

Facets of Psychological Health

One tool frequently used to assess psychological health in a variety of populations, including college students, is the Ryff Scales of Psychological

psychological health A broad dimension of health and wellness that encompasses both mental and emotional health.

mental health The "thinking" component of psychological health that allows you to perceive reality accurately and respond rationally and effectively.

emotional health The "feeling" component of psychological health that influences your interpretation of and response to events.

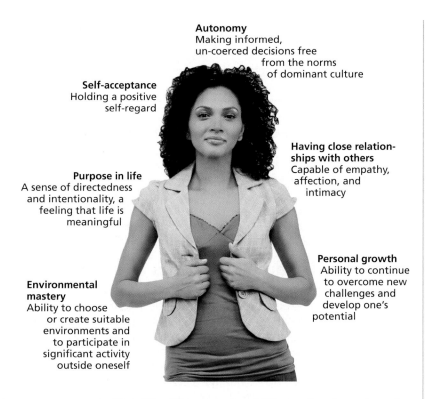

Autonomy
Making informed, un-coerced decisions free from the norms of dominant culture

Self-acceptance
Holding a positive self-regard

Having close relationships with others
Capable of empathy, affection, and intimacy

Purpose in life
A sense of directedness and intentionality, a feeling that life is meaningful

Personal growth
Ability to continue to overcome new challenges and develop one's potential

Environmental mastery
Ability to choose or create suitable environments and to participate in significant activity outside oneself

FIGURE 2.1 Ryff's Facets of Psychological Health. Each of these characteristics is a hallmark of psychological health.

Well-Being. Developed by psychologist Carol D. Ryff, the tool identifies six key facets of psychological health **(Figure 2.1)**.[1]

Self-Acceptance

Ryff states that the characteristic most commonly seen in psychologically healthy people is **self-acceptance** (also called *self-esteem*): having a positive regard for oneself. Self-accepting people tend to respond to challenges in resilient ways, have an optimistic outlook, and even enjoy better physical health.[2] They are realistic, acknowledging their good and bad qualities. They focus on things they can control and accept things they cannot.

Positive Relations with Others

Psychologically healthy people have strong feelings of empathy and affection for all human beings and are concerned about their welfare. Moreover, they are capable of **intimacy;** that is, maintaining close relationships with family members, romantic partners, and/or friends.

Autonomy

Autonomy is your capacity to make informed, un-coerced decisions and to regulate your behavior internally. Autonomous people tend to base their decisions on their own judgment and values. They are also likely to take responsibility for the results of their actions. Autonomy does not devalue the opinions of others. It simply keeps them in perspective.

self-acceptance A sense of positive and realistic self-regard, resulting in elevated levels of self-confidence and self-respect.

intimacy A close relationship with another person.

autonomy The capacity to make informed, un-coerced decisions.

assertiveness The ability to clearly express your needs and wants to others in an appropriate way.

environmental mastery The ability to choose or create environments that suit you.

emotional intelligence (EI) The capacity to perceive, express, and reason accurately with emotion and emotional information.

optimism The psychological tendency to have a positive interpretation of life's events.

Autonomy is expressed in **assertiveness,** or making your decisions clear to others. Unlike anger or aggression, assertiveness means you express yourself calmly and clearly in ways that respect yourself and others.

Environmental Mastery

Your chemistry instructor is a bore. What do you do? **Environmental mastery** is the ability to choose or create environments that suit you. Sometimes, environmental mastery requires you to change your thoughts about a situation; for instance, recognizing that you're not all that happy with your instructor, but accepting that switching out of the course wouldn't be worth the stress, then using other resources to help you succeed.

Purpose in Life

Given that you're in college, you may not feel that you're wandering aimlessly through life. But are your choices—in classes, friendships, and other aspects of your life—aligned with a larger purpose, one you could readily articulate? People who clearly comprehend their life's purpose, and take actions to achieve that purpose, feel productive—that they are actively creating their lives.

Personal Growth

Peak psychological health requires that you continue to grow and expand as a person, opening yourself to new experiences that challenge how you think about yourself and the world. Rather than settling in a fixed state in which all of your problems are solved, you accept a certain level of anxiety as you move outside your comfort zone to accept challenges and develop your full potential.

The Role of Emotional Intelligence

In 1985, Wayne Leon Payne published the first study of **emotional intelligence (EI),** which he defined as the ability to accurately sense, assess, and manage emotions.[3] In the decades since, psychologists have come to characterize EI as encompassing four key abilities:[4]

• To perceive and express emotion

• To incorporate emotion in thought

• To understand and reason with emotion

• To regulate emotion in oneself and others

People with higher levels of EI tend to be both self-aware and socially adept. They conduct themselves in a balanced way, neither denying their emotions nor letting them fly out of control. They also tend to be more productive, less prone to stress, and happier overall than those with lower EI.[5]

Whereas some propose that EI is an inborn trait, others claim that it is a skill anyone can develop by consciously recognizing and naming emotions when you feel them, thinking about other people's feelings and motivations in specific situations, and accepting your emotions without allowing them to control you.

The Value of Optimism

Optimism is the psychological tendency to have a positive interpretation of life's events. Psychologist Martin Seligman explains that optimistic people embrace the belief that positive outcomes are more

Practical Strategies

Building Optimism

- **Notice when things go right.** When something works out for the better, take note. Recognizing when things go well will show you the likelihood of positive outcomes.

- **Learn from mistakes.** Everybody fails to reach a goal at some point. That doesn't mean that failure will happen again next time. Learn from what happened, and decide what you'll do differently in the future.

- **Give yourself time.** When you are first hit with a disappointment, it's not always easy to step back and modify your thoughts. Take time to feel what you feel. Talk with friends, exercise, and get some sleep.

- **Focus on action.** If you're not completely happy with the way things are—congratulations! That means you must have goals you want to reach! Make a list of those goals and then identify the actions you can take today, and in the days and months ahead, to reach them.

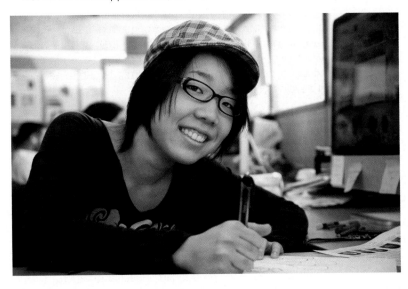

likely to occur than negative ones. People with optimistic outlooks are more likely to view problems as challenges within their power to solve; thus, they are motivated to take action. On the other hand, they are unlikely to see bad events as long-lasting or as capable of damaging other aspects of their lives.[6] In contrast, pessimists tend to believe that bad events will have long-lasting negative effects, undermining everything else they do, and are their own fault. They also give up easily, and have higher rates of depression than optimists.

Optimism helps us in a broad range of situations. Optimists tend to exceed the predictions of aptitude tests, and are more likely than pessimists to succeed academically.[6] Among college students, optimism has been found to be the best predictor of both psychological well-being and reduced levels of psychological distress.[7] Optimism is also a strong predictor of resilience following traumatic stress.[8] It may even reduce pain: In one study, among subjects given a *placebo* (a substance with no active ingredients) for pain, optimists reported greater pain relief.[9] And optimism helps patients fighting serious disease maintain a positive outlook during treatment and avoid anxiety and depression.[10]

You can learn optimism at any age. See **Practical Strategies: Building Optimism** for tips.

≫ **How optimistic are you? Register for a free account on Martin Seligman's website and take the Optimism Test:** www.authentichappiness.com.

Factors Affecting Psychological Health

What makes someone psychologically healthy? Recent genetic studies link certain variants of certain genes directly to specific "psychological resources," including optimism and self-esteem. But researchers acknowledge that these genes are just one factor that influences psychological resources, and that "there is plenty of room for environmental factors as well."[11]

Maslow's Hierarchy of Needs

Humanistic psychologist Abraham Maslow began publishing his ideas about positive psychological health in the 1940s. Maslow proposed that a key factor in achieving psychological health is our drive to meet our needs.[12] That is, people experience increased levels of psychological health as they meet and master ever-higher levels of innate needs via successful interactions with their environment. Maslow modeled this *hierarchy of needs* as a pyramid **(Figure 2.2)**.

The base of Maslow's pyramid represents our physiological needs (for air, food, water, shelter, etc.). If you've ever been truly hungry, or shivered uncontrollably from prolonged exposure to the cold, then you know that your survival needs for food or warmth can become

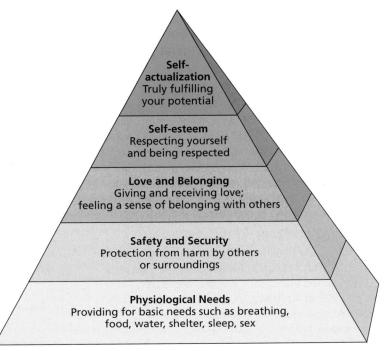

FIGURE 2.2 Maslow's Hierarchy of Needs Pyramid. Basic, physiological needs appear at the base of the pyramid. As you move upward, you address needs that are less urgent to satisfy, developing greater psychological health, until you realize self-actualization.

Source: Maslow, Abraham H.; Frager, Robert D.; Fadiman, James. *Motivation and Personality,* 3rd ed., ©1987. Adapted and electronically reproduced by permission of Pearson Education, Inc., Upper Saddle River, New Jersey.

all-consuming, driving you to meet those needs to the exclusion of almost anything else. Your success or failure will then determine whether or not you progress to perceive—and work on meeting—the next level of needs. This means, of course, that the struggle to put food on the table and pay the rent could block individuals from experiencing peak psychological health.

On the other hand, once your physiological needs are reliably and consistently met, you will experience an inner drive to meet progressively less urgent needs. For instance, whereas a partner in an abusive relationship may be driven to meet the need for safety, those already in loving relationships can work toward self-esteem.

When you finally master the four lower levels, you recognize and work toward fulfilling your need for **self-actualization;** that is, your need to become everything you're capable of becoming—to realize your "full humanness."[12] In later work, Maslow added one higher goal—selfless actualization, or self-transcendence, a "going beyond oneself" to work toward a values-driven goal in service to others or to an altruistic ideal.[13]

Family History

Rejection. Abuse. Abandonment. Shaming. More than a century ago, Sigmund Freud recognized that experiences such as these during childhood could prompt unconscious conflicts that could manifest in adulthood as mental disorders. Today, psychologists theorize that such experiences exert their effect by causing us to develop "early maladaptive" patterns that we then carry into adulthood.[14] We become less successful in meeting our needs, mastering our environment, and learning the appropriate lessons for each stage of life.

In one study, the presence of such patterns among college students was shown to significantly impair their adjustment to college life. It reduced the students' academic success, their social and emotional adjustment, and their attachment to the institution in which they were enrolled.[14]

Social Support

Do you have friends you *know* you could turn to if things ever got really tough? If so, then you have **social support.** A person with social support has a variety of relationships that can and do provide

> " *In a recent study of college students, social support was identified as a significant factor in improving the psychological adjustment of students to college life.*"

self-actualization The pinnacle of Maslow's hierarchy of needs, which indicates truly fulfilling your potential.

social support A sufficient quantity of relationships that provide emotional concern, help with appraisal, information, and even goods and services.

religion A system of beliefs and practices related to the existence of a transcendent power.

emotional concern, assistance with realistic appraisal of situations, information, and even goods and services if necessary. Social support can help by eliminating, changing, or helping you adjust to conditions that cause you distress.

In a recent study of college students, social support was identified as a significant factor in improving the psychological adjustment of students to college life. Students with a lower level of social support were more likely to experience psychological health problems, including a six-fold risk of depression relative to students with a higher level of social support.[15]

The Role of Spiritual Health

Spiritual health contributes to psychological health by providing a sense of connection to a larger purpose coupled with a system of core values that provide direction and meaning in life. For many, that connection takes the form of religion.

Defining Religion

A **religion** is a system of beliefs and practices related to the existence of a transcendent power or presence. Religious beliefs are typically expressed in acts of service and devotion, either through an organized group or independently.

In a 2012 survey, 79% of American adults said that they are affiliated with a particular religion. Here's the breakdown:[16]

- About 73% of respondents identify themselves as Christians.
- About 6% of respondents practice another religion.
- The remaining 21% of respondents identify themselves as atheist, *agnostic* (that is, they claim neither belief nor disbelief in a divine being), nothing in particular, or uncertain.

The statistics for religious affiliation for young adults are somewhat lower: 67% of Americans aged 18–29 say they are affiliated with a particular religion.[16]

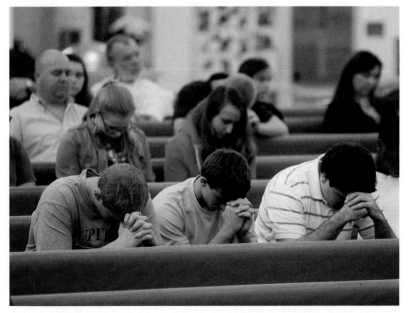

Religion can benefit psychological well-being.

Benefits of Religion

A 2012 Gallup poll found that people who identify themselves as "very religious" have higher levels of well-being than people who describe themselves as only moderately religious or not religious at all.[17] Similarly, in a 2009 study of university students, participants who scored high on "religiousness"—adherence to religious values and practices in daily living—demonstrated higher than average levels of psychological well-being and lower levels of psychological distress.[8]

Defining Spirituality

Affiliation with an organized religion is just one expression of a broader approach to life commonly referred to as **spirituality.** The term is tough to define, in part because spirituality is inclusive of just about everything. As Brian Luke Seaward, a pioneer in the field of health psychology, explains, spirituality is ageless, timeless, knowing no bounds and holding no allegiances.[18] The World Health Organization defines spirituality as "that which is in total harmony with the perceptual and non-perceptual environment."[19] For many, spirituality is a lifelong quest for the answers to life's biggest questions.

Seaward suggests that spiritual well-being rests upon three main "pillars" **(Figure 2.3)**:[18]

- A strong personal value system
- Relationships: connectedness and community
- A meaningful purpose in life

Let's take a closer look at each.

Personal Values. Your term paper is due tomorrow and you haven't even started it. Should you buy one from an online site, stay up all night writing, or go to your instructor's office empty-handed,

apologize, and ask for an extension? Questions like this force us to reflect on our **values,** the internal guidelines we use to make decisions and evaluate the world around us. Building your spirituality starts with knowing your values and putting them into practice. Your answers to the following questions will help reveal your values.

- What is important to me?
- What principles do I want to live by?
- What do I stand for?

Values evolve over the course of a lifetime. Many college students arrive on campus with values very similar to those of their parents. However, with new relationships and experiences, values often change. Throughout adult life, a wide array of influences and circumstances requires you to refine your values repeatedly.

Living your values means reflecting them in the choices you make. For example, if you value the dignity of all human beings, you may be compelled to take action to reduce homelessness in your community. This might lead you to join a homeless outreach program.

Relationships. Your first relationship is with yourself. How comfortable are you with your own company? Through reflection, prayer, or meditation, you can begin to develop a relationship with your "higher self," whatever you conceive this to be.[18] This in turn can help you to see how you relate to everyone and everything in your environment: people, nature, institutions, and even concepts such as principles and laws.

Spiritual well-being also rests upon your connectedness with others. In your life as a college student, peer relationships may be critical, but you may also find spiritual support in your relationships with parents and siblings, old friends, romantic partnerships, or a spouse and children. These loved ones can help you explore your spiritual questions.

As you work to clarify your internal and external relationships, avoid focusing on flaws. Instead, try starting from a place of gratitude. Adopting an "attitude of gratitude" can brighten your outlook on life. This, in turn, can lead to **altruism,** the practice of giving to others out of selfless

---

spirituality That which is in total harmony with the perceptual and nonperceptual environment.

values Internal guidelines used to make decisions and evaluate the world around you.

altruism The practice of helping and giving to others out of genuine concern for their well-being.

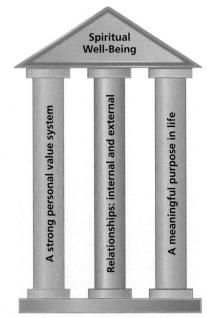

FIGURE 2.3 Seaward's Pillars of Spiritual Well-being. A strong sense of values, meaningful relationships, and a sense of purpose together support spiritual well-being.

Source: Adapted from *Health of the Human Spirit: Spiritual Dimensions for Personal Health*, 2nd ed., by B. L. Seaward, 2013, Burlington, MA: Jones & Bartlett Learning.

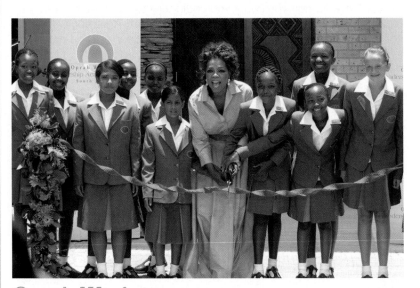

Oprah Winfrey acted altruistically when she started the Leadership Academy for Girls in South Africa.

concern for their well-being. Acts of altruism bring gifts to you: Helping others can help you put your own life in perspective, build self-esteem, manage stress, sleep better, and even live longer.[20]

Purpose. Why do you exist? Thinkers throughout the ages have provided various answers for us, most of which focus on service to humanity. But how would you answer this question? Is it important to you to conduct your life in such a way that you know your living has made some difference? If so, given your unique values and gifts, how will you express your purpose?

Benefits of Spirituality

Studies of the benefits of spirituality on psychological health yield conflicting results. These differences may be due primarily to the way the studies are designed.

Studies that differentiate between religion and spirituality have found that respondents who score high on "religiousness" experience significantly lower rates of psychological distress than average, whereas respondents who score high on "spirituality" tend to have higher rates of psychological distress.[8] This might reflect the potential for people to turn to spirituality as a form of self-treatment for psychological challenges. It's also possible that some people scoring high on spirituality have turned away from organized religion and are thus experiencing psychological distress caused by a "crisis of faith."[8]

Studies that consider "religion and spirituality" as a single variable consistently find it strongly associated with greater psychological health.[21] Moreover, this benefit is not correlated to the frequency of participation in religious activities. Specific effects include decreased anger, anxiety, depression, and substance abuse; and increased hope, optimism, sense of satisfaction with life, and inner peace.[22] Moreover, many studies have associated spirituality with increased physical health and self-healing.[23,24]

Common Psychological Challenges

There may come times when you face challenges to your psychological well-being, just as you do to your physical health. This vulnerability does not mean there is something "wrong" with you. These challenges are common, and some simple strategies can help you overcome them.

Shyness

Shyness is characterized by a feeling of apprehension or intimidation in social situations, especially in reaction to unfamiliar people or new environments. In a survey of more than 25,000 college students, 5% said that the statement "I am shy around others" was extremely like them.[25]

Unlike introverts, who prefer to keep to themselves, shy people want to participate in social interactions, but find it difficult to do so because of self-consciousness, fear of embarrassment, or a negative self-image. Shyness can vary in severity from a slight feeling of discomfort to a pattern of avoidance that can be disabling. It can also lead to *social isolation,* a general withdrawal from or avoidance of social contact or communication.

A common belief is that people are "born" shy, and one variation of a gene that helps regulate brain chemistry has been linked to some cases of shyness.[26] But this "shy" gene doesn't work alone. Life experiences and other environmental factors contribute.

Mild forms of shyness can usually be overcome with practice. Try making small talk with someone you'll probably never see again, like a person in line at the airport. If that feels reasonably comfortable, then try it again with a person you barely know, like the clerk at the bagel shop. In short, ease out of your comfort zone slowly. In addition, cognitive-behavioral therapy, discussed later in this chapter, can help.

Loneliness

Loneliness is not a synonym for being alone. Many people are content to spend much of their time alone. In contrast, **loneliness** is a feeling of isolation from others, a sense that you don't have—and don't know how to make—meaningful connections. In fact, loneliness can be particularly acute when you're with others.

If you feel as though you need more meaningful connections in your life, you have many options:

- **Take advantage of the social and volunteer opportunities offered on campus or in your community.** Seek out groups that share your interests, such as in sports, politics, or theatre, where you are more likely to meet others who share your passions and values—and to form meaningful relationships.

- **Express yourself openly and honestly.** Sharing your true feelings with someone can foster a feeling of connection that mere socializing cannot.

- **Look into college counseling center resources.** Campus counseling centers usually offer a variety of resources that can help you build your social skills and develop more meaningful relationships.

Anger

Anger is a completely normal and even healthy human emotion. Recognizing factors that make you angry can help you understand your values and assert yourself. Expressing anger is an important facet of the communication process.

However, anger that is out of control can be destructive. It can damage your relationships and may make it difficult for you to hold a job or participate in group activities. It can even damage your heart. The exploding rage you feel when you get really angry

shyness The feeling of apprehension or intimidation in social situations, especially in reaction to unfamiliar people or new environments.

loneliness A feeling of isolation from others, often prompted by a real or perceived loss.

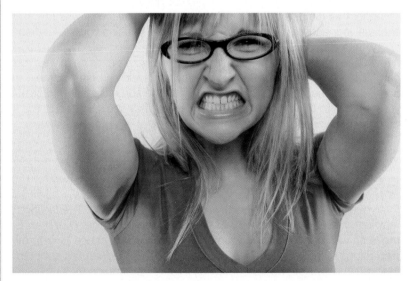

Although it may not feel like it, you can modify anger.

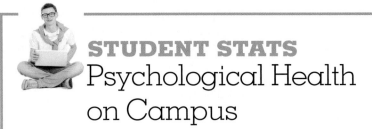

STUDENT STATS
Psychological Health on Campus

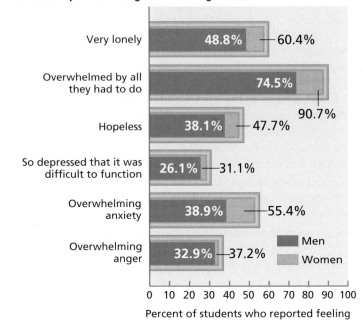

Students reported feeling the following within the last 12 months:

	Men	Women
Very lonely	48.8%	60.4%
Overwhelmed by all they had to do	74.5%	90.7%
Hopeless	38.1%	47.7%
So depressed that it was difficult to function	26.1%	31.1%
Overwhelming anxiety	38.9%	55.4%
Overwhelming anger	32.9%	37.2%

0 10 20 30 40 50 60 70 80 90 100
Percent of students who reported feeling

Data from: *American College Health Association National College Health Assessment (ACHA-NCHA II) Reference Group Executive Summary, Fall 2012,* by the American College Health Association, 2013, retrieved from http://www.acha-ncha.org/reports_ACHA-NCHAII.html.

raises your blood pressure and appears to be associated with abnormal heart rhythms that can lead to sudden cardiac arrest.[27] An analysis of 44 separate studies concluded that anger increases the risk for developing heart disease even in otherwise healthy people.[28]

Anger that remains bottled up can also be harmful. The key is to express your anger in a constructive way. When you find yourself getting angry, take a step back and assess the situation objectively. Try to relax—a few deep breaths can often do the trick. Then explain, as calmly as you can, what's upsetting you. Speak honestly, but avoid criticism, blame, and threats. If necessary, walk away from the person or situation to give yourself time to think. Once you're calmer, you may see solutions to the problem that you didn't notice before.

Mental Disorders in the United States: An Overview

Everyone occasionally feels sad, worried, or "spaced out." The feelings may last a few hours or a few weeks, but eventually we get over it and move on with our lives. In contrast, **mental disorders** cause long-term disruptions in thoughts and feelings that reduce an individual's ability to function in daily life. The American Psychiatric Association (APA) classifies and defines all the mental disorders it currently recognizes in its *Diagnostic and Statistical Manual of Mental Disorders* (DSM). Clinicians are required to use a DSM diagnostic code for reimbursement of mental health services, including prescription of **psychoactive drugs** (drugs that affect the patient's mental state).

Mental disorders are common. The National Institute of Mental Health (NIMH) estimates that more than 1 in 4 Americans over the age of 18 have experienced a DSM-diagnosable mental disorder at some time in the past year—a figure that translates to over 57 million people.[29] Fortunately, most of these cases are mild. Only about 6% of Americans suffer from a *serious mental illness (SMI)*; that is, one that substantially interferes with or limits one or more major life activities. Americans recognized as having an SMI are considered disabled.[30]

College students face distinct academic and social pressures that can challenge their psychological health. In 2012, about 1 in 5 college students in the United States reported being treated for or diagnosed with some type of mental disorder in the past year.[31] However, because many students fail to seek treatment, the actual statistics are thought to be much higher: In one large national survey, almost half of all college students met the DSM criteria for at least one mental disorder in the previous 12 months.[32]

>> This National Public Radio program discusses rising rates of mental health issues on campus: www.npr.org/2011/01/17/132934543/depression-on-the-rise-in-college-students.

A comparison of our rate of mental disorders with that of other countries is troubling. A World Health Organization survey of 17 countries found that the United States has the highest lifetime prevalence of DSM mental disorders: Over 47% of Americans have one or more at some point in their lives. This rate was dramatically higher than the average (27%) of the 16 other countries surveyed.[33]

No one is certain whether the variation reflects cross-cultural differences. For example, sociocultural factors such as stronger family and community ties in some countries could be protective against mental disorders. Or perhaps in the United States, people are more willing to admit to psychological symptoms. Physicians in the United States may also be more likely to diagnose symptoms as a DSM disorder in order to match patients with psychoactive drugs.[34] In the United States, psychoactive drugs became the primary form of treatment for mental disorders as physicians began to accept the *chemical imbalance theory* of mental disorders.[34] The theory arose in the 1950s as drugs initially used to treat certain physical disorders were found to have psychological side effects.[35] Initially, researchers could not explain these effects, but over time, it became clear that the drugs were flooding the brain with chemicals called **neurotransmitters.** These chemicals—including serotonin, dopamine, and others—are called neurotransmitters because they enable the transmission of messages from one nerve cell (called a *neuron*) to another across microscopic gaps called *synapses*.

Researchers theorized that mental disorders might occur because a patient's brain was producing an excess or deficit

mental disorders Significant behavioral and psychological disorders that disrupt thoughts and feelings, impair ability to function, and increase risk of pain, disability, or even death.

psychoactive drugs Drugs that affect the user's mood, perceptions, or other aspects of the mental state.

neurotransmitters Chemicals that enable the transmission of messages from one neuron to another across synapses.

> *A World Health Organization survey of 17 countries found that the United States has the highest lifetime prevalence of DSM mental disorders."*

of neurotransmitters. Thus, psychoactive drugs were prescribed to "correct the imbalance." However, despite decades of research, scientists have failed to find the evidence to support this theory. Neurotransmitter levels and functioning appear to be normal in people with mental disorders before drug treatment.[34,35] Thus, the current edition of the DSM states that the cause of most mental disorders is unknown, and researchers have begun to investigate gene–environment interactions as the source.[35]

We discuss specific medications and other treatment options for the most common mental disorders in the next section.

Mood Disorders

Mood disorders are chronic, pervasive emotional states that significantly alter the person's thoughts, behavior, and normal functioning.

Depressive Disorders

Though most of us have felt sadness from time to time, the feeling is usually temporary and in reaction to a disappointment or loss. However, in a person diagnosed with a **depressive disorder,** the sadness is more profound and long term, and interferes with daily life. Approximately 18 million adult Americans suffer from a depressive disorder every year.[29]

Although the most basic symptom of depressive disorders is persistent sadness, other symptoms include:

- A feeling of being slowed down or lacking energy
- Feelings of helplessness, hopelessness, meaninglessness, or "emptiness"
- Feelings of worthlessness or guilt
- Loss of interest in school, work, or activities once enjoyed
- Social withdrawal
- Difficulty thinking clearly or making decisions
- Sleep disturbances
- Changes in eating habits, eating more or less than formerly
- Restlessness, irritability
- In the most severe cases, recurring thoughts of death or suicide

Depressive disorders also often occur in conjunction with anxiety disorders and substance abuse.[29]

mood disorder Any chronic, pervasive emotional state that significantly alters the person's thoughts, behaviors, and normal functioning.

depressive disorder A mental disorder usually characterized by profound, persistent sadness or loss of interest that interferes with daily life and normal functioning.

major depressive disorder (unipolar depression) A type of depressive disorder characterized by experiencing five or more symptoms of depression, including either depressed mood or loss of interest or pleasure, for at least two weeks straight.

dysthymic disorder (dysthymia) A milder, chronic type of depressive disorder that lasts two years or more.

Types of Depressive Disorders

Two of the most common forms of depressive disorder are major depressive disorder and dysthymic disorder.

Major Depressive Disorder. Also called *unipolar depression*, **major depressive disorder** affects more than 6% of American adults in a given year.[29] It is diagnosed when someone consistently experiences five or more depressive symptoms for at least two weeks straight.[36] These symptoms impair a person's ability to study, work, eat, sleep, maintain relationships, and feel pleasure. An episode of major depression may occur only once in a person's life, or it may occur several times.

Dysthymic Disorder. Also called *dysthymia,* **dysthymic disorder** is characterized by the same depressive symptoms listed earlier; however, the symptoms tend to be milder, and are chronic, occurring on a majority of days for at least two years in adults (one year in children). The person may experience several days or weeks without symptoms, but not longer than two months. Those with dysthymia are more likely to suffer a major depressive episode in their lifetime. This type of depression is less common, affecting about 1.5% of American adults in a given year.[29]

Causes of Depressive Disorders

Although two recent studies have identified the same region of DNA as involved in major depression, genetics alone are not to blame.[37,38] The pattern is likely influenced by the interactions of several genes with environmental factors, such as certain learned behaviors family members pass from one generation to the next. Indeed, the tendency toward depression and other mental disorders in minority groups is thought to be due to social determinants such as discrimination. See the **Diversity & Health** box on page 32 for more information.

Physical factors such as chronic pain can also contribute to depressive disorders. Irregular hormone levels can also be a factor, which is why doctors will often test a patient's thyroid, a gland that secretes regulatory hormones, before diagnosing a depressive disorder. Paradoxically, both antidepressants and anti-anxiety medications can produce major depressive episodes. Even certain medications for physical illnesses can prompt them, and substance abuse is a common trigger.

External events such as the loss of a relationship, financial problems, and academic and career pressures can lead to depression. If a person's network of emotional support is limited, or if it changes following the loss of a loved one, the person may be especially vulnerable.

>> Students and teachers talk about how the pressures of college can lead to depression: www.depressioncenter.org/news-and-publications/video/theviewfromhere.

Depressive Disorders in Men and Women

About twice as many women suffer from depressive disorders as men in any given year.[39] The causes and symptoms may vary between sexes.

Women and Depression. Until adolescence, girls and boys experience depressive disorders at about the same rate.[39] But after puberty,

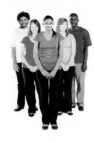

DIVERSITY & HEALTH

Mental Health Through the Lenses of Ethnicity and Sexuality

Race, ethnicity, and sexual orientation can influence a person's risk for developing a mental disorder and the treatment that person receives. In general, minorities have less access to, and less availability of, mental health services.[1]

Although there are not many large-scale studies on mental health in minority populations, it appears that Americans of minority race, ethnicity, or sexual orientation are at greater risk for mental health problems than their Caucasian, heterosexual counterparts. For example, compared with Caucasians, African Americans are 20% more likely to report having serious psychological distress, and Mexican Americans are about 25% more likely to suffer from depression.[1, 2]

The tendency toward depression and other mental illness is no more inborn in minorities than in heterosexual Caucasians, but appears to be related to the obstacles and challenges that they face in society. Many minority groups experience higher rates of certain social factors that can contribute to mental illness, such as discrimination, exposure to violence or trauma, refugee status, and childhood placement in foster care; however, living in poverty has the most measurable effects on the rates of mental illness.[3] Racial and ethnic minorities are overrepresented among the poor. Moreover, the overall rate of poverty within most racial and ethnic minority groups in the United States is much higher than that of Caucasians: More than 20% of Hispanic Americans and African Americans lived at or below the poverty level in 2010, compared with 11% of Asian Americans and 9% of Caucasians.[4] In 2010, adults living below the poverty level were three times more likely to have serious psychological distress and four times more likely to suffer from depression than adults with incomes at or above twice the poverty level.[4]

In addition, discrimination can exacerbate mental health issues. A recent study found that the increased likelihood of mental disorders in Latinos adapting to U.S. society is at least partially due to feelings that they are members of a group that is devalued and discriminated against.[5] Discrimination and violence are also major sources of stress for LGBT (lesbian, gay, bisexual, or transgender) people, while at the same time, discrimination may make it difficult for lesbian, gay, and bisexual people to find support.[6]

To make matters worse, minorities often lack access to culturally or linguistically appropriate mental health services. Minority groups are less likely to have health insurance that would cover the cost of psychotherapy and psychiatric care—for example, in 2010, only 32% of Native Americans, 37% of Hispanic Americans, and 45% of African Americans had private health insurance, compared with 65% of Caucasians.[4] Even when care is available, misdiagnosis of mental health disorders is more common in minorities than in Caucasians, and cultural stigmas against mental illnesses or distrust of mental health care can lead to underreporting of mental health problems or reliance on less-effective traditional remedies rather than medical treatment.

Critical-Thinking Questions

1. What might be some of the barriers to mental health services faced by recent immigrants to the United States? By members of the LGBT community?

2. Statistics show a link between mental illness and poverty. In your opinion, does either directly cause the other, or are there factors that might contribute to the link between them?

>> **Listen to a radio story on mental health in the African American community:** www.npr.org/templates/story/story.php?storyId=87952114&ft=1&f=88201937.

References: **1.** "Mental Health Data/Statistics," by the Office of Minority Health, 2012. Retrieved from http://minorityhealth.hhs.gov/templates/browse.aspx?lvl=3&lvlid=539. **2.** "Depression in the United States Household Population 2005–2006," by the U.S. Department of Health and Human Services, 2008, NCHS Data Brief No. 7. **3.** "Mental Health 101," July 8, 2008. Office of Minority Health. Retrieved from http://minorityhealth.hhs.gov/templates/browse.aspx?lvl=3&lvlid=81. **4.** "Health, United States, 2011," by the National Center for Health Statistics, 2012, p. 38. Available at http://www.cdc.gov/nchs/data/hus/hus11.pdf. **5.** "Attributions to Discrimination Among Latino/as: The Mediating Role of Competence," by L. Torres, 2009, *American Journal of Orthopsychiatry, 79* (1), 118–124. **6.** "Answers to Your Questions for a Better Understanding of Sexual Orientation and Homosexuality," by the American Psychological Association 2008. Available at http://www.apa.org/topics/sexuality/sorientation.pdf.

there is an increased rate in women. One factor may be the hormonal changes women experience in connection with the menstrual cycle, pregnancy, childbirth, the postpartum period, the years just before menopause, and menopause. These hormonal shifts appear to increase the risk of depressive disorders, but no precise cause for this increased risk is known.[39]

A number of social and interpersonal factors increase women's stress, which contributes to depression. Women still tend to play a larger role than men in child care, while also pursuing professional careers. Women also experience higher rates of poverty and sexual abuse than men do.[39]

For about 12–20% of new mothers, the combination of wildly shifting hormonal and physical changes, a radical change in lifestyle, the responsibility for a new baby, and a lack of sleep may contribute to *postpartum depression*. This disorder can make it difficult for a mother to bond with her new baby, or in the most serious cases, can promote thoughts of harming herself or her newborn.[40]

Men and Depression. Depressive disorders in men are often under-diagnosed and under-treated. Because of that, the disparity in rates of depressive disorders between men and women may not be as large as reported. Some of the lack of recognition may arise from the different ways men express their illness. Rather than appearing sad, they may be irritable, angry, or even abusive. Men with a depressive disorder are also prone to physical effects like fatigue and difficulty sleeping.[39]

Depressed men are more likely than women to self-medicate through destructive behaviors such as drug and alcohol abuse, or to engage in reckless, risky behavior.[39] Also, depression is a risk factor for suicide, and although women are more likely to attempt suicide, men are much more likely to succeed.[39] In 2010, 79% of all suicides in the United States were committed by males.[41]

Treatment of Depressive Disorders

For several decades, psychiatrists have acknowledged that many people recover spontaneously from depressive episodes—if given adequate time.[42,43] Still, many people benefit greatly from treatment, and for some, it can be life-saving. One of the first steps in getting treatment

Dealing with Depression

"HI, I'M JAVIER.
I first realized that I had depression when I started taking pills. I suffer from migraines and the pills make me go to sleep so I was kind of addicted to them. I took them all the time and I was practically asleep 24-7. I stopped going to school and I failed a lot of classes because of that. And so I went to a doctor and he told me that I suffer from mild depression and that I needed to do something about it. I needed to stop the medication I was on and take the medication that he prescribed. It was pretty hard for me to accept it. I mean, most guys don't think that there's something wrong with them until, you know, life hits them."

1. Javier self-medicated with his migraine pills when he was depressed. What are some other signs that can indicate depression in men?

2. What options does Javier have to deal with his depression?

3. If you had a friend who was experiencing symptoms like Javier's, would you say something to him? What would you say?

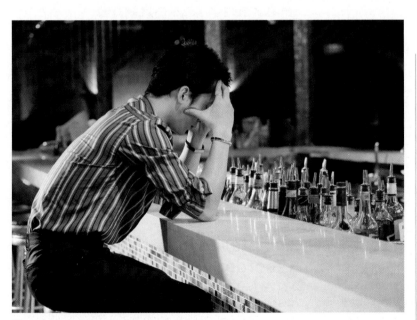

Depressed men are more likely than women to self-medicate through alcohol or drug use.

should be an evaluation by a medical doctor to check for any physical causes. If physical sources have been ruled out, several types of treatment can help depressed people get their lives back on track.

Psychotherapy. Talking with a trained counselor or psychologist can make all the difference for many people with a depressive disorder. Talk therapies (described shortly) encourage depressed people to open up about their thoughts, feelings, relationships, and experiences in order to recognize problems that underlie their depression and work to improve them. Talk therapy may be the best treatment option for mild to moderate depressive disorders.[39]

Antidepressants. For those who are severely depressed or suicidal, the health-care provider may suggest medication as an adjunct to talk therapies. Like most psychoactive drugs, antidepressants prompt a change in the levels of neurotransmitters—typically serotonin—in the brain. Antidepressants do not relieve symptoms immediately, and patients must take regular doses for at least two to four weeks before experiencing an effect.

These medications are not addictive, but abruptly stopping them can cause withdrawal symptoms or lead to a relapse of depression. It's very

Practical Strategies

Questions to Ask Before Starting an Antidepressant

If your doctor thinks you might benefit from taking an antidepressant, discuss the following questions to help you decide whether or not it's the right option for you:

- Why do you believe that an antidepressant is the right choice for me?
- Why do you suggest this particular antidepressant for me?
- How would I know if the antidepressant is really working and I'm not feeling better for other reasons?
- When would I feel its effects?

What should I do while I wait for it to work?

- What are the side effects? Am I at risk for them? What should I do if I decide to take this drug, and start experiencing side effects?
- What is your practice for following up with your patients on the effects of the antidepressants you prescribe?
- When do you anticipate that I could stop taking it? What would the withdrawal process entail?

---

doctor suggests that an antidepressant may help you, check out the **Practical Strategies** box for some important questions to discuss together. If you should decide against medication, talk to your doctor about other treatment options. These are discussed in detail later in this chapter.

Bipolar Disorder

Bipolar disorder, also known as *manic-depressive disorder,* is characterized by occurrences of abnormally elevated mood (or *mania*) alternating with depressive episodes, with periods of normal mood in between. Mania can cause increased energy and decreased need for sleep, an expansive or irritable mood, impulsive behavior, and unrealistic beliefs or expectations. Manic people's thoughts race, their speech is rapid, their attention span is low, and their judgment is poor. Extreme manic episodes can include aggression or delusions and hallucinations. The alternating depressive episodes can lead to thoughts of suicide.

Bipolar disorder affects approximately 5.7 million American adults, about 2.6% of the U.S. population.[29] It occurs equally among both sexes and in all races and ethnic groups.[47] It usually develops in the late teens or early adult years and, until the 1980s, was not recognized in children. Over the last two decades, diagnoses of bipolar disorder in children increased by 4,000%, and the American Psychiatric Association is now urging physicians to curb their use of the diagnosis in children.[48]

Bipolar disorder has a tendency to run in families, and scientists are looking for genes that may increase a person's likelihood of developing the illness. However, most agree that many different genes are likely to act along with environmental factors to produce the illness.

The most common treatment for bipolar disorder is a mood-stabilizing drug such as lithium. Anticonvulsant medications, antidepressants, and antipsychotics may be prescribed as well.

>> **Hear people with bipolar disorder discuss their condition:** www.webmd.com/bipolar-disorder/bipolar-tv/default.htm.

---

important that, if you decide to stop taking antidepressants, you taper them off gradually and under a physician's supervision.

Common side effects of antidepressants include headache, insomnia, tremors, anxiety, and sexual dysfunction. Severe side effects are less common, but include panic attacks, hostility, delusions, and suicidal thoughts. In the 1990s, studies began warning of the increased risk of suicide in young people taking certain antidepressants. The U.S. Food and Drug Administration (FDA) now requires that all antidepressant labels carry a warning that alerts consumers about the suicide risk among teens and young adults up to the age of 24.

Although many experts have concluded that, for people suffering from severe depression, a course of supervised drug therapy can be helpful, many researchers have begun to question the rigor of study data underlying the claims of antidepressants' effectiveness.[44,45,46] They suggest that the best path forward is for psychiatrists and patients to weigh carefully the risk/benefit equation. If your

bipolar disorder (manic-depressive disorder) A mental disorder characterized by occurrences of abnormally elevated mood (or mania), often alternating with depressive episodes, with periods of normal mood in between.

anxiety disorders A category of mental disorders characterized by persistent feelings of fear, dread, and worry.

generalized anxiety disorder (GAD) An anxiety disorder characterized by chronic worry and pessimism about everyday events that lasts at least six months and may be accompanied by physical symptoms.

Anxiety Disorders

Anxiety disorders cover a wide range of conditions characterized by persistent feelings of fear, dread, and worry. They are the most common mental health problems among American adults, affecting over 40 million people each year.[29] They are also the most common mental disorder among college students: Nearly 12% reported being diagnosed or treated for anxiety in 2012.[31] Anxiety disorders frequently occur in conjunction with depressive disorders or substance abuse problems, and anxiety—ranging from nervousness to panic attacks—is a common side effect of many antidepressant medications.[29]

Generalized Anxiety Disorder (GAD)

People who suffer from **generalized anxiety disorder (GAD)** feel chronic anxiety, exaggerated worry, and pessimism, even when there is little or nothing to provoke it. Physical symptoms that often accompany the anxiety include fatigue, headaches,

> **"** *Although people experiencing panic attacks often truly fear that they might die, panic attacks will not kill you.*"

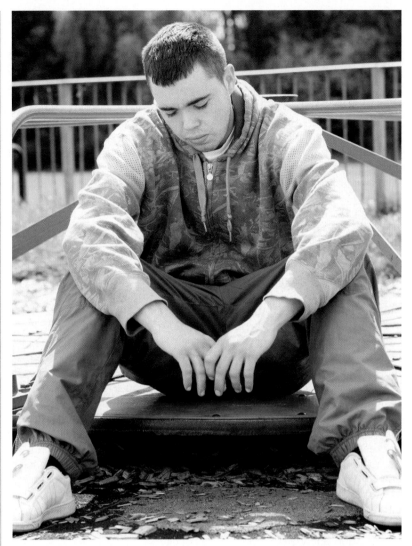

muscle tension, muscle aches, difficulty swallowing, trembling, and nausea. The condition is diagnosed when symptoms last at least six months. GAD affects about 6.8 million adult Americans and about twice as many women as men.[29] It usually develops gradually, and is often accompanied by depression, other anxiety disorders, or substance abuse.

Panic Attacks and Panic Disorder

Panic attacks are sudden feelings of terror that strike without warning. Symptoms include chest pain, shortness of breath, dizziness, weakness, and nausea. Panic attacks usually induce a sense of unreality and fears of impending doom, losing control, or dying, even though there is no rational reason for the person to believe something bad might happen. They usually go away on their own in less than 10 minutes.

Many people have just one panic attack and never have another, but those experiencing repeated panic attacks may have **panic disorder.** Panic disorder affects about 6 million adults in the United States and is twice as common in women as men.[49] It often begins in late adolescence or early adulthood, and the susceptibility appears to be inherited.

About one-third of people who suffer from panic disorder go on to develop *agoraphobia,* the fear of being in places where they cannot quickly leave or get help should they have a panic attack.[29] Agoraphobia can eventually leave victims virtually housebound.

Social Anxiety Disorder

Social anxiety disorder, also called *social phobia,* typically involves an intense fear of being judged by others and of being humiliated by your own actions. It can be accompanied by physical symptoms such as sweating, blushing, increased heart rate, trembling, and stuttering. It may strike only in certain situations—for instance, being called on in class—but in its most severe form a person might experience the symptoms any time he or she is around other people.[50] Social

panic attacks Episodes of sudden terror that strike without warning.

panic disorder A mental disorder characterized both by recurring panic attacks and the fear of a panic attack occurring.

social anxiety disorder (social phobia) An anxiety disorder characterized by an intense fear of being judged by others and of being humiliated by your own actions, which may be accompanied by physical symptoms.

phobia An extreme, disabling, irrational fear of something that poses little or no actual danger.

obsessive-compulsive disorder (OCD) An anxiety disorder characterized by repeated and unwanted thoughts (obsessions) that lead to rituals (compulsions) in an attempt to control the anxiety.

Social anxiety disorder can cause people to isolate themselves from others.

anxiety disorder affects about 15 million adults in the United States, and women and men are equally likely to develop it.[29]

Phobias

Many people have an irrational fear of something—such as mice or spiders—that poses little or no actual danger. A **phobia** is similarly irrational, but so extreme as to be disabling. Phobias are common, and although the average age of onset is 7 years, nearly 9% of American adults experience some type of phobia.[29] The American Psychiatric Association classifies simple phobias into five categories: animal phobias; natural environment phobias (e.g., heights, water); situational phobias (e.g., confined spaces, darkness); blood, injection, or injury phobias; and other phobias.[36]

Obsessive-Compulsive Disorder (OCD)

People with **obsessive-compulsive disorder (OCD)** have repeated and unwanted thoughts (obsessions) that cause them to develop rituals (compulsions) in an attempt to control the anxiety produced by these thoughts. The obsessions tend to be overblown, such as extreme concern about contamination by germs, fear of home intruders, or death of a loved one. The rituals provide brief relief from anxiety, even though the sufferer often knows they are meaningless.

The rituals can end up controlling the person's life. For example, a student obsessed with germs may develop hand-washing rituals that are so extensive that he is unable to leave his apartment to get to class on time. Other common rituals include the compulsion to repeatedly check things, touch things (in a certain order or a certain number of times), or horde unnecessary items. Occurring equally in men and women, OCD affects 2.2 million adults in the United States.[29] First symptoms frequently appear in childhood or adolescence, and it is often diagnosed concurrently with eating disorders, other anxiety disorders, or depression.

>> **Sufferers of OCD tell their stories:** www.nytimes.com/interactive/ 2009/09/24/health/healthguide/TE_OCD.html?ref=health&_r=0.

Post-Traumatic Stress Disorder (PTSD)

After a traumatic event, people sometimes feel recurrent fear, anger, and depression, a condition known as **post-traumatic stress disorder (PTSD)**. Experiences that commonly cause PTSD include child abuse, natural disasters, automobile accidents, being the victim of a violent crime, or serving in the military. Currently, for example, some college campuses are offering veterans specialized counseling services for PTSD.

People with PTSD often startle easily, feel numb emotionally, and can become irritable or even violent. They tend to relive the trauma in flashbacks or dreams, and will avoid places or experiences that might remind them of the traumatic event. PTSD can be accompanied by depression, other anxiety disorders, and substance abuse.

About 7.7 million adults in the United States experience PTSD each year, but it can strike children as well.[29] The condition is more common in women than men. The likelihood of developing PTSD increases with intense, long-lasting trauma involving personal injury or death of a loved one, especially if the victim had little control over the event and received little support afterward.[51]

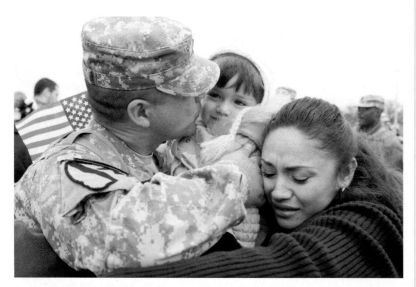

Soldiers returning home from war can often suffer from PTSD.

SELF-ASSESSMENT
Anxiety Assessment

Instructions: How has each of these symptoms disturbed or worried you during the last seven days? Circle the most appropriate score relating to your state.

0 = Never   1 = A little   2 = Moderately   3 = A lot   4 = Extremely

1.	Nervousness or shaking inside	0 1 2 3 4
2.	Nausea, stomach pain, or discomfort	0 1 2 3 4
3.	Feeling scared suddenly and without any reason	0 1 2 3 4
4.	Palpitations or feeling that your heart is beating faster	0 1 2 3 4
5.	Significant difficulty falling asleep	0 1 2 3 4
6.	Difficulty relaxing	0 1 2 3 4
7.	Tendency to startle easily	0 1 2 3 4
8.	Tendency to be easily irritable or bothered	0 1 2 3 4
9.	Inability to free yourself of obsessive thoughts	0 1 2 3 4
10.	Tendency to awaken early in the morning and not go back to sleep	0 1 2 3 4
11.	Feeling nervous when alone	0 1 2 3 4

HOW TO INTERPRET YOUR SCORE
If you indicated scores of 3 or 4 to five or six questions, your anxiety level is significant and you should consider different strategies such as better health practices, or adding relaxation techniques or physical exercise to your daily routine. If you indicated scores of 3 or 4 in all your answers, your level of anxiety is critical and you should consult your doctor.

To complete this Self-Assessment online, visit MasteringHealth™

Source: "Anxiety Self-assessment Questionnaire" used by permission of the Mental Illness Foundation, Montreal.

>> **Listen to soldiers talk about PTSD in their own words:** www.youtube .com/watch?v=bsFg8wZul-4 **and** www.pbs.org/wgbh/pages/frontline/ shows/heart/view.

Treating Anxiety Disorders

Cognitive-behavioral therapy (discussed shortly) is effective at teaching people with anxiety to recognize and redirect anxiety-producing thought patterns. One effective treatment, called *exposure therapy* or *systematic desensitization,* encourages patients to face their fears head-on. For instance, if a student with OCD fears dirt and germs, part of his therapy might involve getting his hands dirty and waiting progressively longer amounts of time before washing them. The therapist will help him work through his anxiety while his hands are dirty, and eventually his reaction will become less severe.

Biofeedback is increasingly being integrated with cognitive-behavioral therapy for patients with anxiety. In biofeedback, patients are connected to a device that provides them with feedback about their muscle tension, breathing rate, and other aspects of their body's functioning. They then make subtle changes, such as

post-traumatic stress disorder (PTSD) An anxiety disorder characterized by recurrent fear, anger, and depression occurring after a traumatic event.

relaxing their muscles or breathing more slowly, that help them manage their symptoms. In a recent study of college students receiving treatment for anxiety, those who had biofeedback as an adjunct to cognitive-behavioral therapy experienced a greater reduction in anxiety symptoms than those who had therapy alone.[52]

Among medications, certain antidepressants are the first choice for most anxiety disorders. Some physicians prescribe a class of medications known as the benzodiazepines (Valium, Xanax, etc.) because they exert a calming effect; however, these medications trigger significant dependence and are not recommended.[53]

Other Disorders

In this section, we discuss just two more of the 365 mental disorders now recognized by the APA. We chose attention disorders because they are common in college students, and schizophrenia because it typically first appears during adolescence or young adulthood.

Attention Disorders

Attention disorders create difficulty with jobs that require sustained concentration, such as completing a single task over a long period of time or sitting still for extended periods. The most common form of attention disorder is **attention deficit hyperactivity disorder (ADHD),** which is characterized by inattention, hyperactive behavior, fidgeting, and poor impulse control.

The APA first identified ADHD as a disorder in 1980. Children diagnosed with ADHD became eligible for special educational services, paid for by federal funds, in 1991, and today the majority of diagnoses are based on teacher complaints.[54] Boys are more than twice as likely as girls to be diagnosed. Although attention disorders usually become evident by age 7, many cases continue into adult life, and ADHD is diagnosed in about 6% of adults.[29] Among college students in the United States, 6.7% reported having ADHD.[31]

Although research hasn't conclusively identified social or psychological effects of ADHD among college students, there is consistent evidence that ADHD reduces academic performance.[55] Those with ADHD can have difficulty following directions, remembering information, and making deadlines; they may be chronically late, anxious, unorganized, or irritable. People with attention disorders are also at higher risk for tobacco use and substance abuse.

Options for treating attention disorders include cognitive-behavioral therapy and prescription stimulants such as methylphenidate (Ritalin or Concerta) or amphetamine/dextroamphetamine (Adderall). These drugs affect how the brain controls impulses and regulates attention.[56] Side effects include

agitation, irritability, and anxiety, as well as insomnia, headache, nausea, and loss of appetite significant enough that children taking the drugs long term commonly experience slowed growth.

In 2009, a national survey found that 6.4% of college students use Adderall nonmedically; that is, without a prescription.[57] Nonmedical use of Ritalin and other ADHD drugs is estimated to be similar or even higher. Typically, students use these drugs to help them study longer; however, research evidence suggests that nonmedical use among college students doesn't confer any substantial academic benefit.[58] In fact, users have lower GPAs on average than nonusers, and are more likely to abuse other drugs as well.[58]

Schizophrenia

Schizophrenia is a severe, chronic, and potentially disabling mental disorder that is characterized by *psychosis*, abnormal thinking and loss of contact with reality. It affects about 1% of adults in the United States, usually appearing in the late teens through early 30s.[29] Research has shown that schizophrenia affects both sexes equally and occurs in similar rates in all ethnic groups. Because it occurs in 10% of people who have a first-degree relative (parent or sibling) with the disorder, and in 40–65% of people whose identical twin has it, researchers are studying the role of genes in the disorder.[59] Although no specific gene or genes have yet been identified, it is known that people with schizophrenia have higher rates of genetic mutations overall. These mutations may disrupt brain functioning.[59] Nevertheless, researchers conclude that it is doubtful that genetics alone are sufficient to cause the disease to develop.

Primary symptoms of schizophrenia include:[59]

- **Delusions.** False beliefs, such as thinking you possess unusual powers or believing that others are plotting against you.
- **Hallucinations.** False perceptions of reality, such as hearing or seeing things that are not there, most often voices.
- **Thought disorders.** Often called *disorganized thinking*—problems with thinking or speaking clearly or maintaining focus.
- **Movement disorders.** Agitated or repetitive body movements, or in some extreme cases becoming catatonic (immobile).
- **Reduction in professional and social functioning.** Social withdrawal, unpredictable behavior, poor hygiene, or paranoia can all impair social and professional function.
- **Inappropriate emotions.** Aloofness, a so-called "flat affect," or inappropriate or bizarre reactions to events.

Any of a variety of antipsychotic medications may be prescribed to manage these symptoms. Their long-term use can be problematic for patients, however, because of a wide range of adverse effects, from weight gain to an inability to control muscle movements. Once schizophrenia patients are stabilized, interpersonal therapy can help. Although schizophrenia has a reputation of being incurable, both historic records and contemporary research studies have shown that many people do recover and go on to lead independent, satisfying lives.[59]

attention disorders A category of mental disorders characterized by problems with mental focus.

attention deficit hyperactivity disorder (ADHD) A type of attention disorder characterized by inattention, hyperactive behavior, fidgeting, and a tendency toward impulsive behavior.

schizophrenia A severe mental disorder characterized by delusions, hallucinations, and other aspects of psychosis.

> *There is consistent evidence that ADHD reduces academic performance."*

>> **People with schizophrenia tell their stories:** www.nytimes.com/interactive/2010/09/16/health/healthguide/te_schizophrenia.html.

A Friend's Suicide

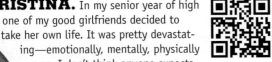

"HI, I'M KRISTINA. In my senior year of high school one of my good girlfriends decided to take her own life. It was pretty devastating—emotionally, mentally, physically even. I don't think anyone expects, as a high-schooler, that one of their peers will commit suicide. At first I felt angry, and then it gradually hit me and I was very upset and cried all the time. I guess, after that all happened, the positive thing that came out of it was I had a closer relationship with my girlfriends and my family; we really watch out for each other and we say "I love you" more.

I just want people to know that nothing is bad enough to take your own life. Even if you feel like nothing's going right in your life, it doesn't mean that you can't turn those negative things into positive things. There are many problems that people have in their teenage years that they can't help, but they end up stronger people because of it."

1. Do you think that Kristina is right that young people don't expect one of their peers to commit suicide? Why or why not?

2. What do you think Kristina means about turning negative things into positive things? Have you ever turned a negative into a positive?

Self-Injury and Suicide

When people experience a deep and persistent anguish, they may consider self-harm. Two common types are non-suicidal self-injury and suicide.

Self-Injury

Non-suicidal self-injury (NSSI) occurs in the form of intentional, self-inflicted cuts, burns, bruises, or other injuries, without the desire to die. Studies suggest that NSSI is used as a means of coping with overwhelming tension, negative, intrusive thoughts, or feelings of dissociation—of being detached from one's body and emotions.[60] Although it provides the injurer with a moment of calm, it is usually followed by feelings of guilt and shame.

NSSI often begins in adolescence. In recent population surveys of adolescents in the United States, Canada, and England, 16–20% admitted to engaging in NSSI.[61,62,63] More than 5% of college students in the United States also report engaging in NSSI in the past year, but this may be an underestimate because many who do injure themselves conceal it.[31]

Therapy and medications can help self-injurers learn to deal with their difficult feelings more appropriately and stop their self-abuse.

On the other hand, the use of certain medications, including some antidepressants and antipsychotics, is associated with an increased risk for self-injury.

Suicide

More than 38,000 people in the United States took their own life in 2011, and for every death there are at least another 11 attempted suicides.[64,65] College students are more likely than the general population to try to take their own lives, and suicide is the second leading cause of death on college campuses. More than 7% of students said they had seriously considered attempting suicide in the past year.[31] Although women attempt suicide more often than men, men are four times more likely to actually die by suicide, possibly because they choose more lethal means.[65] Multiple studies have suggested that lesbian, gay, bisexual, and transgender (LGBT) students have a higher than average risk for suicide.[66] Factors contributing to this risk include experiences of prejudice and discrimination, verbal or physical harassment, violence, and rejection by family members or peers.[65]

Among ethnic groups, Native Americans and Caucasians have a rate of suicide more than double that of other ethnic groups.[65] Another population at increased risk for suicide is older adults. Caucasian males over the age of 85 actually have the highest suicide rate of any group in the United States.[65]

Causes and Warning Signs of Suicide

Several factors clearly play a role in driving up suicide risk. More than 90% of people who commit suicide in the United States have a diagnosable mental health or substance use disorder.[65] In addition, financial problems, serious illness, and the loss of a loved one are frequent catalysts. A family history of suicide, previous suicide attempts, and having access to guns in the home also increase suicide risk.

Signs that a person may be considering suicide include:

- Statements that indirectly imply suicidal thoughts, such as "I don't have much to live for" or "You won't have to worry about me much longer"
- An inability to let go of grief
- Changes in behavior and personality that focus on hopeless, negative thoughts and feelings
- A noticeable downturn in mood within the first few weeks of starting a new antidepressant medication
- Loss of interest in classes, work, hobbies, or spending time with friends and loved ones
- Expressions of self-hatred, excessive risk taking, or apathy toward one's own well-being
- Disregard for personal appearance
- Changes in sleep patterns or eating habits
- A preoccupation with thoughts or themes of death

Preventing Suicide

Don't assume that a person who talks of suicide is just having a bad day or seeking attention. Instead, let the person know you care and that you are there to help. Never be afraid to raise the subject. Offer to call a crisis hotline together, go to a counseling center, or head to the nearest emergency room **(Figure 2.4)**.

≫ **Find links to all of National Public Radio's mental health podcasts at** www.npr.org/sections/mental-health.

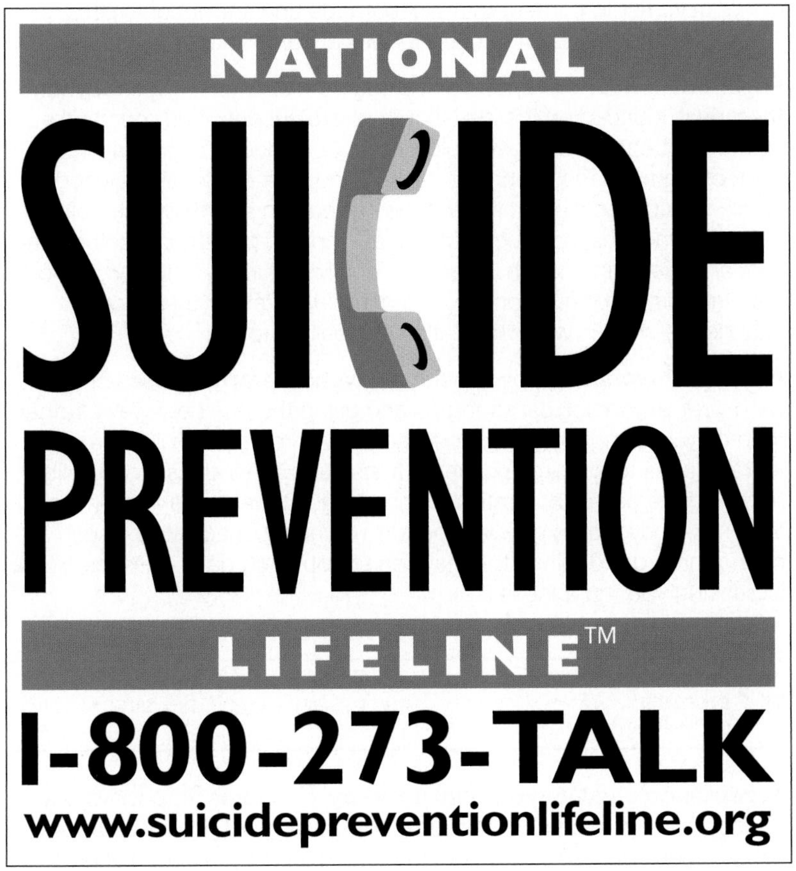

NATIONAL SUICIDE PREVENTION LIFELINE™

1-800-273-TALK

www.suicidepreventionlifeline.org

FIGURE 2.4 National Suicide Prevention Lifeline.

Source: U.S. Department of Health and Human Services, Substance Abuse and Mental Health Services Administration.

Getting Help for a Psychological Problem

A recent survey found that the number-one reason college students fail to get help for a psychological problem is personal *stigma*, an internalized feeling of shame about the condition.[67,68] So if you're in distress, remember that anxiety, depression, and other problems are common among college students, are treatable conditions, and are not a sign of weakness or deficiency! In fact, seeking help is a sign of psychological health—it shows that you esteem yourself enough to reach out, and that you trust your community to respond effectively.

Options on Campus

More than 60% of all students who stop attending college do so because of a mental health–related reason. Of these, half drop out without even trying to access mental health services.[67] Don't be among them. Most campuses offer a range of options to help address the mental and emotional pressures students face. These services may be provided for free or at low cost, or they may be covered by your insurance plan if you have one. Your campus health clinic or counseling center is a good place to start looking for help.

Clinical Options

In addition to campus and community services, it's important to be aware of the full range of your clinical options.

Types of Mental Health Professionals

The following are the types of licensed professionals who most commonly work with people experiencing psychological distress:

- **Counselors.** Counselors have a master's degree in counseling or social work and focus on talk therapy. Counselors may lead group, family, or individual therapy sessions, as well as recommend services available within your community.
- **Psychologists.** Psychologists have a doctoral degree and provide talk therapy. Many have particular specialties, and they may lead group, family, or individual therapy sessions.
- **Psychiatrists.** Psychiatrists have a medical degree and usually focus on the medical aspects of psychological issues. Unlike counselors or psychologists, psychiatrists can prescribe medication and may have admitting privileges at local hospitals. Psychiatrists and psychologists often work together to provide a full range of care.

See the **Consumer Corner** box on page 40 for information about what to discuss before picking a therapist.

Once you have found a mental health professional, the real work begins. Your treatment can succeed only if you are open and honest about your thoughts, emotions, and what is going on in your life. Therapy can sometimes bring up uncomfortable feelings, but that isn't necessarily a bad thing—it can be a sign that you are working through issues. However, if at any point something happens in therapy that you don't like, say so. Therapists should be eager to work with you to resolve any problems that come up.

Types of Therapy

The type of therapy you choose should depend on your specific condition and your preferences. Some people benefit from a combination of several types of therapy.

Cognitive-Behavioral Therapy. According to the National Association of Cognitive-Behavioral Therapists, **cognitive-behavioral therapy (CBT)** is a form of psychotherapy that emphasizes the role of thinking (cognition) in how we feel and what we do. There are many approaches to CBT, but all are based on the idea that our *thoughts* cause our feelings and behaviors, not external things, like people, situations, and events. The benefit of this fact is that when we can change the way we think, we end up feeling and acting better even if our situation does not change.[69]

One premise of CBT is that consistent dysfunctional thinking, sometimes called *cognitive distortion,* results in unwanted feelings and behaviors. See the **Practical Strategies** box on page 41 for tips on how to notice cognitive distortions that you may have.

In CBT, the therapist and patient work collaboratively to identify distorted, negative thinking and replace it with more positive, reinforcing thinking. This occurs within the treatment setting, but the patient is also typically given homework. Gradually, the patient learns to think and behave in more healthful ways. Cognitive therapy is usually short term and focused, and is most effective in treating mood and anxiety disorders.

Behavior Therapy. Either under the umbrella of CBT or alone, **behavior therapy** focuses on

> **cognitive-behavioral therapy (CBT)** A form of psychotherapy that emphasizes the role of thinking (cognition) in how we feel and what we do.
>
> **behavior therapy** A type of therapy that focuses on changing a patient's behavior and thereby achieving psychological health.

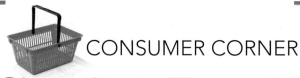

CONSUMER CORNER

Choosing a Therapist Who's Right for You

Therapy can help people with a variety of issues, but it's important to find a therapist with whom you feel comfortable and who is qualified to address your needs. Key points to discuss in your first meeting with a potential therapist are:

- Cost. Make sure you understand what the costs are and how they will be covered. If you are paying for care yourself, therapists will sometimes offer a sliding scale for fees, so be sure to ask.

- The therapist's credentials, education, and approach to therapy.

- Areas of specialization that the therapist has or that you would prefer—for example, specializations in bipolar disorder, childhood trauma, cognitive therapy, and so on.

- An overview of the problems you are experiencing and your goals for therapy.

- The experience the therapist has in helping people with similar problems.

- Whether or not you are taking or are interested in taking antidepressants or other medication. Keep in mind that psychologists and counselors cannot prescribe medication.

- Frequency and length of therapy sessions.

The information that you get from this preliminary conversation, as well as your overall impression of the therapist, will help you determine whether you would like to undertake therapy with that person. Don't be afraid to have an initial consultation with a few different therapists or to switch to someone else if, after a few sessions, you don't feel comfortable.

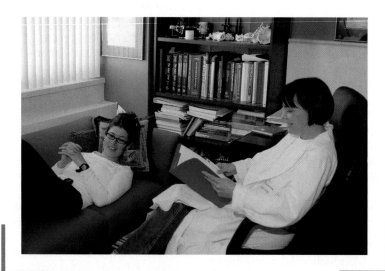

changing learned behaviors as efficiently and effectively as possible. The core idea behind behavior therapy is that, once our behavior changes, our thoughts, feelings, attitudes, and moods will follow. Techniques include exposure therapy, which is gradual exposure to an anxiety-provoking situation paired with relaxation techniques; positive reinforcement, which encourages desired behaviors; and aversion therapy,

or negative reinforcement that discourages unwanted behaviors. Behavioral therapy is often used for anxiety and attention disorders.

Psychodynamic Therapy. Also called *psychoanalysis*, **psychodynamic therapy** is founded on the idea that there are unconscious sources for a person's behavior and psychological state. Although originating in the work of Sigmund Freud about a century ago, contemporary psychodynamic therapy focuses broadly on the exploration and discussion of the patient's emotions, past experiences, and coping patterns. Together, patient and therapist unearth unresolved conflicts buried in the unconscious, then talk through these conflicts in order to understand them and to change the ways in which they affect the patient today.

Positive Psychotherapy. **Positive psychotherapy** focuses on identifying your psychological strengths and using them in new ways, rather than dwelling on "fixing" your psychological problems. This type of therapy aims to nurture in patients traits such as kindness, originality, humor, generosity, and gratitude and to help patients learn optimism. In positive psychotherapy, you perform a variety of activities—such as noting three good things that happen to you each day—with the goal of increasing your happiness.[70]

 Hear prominent positive psychologist Martin Seligman explain his approach: www.ted.com/talks/martin_seligman_on_the_state_of_psychology.html.

Acceptance and Commitment Therapy. In contrast to positive psychology, **acceptance and commitment therapy (ACT)** views happiness not as a goal, but as a byproduct of living according to one's values. An outgrowth of cognitive-behavioral therapy, it uses mindfulness and behavioral techniques to help patients clarify their values, set goals guided by these values, and take committed action to achieve these goals while experiencing difficult thoughts, emotions, or sensations.[71] Although a reduction in symptoms may indeed occur as a result of taking committed action, ACT makes no attempt at symptom control. Rather, it points out that patients' efforts to control their symptoms through alcohol abuse, overeating, and other destructive choices impede achievement of their goals. Thus, patients learn to take action to create a meaningful life while accepting the pain that inevitably accompanies such a pursuit.

Other Clinical Options

One of the most commonly prescribed clinical options is of course, pharmacologic therapy, which we have discussed with each specific disorder. In addition, although you might associate it with horror films, electroconvulsive therapy (ECT) is still sometimes used for severely ill patients who are not responsive to counseling or drug treatment. Formerly called *electroshock therapy*, ECT is administered by devices that transmit a jolt of electricity that induces seizures in the anesthetized patient. No one knows precisely how ECT produces therapeutic effects.

The FDA classifies ECT machines as high-risk devices

psychodynamic therapy A type of therapy that focuses on the unconscious sources for a patient's behavior and psychological state.

positive psychotherapy A new field of psychology that focuses on increasing psychological strengths and improving happiness, rather than on psychological problems.

acceptance and commitment therapy (ACT) An outgrowth of cognitive-behavioral therapy that increases patients' ability to engage in values-based, positive behaviors while experiencing difficult thoughts, emotions, or sensations.

because of the potential for significant adverse effects; most commonly, these are memory loss and cognitive impairment that may last for several months.[72] Despite controversy over ECT, some psychiatrists support its use in patients with resistant suicidal depression and other severe mental disorders.

Change Yourself, Change Your World

There are many steps you can take independently, among friends, and on campus to promote psychological well-being. Let's start with you.

Personal Choices

If you're feeling the need for a little psychological TLC, look no further. This section provides tips for self-care, building self-esteem and optimism, reaching out, and chilling out.

Take Care of Yourself

When you're experiencing mental or emotional distress, the basic tasks of daily life can feel overwhelming. Yet it's at just such times that self-care becomes more important than ever. If you are feeling mentally or emotionally on edge, be sure to:

- **Eat well.** Don't skip meals or binge on junk food. Calming your mind and emotions will be easier if your body isn't nutritionally stressed.

- **Get the right amount of sleep.** Sleeping 7-9 hours every night is important to both physical and mental well-being. In your busy schedule as a college student, make sure you make sleep a priority. (See the electronic Chapter 16.) If you're depressed and find yourself sleeping in, know that the very act of getting out of bed can be an instant boost. Once you're up, open the curtains and windows, as letting in light and air will help improve your mood.

- **Get some exercise.** Exercise releases body chemicals that boost mood. Even a half-hour walk is likely to improve your mood, clear your head, and make you feel better. Daytime exercise will also help make you tired and make it easier to sleep.

- **Set realistic goals.** Don't expect yourself to function at your regular level. Set smaller goals, and break big jobs up into small ones.

- **Take steps to build your self-esteem.** CBT recognizes that there are things you can do to change the way you think and the way you act that will, as a result, change the way you feel. For suggestions, see the **Practical Strategies: Building Self-Esteem** box on page 42.

Reach Out

We discussed earlier how social support contributes to psychological health. Yet feelings of anxiety and despair can often cause you to prefer to be alone. If so, it's important to recognize a desire for isolation as a symptom of your distress. Defy it—and reach out. Talk to someone you trust, or if you'd prefer to confide in a professional, visit your campus counseling center. Support groups are also good options. Often free or low cost, they are usually led by a trained professional who can steer the group's conversations and interactions in positive ways.

 Find online support at one of these websites: www.patientslikeme.com; www.dailystrength.org; www.wellsphere.com/communities.

Chill Out

Psychological health also thrives when you withdraw your thoughts from the chaos of everyday life and spend at least a few minutes in stillness.

Practical Strategies

Spotting Destructive Thoughts

Do you ever find yourself thinking thoughts like, "I *never* get things right!" or "I'm such a failure!"? If so, these cognitive distortions may be the sources of a bad mood or even a serious depression. Here are some thought patterns to watch out for:

- **All-or-nothing thinking.** In all-or-nothing thinking there is no middle ground. You think of situations or yourself as either perfect or a complete failure.

- **Overgeneralization.** You make a general conclusion based on a single event or experience from the past. You see one negative event as a never-ending pattern of defeat.

- **Mental filter.** You dwell excessively on a single negative detail, although everything else is positive.

- **Disqualifying the positive.** You reject positive experiences because they "don't count" for one reason or another.

- **Jumping to conclusions.** Without any definite facts to support it, you assume that other people are thinking or feeling negatively toward you. Or you predict that a situation will turn out badly and feel convinced that it is an already-established fact.

- **Magnification (catastrophizing) or minimization.** You exaggerate the importance of something minor (such as a poor grade on a quiz). Or you minimize a significant positive event (such as acing the final exam), predicting that "it won't make any difference."

- **Emotional reasoning.** You assume that your negative emotions necessarily reflect the way things really are: "I feel it, so it must be true."

- **Should statements.** You tell yourself what you "should" do, and if you don't perform, you feel guilty. This can also be applied to other people; if they don't live up to the "should" statement, you can feel angry, frustrated, or resentful.

- **Labeling and mislabeling.** Instead of thinking of something in a balanced way, you attach labels to yourself or others, such as "I'm a loser," or "He's no good." Mislabeling involves describing an event with highly colored or emotionally loaded language.

- **Personalization.** You think that everything people do or say is in reaction to you; you think you are the cause of a negative external event that, in reality, you had nothing to do with.

Source: Based on *The Feeling Good Handbook,* by D. D. Burns, 1989, New York: William Morrow and Company, Inc.

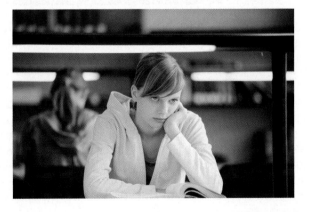

Practical Strategies

Building Self-Esteem

- **Listen to yourself.** What do you really want, need, and value? If you want others to listen to you, you need to understand and respect your own thoughts and feelings first.

- **Stretch your abilities.** Decide to learn something new, whether it's a school subject that seems intimidating or a sport you've never tried. Give yourself time to learn your new skill piece by piece, and then watch your talents grow.

- **Tackle your "to do" list.** Think about tasks you've been putting off, like calling a relative with whom you haven't spoken for a while or cleaning out your closet. Get a couple of them done each week. You'll be reminded of how much you can accomplish, and feel less distracted by loose ends.

- **Pat yourself on the back.** Notice when something you've done turns out well, and take a moment to congratulate yourself.

- **Schedule some fun.** In your drive to finish your "to do" list, make sure to leave time in your schedule for fun. Don't wait for others to invite you to a party or a film—invite them first. If money is tight, suggest hitting the bike paths or hiking trails and get the added feel-good benefit of exercise.

- **Serve others.** There is no simpler, or more generous, way to build self-esteem than by doing something nice for someone else. You'll both benefit.

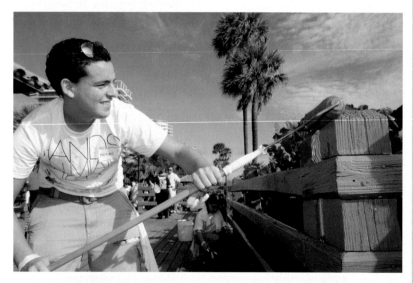

Participating in volunteer activities is a great way to boost self-esteem.

Many people cultivate stillness with meditation. Meditation can have different intended purposes, such as reaching higher states of consciousness, developing greater self-awareness, or simply achieving a more peaceful state of mind.[73] For some, the practice is as simple as sitting quietly and focusing attention on a single idea, word, or symbol, or on their breath. Others find meditative contemplation in nature. This might mean a solitary walk through the park or getting up early to watch the sun rise.

 Don't know how to meditate? Try one of these tools: www.mayoclinic .com/health/meditation/MM00623 **or** http://health.howstuffworks.com/ wellness/stress-management/how-to-relieve-stress-in-daily-life2.htm.

Helping a Friend

Earlier, we discussed what to do if you're concerned that a friend may be contemplating suicide. But how do you support a friend who's just generally feeling sad, anxious, or angry? Or how do you respond if a friend told you he or she was diagnosed with a mental illness?

Get Informed

The first step is to find out about what's going on. Did your friend's arms get scratched when she tried to pet a neighbor's cat, as she claims, or is she cutting herself? Is your friend holing up in his dorm room because he's trying to finish a project, or is he depressed? You might decide to check your own observations against those of mutual friends. If you agree that your friend's behavior is a cause for concern, then you need to have the courage to ask him or her about it.

Listen

That's where the next step comes in: Listen, without judging. Acknowledge that your friend's pain—even if it's difficult for you to understand—is real for him or her. Don't dismiss it with assertions such as, "But your parents seem so understanding!" Such comments might only cause your friend to lose trust in you. On the other hand, if your friend refuses to say what's up, accept that, and simply affirm that you'll be there if needed.

Offer Your Help

Don't put pressure on yourself to fix things. An open-ended question— Is there anything I could do to help?—is fine, or you could offer specific assistance, like driving your friend to a scheduled appointment.

You can also help your friend by modeling healthy behavior (see Chapter 1). Trust that maintaining your own balance will help your friend realize his or her own capacity to navigate life's challenges successfully.

Campus Advocacy

What steps can you take to increase psychological health on your campus and decrease the stigma associated with psychological distress? Active Minds is a student-founded and student-led organization working to change the conversation about mental health on college campuses. Currently, nearly 350 U.S. colleges and universities have chapters of Active Minds.

 To find out if your college has an Active Minds chapter, click on the U.S. map at www.activeminds.org/index.php?option=com_content&task=vi ew&id=27&Itemid=56. **If your campus isn't listed, click on Start a Chapter and find out how to set one up!**

The National Alliance on Mental Illness (NAMI) is an organization founded in 1979 to improve the lives of individuals and families affected by mental disorders. One of its initiatives, NAMI on Campus, supports student-run, student-led clubs that provide mental health support, and work to eliminate the stigma that students with mental disorders face.

 Watch videos of real students discussing psychological health at MasteringHealth™

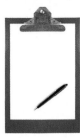

Choosing to Change Worksheet

To complete this worksheet online, visit MasteringHealth™

Part I. Building the Qualities of Psychological Health

Directions: Fill in your stage of behavior change in Step 1 and complete the rest of Part I with your stage of change in mind.

Step 1: *Your Stage of Behavior Change.* Please check one of the following statements that best describes your readiness to improve your psychological health.

_____ I do not intend to improve my psychological health in the next six months. (Precontemplation)

_____ I might improve my psychological health in the next six months. (Contemplation)

_____ I am prepared to improve my psychological health in the next month. (Preparation)

_____ I have been improving my psychological health for less than six months but need to do more. (Action)

_____ I have been improving my psychological health for more than six months. (Maintenance)

Step 2: *Identifying a Facet of Psychological Health to Improve.* The Ryff Scale of Psychological Well-Being identifies six key facets of psychological health (see Figure 2.1 on page 25). With this in mind, think about one facet of your psychological health that is important to you and needs improvement. Write it down.

_____

Step 3: *Making a Plan to Improve Psychological Health.* Keeping your current stage of behavior change in mind, describe what you might do or think about as a "next step" to improve that quality of psychological health. You can use the strategies presented in this chapter for ideas. Also list your timeline for making your next step.

_____

_____

_____

_____

Step 4: *Overcoming Challenges to Psychological Health.* In our daily lives we sometimes experience challenging situations that can put our psychological health to the test. What techniques can you use to counter roadblocks to developing your psychological health to the fullest? Again, you can refer to the information provided in this chapter.

_____

_____

_____

_____

Step 5: *Setting a SMART Goal.* Keeping your current stage of change in mind, set a SMART goal, including a timeline, for improving your psychological health.

Goal: _____

_____

_____

Timeline: _____

Part II. Reducing Cognitive Distortions and Increasing Positive Thinking

Far too often we engage in negative self-talk and destructive thinking patterns. If you have thoughts that consistently weigh you down, work through the steps below to unravel that harmful pattern of thinking.

Step 1: *Identifying Cognitive Distortions.* Take a look at the types of cognitive distortions discussed in **Practical Strategies: Spotting Destructive Thoughts** on page 41. Do any of these thinking patterns sound familiar to you? Write down any negative thoughts you have, and list which category each fits into.

Thoughts   Categories

_____   _____

_____   _____

_____   _____

_____   _____

_____   _____

Step 2: *Disputing Your Negative Thoughts.* Pick one of these thoughts to focus on. Do the facts of your current situation back up your negative perception? Write down all the facts that go against your current negative interpretation.

Example: I received a good grade on my last test, so although I did poorly on this test, I know I can do well at school.

Thought: _____

Facts that go against the negative interpretation: _____

_____

_____

Step 3: *Changing Your Perspective.* Imagine that a friend or a family member was thinking these things. What would you say to cheer that person up? Would things seem so bad if they weren't happening to you?

_____

_____

_____

Step 4: *Creating a More Optimistic Viewpoint.* Taking into account the evidence above that goes against your negative self-talk, can you think about the situation in a more optimistic way?

Example: Instead of thinking "I received a bad grade on this test; I'm going to flunk out of school!" you could think "I did poorly on this test, but I've done well on tests before. Now I know to create a study plan and attend review sessions before the next test."

_____

_____

_____

_____

Chapter Summary

MasteringHealth™

Build your knowledge—and health!—in the Study Area of **MasteringHealth**™ with a variety of study tools.

- Psychological health encompasses both mental and emotional health.

- Six facets of psychological health are self-acceptance, positive relations with others, autonomy, environmental mastery, a sense of purpose in life, and ongoing personal growth.

- Emotional intelligence enables you to process information of an emotional nature and use it to guide your thoughts, actions, and reactions.

- Optimism is the psychological tendency to have a positive interpretation of life's events.

- Psychological health is influenced by complex genetic factors interacting with aspects of our environment.

- Maslow's hierarchy of needs models the theory that people experience higher and higher levels of psychological health as they meet ever-higher levels of needs.

- Experiences of abuse or neglect during childhood can prompt the development of maladaptive coping patterns that are carried through adulthood.

- Your current level of social support can strongly influence your response to psychological challenges. Religion and spirituality can contribute to psychological health. Spiritual well-being is said to rest upon three pillars: a strong personal value system, connectedness and community in relationships, and a meaningful purpose in life.

- Common psychological challenges include shyness, loneliness, and anger.

- Serious mental disorders cause long-term disruptions in thoughts and feelings that reduce an individual's ability to function in daily life.

- The United States has the highest rate of mental disorders in the world. About 1 in 5 college students in the United States reports being treated for or diagnosed with some type of mental disorder; however, the actual prevalence may be much higher.

- The chemical imbalance theory of mental illness arose in the 1950s; however, the American Psychiatric Association acknowledges that the causes of mental disorders are unknown.

- Depressive disorders and bipolar disorder are mood disorders.

- Depression is considered one of the most treatable mental disorders. A variety of forms of psychotherapy are successful in treating depression, and regular exercise can help. Antidepressant medications are often prescribed; however, they can prompt serious side effects and withdrawal from these drugs must be done gradually, under a physician's supervision.

- Bipolar disorder is characterized by periods of mania followed by periods of depression.

- The most common mental disorders among college students are anxiety disorders, such as generalized anxiety disorder, panic disorder, and post-traumatic stress syndrome. Psychotherapy and antidepressant medications are common treatments.

- Other mental disorders common in young adults are attention disorders, such as ADHD, and schizophrenia.

- Non-suicidal self-injury is the act of cutting, burning, bruising, or otherwise injuring yourself in an effort to cope with negative, intrusive thoughts or feelings of dissociation.

- Suicide is the second most common cause of death in young adults. If a friend makes a statement indicating suicidal thoughts, offer to call a crisis hotline together, accompany your friend to your campus health services or a counseling center, or head to the nearest emergency room.

- Common options in psychotherapy include cognitive-behavioral therapy (CBT), behavior therapy, psychodynamic therapy, positive psychotherapy, and acceptance and commitment therapy. Some therapists use a combined approach.

- Self-care can be a good place to start if you are experiencing psychological distress. Self-care includes eating well, getting the right amount of sleep, exercising, setting realistic goals, and taking practical "thought and action" steps to build your self-esteem.

- A desire to isolate yourself is a common symptom of psychological distress, and reaching out is an important coping strategy.

- Meditation can be helpful to chill out and increase positive feelings.

- To help a friend with psychological distress or a diagnosed mental disorder, it's important to listen objectively and compassionately. Don't try to fix things for your friend, but do offer your presence and support.

- There are many ways to promote psychological well-being on campus, from joining an organization such as Active Minds to volunteering to become a peer counselor.

GET CONNECTED

>> Visit the following websites for further information about the topics in this chapter:

- American Psychological Association Help Center
www.apa.org/helpcenter
- National Institute of Mental Health
www.nimh.nih.gov
- Beliefnet
www.beliefnet.com
- ScienceDaily: Mind & Brain
www.sciencedaily.com/news/mind_brain
- Anxiety and Depression Association of America
www.adaa.org
- National Suicide Prevention Lifeline
www.suicidepreventionlifeline.org
- American Psychological Association Psychologist Locator
http://locator.apa.org
- Active Minds
www.activeminds.org

MOBILE TIPS!
Scan this QR code with your mobile device to access additional tips about psychological health. Or, via your mobile device, go to **http://chmobile.pearsoncmg.com** and navigate to Chapter 2.

- Mental Health America
www.mentalhealthamerica.net
- The Jed Foundation
www.jedfoundation.org

Website links are subject to change. To access updated web links, please visit MasteringHealth™

TEST YOUR KNOWLEDGE

1. One of Ryff's six facets of psychological health is
   a. having a romantic relationship.
   b. achieving a fixed state of wellness.
   c. happiness.
   d. environmental mastery.

2. Values, relationships, and purpose are three pillars of
   a. religiosity.
   b. spirituality.
   c. generativity.
   d. ego integrity.

3. Loneliness is
   a. the experience of being alone.
   b. sometimes prompted by a real loss.
   c. rarely experienced when you're with others.
   d. all of the above.

4. Mental disorders are
   a. more common in developing nations than in the United States.
   b. caused by an underlying chemical imbalance in the brain.
   c. classified in the *Diagnostic and Statistical Manual of Mental Disorders* (DSM).
   d. diagnosed in about 6% of Americans.

5. Depressive disorders
   a. are more common in men than in women.
   b. are typically treated by a class of medications called benzodiazepines.
   c. include dysthymic disorder and bipolar disorder.
   d. are none of the above.

6. Anxiety disorders
   a. are often treated with antidepressants.
   b. are the second most common mental health problem among American adults.
   c. are characterized by mania, delusions, and hallucinations.
   d. are classified as mood disorders.

7. Schizophrenia is
   a. a disabling and irrational fear of something that poses little or no actual danger.
   b. associated with compulsive behaviors such as hand washing.
   c. characterized by psychosis.
   d. incurable.

8. A suicidal person
   a. is not making idle threats.
   b. needs help immediately.
   c. wants relief from a situation that feels unbearable.
   d. is all of the above.

9. Psychiatrists
   a. specialize in group therapy.
   b. only see patients with severe mental illness.
   c. can prescribe medication.
   d. are all of the above.

10. Which of the following is a sensible strategy for psychological self-care?
    a. Eat nourishing foods and don't skip meals.
    b. On days when you have no early-morning commitments, get as many hours of sleep as possible.
    c. Allow yourself lots of alone time each day so that you can figure things out.
    d. Do all of the above.

Get Critical

What happened

In December 2011, Facebook announced that it was partnering with the National Suicide Prevention Lifeline to help users in severe distress. The service has two components: users can click a link to have a live chat with a suicide prevention counselor, and users concerned about a friend can request that Facebook send a message encouraging the friend to click on the Lifeline link. In January 2013, Facebook stepped up its suicide prevention efforts by partnering with SAVE (Suicide Awareness Voices of Education) to study how people's social networking behaviors change as depression deepens and they become suicidal. Researchers could then use the data to help Facebook locate and reach out to people in distress before it's too late.

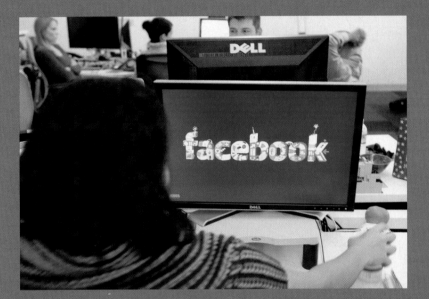

What do you think?

- Given that Facebook is a social media site, is its engagement in suicide prevention appropriate, or not?

- How do you feel about your user data being scanned for warning signs of suicide? Do you think it's an invasion of privacy or a public health service?

- What other steps could social media sites take to help people in distress—whether or not they're suicidal?

STRESS MANAGEMENT

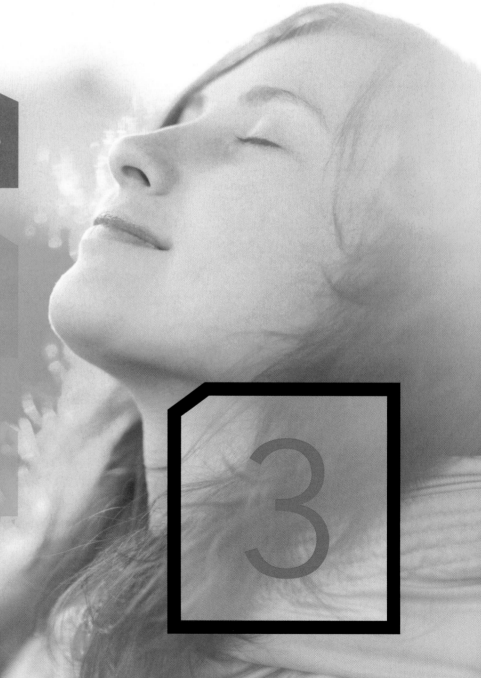

Year after year, college students report **stress** as the number-one **obstacle** to their academic achievement.[i]

Money is the greatest source of stress among adults aged 19-31 in general, and the second greatest **source of stress** (after academics) among college students.[i, ii]

Millennials (those aged 18–33) report some of the highest levels of stress in the United States.[ii]

3

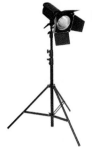

Science Discovers Stress

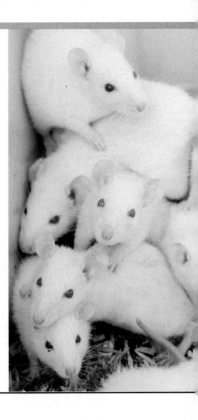

The science of stress studies began by accident. In the 1930s, Hans Selye, a young Hungarian-born endocrinologist, was immersed in a study of hormones at McGill University in Montreal. Selye injected lab rats with a variety of hormones and observed their responses. He found that regardless of which hormone he used, the rats all seemed to demonstrate the same basic physical reactions each time, including enlargement of the adrenal cortex; atrophy of the thymus, spleen, and lymph nodes; and stomach ulcers. This led Selye to wonder if he could be observing something broader than merely the rats' responses to specific hormone injections. Were the rats reacting to something more general—to some other "external pressure" he was applying?

Selye decided to find out, using the simplest and cheapest method he could find. He set the hormones aside, and looked for a different external pressure to apply to the rats. He found inspiration in the frigid weather outside the walls of his laboratory. He placed a group of rats in a box and left them outside on his windowsill overnight. The next morning, the unhappy rats reacted in much the same way as those that had previously been injected with hormones. The rats' overall behavior, Selye surmised, had much more to do with external pressures—introduced hormones, freezing weather—than any one specific substance or force. In short, the rats' response reflected *stress*.

- Tiny hairs stand on end all over your body, a reflection of your heightened state of alarm.
- Your *adrenal glands*, two small organs sitting on top of your kidneys, are stimulated to produce a chemical similar to noradrenaline, called *adrenaline*, which sustains the above reactions.

Within about 15 minutes, a second, hormonal, response begins. **Hormones** are chemicals released by glands into the bloodstream, which transports them to their target organs elsewhere in the body. When hormones reach their target, they act in a way that regulates its activity. Whereas nervous system responses are nearly instantaneous, hormonal responses require some "travel time." The second wave of the alarm phase begins when a region of your brain called the *hypothalamus* signals the nearby *pituitary gland* to release a hormone called ACTH. This travels through your bloodstream to the adrenal glands, where it stimulates the release of an important stress hormone called **cortisol**. The flood of cortisol further increases the amount of glucose in the bloodstream, allowing a sustained response to the threat. It also speeds up the breakdown of the body's nutrient compounds—carbohydrates, fats, and proteins. These actions ensure a supply of fuel to the muscles, should you need to run quickly to escape a real assailant.

Like homeostasis, this complex set of reactions was first described by Walter B. Cannon, who named it the **fight-or-flight response.** Cannon theorized that it evolved as a survival mechanism to help early humans fight an enemy or escape from a predator; probably our ancestors could not have survived in their dangerous "eat-or-be-eaten" world without it. Even today, your fight-or-flight response temporarily boosts your strength and stamina to enable you to fight off a would-be assailant or flee a smoke-filled building.

Despite its continued usefulness in our modern world, the fight-or-flight response can also be unhelpful or even harmful. Most of our day-to-day stressors are not the extreme physical threats that our ancestors faced. Yet a fight-or-flight response kicks in *any* time you face a stressor—even when that stressor is mostly emotional or psychological, such as frustration at being stuck behind a slow driver on the highway, or worry at finding yourself unprepared for mid-term exams. If you experience fight-or-flight reactions too often, or find yourself unable to resist them successfully, then in a sense you remain perpetually in the alarm phase. Such "high-alert" living can take a powerful toll on your body and your health.

>> Stress researcher Robert Sapolsky explains the evolutionary basis of the stress response and how it affects us today: www.youtube.com/watch?v=sPS7GnromGo.

hormone Chemical secreted by a gland and transported through the bloodstream to a distant target organ, the activity of which it then regulates.

cortisol Adrenal gland hormone that is secreted at higher levels during the stress response.

fight-or-flight response A series of physiological reactions to a stressor designed to enable the body to stand and fight or to flee.

Resistance Phase

As a stressor continues, the body mobilizes homeostatic mechanisms that make it more resistant to the stressor. For example, the first time you hike a strenuous trail, you're likely to experience significant physical distress. But if you were to hike that trail twice weekly, you'd soon adapt to its demands and it would no longer set off the alarm phase.

Even with stressors that aren't primarily physical, you can develop strategies that increase your level of resistance and help you adapt. For instance, if you're a college freshman, you might feel stress hormones pouring into your bloodstream as you sit down to take your first mid-term exam. But over time, repetition helps you perceive the situation as more familiar (and thus less like a "change").

Balancing School and Family

"HI, I'M DAVID. As a nontraditional student, some of the things that stress me out are maybe a little bit different than what other students go through. I own a house. I have to pay a mortgage, bills, and taxes. I have to put food on my kids' table, clothing on their backs, and spend time with my wife. These things really stress me out! And on top of all of that, I'm a full-time college student.

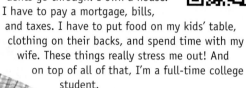

One of the ways that I balance being a family man and college student is to try to keep both worlds separate. I know that when I go to school, that's what I need to concentrate on. I try to do all my homework and everything else at school. And when I go home, I try to leave the school behind. Sometimes the two blend together, but that's a good thing, I think."

1. Identify at least three stressors that David is dealing with. Are these stressors caused by *eustress* or *distress*?

2. How well do you think David is managing his stress load? What negative health effects could he experience if he was unable to manage stress?

Moreover, you learn that, when you study thoroughly, you do well. Building this "track record" of success also helps calm your nerves. Finally, over time, you may learn a set of stretches, breathing techniques, or motivational phrases to keep you relaxed during exams. As a result of your growing familiarity with the situation, your confidence in your preparation, and your use of coping mechanisms, the jolt of stress you feel as you walk toward the exam room is likely to actually improve your performance by keeping you alert and focused. That's right: A little stress actually helps you do better.

This phenomenon was first identified in 1908 by psychologists Robert Yerkes and John Dodson. According to the Yerkes-Dodson law, performance improves with moderate physiological or mental arousal—which today we call stress. Similarly, in 1982, cardiologist Peter Nixon described a human function curve according to which a manageable degree of stress improves a performance . . . but too much stress leads to illness.[3]

Exhaustion Phase and Allostatic Overload

When the degree of stress is not manageable—when stressors are severe and persistent—the homeostatic mechanisms that formerly helped you adapt become depleted. Both Selye and Nixon recognized that, at this point, your body enters an

burnout Phenomenon in which increased feelings of stress and decreased feelings of accomplishment lead to frustration, exhaustion, lack of motivation, and disengagement.

allostatic overload The wear and tear the body experiences as the result of continuous or repeated demands of allostasis.

chronic stress syndrome Collection of symptoms resulting from the long-term effects of prolonged exposure to the body's physiological stress responses.

exhaustion phase and, as a result, you experience stress-related disease and **burnout.**

Recently, some researchers have introduced the term **allostatic overload** to describe the exhaustion phase. The prefix *allo-* means "variability," so an allostatic overload is a harmful state resulting from excessive change.[4] But whether we call it exhaustion or allostatic overload, the result of chronic, excessive stress is always a failure of homeostasis, which is inevitably manifested as disease.[5] If multiple commitments keep cutting into your time for study and sleep, your stress is likely to increase well beyond the point of optimal performance. If it stays elevated for long, you may experience burnout and illness. Scientists currently studying stress now believe that this overwhelmed feeling contributes to many of our major health concerns.[6]

Health Effects of Chronic Stress

Physical symptoms associated with stress include fatigue, lying awake at night, headache, upset stomach, muscle tension, change in sex drive, teeth grinding, dizziness, feeling a tightness in the chest, and change in menstrual cycle (for women). Psychological symptoms of stress include feeling angry, irritable, or overwhelmed.[7]

When your body maintains the fight-or-flight response for extended periods of time, **chronic stress syndrome** can develop. Chronic stress syndrome is a collection of symptoms resulting from the long-term effects of prolonged exposure to the body's physiological stress responses **(Figure 3.3)**. While the specific effects of chronic stress vary from person to person, they can ultimately affect nearly every system of the body.

Effects on the Cardiovascular System

The physical effects of stress touch all parts of your cardiovascular system, from the molecules that shape the health of your blood vessels to the rhythms and function of your heart. Stress, for example, appears to increase the risk of inflammation in blood vessel walls, triggering a cascade of problems that can lead to coronary artery disease.[8] The fight-or-flight response causes the heart to work harder and faster, raising blood pressure. Over time, high blood pressure can damage internal organs, greatly increasing the risk of a heart attack or stroke. Stress can also indirectly affect heart disease incidence by increasing the likelihood of its risk factors. For example, those under chronic stress may overeat and exercise less, thereby increasing their risk of obesity, and may be less likely to follow recommendations on living more healthfully.[9] Obesity increases cholesterol levels and diabetes risk, and both are leading risk factors for heart disease.

Effects on the Digestive System

When the fight-or-flight response constantly directs blood away from the stomach and intestines, the digestive system doesn't get the fuel it needs to do its job. This can result in stomachache, constipation, or diarrhea. Stress hormones can also affect the body's ability to regulate blood sugar levels, which may increase the risk of diabetes. You might be wondering whether or not stress can trigger the formation of ulcers. Check out the nearby **Myth or Fact?** box to find the answer.

Can Stress Give You an Ulcer?

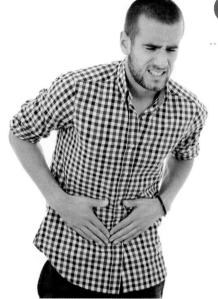

You've got a huge set of lab problems to solve for class, and you're way behind on getting it done. After a quick dinner of extremely cold, old pizza, you head for the library. Your stomach is killing you—again.

Yes, the pizza was kind of nasty. But you still can't help but wonder if all the pressure this term is giving you an ulcer.

Ulcers are lesions in the lining of the stomach or small intestine that can cause pain, bloating, and nausea. But though all the stress you face could indeed be making you feel terrible, it probably isn't directly causing an ulcer. Researchers have found that most ulcers are caused by bacteria called *Helicobacter pylori*. Those ulcers not triggered by bacterial infection are often due to the overuse of painkillers, such as aspirin or ibuprofen, or to alcohol abuse. Smokers also have an increased risk of ulcers, and their ulcers are especially resistant to healing.

Although researchers no longer believe that stress directly causes ulcers, studies have shown that chronic stress can increase stomach acid production, disrupt immune system activity, and make the symptoms of an ulcer worse. If you suffer from ongoing stomach pain, visit your campus health center or personal doctor.

References: **1.** "Peptic Ulcer: Causes," by the Mayo Clinic, 2009. Retrieved from http://www.mayoclinic.com/health/peptic-ulcer/DS00242/DSECTION?causes. **2.** "Peptic Ulcer," 2006, *Merck Manual.* Retrieved from http://www.merckmanuals.com/home/sec09/ch121/ch121c.html.

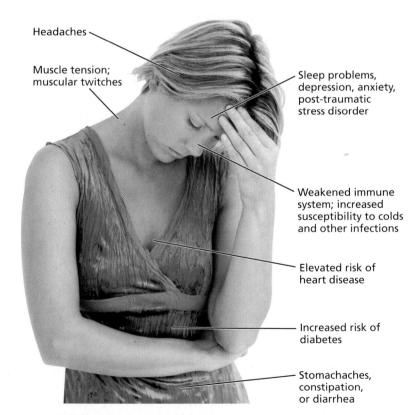

Headaches

Muscle tension; muscular twitches

Sleep problems, depression, anxiety, post-traumatic stress disorder

Weakened immune system; increased susceptibility to colds and other infections

Elevated risk of heart disease

Increased risk of diabetes

Stomachaches, constipation, or diarrhea

FIGURE 3.3 Health Effects of Long-Term Stress. Chronic stress can have long-term health effects, ranging from stomachaches to increased risk of disease.

Effects on Weight

Stress can reduce a person's appetite, or cause an upset stomach or other symptoms that discourage eating. But for many, stress can also induce a longing for sweets, chips, or other "comfort foods" high in calories. Both children and adults can gain weight if they try to cope with stress by overeating. Moreover, researchers have long acknowledged an "income–body weight gradient," in which economic stressors provoke metabolic changes that are associated with increased weight.[10]

In addition, both children and adults who are overweight or obese report that they experience more stress compared with people of normal weight.[11] A much greater percentage of obese adults (29%) than normal-weight adults (20%) report experiencing a very high degree of stress. Obese adults are also much more likely to report physical and emotional symptoms of stress, such as fatigue, irritability, anger, and sadness.[11]

> " *Both children and adults who are overweight or obese report that they experience more stress compared with people of normal weight.* "

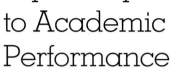

STUDENT STATS
Top 10 Impediments to Academic Performance

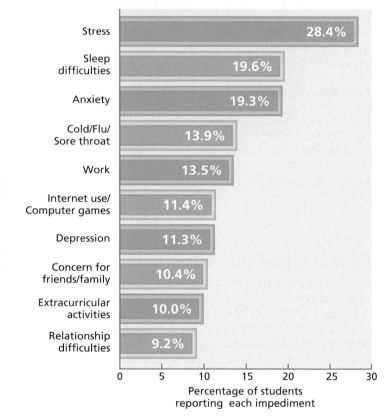

Stress — 28.4%
Sleep difficulties — 19.6%
Anxiety — 19.3%
Cold/Flu/Sore throat — 13.9%
Work — 13.5%
Internet use/Computer games — 11.4%
Depression — 11.3%
Concern for friends/family — 10.4%
Extracurricular activities — 10.0%
Relationship difficulties — 9.2%

Percentage of students reporting each impediment

Data from *American College Health Association National College Health Assessment (ACHA-NCHA II) Undergraduate Students Reference Group Executive Summary, Fall 2012,* by the American College Health Association, 2013, retrieved from http://www.acha-ncha.org/reports_ACHA-NCHAII.html.

In addition, the fear, tension, anxiety, or depression that accompany stress may also increase heart rate or blood pressure, which can compromise your immune system further. Some researchers theorize that chronic stress may suppress some body activities that require a lot of energy—such as the immune response—in order to conserve energy needed to counteract the loss of energy and other physiological resources due to stress.[13]

Even stress caused by relatively minor events such as academic exams can cause temporary increases in white blood cell counts, a sign that the immune system has been activated to ward off a threat.[14] Such demands on the immune system, if frequent, may leave you vulnerable to colds, trigger flare-ups of asthma or cold sores, and put you at risk of developing more serious diseases.

Effects on Sleep

Adequate sleep is essential to conserve body energy; grow, repair, and restore your body's cells and tissues; maintain your immune system; and organize and synthesize new learning and memories. Unfortunately, many college students are not experiencing the benefits of enough sleep: A national survey found that about 6% of college students had been diagnosed with insomnia or a sleep disorder in the past year, and 25% said they had experienced a serious sleep difficulty.[15] Although illness and disability, alcohol and other drug use, and many other factors can interfere with sleep, stress is one of the most common culprits.[16] In turn, not getting enough sleep increases the physical stress placed on your body. (You'll learn more about sleep and its many health benefits in the electronic Chapter 16.)

Effects on Relationships

Our connections with others play a complex role when it comes to the stress in our lives. As you probably know instinctively, and will learn about in more detail later in this chapter, supportive friendships and relationships are often essential in helping us cope with stress. But stress can damage relationships, as those under stress may have less patience or time to be involved and supportive, or appreciative of assistance. Chronic stress, for example, can be a threat to both the happiness and longevity of a marriage.[17] Other research has found that when someone in a marriage is under stress they cannot manage, the person's ability to adjust the daily pressures of a relationship falters, which in turn may lead to more stress.[18] Later in this chapter, you'll learn more about ways to manage stress so that you can shield your friendships and relationships from its corrosive effects.

Effects on the Immune System

Do you always seem to get sick during finals week? At the end of the term, a quarter or semester's worth of stress may weaken your body's ability to fight off viruses and other infections.

Psychoneuroimmunology is the study of interactions among psychological processes, the nervous system, hormones, and the immune system.[12] When acute stress activates the fight-or-flight response, your body releases cortisol and other stress hormones. In the short term, these hormones enable you to effectively respond to stressors and may actually strengthen your immune system. However, long-term overproduction of these hormones due to chronic stressors can suppress the immune system, reducing your ability to fight off infection.[13] Long-term exposure to cortisol can cause immune cells to decrease, promote weight gain, lead to the breakdown of muscle, increase fluid retention, and decrease inflammatory response.

Effects on Mood, Mind, and Mental Health

Chronic stress is an important risk factor for many mental health problems. Stress contributes to the development of depression, panic attacks, anxiety disorders, eating disorders, and post-traumatic stress disorder (PTSD). Unfortunately, stress and these mental health problems often form a vicious cycle where one feeds the other, complicating treatment. People experiencing severe long-term stress may develop depression, for example, only to have their condition create more stress in their lives.[19]

Anxiety is a normal response to stressful situations; however, stress itself may also contribute to the development

psychoneuroimmunology The study of the interactions among psychological processes, the nervous system, hormones, and the immune system.

of anxiety disorders. For example, some researchers theorize that an inappropriate activation of the fight-or-flight response may at least partly explain the experience of a panic attack, a sudden episode of intense fear.[20] In addition, post-traumatic stress disorder (PTSD) can develop when people are exposed to very traumatic forms of stress, such as violence, deadly natural disasters, or combat. Unfortunately, stress and these psychological health challenges can form a vicious cycle in which one feeds the other, complicating treatment. (For more information on psychological health, see Chapter 2.)

As a college student, you're bound to feel some degree of stress. So how do you know whether a few signs and symptoms you might be experiencing are normal—or increase your risk for illness? Check out the nearby **Practical Strategies: Recognizing the Signs of Stress Overload.**

What Influences Our Stress Response?

We said earlier that our perception influences whether or not we experience an event as a stressor. But even two people who perceive the same stressor can have very different responses to it. Why is that the case? Stress researchers believe that personality, sociocultural factors, and past experiences all play a role in how we perceive and respond to stress.

The Role of Personality Types

A **personality type** is a set of behavioral tendencies. For instance, if you tend to analyze situations, someone might refer to you as a left-brain type, as opposed to a right-brain type who leaps to creative solutions. Although many researchers see such distinctions as too broad to help us make predictions about the behavior of individual human beings, they may be useful in helping us to explore aspects of the stress response.

In 1959, cardiologists Meyer Friedman and Ray Rosenman identified a relationship between heart disease and what they referred to as *type A* behavior.[21] Friedman identified three basic characteristics of the type A personality:[22]

- The person is impatient, almost chronically irritated and exasperated, and has a low tolerance for mistakes, whether his or her own or those of others.

- The person exhibits a free-floating hostility; that is, almost anything can provoke a hostile response.

- The person has low self-esteem. Those who interact with the person are not likely to observe this directly; however, the person's competitive, achievement-oriented behavior may be an outward attempt to compensate for low self-esteem.

> **personality type** A set of behavioral tendencies.

In contrast, people with a *type B* personality are typically characterized as patient, tolerant, and friendly, with a realistic sense of self-esteem that may even manifest as humility. These people are thought to have a lower risk of disorders related to stress.

Recently, some researchers have posited the existence of two additional personality types: *Type C* people are said to be stoical

Practical Strategies

Recognizing the Signs of Stress Overload

It's important to be able to recognize the warning signs of too much stress before they add up to a serious health problem. While many people find the following symptoms common, keep in mind that stress affects different individuals in different ways. You may have less-typical signs of stress, but they still merit the same attention.

Emotional warning signs

- Anxiety
- Sleep disruption
- Anger and agitation
- Trouble concentrating
- Unproductive worry
- Frequent mood swings
- Depression

Physical warning signs

- Stooped posture
- Sweaty palms
- Chronic fatigue
- Weight loss or weight gain
- Migraine or tension headaches
- Neck aches

- Digestive problems
- Asthma attacks
- Physical symptoms that your doctor can't attribute to another condition

Behavioral warning signs

- Overreacting to problems or difficult situations
- Increased use of alcohol, tobacco, or drugs
- Unusually impulsive behavior
- Withdrawing from relationships or contact with others
- Feeling "burned out" on school or work
- Frequent bouts of crying
- Feelings of anxiety or panic

If you are experiencing the warning signs of stress overload, be proactive and seek the solutions that are right for you. Use the stress management techniques outlined in this chapter to help you manage your stress load. Also, consult your college health center, which may offer classes, workshops, or individual and group counseling to further help you cope with stress.

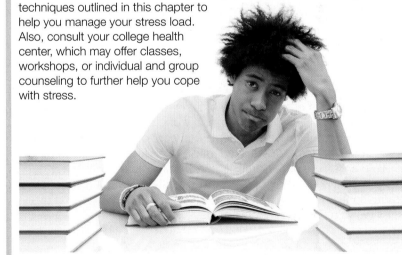

and internalize stress; therefore, they are thought to be at increased risk for immune disorders, including cancer.[23] *Type D* people are described as responding to stressful situations either with resignation or withdrawal, whether from a job or from academic pursuits.[24]

In thinking about these various personality types, it's important to recognize that there is a great deal of debate among researchers as to whether or not they have any real validity. Although they may be useful in theory, they cannot explain the complexity of human personality or behavior, or fully capture how each of us responds to stress over the course of our lives.

The Role of Personality Traits

Some stress researchers have linked certain personality traits to an improved ability to adapt to stress. Primary among these are optimism, hardiness, and resiliency.[25]

- **Optimism.** People who are optimistic are more likely to see stressors as transient and specific, and therefore within their power to change and control. At the same time, they are less likely to view stressors as a consequence of internal faults. (For more on optimism, see Chapter 2.)
- **Hardiness.** Social psychologist Suzanne Kobasa identified a quality she called *hardiness* as important in enabling a person to successfully navigate the resistance phase of stress.[26] Hardiness is an ability to respond to the challenges of life and turn them into opportunities for growth. It includes three dimensions: commitment to relationships and ideals, self-efficacy (belief in your ability to change things) and internal locus of control (belief that you are capable of taking action to improve a stressful situation), and a positive attitude toward change.[26]
- **Resiliency.** Resiliency is an ability to experience success and satisfaction following trauma or other stressors. Resilient people are typically both optimistic and hardy, with an internal locus of control.[25] From an evolutionary perspective, resiliency is an innate capacity to adapt to changes in the environment, and thus to survive.

Although personality traits might seem fixed, by examining your thought patterns and behaviors, you can foster in yourself optimism, hardiness, and resiliency.

Common Causes of Stress

You have assignments to complete, tests to take, and papers to write. You may be juggling school and work, or facing loans and credit card debt. First-year students and sophomores, newer to the pressures of undergraduate academics, often face more schoolwork stress than juniors or seniors.[27] Meanwhile, seniors close to getting their diploma need to grapple with the question of what to do after graduation.

As we've mentioned, any event that triggers your stress response is called a *stressor*. In today's world, many stressors are psychological, emotional, or biological. Some stressors come and go fairly quickly, such as getting called on in class or taking a big exam. Others may have effects that linger much longer, such as a bad breakup or the death of someone you love.

Financial Stressors

The economy is in a slump. Perhaps one or both of your parents are out of a job, and you are starting to worry about how you will pay for tuition next term—not to mention your student loans after you graduate. Maybe you already have credit card debt. Almost everyone must deal with some form of financial stress in their lifetime. **Practical Strategies: Coping with Financial Stress** provides some tips for relieving money-related stress.

Daily Hassles

The school registration office says they can't find the check you sent to cover your tuition this term, even though your bank says the check has been cashed. You've completely gone over your limit of cell phone minutes for the month, and you can't find the research material you need for a class paper because your Internet connection has crashed. These problems may sound small, but daily hassles can add up to a significant source of stress. Complete the **Self-Assessment** on page 58 to rate daily hassles often encountered by college students and gauge the stress load in your own life.

Academic Pressure

College represents a great opportunity—and a big responsibility. To graduate, get good internships, and land a fantastic job, you need to perform. As a student, you probably worry about doing well in school. But studies have shown that too much anxiety about grades, exams, papers, and deadlines can actually prevent you from being successful in college.[28]

Job-Related Stressors

Show up to work on time, excel at your job to get that raise—and try not to think about all the school assignments you have hanging over your head at the same time! Many college students work to ease the financial pressure of school, but earning money brings stress of its own when it cuts into your time for classwork.

Social Stressors

Friends, relationships, and the opinions of others all carry the potential to trigger or reduce stress. Strong, supportive social networks can do a great deal to help carry you through tough times. Researchers have discovered, for instance, that the perceived emotional support college students experience using a social networking site like Facebook can lower their stress levels.[29] In another study, college students in committed romantic relationships were found to experience fewer mental health problems.[30] Social interactions that aren't supportive, on the other hand, increase stress. A national survey of college students found that about 18% reported interpersonal stresses significant enough to affect their academic performance, including relationship difficulties (9.2%), roommate difficulties (4.9%), and homesickness (3.7%).[15]

Different social groups can perceive or experience stress in varying ways. Members of minority groups may perceive discrimination or isolation as sources of stress on campuses.[31] Men, women, and members of different demographic groups feel the stress in their lives differently, as examined in the box **Diversity & Health: Stress Through the Lenses of Gender, Age, and Geography** on page 60.

Practical Strategies

Coping with Financial Stress

Even during the best of financial times, money is usually among the top five stressors reported by students. Financial concerns become even more of a stressor as parents lose jobs or as student work becomes less available and scholarship and loan dollars dry up.

Following are some strategies for coping with financial stress:

- Get a realistic handle on your finances. How much money do you have coming in from your parents, your job, and/or financial aid? How much money does it take to pay your rent, groceries, books and tuition, clothing, transportation, entertainment, and other day-to-day expenses? Try a (free) online budget tracker, such as the ones listed in the **Get Connected** section on page 68, which makes it easy for you to input information and identify where in your budget you can cut back.

- If you are carrying any credit card debt, develop a plan for paying it off. Reserve a set amount of money each month for paying off debt, and *stick to it*. You will feel less stress just by having a plan in place, versus doing nothing and watching your debt mount.

- If you've been completely reliant on your parents for financial support, consider taking on a part-time job—no matter how small. If there are no jobs to be found, get entrepreneurial! Consider your skills and advertise your services—for example, tutoring, babysitting, lawn mowing, car washing, general repairs, moving, housecleaning—you get the picture.

- Take an honest look at your current lifestyle. Do you pay for cable/premium TV or a cell phone plus a land line? How much money do you spend each month on eating out, expensive coffee drinks, or designer clothing? Distinguish luxuries from true necessities and *pare back*. Cancel any subscriptions or services you don't really need. Use public transportation instead of paying for gas and parking. Cut back on the number of times you eat out each month. You'd be surprised at how all of the "little things" can add up to quite a sizeable chunk of change.

- Talk to a financial aid advisor to make sure you've explored all the aid options available to you. Know exactly how much money you will need to pay off when you graduate. Only take on loans that you feel certain you will be able to pay back.

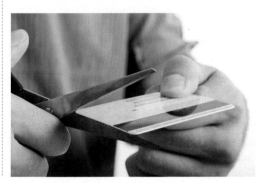

Major Life Events

Traumas such as a bad breakup or a death in the family are obvious stressors. But positive, exhilarating events such as starting college, graduating, or getting married can also bring heavy doses of stress. In 1967, psychiatrists Thomas Holmes and Richard Rahe published what has come to be known as Holmes and Rahe's Social Readjustment Rating Scale (SRRS), an inventory of 43 stressful life events that can increase the risk of illness.[32] The scale assigns "life change units" from 1 to 100 for each stressful event, such as the death of a spouse (100 units), divorce (73 units), imprisonment (63 units), death of a close family member (63 units), personal injury or illness (53 units), marriage (50 units), and job loss (47 units). The scale also includes more minor stressors, such as Christmas (12 units), a change in sleeping habits (16 units), and a change in living conditions (25 units). According to this scale, the higher the number of "life change units" that a person accumulates over a given year, the greater that person's risk of illness.

Environmental Stressors

Environmental stressors are factors in your living or working environments that you find disruptive. Examples of environmental stressors include poor air quality, pollution, noise, toxic chemicals, and severe weather—as well as living in an unsafe neighborhood, having an annoying roommate, and dealing with a long commute. Digital technologies (such as cell phones) that beep to alert you to text messages or voicemails can also be a source of environmental stress.

> " *Digital technologies (such as cell phones) that beep to alert you to text messages or voicemails can also be a source of environmental stress.*"

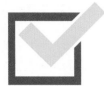

SELF-ASSESSMENT
Negative Event Scale for University Students

Below is a list of items that can be negative events. **Please remember that it is important that you** circle one number for **each item even if there was no hassle** and consider each item with **only the last month in mind**

How much of a *hassle* was this negative event?

0 = Did not occur

1 = Event occurred but there was no hassle

2 = Event occurred and was a little bit of a hassle

3 = Event occurred and was somewhat of a hassle

4 = Event occurred and was a lot of a hassle

5 = Event occurred and was an extreme hassle

In the last month:

Problems with Friends

1. Negative feedback from your friend/s	0	1	2	3	4	5
2. Negative communication with friend/s	0	1	2	3	4	5
3. Conflict with friend/s	0	1	2	3	4	5
4. Disagreement with friend/s	0	1	2	3	4	5

Problems with Your Spouse/Partner (Boy/Girl Friend)

5. Negative communication with your spouse/partner (boy/girl friend)	0	1	2	3	4	5
6. Conflict with spouse/partner (boy/girl friend)	0	1	2	3	4	5
7. Disagreement with spouse/partner (boy/girl friend)	0	1	2	3	4	5
8. Rejection by your spouse/partner (boy/girl friend)	0	1	2	3	4	5
9. Your spouse/partner (boy/girl friend) let you down	0	1	2	3	4	5

Work Problems

10. The nature of your job/work (if employed)	0	1	2	3	4	5
11. Your work load	0	1	2	3	4	5
12. Meeting deadlines or goals on the job	0	1	2	3	4	5
13. Use of your skills at work	0	1	2	3	4	5

Money Problems

14. Not enough money for necessities (e.g., food, clothing, housing, health care, taxes, insurance, etc.)	0	1	2	3	4	5
15. Not enough money for education	0	1	2	3	4	5
16. Not enough money for emergencies	0	1	2	3	4	5
17. Not enough money for extras (e.g., entertainment, recreation, vacations, etc.)	0	1	2	3	4	5

Problems with Children

18. Negative communication with your child(ren)	0	1	2	3	4	5
19. Conflict with your child(ren)	0	1	2	3	4	5
20. Disagreement with your child(ren)	0	1	2	3	4	5

School Problems

21. Your study load	0	1	2	3	4	5
22. Study/course deadlines	0	1	2	3	4	5

23. Time pressures	0	1	2	3	4	5
24. Problems getting assignments/essays finished	0	1	2	3	4	5

Problems with Teachers/Lecturers

25. Negative communication with teacher/s, lecturer/s	0	1	2	3	4	5
26. Negative feedback from teacher/s, lecturer/s	0	1	2	3	4	5
27. Conflict with teacher/s, lecturer/s	0	1	2	3	4	5
28. Disagreement with your teacher/s, lecturer/s	0	1	2	3	4	5

Problems with Other Students

29. Negative communication with other student/s	0	1	2	3	4	5
30. Conflict with other student/s	0	1	2	3	4	5
31. Disagreement with other student/s	0	1	2	3	4	5
32. Doing things with other student/s	0	1	2	3	4	5

Problems with Relatives

33. Negative communication with relative/s	0	1	2	3	4	5
34. Conflict with relative/s	0	1	2	3	4	5
35. Disagreement with relative/s	0	1	2	3	4	5
36. Doing things with relative/s	0	1	2	3	4	5

Health Problems

37. Your health	0	1	2	3	4	5
38. Your physical abilities	0	1	2	3	4	5
39. Your medical care	0	1	2	3	4	5
40. Getting sick (e.g., flu, colds)	0	1	2	3	4	5

Problems with Your Work Supervisor/Employer

41. Negative feedback from your supervisor/employer	0	1	2	3	4	5
42. Negative communication with your supervisor/employer	0	1	2	3	4	5
43. Conflict with your supervisor/employer	0	1	2	3	4	5
44. Disagreement with your supervisor/employer	0	1	2	3	4	5

Hassles Getting a Job

45. Finding a job (e.g., interviews, placements)	0	1	2	3	4	5
46. Finding work	0	1	2	3	4	5
47. Problems with finding a job	0	1	2	3	4	5
48. Employment problems (e.g., finding, losing a job)	0	1	2	3	4	5

Academic Limitations

49. Not getting the marks (results) you expected	0	1	2	3	4	5
50. Your academic ability not as good as you thought	0	1	2	3	4	5
51. Not understanding some subjects	0	1	2	3	4	5

School Interest

52. Courses not relevant to your future career	0	1	2	3	4	5
53. Your courses are boring	0	1	2	3	4	5

HOW TO INTERPRET YOUR SCORE

Any negative events for which you score a 4 or 5 would be considered significant stressors. You can use the **Choosing to Change Worksheet** at the end of the chapter to help you modify your perceptions of these stressors and reduce the amount of hassle you feel.

To complete this Self-Assessment online, visit MasteringHealth™.

Source: "Negative Event Scale" by Dr. Darryl Maybery, Monash University, Melbourne, Australia. Reprinted with permission.

Internal Stressors

Worries, critical thoughts, and the demands we place on ourselves represent some of our most constant stressors. One study of university honors students, for example, found that those highly critical of themselves were more prone to feelings of stress, depression, and hopelessness.[33]

In an era where fewer of our stressors are physical, we assign increasing value to psychological or emotional stressors, and our bodies' stress response kicks in accordingly.[34] Do you find yourself overreacting to small problems? Do you view every task as critical when many of them really aren't? Are you often imagining horrific consequences for your actions that will probably, in reality, never come to pass? Do you procrastinate? These are all examples of situations you have the power to control or minimize, and thereby reduce your stress level.

Getting Help for Managing Stress

Sometimes we face stress that feels truly overwhelming. If you find yourself having trouble managing stress on your own, trained professionals can help.

- **Consider counseling.** Talking with a mental health professional, in either a group therapy or an individual setting, can help you manage the stressors in your life and reframe how you confront them. Talk to a health professional at your student health center about free or low-cost group and individual counseling.

- **Talk with a doctor.** If you are experiencing a serious stress-related condition such as depression or severe anxiety, a doctor may recommend prescription medication to help you get your symptoms under control. A recent report shows that people who do not receive stress or behavioral management help from a health-care provider are more likely to say their stress increased in the past year than those who do get help.[7]

- **Use caution with alternative remedies.** Many herbal supplement and vitamin companies sell products that promise to reduce stress or ease its symptoms. Before you try any of these products, however, talk to a health professional and ask whether these supplements have proven benefits, side effects, or dangers. Some supplements can mix badly with other medications you may be taking, so be sure to also ask about possible drug interactions before taking any supplement.

 View videos of stress management techniques at http://health .howstuffworks.com/wellness/stress-management.

Change Yourself, Change Your World

Stress doesn't have to escalate beyond your control. There's a lot you can do to relax, step back from stressful situations, and face your challenges with renewed energy and confidence. Some of these techniques involve making changes to your lifestyle and cultivating habits that strengthen your resilience and energy. Others give you ways to reframe situations in your mind, gain perspective about your stressors, and switch off your internal alarms. You can also get to work changing stressors that you or other students might face on your campus.

Personal Choices

With a few changes, your life on campus can be more fun, and less stressful. You can't expect to eliminate stress overnight. But by altering

Handling School Stress

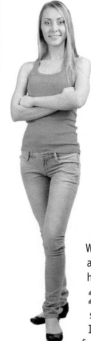

"HI, I'M JESSICA. The biggest source of stress in my life would probably be school and just the pressure to succeed in the future. My family doesn't really put pressure on me but I think I put a lot of pressure on myself, just based on the economy and based on the amount of money I feel I need to make to give myself a good future.

To minimize stress, exercise really is important to me. I don't do it as often as I would like but the days I do it, it does make me feel a lot better. I, unfortunately, relieve stress in other ways like drinking, like a lot of college students do. Not in any dangerous sense or any excess, maybe once a week at most. And, you know, I stress in typical other ways like crying, too."

1. Jessica uses several methods to manage stress. Which are more healthy and which are less so? What advice would you give Jessica about how to handle her stress?

2. Jessica mentions the economy as a source of stress. Does the economy affect your stress levels? If so, what can you do to address that now and in the future? Do you track your spending? How much of what you spend money on are true essentials (versus luxuries)?

---

your daily routine, giving yourself opportunities to relax, and thinking about stress in useful ways, you can reduce and better manage the stressors in your life.

Manage Your Time Effectively

For many students, a 24-hour day seems about 10 hours too short. You may feel like you can't cram your classes, studying, assignments, job, friends, significant others, hobbies, physical activity, chores, and even basic survival needs (remember eating and sleeping?) into a typical day. If this describes you, take heart. Better time management can result in better stress management. The **Choosing to Change Worksheet** at the end of this chapter offers one way to evaluate where your time goes. The following are additional strategies you can employ for better time management:

- **Plan, even just a little.** Use a daily scheduler or planner to remind you of big events and track your to-do list. Even a simple paper-based scheduler can keep important tasks from sneaking up on you.

- **Stay prepared.** When you find out the dates of big assignments and tests at the start of the term, make note of them in your planner so you can prepare ahead of time. Read assignments before class, and review your class notes shortly after class ends. Both strategies will help you get more out of class, and make big study sessions a lot easier.

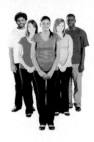

DIVERSITY & HEALTH

Stress Through the Lenses of Gender, Age, and Geography

In 2013, the American Psychological Association released a broad national survey of how Americans perceived the stress in their lives. Among the survey's findings:

Stress

- Stress levels for Americans remain high. Twenty percent of respondents rated their stress levels as an 8, 9, or 10 on a 10-point scale. Thirty-five percent of Americans said their stress had increased in the past year.

Gender

- As in previous surveys, women reported higher levels of stress than men did.
- Thirty-nine percent of men reported doing an excellent or very good job at managing stress, while 34% of women reported the same success. Over the years, men are increasingly reporting that they are doing an excellent or very good job at managing stress.
- Exercise and listening to music are the top two stress management techniques for both men and women, but women are more likely to engage in social or sedentary activities to manage stress, such as reading, spending time with friends or family, shopping, or eating.

Age

- Millennials (those aged 18–33) and Gen Xers (aged 34–47) report the highest levels of stress of all age groups (an average of 5.4 on a 10-point scale for both groups). These groups are also the most likely to report that they engage in unhealthy behaviors because of stress and experience symptoms of stress.
- Growing older appears to mean growing wiser when it comes to managing stress. The percentage of people in each age group who report that they are doing an excellent or very good job of managing their stress increases with age. Millennials: 29%, Gen Xers: 35%, Boomers (aged 48–66): 38%, Matures (aged 67 and older): 50%.
- Boomers and Matures are more likely to go to religious services than are younger generations, while Millennials and Gen Xers are more likely to shop.

Geography

- Americans living in the eastern United States reported the highest levels of stress; however, they also consider a higher level of stress to be healthy compared with people in other parts of the country. Since last year, many more Easterners are placing higher importance on healthy lifestyles for managing stress, although many aren't achieving their healthy living goals.
- Americans in the Midwest report some of the lowest levels of stress in the country, on average. The majority of Midwesterners also say they are doing enough to manage their stress. And fewer Midwesterners report engaging in unhealthy behaviors due to stress.
- Americans in the South report some of the lowest average levels of stress in the country but they report more difficulty in managing their stress in healthy ways. People in the South are less likely to exercise or walk to help manage stress and are more likely to eat to manage stress.
- Adults in the West report the second highest average stress levels in the United States. However, many people in the West believe they are doing enough to manage their stress and are most likely to engage in healthy activities to manage stress.

Critical-Thinking Questions

1. Think about your three closest male friends. What are their major sources of stress, and how do they cope? Then do the same for your three closest female friends. Are the sources of stress and coping mechanisms different for each group? If so, how?

2. What are some of the risks of sedentary stress management techniques? Do you reach for the TV remote, game console, or go online when you are stressed? What is a more active option you could try instead?

3. What are some of the prime stressors on your campus or in your community? Do you see individuals or organizations coming up with effective coping strategies for these local sources of stress? If not, what is one that you'd suggest?

>> **View the results of the complete Stress in America survey at** www.apa.org/news/press/releases/stress/index.aspx.

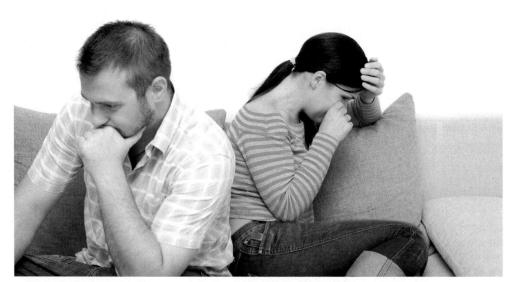

Women, in general, report higher levels of stress than men.

Source: Data from *Stress in America: Missing the Health Care Connection*, by the American Psychological Association, 2013.

- **Break down big jobs.** Remember that a forest consists of individual trees. When a task feels overwhelming, write down all the steps required to get it done, and then tackle them one at a time.
- **Hate it? Do it first.** If you can get the task you like the least out of the way, everything that follows will feel much easier.
- **Leave time for surprises.** Your car breaks down, and you need a couple of hours to get it to the shop, for example. If every hour of your schedule is always booked, you won't have room to deal with the unexpected turns life takes.
- **Reward yourself.** Been wrestling with a challenging assignment for an hour? Take a break. Finish a paper early for a change? Let your laundry slide, and watch a movie. And leave time in your schedule to relax. If you are working hard in college, you've more than earned a reward.

Get Adequate, Restful Sleep

As we discussed earlier, sleep is a naturally restorative process that is essential for healthy physical and psychological functioning—and reducing your body's stress. (For information on how to get a better night's sleep, see electronic Chapter 16.)

Live a Healthier Lifestyle

You can go a long way toward reducing your stress level by practicing the following basic wellness habits:

- **Eat well.** Food and stress have a reciprocal relationship. On the one hand, a nutritious diet allows your body to function smoothly and helps keep your stress responses in balance. On the other hand, chronic stress can lead to unhealthful eating habits.
- **Exercise.** Exercise, especially activities such as walking, cycling, weight training, or running that work your large muscles and build sustained strength, is an effective stress-reducer.[35] Scientists theorize that physical activity allows the body to complete the fight-or-flight response by actually doing what it has been prepared to do. After all, whether you are running around a track or running from a bear, you are still "fleeing" and thereby helping your body return to balance. As little as 20 minutes a day can help.[36] Moreover, even one exercise session can generate post-exercise euphoria that can last anywhere from 90 to 120 minutes.[35] For tips on exercising for stress management, see the **Practical Strategies** box on page 62.
- **Avoid caffeine, alcohol, tobacco, or other drugs.** People under stress may turn to caffeine to help them keep going, but too much caffeine can cause sleep problems and add to the physiological effects of stress.[37] Likewise, drinking, smoking, and recreational drugs can seem to offer a brief vacation from stress. But numerous studies have shown that the long-term health risks of smoking, drugs, or excess drinking far outweigh the few moments of relief they offer. If you find yourself drawn to potentially addictive substances to relieve stress, seek help from your doctor or from a health professional at your student health center.
- **Take time for hobbies and leisure.** It probably feels like you have no time at all right now for hiking, dance class, mountain biking, scrapbooking, or helping design T-shirts for friends' bands. But even small amounts of time spent away from school and work will reduce your stress and give you new energy to face the main tasks at hand. Breaks can also improve learning, giving you time to consider the material you've been studying in new ways.

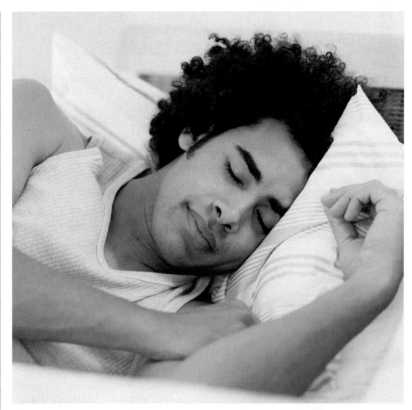

Sleep can refresh and revive you, and help you feel less stressed.

- **Keep a journal.** Make time to record what's going on in your life and how you feel about it. If you don't feel like toting around a traditional diary, online blogs and personal web pages (with privacy controls) are also good ways to keep a journal.

Ask for Help

Ask your professors for help. Find out their office hours and visit them in person to get help on material you don't understand, or to voice your concerns. They might be able to offer you helpful advice about how to approach assignments or prepare for exams. If your stress should start to feel overwhelming, make an appointment at your campus health center to speak to a counselor.

Call your family and make time for your friends, especially old friends from high school who may now be far away. They know you well, and can help you keep the stress in your life in perspective. At the same time, building a new network of college friends through your dorm life or social clubs will let you find and give support in a group that knows the pressures you face firsthand.

Communicate your feelings. For instance, let your roommates know that you have a big test in the morning and need them to wear headphones when the TV is on. Talk with supportive friends and family about the pressures you face and how they can help you cope.

Improve Your Test-Taking Skills

The following steps can help get you ready for success *before* your next test.

- **Learn test-taking skills.** Many colleges offer courses on test-taking skills. Sign up for one!

Practical Strategies

Exercising for Stress Management

Having trouble getting moving? Consider the following tips:

- Think of exercise as "recess"— not as a chore, but as a chance to break up an otherwise routine day with a fun, active, recreational activity.
- Vary your exercise activity. You might go swimming one day and bicycling another day. This way, you will have more options to choose from depending on your mood on any given day.
- Pick activities you genuinely enjoy. If you hate jogging but love to dance, by all means, dance!
- Remember that any activity that gets your body moving can ease stress. If you're not into sports, consider walking around campus just for fun, walking your dog, or

even walking in a shopping center. Any physical activity is better than none!

- Consider exercise classes such as yoga or tai chi that focus on breathing and relaxation.
- Enlist a friend as an exercise partner. You can keep each other encouraged and have more fun while you exercise.
- Make exercise a regular part of your schedule. Prioritize it the same way you would prioritize your schoolwork or a job.
- Exercise releases endorphins in the body, which makes you feel good. So the next time you find yourself resisting the thought of getting up and moving, remind yourself of how great you will feel afterward!

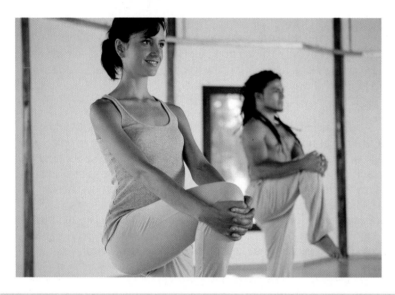

- **Learn about the test ahead of time.** Find out what topics the test will cover and what format it will be in. If your instructor provides practice tests or preparation materials, use them.
- **Schedule your study time.** Study over a series of days or weeks; avoid cramming at the last minute or pulling an "all nighter."
- **Talk with your instructor.** Tell your instructor in advance if you experience test anxiety. He or she may be able to offer suggestions or help.

- **Prepare yourself mentally.** Think positively. In the days leading up to the test, visualize yourself calmly taking the test and knowing the answers.
- **Prepare yourself physically.** Get enough sleep the night before.

When test day arrives, get up early so that you avoid having to rush. Before the test, eat a light meal so you are not hungry. Once you're in the testing room, choose a seat in a place that seems comfortable for you—for instance, near a window so you can get some fresh air, or away from a classmate whose mannerisms you find distracting. During the test, follow these strategies:

- **Read the directions carefully.**
- **Answer the easy questions first.** This will give you confidence and allow you to budget your remaining time on the more difficult questions.
- **If you get stuck, move on.** You can turn back to the question later.
- **Stay calm.** If you find yourself getting anxious: (1) Relax. Remind yourself that you are in control and are well-prepared for this test. (2) Take slow, deep breaths. (3) Concentrate on the questions, not on your fear. (4) Remind yourself that some anxiety is natural.
- **Even if you don't know the final answer, show your work.** Graders may give you partial credit.
- **Don't be alarmed if others turn in their tests before you.** They might have left several questions unanswered. Use all the time you need.
- **When you have finished, check your work.** However, do not second-guess yourself or change an answer unless you have remembered more-accurate information.

What if you've finished the test, and then start to stress out about your grade? Try these three post-test strategies:

- **Focus on the positive.** Think about all the things you did right either before or during the test.
- **Evaluate your test preparation.** Which strategies were helpful and which were not? Did you neglect anything? For instance, perhaps you were distracted because your mouth was dry during the test, and wished you had brought a bottle of water or some mints.
- **Develop a plan for your next test.** Base your new plan on what worked and didn't work for this test.

Loosen Tight Muscles

For centuries, people have practiced a variety of techniques to stretch and relax tense or tired muscles. These include the following:

- **Progressive muscle relaxation (PMR).** This technique helps you relax each major muscle group in your body, one by one, adding up to a powerful reduction in physical tension. Start by choosing one part of your body, such as your left foot. Inhale as you flex and tense it. Then exhale as you relax it. Repeat this once or twice. Then move on to your left leg and repeat the same process. Slowly move through all the major muscle groups of your body, deliberately tensing and relaxing each one, until your whole body relaxes.
- **Yoga.** Fundamental to the ancient Indian healing system called *ayurveda*, yoga is a mind–body practice that includes three main components: physical postures and stretches, breathing techniques, and quiet contemplation. There is growing evidence to suggest that yoga not only relaxes your muscles, but also enhances stress-coping mechanisms and improves the individual's mood and sense of well-being.[38]

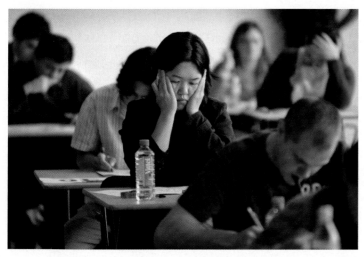

Stress less when preparing for and taking exams.

- **Massage.** A professional massage therapist uses pressure, stretching, friction, heat, cold, and other forms of manipulation to stimulate skin and muscles and relieve tension. Some studies have shown that massage can be helpful in reducing anxiety, decreasing pain, relieving sports-related soreness, and boosting the immune system.[39] Check with your campus wellness center to see if it offers reduced-price massages on campus.

>> This university website offers information about various mind and body relaxation techniques: www.uhs.uga.edu/stress/relax.html.

Explore Other Tension Relievers

Finally, there are three simple, low-cost techniques you can do almost anywhere to bust your stress.

Breathe Deeply. Research suggests that the following breathing exercise can reduce stress:[40]

- Take a slow, deep breath, drawing the breath in through the nose with your mouth closed, and then exhaling through the mouth. Inhaling and exhaling should take about 6 seconds each.
- Rest one hand gently on your abdomen and continue drawing long, slow, deep breaths.
- Notice that, while you are breathing deeply, your chest wall expands and contracts. At the same time, your hand on your upper abdomen should move outward—away from your core—as your chest fills with air, and back in again as you empty your lungs.
- Throughout this exercise, your shoulders should remain stationary. Rising and falling shoulders mean your breathing is high and shallow. If this is happening, just focus on expanding your rib cage outward with each inspiration, and feeling it relax back inward with each exhalation.
- Once you've achieved a slow, steady breathing rate, continue this exercise for several minutes.

Listen to Music. Taking a break can be as close as your MP3 player. Music therapy has been used in clinical settings for many years to control acute and chronic pain, relax tense muscles, reduce fatigue, relieve depression, and increase feelings of comfort.[41] It does this in part by

helping to induce the body's relaxation response—but not all music has the desired effect. When selecting music for relaxation, volume, speed, and style are all important. In one study, college students overwhelmingly preferred low-volume music over medium or loud music for relaxation, and researchers also noted that a soft volume was more effective at reducing heart rate.[42] Another study showed that slow, classical music can be effective at lowering blood pressure after a stressful situation.[43] This effect has also been shown for other types of soothing music, from gentle Celtic music to Indian ragas. In contrast, lively music speeds up heart and breathing rates, and can distract you. So make yourself a relaxation playlist, and listen to it regularly—it doesn't count if you merely put on headphones while cramming for a test.

>> This slideshow provides ideas for stress relief: http://fit.webmd.com/teen/recharge/slideshow/slideshow-teen-relax.

Change Your Thinking

Changing the way you think about the stressors in your life can help hold stress at bay. To keep your everyday stressors from turning into mountains of tension, consider the following:

- **Rewrite internal messages.** How do you talk to yourself? When you have a test coming up, do you tell yourself you can ace it with consistent study ahead of time? Or do you tell yourself that you'll probably fail, so why bother studying? If you tend to tell yourself negative messages, first identify them, then restate them as positive, solution-oriented, constructive messages.

- **Set realistic expectations.** College brings new challenges—and a whole new level of competition. Do you feel disappointed if you don't ace every single course you take? Or do you give yourself permission to feel that your best effort is reward enough? Regardless of how ambitious you are, be honest with yourself and try to set realistic goals in order to keep your stress level manageable.

- **Build your self-esteem.** Increasing your self-worth through positive affirmations and self-talk, replaying compliments in your head, and the other self-esteem-boosting tips we discussed in the psychological health chapter can help you build the inner strength and confidence to handle stressful situations when they come along.

- **Be proactive.** Do you have a professor who enjoys pop quizzes, and does this make you think about skipping class some days? Unfortunately, avoidance is a poor strategy for stress management. Studies have found that trying to avoid stressful scenes ahead of time will only worsen your stress later.[44] If you have a class with a professor who likes surprises, be prepared by keeping up with your studies. A little planning now will mean less stress later on.

- **Tackle problems head-on.** When confronted by a difficult task or situation, do you believe in your ability to find a creative, effective solution? Or do you automatically assume you'll fail from the start? Strong problem-solving skills are closely linked to better health and fewer feelings of stress in college students.[45] If a problem seems overwhelming, try breaking it into pieces and tackling one bit at a time. Ask your professors, classmates, and friends for help. Taking active steps to solve a problem can reduce your feelings of stress.

- **Have a sense of humor.** A little laughter can go a long way toward reducing stress. Laughter increases your intake of oxygen, improves

When you're **stressed**, the way you choose to cope with it can help—
or set you up for more problems. To de-stress in a healthy way:

CHOOSE THIS.

NOT THAT.

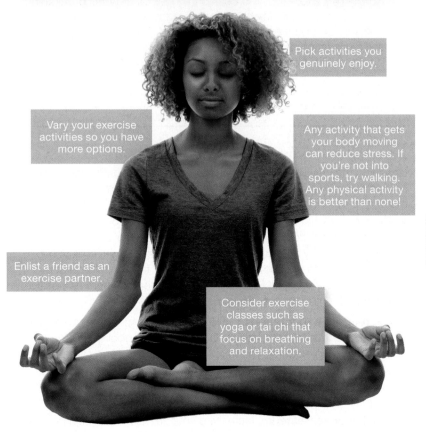

Pick activities you genuinely enjoy.

Vary your exercise activities so you have more options.

Any activity that gets your body moving can reduce stress. If you're not into sports, try walking. Any physical activity is better than none!

Enlist a friend as an exercise partner.

Consider exercise classes such as yoga or tai chi that focus on breathing and relaxation.

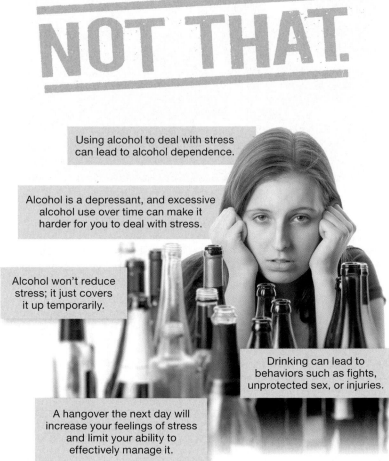

Using alcohol to deal with stress can lead to alcohol dependence.

Alcohol is a depressant, and excessive alcohol use over time can make it harder for you to deal with stress.

Alcohol won't reduce stress; it just covers it up temporarily.

Drinking can lead to behaviors such as fights, unprotected sex, or injuries.

A hangover the next day will increase your feelings of stress and limit your ability to effectively manage it.

⋀ Exercise:

Exercise releases endorphins in the body, which make you feel good and help reduce stress. As little as 20 minutes per day can have an effect on your stress level.

⋀ Alcohol:

You may think that having a drink, or several, is a good stress reliever. But alcohol's negative effects can actually make stress worse.

Reference: **1.** "Bidirectional Interactions between Acute Psychosocial Stress and Acute Intravenous Alcohol in Healthy Men," by E. Childs, S. O'Connor, & H. de Wit, 2011, *Alcoholism: Clinical & Experimental Research, 35* (10), 1794–1803.

your circulation, relaxes your muscles, and reduces tension. So read some cartoons, or watch some funny YouTube videos, or talk to your most hilarious friend. Humor can help you get a better perspective on which stressors are really important and which ones are overblown.

- **Take the long view.** Are most of the stressors in your life right now going to matter to you in a few years? Cultivating patience and a sense of what matters in the long term can help you keep problems in perspective.

- **Accept that you cannot control everything.** Being able to accept that you can't control everything—and being adaptable to less-than-ideal situations—can make a big difference in how well you deal with stress. For instance, if you play team sports, consciously

acknowledge that the final score or season ranking isn't up to you alone.

Create a Personalized Stress Management Plan

As we have discussed throughout this chapter, many common stressors are either emotional or psychological in nature. Nonetheless, these stressors still trigger a physical stress response, and over time, the stress response itself can negatively affect your health. A growing number of researchers believe that managing stress effectively is an important aspect of staying healthy. You can start creating your own stress management plan by first identifying and examining the stressors in your own life. By writing them down and spelling them out, you can then think about ways to reduce their occurrence, or to mentally reframe them in ways that can lessen your stress response.

The first step is to realistically assess the stressors in your own life. Begin with the following:

- Complete the **Self-Assessment** on page 58 to assess your current stressors.
- Complete the **Choosing to Change Worksheet** found at the end of this chapter to evaluate your readiness for behavior change, and take steps to reduce the controllable stressors.

Once you have done everything you can to minimize the controllable stressors in your life, it's time to think about how you can better respond to (and manage) the stress that remains. Review the section on strategies for managing stress. Which techniques seem like the best fit for your life and personality? Select the options you find the most comfortable and natural for you. Keep the following guidelines in mind:

- Remember that not all stress is harmful. You may find one of your classes tough, for example, but intellectually fun and challenging. Focus on changing your response to stressors that leave you exhausted, irritable, anxious, or sick.
- If the stress management technique that you pick requires adjustments to your schedule, take action to make room for it. For example, if school stress leaves you feeling anxious, and you've resolved to shake some of that stress through more exercise, prioritize time for workouts into your schedule.
- Decide how long you will try the stress management technique to see if it is working. Remember that managing stress is a long-term commitment. Tackle your stressors little by little, rather than trying to eliminate all of your stress at once.

>> This video from Dartmouth College provides tips for students on how to incorporate stress management into their lives: www.dartmouth .edu/~acskills/videos/video_sm.html.

Helping a Friend

When friends are stressed, even a friendly text or a supportive email can make a big difference. Invite someone to take a break for coffee or play a fast pickup game of hoops. If you see someone drowning in schoolwork, help them talk through the project to set priorities and break the work down into manageable pieces. And if a friend seems dangerously stressed, help them find professional support through your campus health center.

When you are under stress yourself, it may seem impossible to fit in time for others. But taking even a few minutes each day to support a friend can have an equal effect on you. When it comes to stress, social support is just about the best medicine: One study of college students found that while unhealthful coping mechanisms like drinking or drug use harm well-being, positive social support brings a major boost.[46]

Campus Advocacy

When you feel stressed out on campus, look around and you'll realize very quickly that you aren't alone. Talk to your friends, classmates, and roommates about how you are feeling. Many student organizations and student health centers also offer support groups where you can vent about stress, hear what others are going through, and swap suggestions for coping. Find out what's happening on your campus, and get involved! Here's a sampling:

- **Transitioning.** Many researchers believe that the first year of college is the toughest.[47] Making the transition from home to campus can be easier if students have access to stress management information and supportive services. A new campaign aims to give students exactly that. Called *The Transition Year*, it's jointly sponsored by the American Psychiatric Association and the Jed Foundation, a nonprofit established in 2000 by Donna and Phil Saltow, who lost their son Jed to suicide.[47] The campaign includes a website that offers tools and links to help students navigate all kinds of issues, from homework to dorm life.

>> Check out the foundation's website at www.transitionyear.org.

- **Debt.** Some campus financial aid departments are sponsoring informational websites and free crash courses to help students avoid or reduce their credit card debt. Some even offer short-term, emergency loans to help students pay off their high-interest consumer debt and get on a manageable payment plan. If your campus doesn't offer such a service, contact your local consumer credit counseling agency and suggest that it offer its services on your campus.

>> For a list of approved consumer credit counseling agencies by state and district, see www.justice.gov/ust/eo/bapcpa/ccde/cc_approved.htm.

- **Grades.** Most colleges and universities have academic advising offices where students can go to get help with academic challenges. Many also have peer tutoring services. Don't hesitate to take advantage of these services—it's more effective to use them as soon as you realize there's a problem.

>> Watch videos of real students discussing stress management at MasteringHealth™

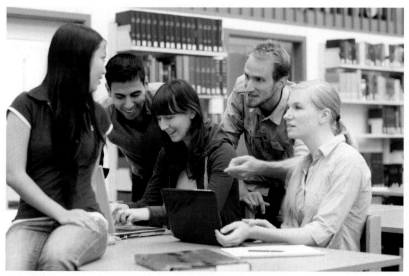

College brings many opportunities for stress, but with effective stress management, it can be a time of great growth and fun as well.

Choosing to Change Worksheet

To complete this worksheet online, visit MasteringHealth™

You have acquired extensive information from this chapter about stressors and how to manage them. You had the opportunity to make observations about whether or not your perceptions of negative events in your life may be contributing to making you feel distressed by completing the **Negative Event Scale for University Students** Self-Assessment on page 58.

Directions: Fill in your stage of change in Step 1 and complete the remaining steps with your stage of change in mind.

Step 1: *Your Stage of Behavior Change.* Please check one of the following statements that best describes your readiness to adopt stress management techniques.

_____ I do not intend to adopt stress management techniques in the next six months. (Precontemplation)

_____ I might adopt stress management techniques in the next six months. (Contemplation)

_____ I am prepared to adopt stress management techniques in the next month. (Preparation)

_____ I have been adopting stress management techniques for less than six months. (Action)

_____ I have been adopting stress management techniques for more than six months. (Maintenance)

Step 2: *Recognizing Chronic Stress.* It is important to identify the warning signs of chronic stress to assess whether or not your health may be at risk. The following table lists some of the common warning signs and symptoms of stress overload. Check whether or not you have experienced any of these within the last month.

Recognizing Warning Signs and Symptoms of Stress Overload

Emotional	Yes	No	Physical	Yes	No	Behavioral	Yes	No
Anxiety			Stooped posture			Overreacting to problems or difficult situations		
Sleep disruption			Sweaty palms			Increased use of alcohol, tobacco, or other drugs		
Anger and agitation			Chronic fatigue			Unusually impulsive behavior		
Trouble concentrating			Weight loss or weight gain			Feeling "burned out" on school or work		
Unproductive worry			Migraine or tension headaches			Withdrawing from relationships or contact with others		
Frequent mood swings			Neck aches			Frequent bouts of crying		
Depression			Digestive problems					
			Asthma attacks					
			Physical symptoms that your doctor can't attribute to another condition					
			Feelings of anxiety or panic					

The more signs and symptoms you notice, the closer you may be to allostatic overload or excessive stress. Be mindful that the signs and symptoms of stress can also be caused by other psychological and physiological medical problems. If you're experiencing any of the warning signs of stress overload, it's important to see a health-care professional for a full evaluation.

Step 3: *Identifying Stressors.* What were your top five stressors based on your completion of the **Negative Event Scale for University Students** Self-Assessment on page 58? Choose those that you scored as a 4 (a lot of a hassle) or 5 (an extreme hassle).

My Top 5 Stressors	How Much of a Hassle Was This Stressor? (4 or 5)
1.	
2.	
3.	
4.	
5.	

Now that you have completed Steps 2 and 3 you can begin to take action about changing the way you think about the primary stressors in your life and reduce or eliminate stress by completing Steps 4 and 5.

Step 4: *Choosing Stress Management Techniques.* For each of the stressors listed in Step 3, write down a stress management technique from the **Change Yourself, Change Your World** section of the chapter that can reduce this stressor. On a scale of 1–5 (1 being the lowest and 5 the highest), what is your confidence in your ability to implement the stress management technique the next time you experience the stressor?

Stressor	Stress Management Technique	How Confident Are You in Your Ability to Employ This Technique?				
		Low Confidence (1)			High Confidence (5)	
1.		1	2	3	4	5
2.		1	2	3	4	5
3.		1	2	3	4	5
4.		1	2	3	4	5
5.		1	2	3	4	5

Step 5: *Using Effective Time Management to Reduce Daily Hassles.* You can reduce some of your daily stress, and handle the hassles in your life more effectively, by rethinking how you use your time. Start by taking a closer look at your schedule. Using the following chart, fill in your activities every day for a week.

Time	Monday	Tuesday	Wednesday	Thursday	Friday	Saturday	Sunday
5:00 a.m.							
6:00 a.m.							
7:00 a.m.							
8:00 a.m.							
9:00 a.m.							
10:00 a.m.							
11:00 a.m.							
12:00 p.m.							
1:00 p.m.							
2:00 p.m.							
3:00 p.m.							
4:00 p.m.							
5:00 p.m.							
6:00 p.m.							
7:00 p.m.							
8:00 p.m.							
9:00 p.m.							
10:00 p.m.							
11:00 p.m.							
12:00 a.m.							
12 a.m.–5 a.m.							

Now, examine the chart and consider the following: Which tasks are most important to your goals in school and in your personal life? Which tasks are needed to keep you healthy, such as eating, sleeping, and making time to relax? Which tasks are unnecessary time-busters—that is, activities that eat away at your time, or waste it (be honest)? Decide how you can kick a time-buster or two out of your schedule. Mark these areas with red pencil, and see how much more time you have for important tasks.

Step 6: Set a SMART goal for how you can manage stress, including a timeline.

_____

_____

_____

Chapter Summary

- *Stress* is the collective psychobiological condition that occurs in reaction to a disruptive, unexpected, or exciting stimulus.

- *Eustress* is stress resulting from positive stressors; *distress* is stress resulting from negative stressors.

- The *stress response* is the set of specific psychobiological changes that occurs as the body attempts to cope with a stressor and return to *homeostasis* (a balanced state).

- The *general adaptation syndrome (GAS)* is a theory developed by Hans Selye that attempts to explain the biology of the stress response. It consists of three stages: alarm, resistance, and exhaustion.

- The *fight-or-flight response* is a component of the alarm phase of the stress response. It is an instantaneous set of reactions prompted by the nervous system's release of noradrenaline, which temporarily boosts strength and reflexes to physically prepare the body to deal with a stressor. This is followed by a hormonal response, including the secretion of cortisol, that sustains the initial nervous system response.

- *Allostatic overload* is the long-term wear and tear experienced by the body as a result of continuous or repeated reactions to stressors.

- Chronic stress can increase your risk of heart disease and stroke, result in digestive problems, promote weight gain, weaken your immune system, disturb your sleep, compromise your mental health, and negatively affect your relationships.

- Common sources of stress include daily hassles, academic pressure, job-related issues, social stressors, major life changes, environmental stressors, and internal stressors.

- How you view, think about, and manage your stress can have a critical impact on how stress affects your health. Part of your individual response may be related to your personality type, although anyone can feel stress—and can learn to manage it effectively.

- General strategies for reducing stress include getting enough sleep, eating well, exercising, strengthening your support network, communicating, taking time for hobbies, keeping a journal, practicing relaxation techniques, changing your thinking, and seeking help.

GET CONNECTED

≫ Visit the following websites for further information about the topics in this chapter:

- American Psychological Association
  www.apa.org
- Time Management for Students
  www.dartmouth.edu/~acskills/success/time.html
- Stress Management Techniques
  www.mindtools.com/pages/main/newMN_TCS.htm
- Budget Worksheet for College Students
  http://financialplan.about.com/od/moneyandcollegestudents/l/blcollbudget.htm

MOBILE TIPS!

Scan this QR code with your mobile device to access additional tips about stress management. Or, via your mobile device, go to **http://mobiletips.pearsoncmg.com** and navigate to Chapter 3.

- Kiplinger.com Budget Worksheet
  www.kiplinger.com/article/saving/T007-C000-S001-build-your-budget.html

Website links are subject to change. To access updated web links, please visit MasteringHealth™

TEST YOUR KNOWLEDGE

1. The stress that results from positive experiences (such as graduating from college or getting married) is called
   a. eustress.
   b. distress.
   c. homeostasis.
   d. allostasis.

2. The fight-or-flight response
   a. is characteristic of the resistance phase.
   b. can take a toll on your body.
   c. is a sign of allostatic overload.
   d. All of the answers are correct.

3. In the "alarm" phase of the general adaptation syndrome
   a. the adrenal glands release cortisol.
   b. the stomach releases glucose.
   c. the heart rate slows.
   d. All of the answers are correct.

4. The long-term wear and tear on the body that results from continuous or repeated responses to stress is termed
   a. homeostasis.
   b. allostasis.
   c. allostatic overload.
   d. eustress.

5. The effects of chronic stress can include
   a. increased risk of heart disease.
   b. stomachache, constipation, or diarrhea.
   c. a weakened immune system.
   d. All of the answers are correct.

6. Worries, critical thoughts, and the demands we place upon ourselves are examples of
   a. environmental stressors.
   b. internal stressors.
   c. social stressors.
   d. post-traumatic stress disorder.

7. An example of an ideal exercise program for consistent stress reduction consists of
   a. 1 hour of high-intensity cardiovascular activity per month.
   b. 20 to 30 minutes of walking at a brisk pace 5 days a week.
   c. 45 minutes of strength training every weekend.
   d. light activity such as shopping or cleaning your room.

8. Progressive muscle relaxation involves
   a. systematically contracting and relaxing muscle groups.
   b. taking naps of longer and longer lengths.
   c. stretching your muscles a little more each day.
   d. quietly focusing on relaxing only your body's tiniest muscles.

9. In stressful situations, a "type C" personality
   a. is likely to respond in an aggressive, hostile manner.
   b. will keep problems and pressures in perspective.
   c. may tend to be very passive and indifferent.
   d. may respond stoically and internalize stress.

10. A feeling that you are able to improve a stressful situation is
   a. part of the personality trait of hardiness.
   b. one of the benefits of social support.
   c. one of the basic elements of psychoneuroimmunology.
   d. not going to truly help you manage stress.

Get Critical

What happened

On October 13, 2010, 33 Chilean miners who had been trapped more than 2,000 feet underground for 69 days were pulled out of the earth. As people around the world watched, the miners, once thought dead, emerged one by one. All but one—a miner suffering from pneumonia—were found to be in "more than satisfactory health." In the days following their rescue, many observers marveled that the miners had not simply managed to survive their ordeal, but had transformed it into a triumph.

How did they do it? During their first 17 days before contact with rescuers above, the miners met their physical needs by rationing their food, establishing a duct for potable water, and setting up a chemical toilet. They exerted what control they could over their confined living space by creating areas for eating, sleeping, and praying, and they chose unique roles for each miner according to his skills. They also mutually supported and encouraged one another.

Once they were discovered, the rescue team kept them busy with a variety of important tasks: transmitting information about the conditions underground, providing input on certain decisions, establishing and maintaining lighting that mimicked day and night, clearing away debris, and keeping themselves fit with obligatory exercise. Rescuers also provided the miners with supplies to keep them physically and emotionally healthy. They even sent down a video showing the birth of one of the miner's daughters, whose mother named her Esperanza, meaning "Hope."

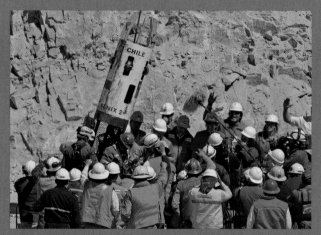

The Chilean miners were rescued through a narrow tube that lifted them 2,000 feet to the surface.

What do you think?

- Which phase of the stress response were the miners most likely to have experienced in the initial moments after the mine collapsed? What physical signs and symptoms did the miners probably experience during this phase?

- As the miners' time underground expanded from days to weeks to months, what environmental, social, and internal stressors did they face?

- How did they resist these stressors so successfully? Identify several resources the miners already had in place, as well as new coping techniques that they developed independently or that their rescuers initiated.

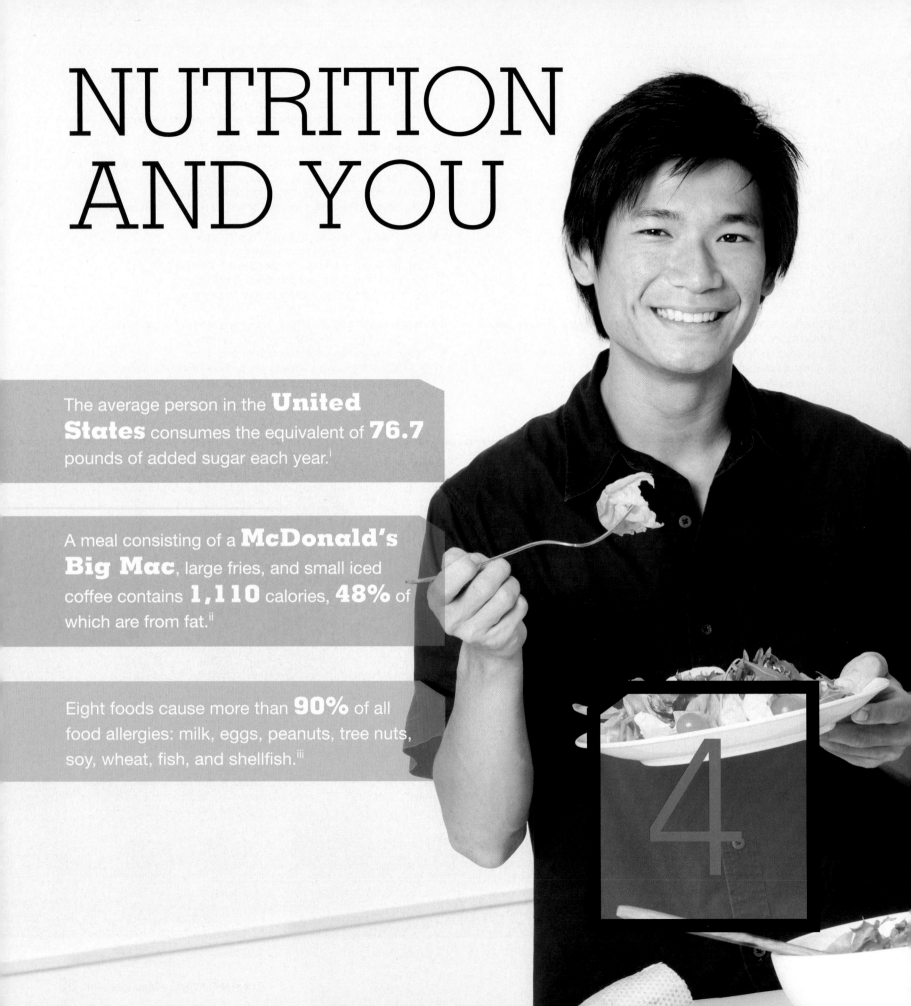

NUTRITION AND YOU

The average person in the **United States** consumes the equivalent of **76.7** pounds of added sugar each year.[i]

A meal consisting of a **McDonald's Big Mac**, large fries, and small iced coffee contains **1,110** calories, **48%** of which are from fat.[ii]

Eight foods cause more than **90%** of all food allergies: milk, eggs, peanuts, tree nuts, soy, wheat, fish, and shellfish.[iii]

4

Learning Objectives

IDENTIFY the six classes of nutrients and explain their functions in the body.

DESCRIBE the importance of fiber, phytochemicals, antioxidants, probiotics, and prebiotics in foods.

DEMONSTRATE how to use the DRIs, MyPlate, and other resources to design a healthful diet.

EXPLAIN how nutrition guidelines vary according to age, gender, activity level, and dietary preferences.

SUMMARIZE four steps for handling food safely.

IDENTIFY strategies for making nutritious, inexpensive choices when shopping, cooking for yourself, and eating out.

Why is orange juice more nutritious than orange soda?

Why does a baked potato beat French fries? Why is fat from a fish better than fat from a cow? In short, what foods should you limit, and what foods should you favor? Most importantly, why does it matter?

The science of **nutrition** examines how the foods you eat affect your body and health. A nutritious **diet** provides you with energy, helps you stay healthy, and allows you to function at your best. Diets lacking in nutrition can drain your energy and decrease your sense of well-being, as well as increase your risk for developing chronic health problems such as high blood pressure, heart disease, type 2 diabetes, and obesity. Whether you're in line at the deli or your dining hall, knowing the basic principles of good nutrition can help you make choices that will benefit your health for a lifetime.

What Are Nutrients?

Your body relies on food to provide chemical compounds called **nutrients.** In a process called digestion, the food you eat is broken down into nutrients that are small enough to be absorbed into your bloodstream **(Figure 4.1)**. Once in your body, nutrients work together to provide energy; support growth, repair, and maintenance of body tissues; and regulate body functions.

Six major classes of nutrients are found in food:

- Carbohydrates
- Fats (more appropriately called *lipids*)
- Proteins
- Vitamins
- Minerals
- Water

Within these six classes are about 45 specific nutrients that your body is unable to make or can't make in needed quantities to support health. These are called **essential nutrients.** You must obtain essential nutrients from food, beverages, and/or supplements.

Nutrients your body needs in relatively large quantities are called *macronutrients* (*macro-* means "large"). These are carbohydrates, fats, proteins, and water. Nutrients you need in relatively small quantities are called *micronutrients* (*micro-* means "small"). These are vitamins and minerals.

Energy and Calories

Three of the four macronutrients—carbohydrates, fats, and proteins—are also known as *energy-yielding nutrients* because the body breaks them down to provide you with the energy you need to move, to think, and simply to survive. Although vitamins, minerals, and water assist this process, they don't supply you with energy.

If you've ever thought that you felt warmer after eating a meal, you weren't imagining it! Scientists determine the amount of energy that a food

---

nutrition The scientific study of food and its physiological functions.

diet The food you regularly consume.

nutrients Chemical substances in food that you need for energy, growth, and survival.

essential nutrients Nutrients you must obtain from food or supplements because your body either cannot produce them or cannot make them in sufficient quantities to maintain health.

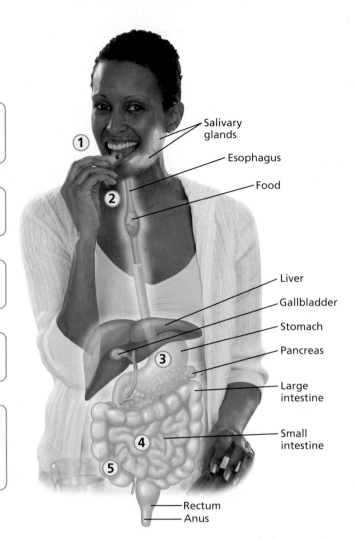

1 Digestion begins in the mouth. Chewing mixes saliva with food and begins to break it down.

2 The food travels from the mouth to the stomach through the esophagus.

3 The stomach mixes food with chemicals that break it down further.

4 Most digestion and absorption occurs in the small intestine.

5 Water, vitamins, and some minerals are absorbed in the large intestine. The remaining wastes are passed out of the body in stool.

Salivary glands
Esophagus
Food
Liver
Gallbladder
Stomach
Pancreas
Large intestine
Small intestine
Rectum
Anus

FIGURE 4.1 The Digestive Process. Digestion is the process of breaking food down into nutrients that can be used by the body for energy.

Source: Adapted from Thompson, Janice, and Melinda Manore. *Nutrition: An Applied Approach,* 3rd Ed., © 2012, p. 81. Reprinted and Electronically reproduced by permission of Pearson Education, Inc., Upper Saddle River, New Jersey.

provides by measuring how much heat it generates. They calculate that heat in units called *kilocalories*. You're probably more familiar with the simpler term **calorie,** and we will use the term *calorie* throughout this text.

The energy-yielding nutrients differ in their calorie content. Carbohydrates and proteins each provide 4 calories per gram. (A gram is a very small amount; for instance, a standard packet of sugar contains about 3 grams.) Fats provide 9 calories per gram—more than twice the amount in carbohydrates or proteins. Alcohol is not a nutrient because it doesn't provide any substance you need to grow or survive. However, alcohol does provide energy, 7 calories per gram, which explains why consuming alcohol regularly can pack on the pounds. Regardless of their source, calories consumed in excess of energy needs are converted to fat and stored in the body.

Vitamins, minerals, and water provide no energy, but they are essential to **metabolism,** the process by which your body breaks down foods into molecules small enough to absorb, and then converts those molecules into energy.

People vary in how many calories they need to eat each day to meet their energy needs, yet avoid gaining weight. For instance, women, on average, need fewer calories than men. And because vigorous activity burns more calories than sitting still, athletes need many more calories

than people who spend hours every day watching TV, surfing the Internet, and, yes, sitting in the library studying.

>> How many calories do *you* need each day? Find out in seconds using this simple tool: www.cancer.org/healthy/toolsandcalculators/calculators/app/calorie-counter-calculator.

Carbohydrates

Carbohydrates are compounds that contain three common elements: carbon, hydrogen, and oxygen. Plants manufacture carbohydrates using energy from the sun, and we derive the carbohydrates in our diets predominantly from plant foods. Milk and other dairy products are the exception, but even the carbohydrates in these foods come from the plants that the cow, goat, or sheep consumed.

calorie Common term for *kilocalorie.* The amount of energy required to raise the temperature of 1 kilogram of water by 1 degree Celsius.

metabolism The sum of all chemical reactions occurring in body cells, including those that break large molecules down into smaller molecules.

carbohydrates A macronutrient class composed of carbon, hydrogen, and oxygen, that is the body's universal energy source.

> ❝ *Some body cells, including those in your brain, can use only carbohydrates for fuel.*"

Carbohydrates are sometimes called the body's universal energy source because most body cells, especially during high-intensity activities, prefer carbohydrates for energy. Some body cells, including those in your brain, can use only carbohydrates for fuel.

There are two categories of carbohydrates: *simple carbohydrates* and *complex carbohydrates*. Both are composed of the same basic building blocks: sugar molecules, whose names usually end in "ose."

Simple Carbohydrates

Simple carbohydrates are constructed from just one or two sugar molecules. That means they are easily digested. We commonly refer to simple carbohydrates as *sugars*, and six are important in nutrition: glucose, fructose (fruit sugar), galactose, maltose (malt sugar), sucrose (table sugar), and lactose (milk sugar). Of these, the most important is glucose. It is the most abundant sugar in foods and in our bodies, and it is our most important energy source.

Sugars provide much of the sweetness found naturally in fruits, some vegetables, honey, and milk. They are also added to beverages, desserts, and even some peanut butters, soups, and other foods you might not normally think of as sweet. And of course we sprinkle sugar on our cereal and into our coffee and tea. In fact, studies indicate that adults in the United States consume an average of 76.7 pounds of added sugars a year.[1]

As it breaks down, absorbs, burns, or stores the simple carbohydrates you eat, your body is unable to distinguish between those that came naturally from whole foods and those that were added to foods as sweeteners. The fructose present in an orange is the same, chemically, as the fructose in the high-fructose corn syrup (HFCS) that is used to sweeten orange soda. This doesn't mean, however, that drinking fresh-squeezed orange juice is the same as drinking orange soda! Foods with naturally occurring sugars contain many vitamins, minerals, and other substances that promote health. Foods high in added sugars generally provide empty calories and few, if any, health-promoting benefits.

Complex Carbohydrates

Complex carbohydrates are made up of long chains of multiple sugar molecules; therefore, they take longer to digest. Commonly called *starches*, they are found in a variety of plants, especially grains (oats, rice, wheat, etc.), legumes (dried beans, lentils, and peas), other vegetables, and many fruits.

There are two non-starch forms of complex carbohydrate. *Glycogen* is a storage form of glucose in animal tissues, including the liver and muscles. We consume very little glycogen from meat, however, because it typically breaks down when an animal is slaughtered. **Fiber** is a tough (fibrous) complex carbohydrate that gives structure to plants. Although it's not a nutrient, it's a very important component of a healthy diet. Let's see why.

simple carbohydrates The most basic unit of carbohydrates, consisting of one or two sugar molecules.

complex carbohydrates Contain chains of multiple sugar molecules; commonly called *starches* but also come in two non-starch forms: *glycogen* and *fiber*.

fiber A nondigestible complex carbohydrate that aids in digestion.

whole grains Unrefined grains that contain bran, germ, and endosperm.

Facts About Fiber

Whereas starch is readily digested and its components absorbed, fiber passes through the intestinal tract without being digested or absorbed. Nevertheless, it has many health benefits:

- **Weight control.** Fiber can make you feel full before you've consumed lots of calories. In this way, a high-fiber diet can help you avoid weight gain.
- **Bowel health.** As it moves through your large intestine, fiber provides bulk for feces. Because it absorbs water along the way, it also softens feces, making stools easier to pass. A diet rich in fiber can help you to avoid hemorrhoids, constipation, and other digestive problems.
- **Heart health.** No doubt you've heard of cholesterol, an oily substance that can clog your blood vessels and increase your risk for heart disease. A diet rich in fiber can help lower the level of cholesterol in your blood. It's thought that this happens because fiber binds to bile, a cholesterol-containing substance that your liver makes. When fiber is excreted from your body in feces, bile—and its cholesterol load—is excreted along with it. This leaves less cholesterol in your bloodstream.
- **Blood glucose control.** Finally, by slowing the transit of foods through your intestinal tract, fiber promotes a more gradual absorption of their nutrients, including glucose, into your bloodstream. This can help prevent wide fluctuations in glucose levels in your blood, which is important in managing diabetes.

For all these reasons, it's recommended that you maintain a high-fiber diet. Men need 38 grams of fiber per day, and women need 25 grams per day. For men and women 50 years or older, the recommendations are 30 and 21 grams, respectively.[2] Remember we said that fiber absorbs water, so a high-fiber diet should be accompanied by plenty of fluids to keep the fiber moving along the intestinal tract.

Fiber is plentiful in legumes and other vegetables, many fruits, nuts, and seeds, as well as whole grains. But what exactly qualifies as a whole grain food?

Choose Whole Grains

Unrefined grains, or **whole grains,** include three parts—bran, germ, and endosperm—and generally can be sprouted **(Figure 4.2)**. Common examples are whole wheat, whole oats, popcorn, brown rice, millet, and quinoa. Whole grains are especially nutritious because the bran and germ provide valuable vitamins, minerals, and fiber. Like any fiber-rich food, whole grains are bulky, and the body digests them slowly, using the energy they provide more efficiently, and helping people to feel full sooner and for a longer time.

In contrast, refined grains are stripped of their bran and germ during processing, reducing both their fiber and nutrients. Only the starchy endosperm is retained. Examples are white bread, white rice, crackers, and most baked goods such as cookies and pastries. Despite having fewer nutrients, these products usually retain all the calories of their unrefined counterparts.

Many refined carbohydrates, including white bread, are "enriched" after processing, meaning that some of the lost vitamins and minerals are replaced. However, many other important nutrients are not replaced, nor is the fiber.

Practical Strategies

Choosing Complex Carbohydrates

A diet high in complex carbohydrates provides a wide variety of essential nutrients. It's also rich in fiber, a non-nutrient substance that keeps your digestive tract running smoothly. Maintaining a high-complex-carbohydrate diet also reduces your risk of obesity, heart disease, and type 2 diabetes. So

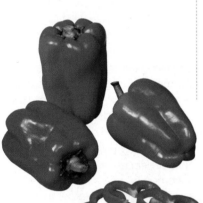

how can you choose more complex carbohydrates? Here are some tips:

- Start your day with whole grain cereal and a piece of fresh fruit.
- Switch to whole grain bread for morning toast and lunchtime sandwiches.
- Choose vegetarian chili or a bean burrito for lunch.
- Instead of a side of French fries or potato chips, choose a small salad, carrot sticks, or slices of sweet red pepper.
- For an afternoon snack, mix dried fruits with nuts, sunflower seeds, and pieces of whole grain cereal.
- If dinner includes rice, pasta, pizza crust, or tortillas, choose whole grain versions.
- Include a side of beans, peas, or lentils with dinner, along with a leafy green vegetable, sweet potato, or vegetable soup.
- For an evening snack, choose popcorn, popcorn cakes, a whole grain toaster pastry, low-fat oatmeal cookies, or a bowl of whole grain cereal with milk.

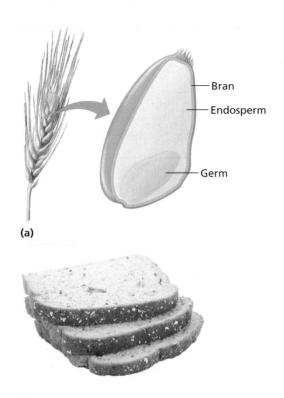

(a)

(b)

FIGURE 4.2 Whole Grains. **(a)** A whole grain includes the bran, endosperm, and germ. **(b)** Whole wheat bread is an excellent source of whole grain.

In contrast, when you eat low-glycemic-index foods, glucose seeps more slowly into your bloodstream, and your pancreas releases a smaller amount of insulin to move it into your cells. As a result, your blood glucose level falls gradually, and you feel satiated (full) much longer.[5]

Foods with a high glycemic index include white potatoes, white bread, pastries, white rice, sweetened soft drinks, and candies. Foods with a low glycemic index include legumes and most other vegetables, most fruits, and most foods made with whole grains.

>> For an online list of the glycemic index of over 100 foods, go to www.health.harvard.edu/newsweek/Glycemic_index_and_glycemic_load_for_100_foods.htm.

Recommended Carbohydrate Intake

Adults 19 years of age or older should consume an absolute minimum of 130 grams of carbohydrates each day.[2] This amount—which you'd get from eating about three slices of whole wheat bread—is estimated to supply adequate fuel to your brain. But you also need carbohydrates to fuel physical activity, and they're an excellent source of other nutrients, as well as fiber. For these reasons, nutrition experts recommend that you consume about half (45–65%) of your total daily calories as carbohydrates. Focus on getting the majority of your carbohydrates from whole grains, fruits, and legumes and other vegetables. The **Practical Strategies** box shows you how.

Most people in the United States eat less than one serving of whole grains a day.[3] If you're among them, you may be missing out on essential nutrients and fiber, while overconsuming calories. So the next time you're debating between the plain bagel or the whole grain toast, go for the whole grain.

Does Glycemic Index Matter?

The **glycemic index** refers to the potential of foods to raise the level of the simple sugar glucose in your bloodstream. When you eat foods with a high glycemic index, they're quickly broken down into glucose, which then flows rapidly from your intestinal tract into your bloodstream. Your pancreas detects this excessive blood glucose and, in response, releases a flood of insulin, a hormone that acts to get the glucose out of your blood and into your cells. This stresses your pancreas and may contribute to the development of type 2 diabetes. Moreover, that surge in insulin prompts a dramatic clearing of glucose out of your bloodstream, leaving you feeling hungry again very quickly. This may lead to overeating and weight gain. Interestingly, a 2013 review study also suggests that a high-glycemic-index diet aggravates acne![4]

glycemic index Value indicating the potential of a food to raise blood glucose.

Fats

Fats are one type of a huge group of compounds called *lipids* that are found throughout nature. Like carbohydrates, lipids are made up of carbon, hydrogen, and oxygen. But these elements are arranged in very different ways that give lipids their key characteristic: They are not soluble in water. Olive oil will float to the top of your salad dressing because it's a lipid. This insolubility is required for some of your body's tissues and chemicals to function, so in moderate amounts, lipids are essential to your health. They cushion and insulate your organs, for example, and they enable your body to absorb fat-soluble vitamins. They are also the most concentrated energy source in your diet, supplying 9 calories per gram. In fact, lipids supply your body with energy both while you are active and while you sleep.

Fats Are One of Three Types of Food Lipids

Three types of lipids are present in foods.

Phospholipids. The least common dietary lipids are phospholipids. They are found only in peanuts, egg yolk, and a few processed foods such as salad dressing. Phospholipids are made up of lipid molecules attached to a compound called phosphate. They're a key component of the cell membrane—the flexible "wall" that keeps the contents of your cells in place. But your body can make them from other substances, so you don't need to consume them.

Cholesterol. *Sterols* are ring-shaped lipids found in both plant- and animal-based foods. Plant sterols are not very well absorbed by the body, but are thought to have an important health benefit: They appear to block the absorption of **cholesterol,** the animal sterol most common in the American diet. Cholesterol is found in animal-based foods such as meats, eggs, shellfish, butter, lard, and whole milk. As we mentioned earlier, cholesterol that circulates in your bloodstream can accumulate along the lining of your blood vessels, increasing your risk for a heart attack or stroke. Still, some cholesterol is essential for your survival because it's a component of cell membranes and many important compounds. But you don't have to consume it because the liver can make all the cholesterol you need.

Fats. The lipid found most abundantly in your diet, **fats** are present in a wide variety of plant and animal foods. Food scientists refer to dietary fats as *triglycerides*, because they are made up of three fatty acid chains (*tri-* means "three") attached to a compound called glycerol (a type of alcohol). Depending on the structure of the fatty acid chains, one of three different types of fats is formed: saturated, monounsaturated, or polyunsaturated. As we explain next, each type has different characteristics and different effects on your health.

Saturated Fats

Saturated fats got their name because their fatty acid chains are "saturated" with hydrogen. This makes them solid at room temperature, and stable, so they tend to have a long shelf life.

A diet high in saturated fats is associated with an increased risk for cardiovascular disease.[6] So what foods should you avoid? Saturated fats generally are found in animal products such as meat, cream, whole milk, cheese, lard, and butter. Red meats tend to have more saturated fat than poultry or fish, and fried meats have more than meats that are broiled, grilled, or baked. Processed foods, including pastries, chips, French fries, and prepared meals are often loaded with saturated fat. Palm, palm kernel, and coconut oils, although derived from plants, also are highly saturated.

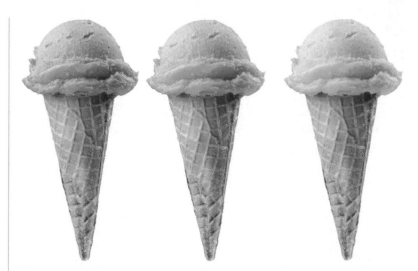

Ice cream, unfortunately, is loaded with saturated fat.

Unsaturated Fats

Unsaturated fats got their name because their fatty acid chains have one or more areas that are not "saturated" with hydrogen. This makes them more flexible, and they are typically liquid at room temperature. Unsaturated fats are abundant in plant oils and fish oils. Replacing saturated fats with unsaturated fats can lower your blood cholesterol level and helps reduce your risk for heart disease.[7]

The two types of unsaturated fats are monounsaturated and polyunsaturated. *Mono-* means "one," and monounsaturated fats have fatty acid chains with one unsaturated region. Sources of monounsaturated fats include canola oil, olive oil, peanut oil, nuts, avocado, and sesame seeds. *Poly-* means "many," and polyunsaturated fats have fatty acid chains with two or more unsaturated regions. Sources of polyunsaturated fats include corn oil, soybean oil, safflower oil, non-hydrogenated margarines, salad dressings, mayonnaise, nuts, and seeds.

cholesterol An animal sterol found in the fatty part of animal-based foods such as meat and whole milk.

fats (triglycerides) Lipids made up of three fatty acid chains attached to a molecule of glycerol; the most common types of food lipid.

saturated fats Fats that typically are solid at room temperature; generally found in animal products, dairy products, and tropical oils.

unsaturated fats Fats that typically are liquid at room temperature; generally come from plant sources.

essential fatty acids (EFAs) Polyunsaturated fatty acids that cannot be synthesized by the body but are essential to body functioning.

Two polyunsaturated fats have been getting a lot of media attention lately. These are *omega-6 fatty acids* and *omega-3 fatty acids*. Both are essential to your body's functioning and are thought to provide some protection against heart disease. As they cannot be assembled by your body and must be obtained from your diet or from supplements, they are also known as the **essential fatty acids (EFAs).**

Most people in the United States get plenty of omega-6 fatty acids from plant oils, seeds, and nuts. However, most people need to increase significantly their consumption of omega-3 fatty acids, which are found in fatty fish (like salmon and mackerel), walnuts, flaxseed, canola oil, and dark green, leafy vegetables. Two types of long-chain omega-3 fatty acids found in fish, EPA and DHA, are thought to be particularly effective in reducing your risk for cardiovascular disease. Eating fish twice a week (a total of 8 ounces) provides an appropriate level of EPA and DHA for most adults.[8] If you never eat fish, ask your doctor for advice about taking a fish-oil supplement.

Practical Strategies

Choosing Healthful Fats

To choose healthful fats, start by sorting the good guys from the bad. Make it a standard practice to pick foods with zero *trans* fats, and replace saturated fats with unsaturated fats. Consume small amounts of vegetable oils, walnuts, flaxseed, leafy green vegetables, and/or fish daily to meet your essential fatty acid needs. Here are some additional tips:

- Instead of butter or a margarine made with hydrogenated oils, spread your toast with a non–*trans* fat margarine or peanut, almond, cashew, or walnut butter.

- If you normally eat two eggs for breakfast, discard the yolk from one. Do the same when making egg dishes such as quiches or casseroles, and in baking.

- Make low-fat foods a priority at each meal. Choose whole grain foods, legumes, fruits, vegetables, non-fat or low-fat dairy products, lean red meats (rump, round, loin, and flank), skinless poultry, and fish.

- Trim all visible fat from red meat and poultry. Instead of choosing fried meats, poultry, or fish, choose baked or broiled. Finally, remove the skin from poultry before eating it.

- Skip the French fries. Opt for a baked potato or side salad instead.

- Make sure that any cookies or other baked goods you buy are *trans* fat free.

- Instead of ice cream, which is high in saturated fat, choose ice milk, sorbet, or low-fat or non-fat frozen yogurt.

- When the munchies hit, go for air-popped popcorn, pretzels, rice cakes, or dried fruit instead of potato chips.

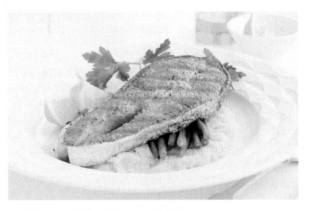

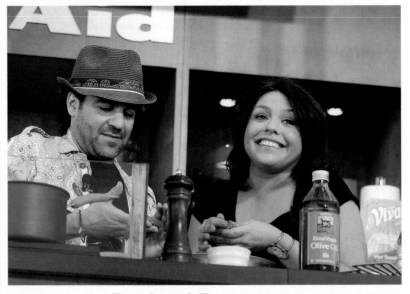

Celebrity cook Rachael Ray popularized the use of "EVOO": extra-virgin olive oil, a monounsaturated fat.

Avoid *Trans* Fats

So far, we've been discussing fats that occur naturally in foods. Now let's turn our attention to a particularly harmful form of fat that occurs almost exclusively in processed foods.

During food processing, an unsaturated fat such as corn oil may undergo a chemical process called *hydrogenation.* To "hydrogenate" means to saturate with hydrogen, so, as you've probably guessed, hydrogenation changes oils into more stable, saturated, solid fats that are less likely to spoil.

trans fat A type of fat that is produced when liquid fat (oil) is turned into solid fat during food processing.

Hydrogenation creates a unique type of fatty acid chain called a **trans fat** that is worse for your health than saturated fats! *Trans* fats have been implicated in high blood pressure, heart disease, stroke, diabetes, and other chronic conditions.[9] Even small amounts can be harmful: For every 2% increase of calories from *trans* fats daily, the risk of heart disease increases by 23%.[9]

Most *trans* fats in your diet come from vegetable shortenings, some margarines, processed foods, and other foods made with or fried in partially hydrogenated oils. You can find out the *trans* fat content of any packaged food by reading the label. However, foods containing half a gram of *trans* fat or less per serving can claim to be "*trans* fat free," so look for the words "hydrogenated" or "partially hydrogenated vegetable oil" in the ingredients list. If they're present, the food contains *trans* fats.[6]

Recommended Fat Intake

Dietary recommendations for fats have changed in recent years, shifting the emphasis from lowering total fat to limiting saturated and *trans* fats. Current recommendations suggest carefully replacing the saturated fats with monounsaturated and polyunsaturated fats and enjoying them in moderation.[7] Here are some specific recommendations:[2]

- In general, fats should make up between 20% and 35% of your total calories to meet daily energy and nutrition needs while minimizing your risk for chronic disease.

- *Trans* fat intake should be kept to an absolute minimum.

- Saturated fats should be less than 7–10% of total calories, or about 140–200 calories for someone consuming 2,000 calories per day.

- Omega-6 fatty acid intake should be about 14 to 17 grams per day for men and about 11 to 12 grams per day for women.

- Omega-3 fatty acid intake should be about 1.6 grams per day for men and about 1.1 grams per day for women. Eating 8 ounces of fish per week is recommended to meet your needs for EPA and DHA.

Because most college students don't monitor their diets closely every day, a good habit is to choose unsaturated fats over saturated and *trans* fats whenever possible. You can do this by adopting the habits described in the **Practical Strategies** box on page 76.

Proteins

Dietary **protein** is a macronutrient available from both plant and animal sources. Although it's one of the energy nutrients, protein is used for fuel only if your body does not have adequate amounts of carbohydrate and fat to burn. Assuming you're well nourished, your body uses the protein you eat to build biological compounds, cells, and tissues.

The Role of Amino Acids

Some misconceptions surround the roles of protein in the diet and in the body. For instance, people who associate meat with protein and protein with strength may eat lots of meat to build their muscles. This is unnecessary: Whenever you consume proteins, whether they come from meats or plants, your body breaks them apart into their component building blocks, which are nitrogen-containing compounds known as **amino acids.** Once absorbed through the intestinal tract, amino acids enter the bloodstream and become part of the amino acid pool. Just as you might go to an auto parts store to buy an air filter or some spark plugs for your car, your body cells draw from the amino acid pool the precise amino acids they need to build or repair a wide variety of body proteins. These include muscle and other body tissues as well as chemicals such as enzymes, which speed up metabolic reactions in your body. In short, you consume dietary protein primarily to maintain your stock of amino acids for your body cells to generate whatever proteins they need.

Complete and Incomplete Proteins

Although all of the 20 amino acids your body needs are available in foods, you don't have to consume them all. That's because your body can produce ample amounts of 11 of them independently. The other nine are called *essential amino acids* because your body either cannot make them or cannot make sufficient quantities to maintain your health. Thus, you need to consume these amino acids in your diet.

Dietary proteins are considered *complete proteins* if they supply all nine essential amino acids in adequate amounts. In contrast, *incomplete proteins* are lacking one or more of the essential amino acids. Meat, fish, poultry, dairy products, soy, and quinoa provide complete proteins. Most plant sources provide incomplete proteins. However, combinations of plant proteins—peanut butter on whole grain bread, for instance, or brown rice with lentils or beans—can complement each other in such a way that the essential amino acids missing from one are supplied by the other. The combination yields complete proteins. Incidentally, foods with complementary amino acids don't have to be consumed at the same meal. People following a plant-based diet simply need to consume a variety of plant proteins throughout the day.

Recommended Protein Intake

For good health, experts recommend that adults consume between 10% and 35% of their calories as protein.[2] Staying within this range can provide adequate protein and other nutrients while reducing the risk for chronic diseases such as type 2 diabetes, heart disease, and cancer. When an individual's protein intake falls above or below this range, the risk for development of these chronic diseases appears to increase.[2]

How much protein *you* need largely depends on your body weight and level of activity. Healthy adults typically need 0.36 grams of protein per pound (0.8 grams per kilogram) of body weight, equaling 54 grams per day for a 150-pound person.[2] Runners and other athletes in aerobic sports can require one-and-a-half times as much protein, and strength athletes, such as bodybuilders, can require up to twice as much.[10] Few people in the United States suffer from protein deficiencies. Research indicates that even athletes, on average, consume protein well in excess of their needs.[11] Don't fall for the myth that consuming excessive protein—whether from foods or expensive supplements—will help you build muscle. Any protein you consume beyond your body's needs is stored as fat.

Unfortunately, many animal sources of protein are high in cholesterol and saturated fat. Follow these tips to go lean with protein:[12]

- Choose lean cuts of meats such as rump, round, loin, and flank. Better yet, choose poultry (remove the skin). Best of all, choose fish.
- Avoid fried meats, as this cooking method adds fat. Choose baked, broiled, or grilled.
- For a lunchtime sandwich, choose turkey, roast beef, canned tuna or salmon, or peanut butter. Avoid deli meats like bologna or salami, which are high in saturated fat and sodium.
- Vary your protein sources by consuming vegetarian meals several times a week. Choose legumes, soy products such as tofu dogs and burgers, nuts, and seeds.
- Don't forget eggs: On average, one egg a day doesn't increase your risk for heart disease, and only the yolk contains cholesterol and saturated fat, so make an omelet with one whole egg and two egg whites.
- Choose a small portion of nuts or seeds as a snack, on salads, or in main dishes to replace meat or poultry.

Vitamins

Vitamins are carbon-containing compounds required in small amounts to regulate body functions and help chemical reactions take place. For example, although not an energy nutrient, vitamins do help your body to break down carbohydrates, fats, and proteins for energy.

Humans need 13 vitamins. Four of these—vitamins A, D, E, and K—are *fat soluble*, meaning they dissolve in fat and can be stored in your body's fatty tissues. Because your body can store them, consuming the fat-soluble vitamins two to three times a week is adequate. Nine vitamins—vitamin C and the eight B-complex vitamins (thiamin, riboflavin, niacin, pantothenic acid, B_6, biotin, folic acid, and B_{12})—are *water soluble*. They dissolve in water, and excesses are generally excreted from the body in urine. Your body can store vitamin B_{12} in the liver, but you cannot store any of the other water-soluble vitamins. Thus, it's important that you consume adequate amounts daily.

Sources of Vitamins

Selected vitamins are listed in **Table 4.1**, along with their food sources. As you can see, many vitamins are abundant in fruits, vegetables, and whole grains. Others are more plentiful in animal-based foods. Vitamin B_{12} is available naturally only from animal foods, so strict vegetarians have to get it from supplements or from eating processed foods to which B_{12} has been added.

protein A macronutrient that helps build many body chemicals and tissues, including muscle, bone, skin, and blood.

amino acids Nitrogen-containing compounds that are the building blocks of proteins.

vitamins Compounds, with no energy value of their own, needed by the body in small amounts for normal growth and function.

TABLE 4.1 Key Facts About Vitamins

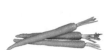 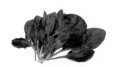 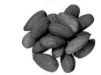   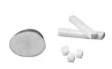

Fat Soluble	**Fat Soluble**	**Fat Soluble**	**Fat Soluble**	**Water Soluble**	**Water Soluble**	**Water Soluble**
Vitamin: A	**Vitamin:** D	**Vitamin:** E	**Vitamin:** K	**Vitamin:** B_1 (Thiamin)	**Vitamin:** B_2 (Riboflavin)	**Vitamin:** B_6
Functions: Required for vision, cell differentiation, reproduction; contributes to healthy bones and a healthy immune system	**Functions:** Regulates blood calcium levels; maintains bone health; assists in cell differentiation	**Functions:** Protects white blood cells, enhances immune function, improves absorption of vitamin A; protects cell membranes, fatty acids, and vitamin A from oxidation	**Functions:** Needed for the production of proteins that assist in blood clotting and maintenance of healthy bone	**Functions:** Needed for carbohydrate and amino acid metabolism	**Functions:** Needed for carbohydrate and fat metabolism	**Functions:** Needed for carbohydrate and amino acid metabolism; synthesis of blood cells
Food Sources: Beef, chicken liver, egg yolk, milk, spinach, carrots, mango, apricots, cantaloupe, pumpkin, yams	**Food Sources:** Canned salmon and mackerel, fortified milk or orange juice, fortified cereals	**Food Sources:** Sunflower seeds, almonds, vegetable oils, fortified cereals	**Food Sources:** Kale, spinach, turnip greens, brussels sprouts	**Food Sources:** Pork, fortified cereals, enriched rice and pasta, peas, tuna, beans	**Food Sources:** Beef liver, shrimp, dairy products, fortified cereals, enriched breads and grains	**Food Sources:** Chickpeas (garbanzo beans), red meat/fish/poultry, fortified cereals, potatoes

One vitamin with a unique source is vitamin D, which has many functions in your body, but is best known for its role in bone health. Your body is able to manufacture vitamin D from a cholesterol compound in your skin if you have adequate exposure to sunlight. For most people, this means about 5 to 30 minutes between the hours of 10 a.m. and 3 p.m. twice a week, on bare arms and legs, without sunscreen.[13] If you cannot get this much average sun exposure each week—for instance, during the winter in a cold climate, or year-round if you live in an area with heavy smog, then you need to make sure you consume enough vitamin D either in foods such as oily fish and fortified milks, or in supplements.

Vitamin Deficiencies and Toxicities

Because vitamins are readily available from the U.S. food supply, deficiencies among people in the United States are rare. However, there are exceptions. For example, people with dark skin need longer sun exposure to synthesize vitamin D, and consistently have lower levels of vitamin D in their blood than people with light skin. As noted earlier, people who avoid all animal-based foods are at increased risk for vitamin B_{12} deficiency. Finally, a deficiency of folate may develop in people who don't consume dark green vegetables, legumes, or fortified commercial breads and breakfast cereals. Women who don't get adequate folate in their diet before and after becoming pregnant are at increased risk for giving birth to a newborn with a neural tube defect, a serious and sometimes fatal birth defect in which the spinal cord fails to close properly. The critical period for healthy development of the neural tube is the first four weeks after conception, typically before a woman even realizes she is pregnant. For this reason, all women of childbearing age, whether or not they intend to become pregnant, are advised to consume 400 micrograms of folic acid daily either from a supplement or from fortified foods.[14]

The likelihood of consuming too much of any vitamin from food is remote. However, the amount in high-potency single-vitamin supplements can reach toxic levels. In contrast, a general multivitamin/

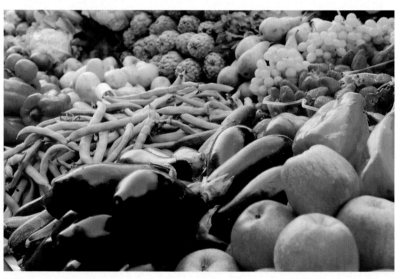

Vitamins and minerals are abundant in fruits and vegetables.

>> **For more detailed information on specific vitamins and minerals, visit Oregon State University's Micronutrient Information Center at** http://lpi.oregonstate.edu/infocenter/vitamins.html.

mineral supplement is often prescribed as "insurance" for children and teens, pregnant women, the elderly, and people with certain illnesses.

Minerals

Minerals are elements that cannot be made or broken down. Minerals in your diet come from a wide variety of plant and animal foods, and even from the water you drink.

minerals Elements, with no energy value of their own, that regulate body processes and provide structure.

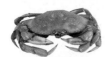 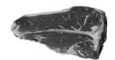

Water Soluble

Vitamin: B$_{12}$

Functions:

Assists with formation of blood; required for healthy nervous system

Food Sources:

Shellfish, red meat/fish/poultry, dairy products, fortified cereals

Water Soluble

Vitamin: Niacin

Functions:

Needed for carbohydrate and fat metabolism; assists in DNA replication and repair; assists in cell differentiation

Food Sources:

Beef liver, red meat/fish/poultry, fortified cereals, enriched breads and grains, canned tomato products

Water Soluble

Vitamin: Pantothenic acid

Functions:

Assists with fat metabolism

Food Sources:

Red meat/fish/poultry, mushrooms, fortified cereals, egg yolk

Water Soluble

Vitamin: Biotin

Functions:

Involved in carbohydrate, fat, and protein metabolism

Food Sources:

Nuts, egg yolk

Water Soluble

Vitamin: Folate (Folic acid)

Functions:

Needed for amino acid metabolism and DNA synthesis

Food Sources:

Fortified cereals, enriched breads and grains, legumes (lentils, chickpeas, pinto beans), spinach, romaine lettuce, asparagus, liver

Water Soluble

Vitamin: C

Functions:

Antioxidant; enhances immune function; assists in synthesis of important compounds; enhances iron absorption

Food Sources:

Sweet peppers, citrus fruits and juices, broccoli, strawberries, kiwi fruit

Source: Adapted from Thompson, Janice, and Melinda Manore, *Nutrition: An Applied Approach*, 3rd Ed., © 2012, pp. 218–219. Reprinted and Electronically reproduced by permission of Pearson Education, Inc., Upper Saddle River, New Jersey.

Your body relies on more than a dozen essential minerals each day to function, and many minerals provide structure. The *major minerals* are those your body needs in amounts greater than 100 milligrams daily. These include sodium, potassium, chloride, calcium, phosphorus, sulfur, and magnesium. You need *trace minerals* in much smaller amounts, typically less than 10 milligrams daily. The trace minerals include iron, fluoride, iodine, selenium, zinc, copper, manganese, and chromium. **Table 4.2** provides more information about selected minerals.

A varied and balanced diet provides most people with all the minerals they need in adequate amounts—not too low or too high. Single-mineral supplements are not recommended for most healthy people.

However, physicians sometimes prescribe iron supplements for patients at risk for iron-deficiency anemia, or fluoride drops to promote healthy tooth development for infants and toddlers who do not drink fluoridated water. Calcium supplements are often prescribed to help patients maintain healthy bone. For more on nutrition for bone health, see the **Spotlight** on page 80.

One major mineral commonly found to excess in the American diet is sodium. Although the recommended intake is about one teaspoon of salt per day, most Americans are thought to consume much more, largely through processed foods. This is a concern because some Americans are sodium sensitive, and high blood pressure is more

TABLE 4.2 Key Facts About Selected Minerals

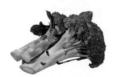 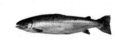

Mineral:

Calcium

Functions:

Primary component of bone; needed for acid-base balance, transmission of nerve impulses, and muscle contraction

Food Sources:

Dairy products, fortified juices, fish with bones (such as sardines or salmon), broccoli, kale, collard greens

Mineral:

Iron

Functions:

Helps transport oxygen in blood cells; assists many functional systems

Food Sources:

Clams, chicken, turkey, fish, ham

Mineral:

Magnesium

Functions:

Component of bone; aids in muscle contraction; assists many functional systems

Food Sources:

Oysters, beef, pork, chicken, turkey, tuna, lobster, shrimp, salmon, milk, yogurt, whole grain cereals, almonds, walnuts, sunflower seeds, beans

Mineral:

Potassium

Functions:

Needed for fluid balance, transmission of nerve impulses, and muscle contraction

Food Sources:

Fruits (bananas, oranges, grapefruit, plums), vegetables (spinach, beans)

Mineral:

Zinc

Functions:

Assists many functional systems; aids in immunity, growth, sexual maturation, and gene regulation

Food Sources:

Red meat, poultry, seafood (oysters, tuna, lobster)

Source: Adapted from Thompson, Janice, and Melinda Manore, *Nutrition: An Applied Approach*, 3rd Ed., ©2012. Reprinted and Electronically reproduced by permission of Pearson Education, Inc., Upper Saddle River, New Jersey.

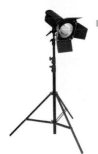

Feeding Your Bones

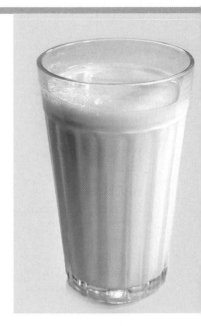

Osteoporosis is a disease characterized by brittle bones and decreased bone mass. You probably think of osteoporosis as a disease of the elderly, but even young adults can start to develop this disorder if they fail to nourish their bones.

Calcium is the main component of the mineral crystals that make up healthy bone. As you age from childhood to adulthood, your bones are not only lengthening, they're increasing in density. They do this by depositing calcium-containing crystals on a protein "scaffold" in the bone interior. If you don't consume enough calcium during these critical years, the supply will run short, and your bones won't be able to increase their density. From age 9 to 18, you should consume at least 1,300 milligrams of calcium a day. If you consider that an 8-ounce glass of milk contains about 300 milligrams of calcium, you can easily see that this level of daily calcium intake can be challenging to meet. After the age of 18, the requirement drops to 1,000 milligrams per day. Calcium is available in dairy foods such as milk, yogurt, and cheese; in green, leafy vegetables; and in fortified tofu, soy milk, rice milk, almond milk, and some juices.

Vitamin D is another important nutrient for bone health. Your body can absorb only a small fraction of the calcium you consume if your level of vitamin D is inadequate. Recall that you synthesize vitamin D in your skin if you have adequate exposure to sunlight. If you do not spend much time in the sun, you will need to obtain vitamin D through your diet or supplements. Food sources of vitamin D include fatty fish, and milk and other fortified foods.

What else can you do to keep your bones strong? Stay active. Any weight-bearing activity, from jumping rope to jogging to carrying textbooks up a flight of stairs, places positive stress on your skeleton and encourages your bones to increase their density.

---

common in these people if they consume a high-sodium diet. (See Chapter 12 for more information on high blood pressure.)

Water

You may be able to survive for weeks or even months without food, but you can live for only a few days without water. **Water** is dispersed throughout your body and is the medium in which most chemical reactions take place. It is vital, for instance, to nutrient digestion, absorption, and transportation. It also lubricates tissues, regulates body temperature, provides moisture to skin and other tissues, carries wastes out of the body, and contributes to a feeling of fullness when consumed with a meal.

Sources of Water

Nearly all foods contain water. On average, foods provide about 20% of an adult's total water intake. Beverages provide the remaining 80% of total water intake. Let's take a look at some commonly consumed beverages:[15]

- **Bottled water.** Plain drinking water hydrates your body and does not contribute calories that can lead to weight gain. Although it may be convenient, bottled water is typically no safer or more healthful than plain tap water, and its bottling and packaging takes a greater toll on the environment than filling your own reusable bottle or cup from the faucet.

- **Sports beverages.** Traditional sports drinks provide water, some minerals, and a source of carbohydrate. They can help athletes and manual laborers avoid fluid imbalances during strenuous physical activity lasting an hour or longer.

- **Milk and milk substitutes.** Soy milk and low-fat and skim cow's milk are healthful beverage choices, providing protein, calcium, vitamin D, and several other vitamins and minerals.

water A liquid composed of hydrogen and oxygen that is necessary for life.

- **Sweetened beverages.** In 2012, the New York City Board of Health approved a ban—subsequently overturned—on the sale of all sugary drinks larger than 16 ounces at city restaurants, movie theatres, and stadiums. Why? Most such beverages are loaded with added sugars, which some nutrition experts claim have contributed greatly to America's obesity problem. Whether in the form of high-fructose corn syrup, "pure cane sugar," honey, or "fruit juice concentrate," the added sugar provides the same 4 calories per gram, and as package sizes continue to increase, the calorie count for such beverages can be astronomical. Some registered dietitians are advising their overweight clients that their first step toward weight loss should be to entirely eliminate these products from their diet. Think this is a little extreme? Visit the **Consumer Corner** and check out the sugar and calorie contents of some popular beverages.

- **Beverages containing caffeine.** Coffee, tea, and hot cocoa all provide caffeine, a stimulant that can interfere with sleep. (See the electronic Chapter 16.) However, they can be healthful beverage choices if consumed in moderation, early in the day. Energy drinks vary greatly in their caffeine content, but on average contain as much as a strong cup of brewed coffee—about 150 milligrams.[16] Many contain far more, from 200 to as much as 500 milligrams per serving. Most also contain guarana, another source of caffeine. And whereas coffee is usually hot and must be sipped slowly, you can chug an energy drink, dumping a load of caffeine into your bloodstream. In 2012, the U.S. Food and Drug Administration (FDA) released a warning linking the consumption of energy drinks to thousands of emergency room visits and at least five deaths.[17]

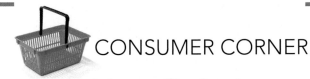

CONSUMER CORNER
Drinking Calories: What's in Your Bottle?

When you choose a beverage, whether from a vending machine or at the dining hall or deli, do you ever stop and read the Nutrition Facts panel on the bottle? If you did, you might be shocked to learn what's inside. Here are the sugar and calorie counts of some popular beverages. All product sizes are 16 ounces.

Snapple Lemon Iced Tea	11 ½ teaspoons of sugar	200 calories
Pepsi Cola	13 teaspoons of sugar	200 calories
Minute Maid Orange Juice	12 teaspoons of sugar	220 calories
Rockstar Energy Drink	15 ½ teaspoons of sugar	248 calories
Ocean Spray Cran-Apple Drink	16 teaspoons of sugar	260 calories
Nesquik Chocolate Milk	14 ½ teaspoons of sugar	400 calories

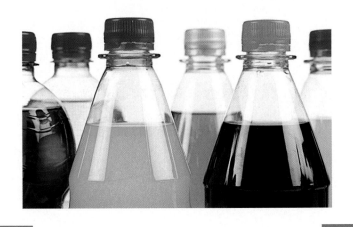

>> **Think you already know all there is to learn about caffeine? Take this test from Consumer Reports and find out!** www.consumerreports.org/cro/food/beverages/coffee-tea/test-your-caffeine-iq/index.htm.

Recommended Water Intake

You lose water every day through sweat, urine, feces, evaporation off your skin, and exhalation of breath from your lungs. Moreover, when you're feverish, or suffering from a runny nose, coughing, diarrhea, or vomiting, you lose more water. This explains why doctors advise you to drink plenty of fluids when you're sick.

Most adult women can maintain an adequate water intake by drinking 9 cups (2.2 liters) of beverages daily and men by drinking 13 cups

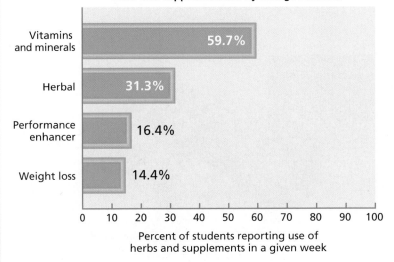

STUDENT STATS
Top Supplements Used by Students

Herb and supplement use by college students

- Vitamins and minerals: **59.7%**
- Herbal: **31.3%**
- Performance enhancer: **16.4%**
- Weight loss: **14.4%**

(x-axis: 0 10 20 30 40 50 60 70 80 90 100)

Percent of students reporting use of herbs and supplements in a given week

Data from *Over-the-Counter Medication and Herbal or Dietary Supplement Use in College: Dose Frequency and Relationship to Self-Reported Distress,* by M. Stasio, K. Curry, K. Sutton-Skinner, & D. Glassman, 2008, *Journal of the American College Health Association, 56* (5), pp. 535–547.

(3 liters) of beverages daily.[18] If you are physically active or live in a very hot climate, you may require more total water.

What About Dietary Supplements?

Do you regularly take dietary supplements? According to a survey of college students, about 70% used a dietary supplement in a given week.[19] Although supplements are popular, they are not without risk.

Dietary supplements are products taken by mouth that include ingredients such as vitamins, minerals, amino acids, herbs, or other compounds that are intended to supplement the diet. They are occasionally prescribed by an M.D.; for example, a doctor may prescribe iron supplements to a pregnant woman or fish-oil capsules to reduce a patient's risk for heart disease. However, "holistic" physicians such as osteopaths and naturopaths are more likely to prescribe a wider variety of dietary supplements, including herbs.

Types of Supplements

Certainly the most popular class of dietary supplements among Americans is multivitamin/mineral supplements (MVMs). More than one out of three Americans takes at least one MVM, and many people take more than one.[20]

dietary supplements Products taken by mouth that include ingredients such as vitamins, minerals, amino acids, or herbs intended to supplement the diet.

When you're **hungry**, nutrition may not be the first thing on your mind, but making healthful choices is still important. To eat well in a healthy way:

CHOOSE THIS.   NOT THAT.

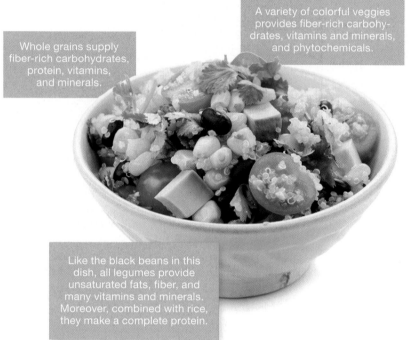

Whole grains supply fiber-rich carbohydrates, protein, vitamins, and minerals.

A variety of colorful veggies provides fiber-rich carbohydrates, vitamins and minerals, and phytochemicals.

Like the black beans in this dish, all legumes provide unsaturated fats, fiber, and many vitamins and minerals. Moreover, combined with rice, they make a complete protein.

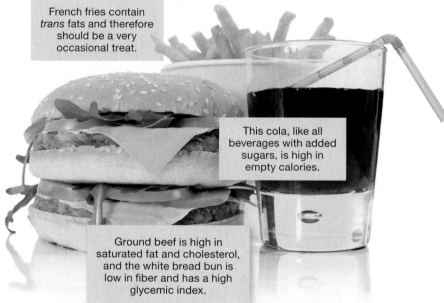

French fries contain *trans* fats and therefore should be a very occasional treat.

This cola, like all beverages with added sugars, is high in empty calories.

Ground beef is high in saturated fat and cholesterol, and the white bread bun is low in fiber and has a high glycemic index.

A Healthful Lunch:

Plant-based meals are naturally rich in healthful unsaturated fats, fiber, and micronutrients. They provide plenty of protein, and have a low glycemic index. And they're delicious!

A High-Fat Lunch:

The foods in this meal are full of empty calories and provide very few healthful nutrients and little fiber.

As shown in the **Student Stats** on page 81, MVMs are also the most popular type used by college students.

Botanical supplements, commonly referred to as *herbs*, are also popular. These are plants or plant parts used for their therapeutic properties. Common preparations include capsules, teas, and extracts. Botanical supplements vary greatly in their potency and safety. For example, ginger, chamomile, and peppermint taken as teas to aid digestion are considered mild and generally safe. In contrast, peppermint oil can be toxic. The fact that a product is manufactured from a plant does not necessarily mean it is "natural" or safe to consume. In fact, several botanical supplements can have harmful effects.

Another popular class of supplements is known as *ergogenic aids*. These are substances used to enhance exercise and athletic performance. If you're considering using such a product, consult with your team physician or regular physician before investing your money. Most are a waste of money and some are even dangerous. Some ergogenic aids are used to increase energy during training and competition, usually by optimizing the body's fuel use. Carnitine, chromium, and ribose are among the most popular of this group, and research results indicate that none of the three have been found to have any benefit.[21] Steroids, another class of ergogenic aids, increase the risk of cardiovascular disease, cancer, liver damage, and other disorders, and can lead to masculinization in women and feminization in men.[21] (To learn more about steroids and other performance-enhancing drugs, see Chapter 5.)

How can ineffective or even dangerous supplements make their way onto the market? Doesn't the FDA regulate supplement safety? The short answer is no. Whereas the FDA requires extensive research supporting a prescription or over-the-counter (OTC) drug's safety and efficacy before it can be sold, supplements do not get this same scrutiny. Federal laws bar supplement advertisements from making specific claims about benefits that haven't been proven (supplement advertisements, for example, cannot promise the product will cure cancer). But there are no regulations for the general claims these ads can make. You may commonly come across supplement advertisements featuring vague statements or leading questions such as "Stay healthy!" or "Need more energy?" There may be no scientific research to back up such language. Also, be aware that a supplement may tout itself as free of one risky ingredient, but that doesn't mean it is free of other harmful substances. Finally, the FDA has the authority to remove a supplement from the market only after it has proven that the supplement is unsafe.

Before taking any dietary supplements, consider these guidelines:

- Talk with your doctor first—especially if you are currently taking any medications, are pregnant, are trying to become pregnant, or have any chronic medical conditions. Some supplements can be inappropriate or even harmful for certain populations. Factors such as your diet, age, health status, and use of prescription and OTC drugs can all affect whether or not a dietary supplement is appropriate for you.

- Look for the USP verification mark. This symbol on the label doesn't guarantee that the supplement has any particular therapeutic action, but it does indicate that the product meets minimum safety and purity standards as set forth by U.S. Pharmacopeia, a nonprofit organization.

- Choose brands made by nationally known manufacturers. These products likely have higher processing and production standards.

- Avoid supplements that contain high doses of a single vitamin or mineral, unless prescribed. Some products containing such "mega-doses" may be toxic. This is especially true for the fat-soluble vitamins A, D, E, and K, as excesses are stored in body fat and can build up over time to harmful levels. Vitamin A is especially toxic: Excessive intakes can cause organ damage and, during pregnancy, can result in birth defects or spontaneous abortion.

 For additional tips on evaluating dietary supplements, visit the FDA's website at www.fda.gov/Food/DietarySupplements **or the National Center for Complementary and Alternative Medicine's "Herbs at a Glance" page:** http://nccam.nih.gov/health/herbsataglance.htm.

Other Healthful Substances in Foods

Today, people are increasingly interested in consuming *functional foods*; that is, foods that confer some kind of health benefit in addition to the benefits provided by their basic nutrients. For example, researchers are studying non-nutrient substances in food that may improve your digestion, boost your immunity, delay aging, or prevent heart disease or cancer. Although many such non-nutrient substances are currently under investigation, we'll limit our discussion to those you're most likely to hear about—these are phytochemicals, antioxidants, probiotics, and prebiotics.

Phytochemicals

Phytochemicals are naturally occurring chemicals in plants (*phyto-* means "plant") that may have health benefits, but are not considered essential nutrients. Sources of phytochemicals include fruits, legumes and other vegetables, nuts, seeds, and grains. Phytochemicals include:

- Carotenoids, which may help reduce the risk of cardiovascular disease, certain cancers, and age-related eye diseases. Carotenoids are found in red, orange, and deep-green foods such as tomatoes, carrots, and kale.

- Flavonoids, which may help reduce the risk of cardiovascular disease and cancer. They are found in foods like berries, black and green tea, chocolate, and soy products.

- Organosulfur compounds, which may help protect against cancer. They are found in foods like garlic, onions, broccoli, cauliflower, and cabbage.

It is likely that the health benefits of phytochemicals are the result of many of them working together along with other substances in foods.[22] Phytochemical supplements (that is, those found in pill form) can't begin to imitate the qualities of natural foods, have not been shown to be beneficial, and may even be dangerous.

In addition to phytochemicals, of course, fruits and vegetables provide fiber and many different vitamins and minerals. So it's no wonder that many nutrition experts recommend that you consume 5 to 9 servings of fruits and vegetables a day. How many college students actually do that? In a 2012 survey, fewer than 6% of college students said that they usually eat at least 5 servings of fruits and vegetables a day.[23]

Antioxidants

As part of your day-to-day body functioning, chemical reactions called *oxidation reactions* continually occur. Although normal, oxidation reactions commonly produce harmful chemicals called *free radicals*, which start chain reactions that can damage cells. Environmental factors such as pollution, sunlight, and cigarette smoke also contribute to free radical production. Damage from free radicals has been linked to cancer, cardiovascular disease, Alzheimer's dementia, and other disorders.

 Want to find out how many fruits and veggies you should eat each day, in cups? Or find recipes to help you increase your fruit and veggie intake? Check out the activities on Fruits & Veggies: More Matters, at www.fruitsandveggiesmorematters.org.

It is impossible for you to avoid producing free radicals; however, certain components of foods can help neutralize them. These substances are generally referred to as **antioxidants** because they work against oxidation. Some antioxidants are nutrients: These include vitamins C and E, beta-carotene (a form of vitamin A), and the mineral selenium. Many other antioxidants are phytochemicals.

Antioxidants are plentiful in fruits, legumes and other vegetables, whole grains, and nuts. Some processed foods are great sources. Commercial

phytochemicals Naturally occurring plant substances thought to have disease-preventing and health-promoting properties.

antioxidants Compounds in food that help protect the body from harmful molecules called free radicals.

Fixing a Poor Diet

"HI, I'M PETER. I was raised on Wonder bread, soda, and a lot of fast food. I didn't think much about what I ate—everyone I knew ate the same way. Now that I'm in college, I have some friends who are super health-conscious. One is a vegetarian, and another will only eat organic food from crazy expensive supermarkets. I like meat too much to ever become vegetarian, and I don't have the money to buy fancy food. But my doctor recently told me I am at risk of becoming diabetic, because of my diet and my weight. I want to change my diet, but I need it to work for me. What should I do?"

1. Given what you've learned, how would you advise Peter? What are examples of foods in each of the six classes of nutrients that you would encourage him to eat?

2. What are examples of foods you would encourage Peter to avoid or minimize in his diet? Why are those foods poor choices?

3. Eating on a budget is an issue for most college students. How can Peter eat nutritiously without spending a fortune?

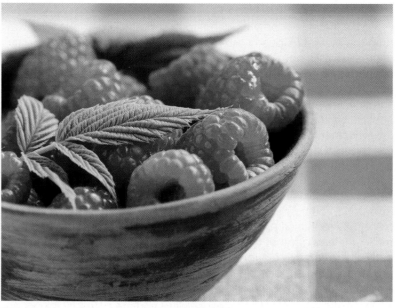

Raspberries are a rich source of antioxidants.

Probiotics and Prebiotics

Probiotics are living, beneficial microbes that develop naturally in fermented dairy foods such as yogurt, buttermilk, and kefir, as well as in fermented vegetable foods such as sauerkraut, miso, and tempeh (fermented tofu). The most common are types of bacteria. If deliberately consuming foods full of live bacteria sounds less than appealing to you, consider that your body already contains at least ten times more bacterial than body cells, and that the vast majority of these bacteria are either harmless or make important contributions to your health. In fact, *probiotic* means "pro-life."

Research into our body's resident bacteria indicates that they promote good health by crowding out harmful bacteria, viruses, and yeasts; producing nutrients, including certain vitamins; promoting bowel regularity; assisting your immune system; degrading potential carcinogens (cancer-causing agents); and helping the body use energy and avoid building up body fat.[25, 26] The bacteria you consume in probiotic foods are thought to exert similar beneficial effects.

Bear in mind that, when you consume a probiotic food, the bacteria adhere to the lining of your intestinal tract for only a few days, so it is important to eat them regularly. They are available in supplements, too.

Another way to increase your population of beneficial bacteria is to consume foods containing **prebiotics.** These are nondigestible food ingredients (typically carbohydrates) that stimulate the growth and/or activity of beneficial bacteria in the large intestine (the colon).[27] An example is inulin, a carbohydrate found in a few fruits, onions, green vegetables, and grains, and added to some processed foods. Prebiotics don't feed you, because they pass through the GI tract without being digested or absorbed. Rather, when they reach the large intestine, they "feed" the helpful bacteria there.

tomato sauce, for instance, is higher in antioxidant phytochemicals than fresh tomatoes, and brewed coffee and tea are both rich in antioxidants.

Although you have numerous choices for antioxidant-rich foods, the United States Department of Agriculture (USDA) has found the following foods to be highest in antioxidants:[24]

- **Fruits.** Wild blueberries top the list, but other berries, cherries, apples, plums, and prunes are included, too.
- **Legumes and other vegetables.** Several types of beans are in this category, as well as artichoke hearts and russet potatoes.
- **Other foods.** Pecans make the list. Also, many cocoa products, especially dark (bittersweet) chocolate, retain a high level of antioxidants.

Fruits and vegetables not on the USDA's list also provide antioxidants—just in smaller amounts. To retain the antioxidants in cooked vegetables, don't boil them. Instead, steam or stir-fry. These cooking methods also preserve more of the vegetable's vitamins.

> **To find out what fruits and veggies are in season this month in your area, click on the U.S. map at** www.epicurious.com/articlesguides/seasonalcooking/farmtotable/seasonalingredientmap.

probiotics Living, beneficial microbes that develop naturally in food and that help maintain digestive functions.

prebiotics Nondigestible food ingredients that benefit human health by stimulating the growth and/or activity of beneficial bacteria in the large intestine.

Tools to Help You Eat Right

You've learned how nutrients and other health-promoting substances function in your body. But how much of each nutrient do you need each day, and how do you choose real foods to meet those nutrient needs? In this section, you'll learn how to use four tools to help you eat right.

Learn About the Dietary Reference Intakes (DRIs)

For more than 50 years, scientists have provided consumers with a set of energy and nutrient standards to protect against nutrient deficiencies, support healthy functioning, and prevent chronic diseases. These recommendations are called the **Dietary Reference Intakes (DRIs).** The DRIs include six groups of recommendations **(Figure 4.3)**:[2]

- **Estimated Average Requirement (EAR).** The amount of a nutrient that meets the needs of half the people of a given age and gender. EARs are not very useful for consumers, but food scientists use them to calculate the RDAs.

- **Recommended Dietary Allowance (RDA).** The intake of a nutrient that is proposed to meet the needs of 98% of all healthy people of similar age and gender.

- **Adequate Intake (AI).** The amount of a nutrient that appears to be sufficient to maintain health. The AI is used as a guide to nutrient intake when an RDA cannot be determined. In other words, a nutrient has either an RDA or an AI, but not both.

- **Tolerable Upper Intake Level (UL).** The maximum amount of a nutrient that appears to be safe for most healthy people to consume daily. This level is not, however, the recommended intake.

- **Estimated Energy Requirement (EER).** The average number of calories needed per day to maintain health and neither gain nor lose weight. Obviously, this will vary according to your gender, age, height, weight, and level of physical activity.

- **Acceptable Macronutrient Distribution Range (AMDR).** This DRI is specific to the energy-yielding nutrients. It defines a healthful range of carbohydrate, fat, or protein intake expressed as a percentage of your total daily calories **(Table 4.3)**. As an example, the AMDR for fat is 20–35%, so if you typically consume 2,000 calories per day, a healthful fat intake would range between 400 and 700 calories.

 You can access DRI tables online at the USDA's Food and Nutrition Information Center at http://fnic.nal.usda.gov/dietary-guidance/dietary-reference-intakes.

Do all these values seem confusing? For most people, they are. That's why many government agencies have developed tools that present the DRIs in more meaningful ways. One such tool is the food label found on nearly all packaged foods sold in the United States.

Read Food Labels

Food labels provide a lot of helpful information—if you read them! In addition to identifying the product and manufacturer, they include a list of all ingredients in the food in descending order by weight. So if you're considering buying a carton of yogurt and notice that sugar is the third ingredient on the list, you might want to choose another brand.

Nutrition Facts Panel

An especially helpful part of food labels is the *Nutrition Facts* panel, which provides nutrient information required by the FDA (see **Figure 4.4** on page 86). On the panel you'll find the recommended serving size for this food, as well as the number of servings per package, the calories, and the calories from fat per serving. If you're watching your calorie intake, you should know that a food that has about 40 or fewer calories per serving is considered low in calories, and 400 or more is high.[28]

Beneath this line, the panel identifies the macronutrients, sodium, and fiber found in a serving of the food. Notice that both saturated fat and *trans* fat are listed to inform you of the quantity of these unhealthful fats provided by this food.

Percent Daily Value

If you wanted to compare the amount of fiber in two different breakfast cereals you were

> **Dietary Reference Intakes (DRIs)**
> A set of energy and nutrient recommendations for supporting good health

Dietary Reference Intakes (DRIs)	
DRIs for most nutrients	**DRIs for energy and macronutrients**
Estimated Average Requirement (EAR)	Estimated Energy Requirement (EER)
Recommended Dietary Allowance (RDA)	Acceptable Macronutrient Distribution Range (AMDR)
Adequate Intake (AI)	
Tolerable Upper Intake Level (UL)	

FIGURE 4.3 Dietary Reference Intakes (DRIs). Most of the DRIs recommend specific amounts to consume, but the AMDR recommends a percentage of your daily calories that should be consumed as carbohydrate, fat, or protein.

Source: Adapted from Thompson, Janice, and Melinda Manore, *Nutrition: An Applied Approach,* 3rd Ed., © 2012, p. 16. Reprinted and Electronically reproduced by permission of Pearson Education, Inc., Upper Saddle River, New Jersey.

TABLE 4.3 Acceptable Macronutrient Distribution Range (AMDR)

Nutrient	AMDR*
Carbohydrate	45–65%
Fat	20–35%
Protein	10–35%

*AMDR values are expressed as percentages of total energy or as percentages of total calories.

Data from *2005 Dietary Reference Intakes for Energy, Carbohydrates, Fiber, Fat, Fatty Acids, Cholesterol, Protein, and Amino Acids (Macronutrients),* by the Institute of Medicine, Food and Nutrition Board, 2005, Washington, DC: National Academies Press.

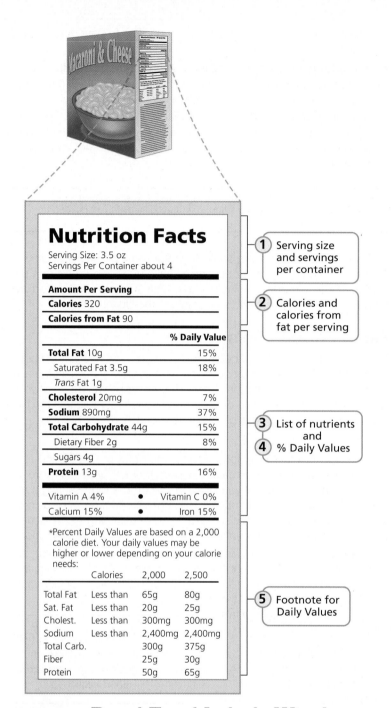

Nutrition Facts

Serving Size: 3.5 oz
Servings Per Container about 4

Amount Per Serving

Calories 320

Calories from Fat 90

	% Daily Value
Total Fat 10g	15%
Saturated Fat 3.5g	18%
Trans Fat 1g	
Cholesterol 20mg	7%
Sodium 890mg	37%
Total Carbohydrate 44g	15%
Dietary Fiber 2g	8%
Sugars 4g	
Protein 13g	16%

Vitamin A 4%	•	Vitamin C 0%
Calcium 15%	•	Iron 15%

*Percent Daily Values are based on a 2,000 calorie diet. Your daily values may be higher or lower depending on your calorie needs:

	Calories	2,000	2,500
Total Fat	Less than	65g	80g
Sat. Fat	Less than	20g	25g
Cholest.	Less than	300mg	300mg
Sodium	Less than	2,400mg	2,400mg
Total Carb.		300g	375g
Fiber		25g	30g
Protein		50g	65g

1. Serving size and servings per container
2. Calories and calories from fat per serving
3. List of nutrients and
4. % Daily Values
5. Footnote for Daily Values

FIGURE 4.4 Read Food Labels Wisely. When reading a Nutrition Facts panel, note the serving size, calories (and calories from fat) per serving, and the nutrients contained per serving.

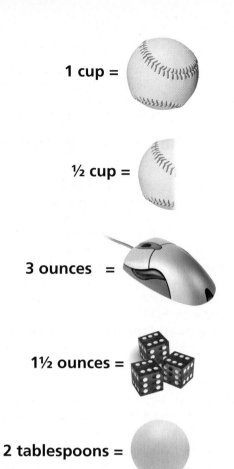

1 cup =

½ cup =

3 ounces =

1½ ounces =

2 tablespoons =

FIGURE 4.5 Estimating Serving Sizes. Comparing food amounts to common household items can help you estimate the serving sizes of your foods.

in this column give you a rough estimate of how much a serving of the food contributes to the overall intake of nutrients in a "typical" 2,000-calorie diet.[28] So if you usually eat about 2,000 calories a day, and your favorite brand of corn flakes provided just 4% of your % DV for fiber, another cereal might be a better choice.

Even if your daily calorie needs are higher or lower than 2,000, you can still use the % DV to help you judge the nutritional quality of a food: 5% DV or less is a low level for that nutrient, whereas 20% or more is high. So a frozen veggie burger that provided 5% of the DV for saturated fat, 0% for cholesterol, and 24% for protein would be a nutritious choice.

If the package is large enough, the bottom of the Nutrition Facts panel will include a footnote identifying the recommended daily intake of six nutrients, plus fiber, for adults eating either a 2,000- or a 2,500-calorie diet. For example, you should keep your daily sodium intake below 2,400 milligrams, but you notice that a small serving of this packaged mac and cheese dinner would provide more than a third of your daily limit! Would you purchase this food?

Use the % DV whenever possible. Consider not only the serving size, but also how many servings you will actually consume. If you will eat double the serving size listed on the package, then you must also double the calories, nutrients, and % DV. To help you interpret the serving sizes listed on food labels, see **Figure 4.5**.

considering buying, all you'd need to consider is the number of grams of fiber per serving on each label. But let's say you wanted to make sure that you meet your need for fiber each day, and would like to find out what *percentage* a serving of your favorite breakfast cereal would contribute toward your daily need. For that, you'd look at the right-hand column of the Nutrition Facts panel to find the **percent Daily Value (% DV).** The percentages

percent Daily Value (% DV)
Nutrient standards that estimate how much a serving of a given food contributes to the overall intake of nutrients listed on the food label.

Label Claims

Milk is milk, right? So how come one carton just identifies the name of the farm, whereas another claims, "Excellent source of calcium!" And would that claim influence you to choose that brand of milk, even if a comparison of the Nutrition Facts panels showed that both brands provide the identical 30% DV for calcium? Food marketers are hoping it would. Are such ploys legal? Actually, they are.

The FDA allows food companies to put two types of claims on food labels:

- **Nutrient claims.** These draw your attention to the amount of a given nutrient in the food. For instance, a brand of soup may boast that it's "low sodium" and "a good source of fiber." Nutrient claims must be supported by the DV identified on the Nutrition Facts panel. For example, a juice cannot claim "Excellent source of calcium!" unless it provides 20% or more of the DV for calcium.

- **Health claims.** The FDA also allows food labels to include a small number of strictly worded claims related to dietary influences on human health. These claims cannot, however, suggest that eating the given product will improve the consumer's health. For example, an approved health claim on a low-fat, high-fiber, whole oat cereal might state: "Three grams of soluble fiber from oatmeal daily in a diet low in saturated fat and cholesterol may reduce the risk of heart disease. This cereal has 2 grams per serving."[29]

The FDA allows, but does not regulate, a third type of claim related to a product's contribution to human structure or function. Examples of such structure/function claims are "Builds stronger bones" and "Immune system support." When you see such claims on food labels, bear in mind that there's no guarantee they're true.

Follow the *Dietary Guidelines for Americans*

The *Dietary Guidelines for Americans* has been published jointly every five years since 1980 by the U.S. Department of Health and Human Services (HHS) and the U.S. Department of Agriculture (USDA). The 2010 Guidelines provide expert advice for achieving and maintaining a healthy weight, and reducing your risk for chronic disease. See page 88 for the key messages.

Log Onto MyPlate

In May 2011, the USDA released an interactive, personalized guide to healthy eating called MyPlate. When you log onto **www.choosemyplate.gov,** you can:

- Learn about different foods and food groups
- Analyze your current diet and physical activity level
- Get a personalized daily food plan
- Find tips for healthy eating and for increasing physical activity
- Learn how to plan healthy menus
- Get information on how to lose weight

MyPlate also includes a simple but vibrant graphic representing the recommended types and amounts of foods you should eat at each meal. The relative portion sizes of each of the five food groups—vegetables, fruits, grains, protein foods, and dairy—are indicated in the plate graphic with segments of five different sizes and colors **(Figure 4.6)**.

Food Groups in MyPlate

What foods are in each of the five groups? Let's take a look.[30]

Vegetables. As you can see in Figure 4.6, the vegetable group is the largest of the five. In fact, fruits and vegetables together should make up half your plate! Any vegetable or 100% vegetable juice counts as

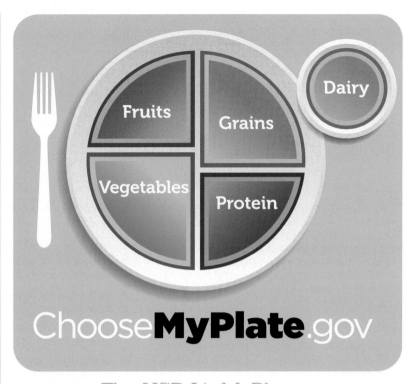

FIGURE 4.6 The USDA's MyPlate. To generate your personalized MyPlate plan, visit www.choosemyplate.gov.

Source: U.S. Department of Agriculture, 2011. www.choosemyplate.gov.

a member of the vegetable group. Vegetables may be raw or cooked, fresh, frozen, canned, or dried. Common examples are dark green vegetables like broccoli and collard greens; red-orange vegetables such as carrots and red peppers; starchy vegetables like corn and potatoes; and miscellaneous others such as beets, mushrooms, and onions.

The fifth subset of the vegetables group is legumes, which include beans, peas, and lentils. Legumes are in the vegetable group because they're excellent sources of the dietary fiber and micronutrients available from other vegetables. However, they're also included in the protein foods group because they provide abundant plant protein as well as two minerals—iron and zinc—that we normally associate with meat. In fact, many people consider legumes the vegetarian alternative for meat. In recognition of their abundant protein, micronutrients, and fiber—not to mention the fact that they're naturally low in fat—the USDA recommends that everyone, including meat eaters, consume legumes at least a few times a week, if not every day.

Fruits. Both whole fruit and 100% fruit juice count as fruit choices. Fruit can be canned, frozen, puréed, or dried. Berries, citrus fruits, apples, bananas, grapes, raisins, and fruit cocktail are common choices.

Grains. Any food made from wheat, rice, oats, cornmeal, barley, or another cereal grain is a grain product. Bread, pasta, oatmeal, breakfast cereals, tortillas, and grits are examples of grain foods. The USDA recommends that you make at least half of your daily grain choices whole grains.

Protein Foods. Meats, poultry, seafood, eggs, legumes, processed soy products, nuts, and seeds are considered part of the protein foods group. Meat should be lean, and you should avoid eating the skin of poultry. Include at least 8 ounces of seafood a week (typically, two servings). Everyone, not just vegetarians, should choose legumes at least a few times a week in place of animal-based proteins.

Dietary Guidelines: A Blueprint for Better Nutrition

The *Dietary Guidelines for Americans, 2010*, are intended to help Americans achieve and sustain a healthy weight, and to focus on consuming foods and beverages high in nutrients and low in empty calories. These actions can reduce the risk of chronic disease and promote overall health. The following tips can help you incorporate the Guidelines into your life.

Build a Healthy Plate

Before you eat, think about what goes on your plate or in your cup or bowl. Foods like vegetables, fruits, whole grains, low-fat dairy products, and lean protein foods contain the nutrients you need without too many calories. Try some of these options.

Make Half Your Plate Fruits and Vegetables

- Eat red, orange, and dark green vegetables, such as tomatoes, sweet potatoes, and broccoli, in main and side dishes.
- Eat fruit, vegetables, or unsalted nuts as snacks—they are nature's original fast foods.

Switch to Skim or 1% Milk

- They have the same amount of calcium and other essential nutrients as whole milk, but less fat and fewer calories.
- Try calcium-fortified milk alternatives.

Make at Least Half Your Grains Whole

- Choose 100% whole grain cereals, breads, crackers, rice, and pasta.
- Check the ingredients list on food packages to find whole grain foods.

Vary Your Protein Food Choices

- Twice a week, make seafood the protein on your plate.
- Choose beans or lentils daily.
- Keep meat and poultry portions small and lean.

Cut Back on Foods High in Solid Fats, Added Sugars, and Salt

Many people eat foods high in solid fats, added sugars, and salt (sodium). Added sugars and fats load foods with empty calories. Too much sodium may increase your blood pressure.

- Make major sources of saturated fats—such as cakes, cookies, ice cream, pizza, cheese, sausages, and hot dogs—occasional choices, not everyday foods.

- Select lean cuts of meat or poultry and fat-free or low-fat milk, yogurt, and cheese.
- Switch from solid fats to oils when preparing food.*
- Drink water instead of sugary drinks. There are about 10 packets of sugar in a 12-ounce soda.
- Select fruit for dessert. Eat sweets less often.
- Choose 100% fruit juice instead of fruit-flavored drinks.
- Compare sodium in foods like soup, bread, and frozen meals—and choose the foods with lower numbers.
- Add spices or herbs to season food without adding salt.

Eat the Right Amount of Calories for You

Everyone has a personal calorie limit. Staying within yours can help you maintain a healthy weight. People who are successful at managing their weight have found ways to keep track of how much they eat in a day, even if they don't count every calorie. Try these tips.

- Get your personal daily calorie limit at **www.choosemyplate.gov** and keep that number in mind when deciding what to eat.
- Think before you eat . . . is it worth the calories?
- Avoid oversized portions.
- Use a smaller plate, bowl, and glass.
- Stop eating when you are satisfied, not full.
- Cook more often at home, where you are in control of what's in your food
- When eating out, choose lower calorie menu options, such as dishes that include vegetables, fuits, and whole grains.
- Order a smaller portion or share when eating out.
- If you drink alcoholic beverages, do so sensibly—1 drink a day for women or 2 drinks a day for men.

Be Physically Active Your Way

Pick activities that you like and start by doing what you can, at least 10 minutes at a time. Every bit adds up, and the health benefits increase as you spend more time being active.

Use Food Labels to Help You Make Better Choices

- Most packaged foods have a Nutrition Facts label and an ingredients list. For a healthier you, use this tool to make smart food choices quickly and easily.
- Check for calories. Be sure to look at the serving size and how many servings you are actually consuming. If you double the servings you eat, you double the calories.
- Choose foods with lower calories, saturated fat, *trans* fat, and sodium.
- Check for added sugars using the ingredients list. When a sugar is close to first on the ingredients list, the food is high in added sugars. Some names for added sugars include sucrose, glucose, high-fructose corn syrup, corn syrup, maple syrup, and fructose.

 To view the full set of 2010 *Dietary Guidelines for Americans,* **visit** www.health.gov/dietaryguidelines**.**

Source: Adapted from *Let's Eat: For the Health of It,* by the U.S. Department of Agriculture, June 2011. USDA Publication number: Home and Garden Bulletin No. 232-CP; HHS Publication number: HHS-ODPHP-2010-01-DGA-B.

* Examples of solid fats: Beef, pork, and chicken fat; butter, cream, and milk fat; coconut, palm, and palm kernel oils; hydrogenated oil; partially hydrogenated oil; shortening; stick margarine. Examples of oils: Canola oil; corn oil; cottonseed oil; olive oil; peanut oil; safflower oil; sunflower oil; tub (soft) margarine; vegetable oil.

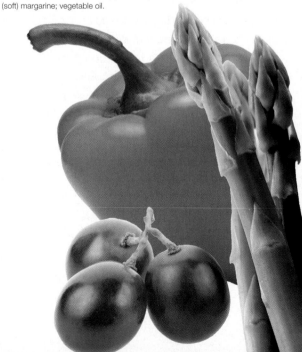

Dairy. Both cow's milk and calcium-fortified milk alternatives are dairy choices, as are cheeses, yogurt, and milk-based desserts such as frozen yogurt, ice cream, and pudding. The USDA recommends low-fat or skim dairy choices.

What About Oils? Although they are not one of the five food groups, oils—fats that are liquid at room temperature—provide essential nutrients, and you should consume them daily. If you eat nuts (including peanut butter), fish, and/or salad dressings, or cook with oils, you are probably already meeting your needs.

Empty Calories

You've probably heard the recommendation to consume **nutrient-dense foods.** These are foods that provide a high level of healthful nutrients for a low number of calories. Peanut butter on whole grain bread is a nutrient-dense snack because it provides abundant plant protein, plant oils, complex carbohydrates, and micronutrients (not to mention fiber and antioxidant phytochemicals) for a relatively low number of calories.

Notice that a peanut butter sandwich is also very low in saturated fat, has no cholesterol, and although it has a few grams of natural sugar, contains no added sugars. In other words, it is free of **empty calories.** These are calories from solid fats and/or added sugars that provide few or no nutrients. The USDA recommends that you limit the empty calories you eat. Examples of foods loaded with empty calories are cookies, cakes, doughnuts, candies, alcohol, soft drinks, sausages, hot dogs, bacon, and ribs.

How Much of Each Group Do You Need?

Now that you know what the five food groups are, you might be wondering *how much* of each food group you should eat. There's no one-size-fits-all answer: The amounts you need are determined according to your age, gender, height, current weight, and activity level. To learn your unique needs, log onto **www.choosemyplate.gov** and click on "Get a personalized plan." Fill out the information requested, and in seconds you'll learn not only how much of each food group you need, but also how many calories you should consume daily, including your allotment of empty calories. The program will also let you know if you're currently underweight or overweight, and offer advice for moving toward a healthier weight.

When your plan appears, you'll notice that the recommended daily intakes of vegetables, fruits, and dairy are given in cups. For example, 1 cup of carrot juice, orange juice, or milk qualifies as a cup, as does 1 cup of sliced carrots, orange wedges, or yogurt. In a few cases, however, a cup is not a cup! Lettuce and other leafy green vegetables are high-volume items: 2 cups is equivalent to a 1-cup serving. In contrast, dried fruits are dense, so ½ cup counts as a 1-cup serving. And what about cheese? Two cups of cottage cheese, 1 ½ ounces of hard cheese, and ⅓ cup of shredded cheese all count as 1-cup servings.

Recommended amounts of grains and protein foods are given in ounces and *ounce-equivalents*, which, as their name implies, are serving sizes that are equivalent to an ounce. For instance, an egg, 3 cups of popcorn, ½ cup of cooked pasta, and ½ ounce of sunflower seeds all qualify as ounce-equivalents. For more examples, see **Figure 4.7.**

nutrient-dense foods Any food in which the proportion of healthful nutrients is high relative to the number of calories.

empty calories Calories from solid fats, alcohol, and/or added sugars that provide few or no nutrients.

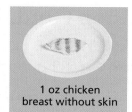
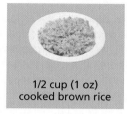
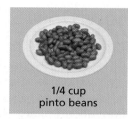

1 oz pork loin chop | 1 oz chicken breast without skin | 1/4 cup pinto beans

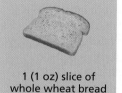
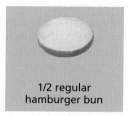

1 (1 oz) slice of whole wheat bread | 1/2 cup (1 oz) cooked brown rice | 1/2 regular hamburger bun

FIGURE 4.7 What's an "Ounce-equivalent"?
Here are sample 1-"ounce-equivalent" servings of various meats, beans, and grains.

>> When you visit www.choosemyplate.gov, you'll be guided to develop an eating plan tailored to your specific sex, age, current weight, and level of activity. You can also enter the foods you've eaten over one or more days and find out how closely your diet corresponds to the *Dietary Guidelines for Americans*.

Why I'm Vegetarian

"HI, I'M NIDYA. I am a vegetarian and I decided to become one basically because of my cousin. She's also a vegetarian and she showed me a PETA video that showed how they treated animals when they kill them for food. So I guess ever since then I've been kind of traumatized and I stopped eating meat. That was about two years ago.

In my household, since my family is Mexican, there's meat every day. So instead I eat a lot of beans and rice and fish and also vegetables, fruits, and salads, so I usually get all my nutrients."

1. What type of vegetarian is Nidya, as her diet includes fish?

2. Is Nidya eating any complementary proteins? If so, what are they?

3. What are the benefits and drawbacks of Nidya's diet?

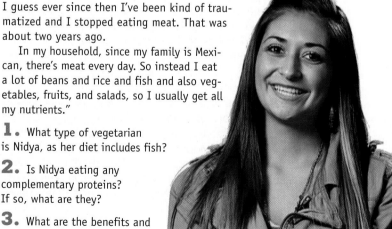

How Do Nutrition Guidelines Vary for Different Groups?

Because of our age, gender, level of physical activity, or diet preferences, we all have unique nutrition needs. The DRIs for all nutrients and all life stages can be found at **http://ods.od.nih.gov/Health_Information/Dietary_Reference_Intakes.aspx**. Here, we discuss a few of the key differences.

At different ages, people need different amounts of nutrients. For example, to promote bone density, children and teens aged 9 to 18 actually need more calcium (1,300 mg/day) than adults do (1,000 mg/day). In fact, calcium needs are never higher, even during pregnancy. Older adults, in contrast, need to consume more vitamin B_6 and vitamin D, but have slightly decreased needs for iron and fiber. Moreover, many mature adults have a reduced ability to absorb naturally occurring vitamin B_{12}, but are able to absorb the synthetic form. For this reason, although the recommended amount of B_{12} intake doesn't change, the source does: Older adults are encouraged to eat foods with added vitamin B_{12} or take the vitamin as a supplement.

Because most men are larger, taller, and have more muscle mass (lean muscle tissue) than most women, they require more calories. For the same reason, men and women also have somewhat different needs for many vitamins and minerals.

Athletes and others who engage in regular, vigorous exercise require the same micronutrients as non-athletes, but need to pay more attention to meeting energy needs and consuming fluids.[31] Although they have the same AMDR for the macronutrients as sedentary adults, they may need somewhat more protein per pound (or kilogram) of body weight, and more total energy. The precise recommendations vary according to the intensity, frequency, and duration of activity.

Fluids, especially water, are important to health and athletic performance. Drink plenty of fluids before, during, and after exercise or competition. If you work out vigorously for longer than one hour, drinking a sports beverage rather than plain water is recommended.

People who follow a **vegetarian** diet may also have unique nutrition needs. See the **Diversity & Health** box on the next page for more details.

>> The MyPlate site provides some tips and resources for vegetarians: www.choosemyplate.gov/healthy-eating-tips/tips-for-vegetarian.html.

Is Our Food Supply Safe?

In early 2009, a nationwide outbreak of illness caused by contaminated peanut products killed 9 people in the United States and sickened over 700 more.[32] In response to this and other outbreaks, the U.S. Congress passed legislation that would require more frequent inspections of food processing plants and would give the FDA greater authority to order the recall of tainted food. Later that year, a new national website, **www.foodsafety.gov**, was launched to provide Americans with a "gateway" to food safety tips, alerts, and instructions for reporting food poisonings and other food problems. Then, in 2011, Congress passed into law the Food Safety Modernization Act, which included new food safety measures for industry and new enforcement tools for the FDA.[33] These measures are important in reducing the estimated 48 million cases of foodborne illness that occur in the United States each year.[34]

Foodborne Illness

Foodborne illness, which most people call *food poisoning,* generally refers to illnesses caused by microbes consumed in food or beverages, or by the toxins that certain microbes secrete into food that has not been properly preserved or stored. In otherwise healthy adults, foodborne illness often resolves in a few days without treatment. However, infants and toddlers, pregnant women and their fetuses, the elderly, and those with weakened immune systems, such as people with HIV infection, cancer, or diabetes, are more at risk for severe complications and death.

Pathogens Involved in Foodborne Illness

Pathogens are disease-causing agents (*patho-* indicates "disease"). Viruses and bacteria are the two types of microbial pathogens most commonly responsible for foodborne illness. The culprit responsible for the most cases, by far, of foodborne illness, hospitalization, and death is norovirus.[35] This highly contagious virus is transmitted from person to person in places like restaurants, hotels, cruise ships, and, yes, on many college campuses. The hepatitis A virus is another common cause of viral foodborne illness. Infection with either of these viruses causes stomach cramps, vomiting, and diarrhea. The microbe responsible for most bacterial foodborne illnesses is *Salmonella.* Infection, called *salmonellosis*, causes fever, diarrhea, abdominal cramps, nausea, and vomiting. Any raw food of animal origin, such as meat, poultry, dairy products, eggs, and seafood, and some fruits and vegetables may carry *Salmonella* bacteria.[36] Other common bacterial causes of bacterial foodborne illness are *Campylobacter* and *Escherichia coli* (*E. coli*). Although responsible for fewer cases of foodborne illness, *Clostridium botulinum* produces a nerve toxin that is one of the most deadly substances known. A potentially fatal poisoning, called *botulism*, can develop after ingesting even a microscopic amount of contaminated food. Botulism is commonly linked to improperly canned foods. If you're shopping for groceries and see a dented or bulging can, bring it to the store manager.

Microscopic worms and other parasites, as well as nonliving protein particles called *prions* can contaminate food. Prions in the nervous tissue of infected cows cause *bovine spongiform encephalitis*, commonly called "mad cow disease." Humans who consume the contaminated tissue are at risk for a variant form of this disease, which causes progressive loss of nervous system functioning and eventually death.

Reducing Your Risk for Foodborne Illness

Generally, pathogenic microbes spread easily and rapidly, requiring only nourishment, moisture, a favorable temperature, and time to multiply. Almost any food can harbor microbes. So, of course, can unwashed hands, as well as sponges, dish towels, cutting boards, and kitchen utensils.

So what can you do to keep food safe? Check out these steps:[37]

1. **Clean.** Wash your hands, kitchen items, and fruits and veggies. Here's how:
   - Wash your hands for at least 20 seconds with soap and running water. Do it before you eat any meal or snack, as well as before, during, and after preparing food.
   - Wash utensils and small cutting boards with hot soapy water after each use. To clean surfaces and larger cutting boards that won't fit in the sink, mix 1 teaspoon of bleach with 1 quart of water,

vegetarian A person who avoids some or all foods from animal sources: red meat, poultry, seafood, eggs, and dairy products.

foodborne illness (food poisoning) Illness caused by pathogenic microorganisms consumed through food or beverages.

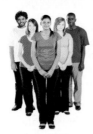

DIVERSITY & HEALTH

Vegetarian Diets

Broadly speaking, being a vegetarian means avoiding foods from animal sources. But the term has many subcategories:

- *Vegans* consume nothing derived from an animal—no meat, poultry, seafood, eggs, milk, cheese, or other dairy products, and typically no gelatin or honey. Many vegans also avoid products made from or tested on animals.
- *Lacto-ovo-vegetarians* avoid meat, poultry, and seafood but will consume dairy products and eggs.
- *Pesco-vegetarians* avoid red meat and poultry but will eat seafood (*pesce* means "fish"), dairy products, and eggs.
- *Semivegetarians* (also called *flexitarians*) may avoid only red meat, or may eat animal-based foods only once or twice a week.

Except for fruit, every edible plant contains protein, so well-planned vegan and vegetarian diets do provide enough. When meals and snacks contain a variety of plant-based foods and caloric intake is sufficient to meet energy needs, protein needs can be met easily.

Vegetarians who consume dairy products and eggs don't have different nutrient needs from their nonvegetarian counterparts. But for vegans, nutrition requires special attention. They may not get enough vitamin B_{12}, which is available only from animal sources or fortified foods or supplements. Other nutrients of concern include riboflavin, vitamin D, vitamin A, calcium, iron, and zinc. Even so, planned wisely, a vegan diet can provide adequate nutrients for overall good health.

Although health experts don't necessarily recommend that everyone become a vegetarian, they are increasingly suggesting that you adopt a plant-based diet, in which most of the meals you consume are vegetarian. Why? Plant-based diets tend to be lower in saturated fat and cholesterol, and higher in healthful unsaturated fats, many vitamins and minerals, fiber, and phytochemicals than the typical American diet. Studies show that such diets can reduce your risk for obesity as well as several chronic diseases and some forms of cancer.[1] What steps can you take to move toward a plant-based diet? Build your meals

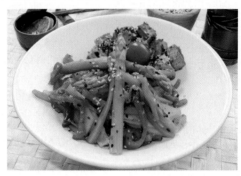

around legumes or other vegetables and whole grains. Think lentil soup with barley, a bean burrito on a whole grain tortilla, or mixed vegetables over quinoa pasta. Switch to veggie versions of your favorite foods, from pizza to tacos to chili. Most importantly, have confidence that nonmeat meals will provide you with all the nutrition that your body needs.

Critical-Thinking Questions

1. Let's say you weigh 145 pounds (about 68 kilograms) and are not an athlete. How much protein do you need each day? Would the following vegetarian foods provide enough protein for one day? Whole grain breakfast cereal with one cup soy milk: 12 grams; peanut butter sandwich on whole grain bread: 18 grams; snack of pumpkin seeds: 10 grams; and vegan black bean enchiladas: 13 grams.

2. Why do vegans have to consume vitamin B_{12} in fortified foods or supplements?

Reference: **1.** "Position of the American Dietetic Association: Vegetarian Diets," by W. J. Craig & A. R. Mangels, 2009, *Journal of the American Dietetic Association, 109*, pp. 1266–1282.

flood the surface, and let it sit for 10 minutes before rinsing with clean water and allowing to air dry.
- Before you cut or peel them, wash fruits and vegetables. If they're delicate, rinse them under running water.

2. **Separate.** Use different cutting boards for bread, produce, and raw meats, poultry, and seafood. At the grocery store, keep meats, poultry, and seafood separate from all other foods in your shopping cart. Keep them wrapped in your fridge, or if you don't plan to use them for a few days, freeze them. Keep eggs in their packaging, and put them in the main compartment of the fridge where they'll stay cooler, not in the door.

3. **Cook.** The bacteria that cause food poisoning multiply quickest in the **danger zone** between 40°F and 140°F. Cook meats, poultry, seafood, and egg dishes until they are at or above 140°F. Use a food thermometer.

>> **To find safe minimum cooking temperatures for various types of foods, visit** www.foodsafety.gov/keep/charts/mintemp.html.

4. **Chill.** Notice that "room temperature" is right in the middle of the danger zone. In fact, bacteria can reproduce—and secrete their toxins—in foods left at room temperature within 2 hours. On a hot day, that time can be as short as an hour! So always refrigerate or freeze foods, including leftovers, within 2 hours. If you're not sure whether a food has been prepared, served, and/or stored safely, don't risk it. Heed the advice, "When in doubt, throw it out!"

danger zone Range of temperatures between 40° and 140° Fahrenheit at which bacteria responsible for foodborne illness thrive.

Food Allergies and Intolerances

Although allergies to pollen, grass, or other environmental sources typically cause discomfort during spring and fall, food allergies know no season. Although the precise incidence in the United States is not known, the FDA estimates that millions of Americans have allergic reactions to foods each year.[38, 39]

Broadly speaking, we can describe a **food allergy** as an adverse reaction of the body's immune system to a food or food component, usually a dietary protein. The body's immune system recognizes a food allergen as foreign and, in an attempt to combat the invasion, produces symptoms of inflammation. These may include swelling of the lips or throat, digestive upset, skin hives or rashes, and breathing problems. The most severe response, called *anaphylaxis,* includes most of these symptoms within minutes of exposure to the allergen. If not treated quickly, it can progress to anaphylactic shock, in which the cardiovascular and respiratory systems become overwhelmed. Without immediate treatment, anaphylactic shock is usually fatal.

Eight foods cause more than 90% of all food allergies: milk, eggs, peanuts, tree nuts (such as almonds, Brazil nuts, cashews, hazelnuts, pine nuts, and walnuts), soy, wheat, fish, and shellfish (such as lobster, crab, and shrimp).[39] The FDA requires that food labels clearly identify the presence of any of these eight allergens. The only known "treatment" for food allergies is avoidance of the offending food; however, some medical researchers have had success with a program of progressive introduction of the food into the patient's diet—under close supervision.

An adverse food reaction that doesn't involve the immune system is known as a **food intolerance.** This type of reaction generally develops within a half hour to a couple of days after eating the offending food. The most common example is *lactose intolerance,* an inability to properly digest the milk sugar lactose. Symptoms, which occur within about 30 minutes of consuming dairy products, include abdominal bloating, painful intestinal cramps, and diarrhea. Food intolerances have also been reported to wheat and to gluten, a protein present in wheat, rye, and barley. Gluten intolerance should not be confused with celiac disease, an immune system disorder in which consumption of gluten prompts inflammation and destruction of the lining of the small intestine.

Food Residues

Food residues are chemicals that are not naturally part of the food, but remain in the food despite cleaning and processing. Two residues of concern to consumers are pollutants and pesticides.

Many different chemicals are released into the air, soil, and water as a result of industry, agriculture, automobile emissions, and improper waste disposal. If a pollutant gets into the soil, a plant can absorb it, and then you can ingest it when you eat the plant. The plant can also

pass it on to food animals that feed on it. Fish and land animals can also absorb pollutants directly into their tissues as well as ingest them when they eat other animals that are contaminated. Pollution residues have been found in virtually all categories of foods.

Pesticides are chemicals used in the field and in storage areas to help protect crops from weeds, insects, fungus, and birds and mammals. When pesticide residues are not effectively removed, they can build up and damage body tissues. The health effects depend on the type of pesticide. Some cause disorders of nerves, others affect glands, and still others can increase the risk of cancer.

The U.S. Environmental Protection Agency (EPA) provides the following tips to reduce your exposure to pesticides:[40]

- Scrub all fresh fruits and vegetables thoroughly under running water.
- Peel fruits and vegetables whenever possible and discard the outer leaves of leafy vegetables.
- Trim the fat from meat and the skin from poultry and fish.
- Eat a variety of foods from various sources.

Considering the harmful effects of pollution and pesticides, are foods produced locally better? What about foods labeled "Organic," "All natural," or "Fair Trade"? To find out, see the **Consumer Corner: Organic, Local, All Natural, and Fair Trade: What to Choose?**

>> For more information on genetically modified foods, check out this special report from PBS's *Nova/Frontline:* www.pbs.org/wgbh/harvest.

Genetically Modified Foods

Scientists create genetically modified fruits and vegetables by altering the genetic material inside the cells of plants, then cultivating their seeds for agricultural production. For example, the process is used to produce food plants that resist heat or pests, tolerate poor soils, or have a higher yield. **Genetic modification** is also used on animals, to produce meat or poultry products with lower fat, for instance.

Supporters of genetically modified foods say that their use increases agricultural productivity, decreases the level of pesticides used, and can improve nutrient content. Opponents express concern about environmental hazards, such as loss of biodiversity, or unintended transfer of modified genes to other crops when pollen is spread on the wind or by bees or birds. The debate continues to this day.

Change Yourself, Change Your World

Armed with the information in this chapter, you're ready to improve your own diet, advocate for healthier food choices on campus, and take action to improve the safety of your community's food supply.

food allergy An adverse reaction of the body's immune system to a food or food component.

food intolerance An adverse food reaction that doesn't involve the immune system.

pesticides A chemical used to kill pests, including agricultural chemicals used to help protect crops from weeds, insects, fungus, slugs and snails, birds, and mammals.

genetic modification Altering a plant's or animal's genetic material in order to produce desirable traits such as resistance to pests, poor-soil tolerance, or lower fat.

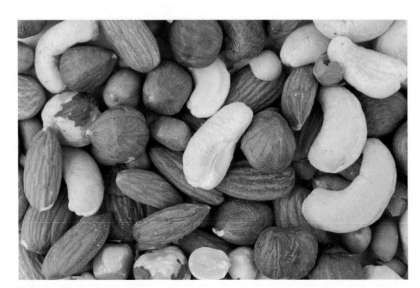
Nuts are a common source of food allergies.

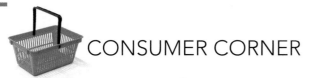

CONSUMER CORNER

Organic, Local, All Natural, and Fair Trade: What to Choose?

You're at the deli, waiting for your sandwich, and debating between several choices of beverage. You could go with a bottle of the "all natural" apple juice made with "Locally Grown!" apples from an orchard right in your county. Or what about a carton of "organic" milk "with no rBGH." Then again, the "fair trade" coffee at the self-serve counter smells divine. Although you're not exactly sure what any of these terms specifically means, they all sound good. So which should you buy?

Organic foods are grown without the use of toxic and persistent fertilizers or pesticides, genetic modification, or irradiation (exposing a food to radiation as a means of preservation). Red meat, poultry, eggs, and dairy products that are certified organic come from animals fed only organic feed and not given growth hormones—including recombinant bovine growth hormone (rBGH)—or antibiotics. To earn the USDA organic seal, a food must contain 95% organically produced ingredients by weight, excluding water and salt. Farms must be certified as organic by the USDA, and any companies that handle the food after it leaves the farm must also be certified. In contrast, the claim "all natural" has no regulated definition, so it can mean pretty much anything the food producer wants it to mean.

Are organic foods safer choices than foods grown with pesticides? That depends. If a conventionally grown fruit or vegetable can be thoroughly scrubbed or peeled, or if it tends to have a low pesticide residue anyway, then its safety is probably comparable to that of organically grown versions. Foods that don't tend to absorb pesticides include onions, corn, peas, pineapples,

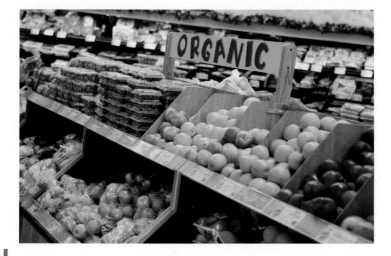

grapefruit, and several others. Foods that have tended to show a high level of pesticides include apples, celery, sweet bell peppers, peaches, nectarines, and carrots, among others.[1] Notice that apples top the list for level of pesticide residue, so despite the fact that the juice in the deli is from a local orchard, if it isn't organic, you might want to give it a miss.

Are organic foods more nutritious? To date, research does not support this. Keep in mind that the term "organic" refers only to how food has been farmed and produced. It is not synonymous with "nutritionally better for you." As a consumer, it's up to you to weigh the pros and cons of organic versus conventional foods. Before you entirely rule out the apple juice, remember that it's locally grown. Why is that important?

There's no universally accepted definition of a "local food."[2] Still, a popular conception is that it refers to a food produced within a 100-mile radius of the consumer. In contrast, produce in the conventional market system in the United States is thought to travel, on average, about 1,500 miles from farm to consumer. This transport requires huge refrigerated trucks to haul the food, using energy not only for transportation but also for refrigeration, at the same time emitting pollution all along the way. However, mileage is only part of the story, since moving foods by freight train is about 10 times more efficient than moving them by truck. This means that an orange shipped by rail from Florida to Maine might have a smaller environmental impact than an apple trucked in from New York.

At this point, you may be thinking that the carton of milk is your best bet. But consider the problem of dairy. It requires far more energy, and produces far more pollution, to feed and maintain dairy cows to produce milk for human consumption than it does to produce plant-based foods and beverages.[2]

So how about that coffee? It was shipped to a local distributor from Columbia, so it's far from locally grown, but it does claim to be "fair trade." What does this mean? Well, many coffee farmers receive prices for their crop that are less than the costs of production, keeping them trapped in a cycle of debt. Moreover, their laborers often work in abysmal conditions for wages that cannot sustain them, even when they bring their children as young as six years old into the fields to pick with them.[3] In contrast, fair trade coffees (and other goods) are produced and sold in international partnerships between growers and buyers that promote sustainability and secure the rights of marginalized farmers and laborers.

So which beverage should you buy? There's no right answer, of course. Each has its merit and costs in terms of its nutritional quality, safety, environmental effects, and impact on the lives of others. As you weigh each choice, it's okay to feel a little intimidated. It's not often that we stop to consider that our day-to-day choices, like what we drink with lunch, can help change ourselves and our world.

References: **1.** "EWG's 2012 Shopper's Guide to Pesticides," by the Environmental Working Group, retrieved from http://www.ewg.org/foodnews. **2.** "Is Local Food Better?" by Sarah DeWeerdt, *Worldwatch Magazine*, May/June 2011, vol. 22, no. 3. **3.** "Coffee FAQs," by Global Exchange, 2011, retrieved from http://www.globalexchange.org/fairtrade/coffee/faq.

Personal Choices

Maintaining a healthy diet is easier than you might believe. Start by visiting **www.choosemyplate.gov** for a step-by-step guide to healthful eating and physical activity that's tailored to your age, gender, height, current weight, lifestyle, and calorie needs. Then choose "Analyze my diet" to find out how well a day's or week's food choices are meeting your needs. What food groups should you eat more of? What do you need to decrease? Are you eating too many calories overall, or too few? For a quick assessment of your diet, see the **Self-Assessment** on the next page.

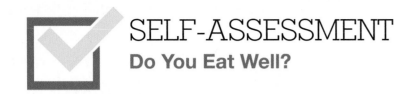

SELF-ASSESSMENT
Do You Eat Well?

The following 13 descriptions of healthy eating behaviors are based on the 2010 *Dietary Guidelines for Americans* recommendations regarding the foods and nutrients all Americans should increase or reduce. Next to each statement, check how often each applies to you.

1. I eat a variety of vegetables, especially dark green, red, and orange vegetables, and beans and peas.
   ☐ Always ☐ Sometimes ☐ Never

2. I consume at least half of all grains as whole grains and/or increase whole grain intake by replacing refined grains with whole grains.
   ☐ Always ☐ Sometimes ☐ Never

3. I consume fat-free or low-fat milk and milk products, such as milk, yogurt, cheese, or fortified soy beverages.
   ☐ Always ☐ Sometimes ☐ Never

4. I choose a variety of protein foods, which include seafood, lean meat and poultry, eggs, beans and peas, soy products, and unsalted nuts and seeds.
   ☐ Always ☐ Sometimes ☐ Never

5. I increase the amount and variety of seafood consumed by choosing seafood in place of some meat and poultry.
   ☐ Always ☐ Sometimes ☐ Never

6. I replace protein foods that are higher in solid fats with choices that are lower in solid fats and calories and/or are sources of oils. (The fats in meat, poultry, and eggs are considered solid fats, while the fats in seafood, nuts, and seeds are considered oils. Meat and poultry should be consumed in lean forms to decrease intake of solid fats.)
   ☐ Always ☐ Sometimes ☐ Never

7. I use oils to replace solid fats where possible.
   ☐ Always ☐ Sometimes ☐ Never

8. I choose foods that provide more potassium, dietary fiber, calcium, and vitamin D, which are nutrients of concern in American diets. These foods include vegetables, fruits, whole grains, and milk and milk products.
   ☐ Always ☐ Sometimes ☐ Never

9. I choose and prepare foods with little salt and consume less than 2,300 milligrams (mg) of sodium per day.
   ☐ Always ☐ Sometimes ☐ Never

10. I consume less than 7% of calories from saturated fats by replacing them with mono-unsaturated and polyunsaturated fatty acids.
    ☐ Always ☐ Sometimes ☐ Never

11. I keep *trans* fatty acid consumption as low as possible by limiting foods that contain synthetic sources of *trans* fats, such as partially hydrogenated oils, and by limiting other solid fats.
    ☐ Always ☐ Sometimes ☐ Never

12. I limit the consumption of foods that contain refined grains, especially refined grain foods that contain solid fats, added sugars, and sodium.
    ☐ Always ☐ Sometimes ☐ Never

13. If I consume alcohol, I consume it in moderation—up to one drink per day for women and two drinks per day for men—and only because I am of legal drinking age.
    ☐ Always ☐ Sometimes ☐ Never

HOW TO INTERPRET YOUR SCORE

The more "Always" responses, the better. Focus on improving the eating behaviors for which you selected "Never" or "Sometimes." The **Choosing to Change Worksheet** at the end of the chapter will assist you in improving these areas.

Take this Self-Assessment online at **MasteringHealth™**

Once you've identified your dietary drawbacks, you're ready to create a practical plan for improving your nutritional health. The **Choosing to Change Worksheet** at the end of this chapter will help you generate a plan that fits your food preferences, your goals—your life! But even with a plan in place, how do you put it into action? Follow the suggestions ahead.

Think Smart When Making Choices

You understand the reasons why it's better to choose a black bean burger over a hamburger, but will you do it when you're in the dining hall—today? By adopting a smart thinking style, you'll find it easier not just to understand nutrition guidelines, but to embrace them. Here are some strategies:

- **Be realistic.** Make small changes consistently over time. If your fruit intake is low, try adding a serving to one of your meals each day or as a snack. Or if you need to increase your calcium intake, start having a cup of yogurt every day as your afternoon snack.

- **Be sensible.** Pay attention to portion sizes and try to minimize your intake of empty calories.

- **Be adventurous.** Expand your tastes to include a variety of fruits, legumes and other vegetables, and whole grains. Have fun trying a new healthful food once a week.

- **Be flexible.** If you happen to overeat for one meal, let it go. Get back on track the next meal.

- **Be active.** You don't need to run 10 miles a day. You just need to be physically active. Consistently choose the stairs instead of the elevator. Walk over to your friends' dorm rather than calling them on your cell phone. Every step counts—just get moving. (For more tips, see Chapter 5.)

Eat Smart When Eating Out

If you're like most college students, you get a lot of your meals from the campus dining hall, food kiosks, and fast food outlets. But you can still make smart choices. For instance, compare these two fast food meals:

- A McDonald's Big Mac, large fries, and small iced coffee contain about 1,110 calories, a whopping 48% of which come from fat.

- A McDonald's Premium Grilled Chicken Classic Sandwich, side salad, and black coffee contains 370 calories and 22% of its energy as fat.

As you can see, small choices you make every day can make a big difference in your nutrition, weight, and health. For some tips for eating at fast food restaurants, see the **Practical Strategies** box on page 95.

>> This site compares serving sizes, calories, saturated fat, *trans* fat, and sodium content for several popular fast foods: www.acaloriecounter.com/fast-food.php.

Shop Smart When Money's Tight

You might believe that it costs more to eat right, but in fact, some of the cheapest foods in your supermarket are also among the most healthful. Here are some smart choices:

- **Legumes.** Dried beans, peas, and lentils are a must-have staple. If you don't have the time to cook them, stock up on canned beans. They still cost less than 50 cents per serving, and provide 7 grams of protein, 7 grams of fiber, calcium, and iron.

- **Canned tuna.** A small can provides two servings, each of which should cost you less than 75 cents, while providing 12 grams of protein and about 250 milligrams of omega-3 fatty acids.

- **Lean meats, poultry, and fish.** Fill most of your plate with veggies and grains, accompanied by a small portion of high-quality lean meat, poultry, or fish. You'll save money and reduce your intake of saturated fat and cholesterol, not to mention calories.

- **Whole grains.** Choose brown rice, whole oats, and whole wheat bread. These foods are all inexpensive and are loaded with nutrients and fiber.

- **Frozen vegetables.** These are just as nutritious as fresh vegetables, less expensive, and quick to prepare: Pour the amount you want into a bowl with a tablespoon of water, and microwave.

- **Fresh and frozen fruits.** Buy fruits in season, or buy frozen fruit.

The bottom line? Make smarter food choices every day. Over time, these little changes can have an enormous impact on your health and well-being.

Campus Advocacy

Whenever you make a food choice, you're promoting that food. So whether you're buying frozen blueberries in your supermarket, or ordering the bean burrito at your favorite Mexican hangout, you're sending the message that consumers value healthful foods and that it's profitable to offer them. At the same time, avoiding foods with empty calories limits their profitability and discourages their production.

On campus, make friends with the staff at your dining hall. Provide feedback—positive and negative—about the nutritional quality of the selections offered, and ask for more plant-based meals. Find out where the food they serve comes from—is produce locally grown when possible, and what food safety measures are in place? Check out the vending machines on campus, too. Do they offer nutritious snacks and beverages, or junk? Who decides what's sold, and how can you improve the choices?

>> The USDA created the MyPlate on Campus program to empower college students to work with their campuses to promote healthy lifestyles. Visit the site to sign up as a MyPlate on Campus Ambassador, find a MyPlate on Campus Toolkit, and access other resources designed specifically for college students: www.choosemyplate.gov/MyPlateOnCampus.

And while you're advocating for more healthful food choices for yourself and other students, don't forget those less fortunate. One way to help is to join a branch of the National Student Campaign Against

Practical Strategies

Eating Right While on the Run

You're a college student, right? So almost by definition, you eat lots of your meals on the run. Fortunately, healthful choices are available, even from fast food restaurants. Here are some tips:

- Order a vegetarian version of popular fast foods, such as burgers, pizzas, tacos, burritos, or subs.

- When ordering meat, choose chicken, turkey, or fish instead of beef or pork.

- Order your burger or sub without cheese.

- Don't super-size it! Instead, order the smallest size of burger or sandwich available, or cut it in half and share it with a friend.

- Order a side salad instead of fries.

- If you crave fries, order the smallest serving size.

- Order a carton of low-fat or skim milk, a bottle of water, or a diet soda instead of a regular soda or a milkshake.

- Skip dessert or order a piece of fruit instead. Watch out for those "yogurt parfaits" now offered at many fast food restaurants. They're typically loaded with saturated fat, added sugars, and calories.

- Monitor your sensations of fullness as you eat, and stop as soon as you're satisfied.

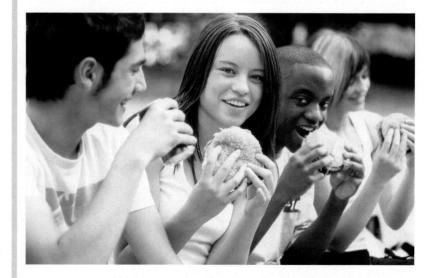

Hunger and Homelessness. For more than 25 years, this organization has fought hunger and homelessness by educating, engaging, and training college students to directly meet individuals' immediate needs while advocating for long-term systemic solutions. For a list of participating colleges and universities, go to **www.studentsagainsthunger.org/page/hhp/participating-schools**. If you find out that your campus doesn't have a branch, start one yourself!

>> Watch videos of real students discussing their nutrition at MasteringHealth™

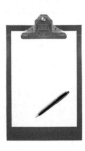

Choosing to Change Worksheet

To complete this worksheet online, visit MasteringHealth™

To conduct a self-assessment of your diet, log on to **www.supertracker.usda.gov** and select the interactive tool **Food Tracker.** To use the Food Tracker you must keep track of everything you eat and drink for at least one *typical* day and enter the information into the website. For more accurate results, enter your food and drink information for three days—two typical week days and one typical weekend day. After you have completed entering all food and drink, under the 'My Reports' drop-down menu, select 'Food Groups & Calories' and print your report. You are ready to evaluate the quality of your current diet based on the daily food group targets.

Directions: Fill in your stage of behavior change in Step 1 and complete the rest of the worksheet with your stage of change in mind.

Step 1: *Your Stage of Behavior Change.* Please check one of the following statements that best describes your readiness to improve your diet.

_____ I do not intend to improve my diet in the next six months. (Precontemplation)

_____ I might improve my diet in the next six months. (Contemplation)

_____ I am prepared to improve my diet in the next month. (Preparation)

_____ I have been improving my diet for less than six months. (Action)

_____ I have been improving my diet for more than six months. (Maintenance)

Step 2: *Analyze Your Diet.* Review your Food Groups & Calories Report from the Food Tracker. Let's start with a comparison of your intake with MyPlate recommendations. Below, list the food groups for which your intake did and did not meet the target.

Food groups that met target intake: _____

Food groups that didn't meet target intake:_____

Next, look at the section on the bottom called "Limits." How does your intake of empty calories from consuming solid fats and added sugars compare with the Allowance listed? What contributed most to your empty calorie intake (solid fats or added sugars)?

_____

Step 3: *Plan to Improve Your Diet.* Next, jot down a plan for *increasing* your intake of the food groups that didn't meet your target intake, and for *decreasing* your intake of the less healthful items such as empty calories, oils, and refined grains. An example is provided.

Food Group	**Plan for Change**
Dairy	*By the end of this semester, I'll be consuming at least three servings of dairy every day.*

_____

_____

_____

Step 4: *Anticipate Obstacles.* Finally, write below about any obstacles that might interfere with your ability to meet your goals. For instance, are you concerned that you won't have enough money to purchase fresh fruits and vegetables? Or that your lunch break is so short that you have no time for anything but fast food? For each obstacle, jot down a strategy to get around it.

_____

_____

_____

Step 5: *Work Within Your Stage of Change.* Given your stage of change, how likely do you think it is that you will implement the plan in Step 3? What might encourage you to complete your plan?

_____

_____

Chapter Summary

- The science of nutrition explores how the foods you eat and the beverages you drink affect your body and your health.

- There are six major classes of nutrients found in foods: carbohydrates, proteins, fats, vitamins, minerals, and water. Within these classes are essential nutrients, or substances that must be obtained from the diet because the body either cannot make them or cannot make sufficient quantities to support health.

- Carbohydrates and proteins contain 4 calories per gram. Fats contain 9 calories per gram. Alcohol contains 7 calories per gram. Vitamins, minerals, and water are calorie free.

- Glucose derived from the breakdown of carbohydrates is a key energy source during physical activity. Brain and blood cells can only use glucose for energy.

- Fiber is a non-nutrient, nondigestible component of plant foods that helps maintain health and may prevent digestive and some chronic diseases.

- Fats are the most concentrated energy source and the primary source of energy for the body at rest. Unsaturated fats are the most healthful.

- Proteins are made up of different combinations of 20 building blocks called amino acids. Proteins can be used for fuel, but their primary role is in building and repairing body tissues and functional compounds.

- Vitamins are compounds that facilitate many of the body's functions, from metabolism to nerve function.

- Minerals are discrete elements that regulate body processes and provide structure to the body.

- Water is vital to nutrient digestion, absorption, and transportation. It serves as a lubricant, regulates body temperature, and is the medium in which the body's chemical reactions take place.

- Multivitamin/mineral supplements, herbs, and ergogenic aids are all popular among college students, but the FDA doesn't regulate the safety and effectiveness of dietary supplements. Therefore, you should check with your healthcare provider before using them.

- Phytochemicals, antioxidants, probiotics, and prebiotics are not nutrients, but are thought to have health-promoting properties.

- Strategies for eating right include learning about the Dietary Reference Intakes, reading food labels, following the *Dietary Guidelines for Americans*, and using MyPlate to help you evaluate your current diet and develop and follow a diet plan that's right for you.

- Your age, gender, level of physical activity, and many other factors influence your nutrient needs.

- Well-planned vegetarian diets provide ample protein. Vegans need to be especially careful that they are getting enough vitamin B_{12} from fortified foods and supplements.

- Foodborne illness occurs when microbes, such as viruses and bacteria, contaminate foods.

- You can reduce your risk of foodborne illness by following four steps: clean, separate, cook, and chill.

- Food allergies and intolerances are best prevented by identifying and avoiding the offending foods.

- Food residues of concern include pollutants and pesticides. All produce should be washed thoroughly before consumption.

- The benefits and risks of genetically modified foods are the subject of considerable debate.

- Creating a personalized nutrition plan that includes smart food choices can improve your health and well-being.

GET CONNECTED

>> Visit the following websites for further information about the topics in this chapter.

- MyPlate
  www.choosemyplate.gov
- Foodsafety.gov
  www.foodsafety.gov
- Dietary Guidelines for Americans
  www.health.gov/dietaryguidelines
- Food and Drug Administration: For Consumers
  www.fda.gov/ForConsumers/default.htm
- Academy of Nutrition and Dietetics
  www.eatright.org

MOBILE TIPS!
Scan this QR code with your mobile device to access additional nutrition tips. Or, via your mobile device, go to **http://chmobile.pearsoncmg.com** and navigate to Chapter 4.

- The Center for Science in the Public Interest
  www.cspinet.org

Website links are subject to change. To access updated web links, please visit MasteringHealth™.

TEST YOUR KNOWLEDGE

1. Which of the following substances contributes the most calories?
   a. alcohol
   b. proteins
   c. carbohydrates
   d. vitamins

2. Which of the following is characteristic of an essential nutrient?
   a. It cannot be found in food.
   b. It cannot be degraded by the body.
   c. It cannot be made in sufficient quantities by the body.
   d. It cannot be used to manufacture other compounds in the body.

3. Dietary supplements
   a. do not need FDA approval before they are marketed.
   b. cannot be removed from the market by the FDA.
   c. are generally safe if the label identifies the product as "all natural."
   d. are safe and effective if the product label shows the USP mark.

4. Prebiotics are
   a. helpful bacteria found in yogurt and certain other fermented foods.
   b. non-nutrient food components that stimulate the growth of bacteria in the large intestine.
   c. antioxidant phytochemicals found in cocoa.
   d. types of fatty acids thought to be protective against heart disease and cancer.

5. Which of the following statements about the DRIs is true?
   a. The AMDR identifies the amount of protein, fat, and carbohydrate that an average adult should consume each day.
   b. The AI designates a nutrient intake level when an RDA cannot be determined.
   c. The DRIs include the RDA, the AI, and the % DV.
   d. The UL is the ideal intake recommended to promote health.

6. Which of the following is true of the *Dietary Guidelines for Americans*?
   a. It recommends that you consume no more than 2,000 calories a day.
   b. It recommends that you drink water instead of milk.
   c. It recommends that you be physically active at least 10 minutes at a time.
   d. It recommends that you adopt a vegetarian diet.

7. Athletes typically need
   a. more then twice as much protein as non-athletes.
   b. about the same level of carbohydrates as non-athletes.
   c. somewhat more fat than non-athletes.
   d. All of these answers are true.

8. Most foodborne illnesses
   a. are deadly.
   b. are due to overcooking meat.
   c. can be prevented by using safe food-handling practices.
   d. can be prevented by choosing genetically modified foods.

9. Which of the following would be considered a food residue?
   a. phytochemicals
   b. probiotics
   c. preservatives
   d. pesticides

10. Which of the following is a healthful, inexpensive choice for improving your nutrition?
    a. Shop for, cook with, and order menu items containing legumes.
    b. Maximize your intake of foods with empty calories because they are less likely to cause you to gain weight.
    c. Avoid all genetically modified foods.
    d. If your food budget is tight, purchase a variety of dietary supplements to make sure you get the nutrition you need.

Get Critical

What happened

In 2009, eight-time NBA all-star Steve Nash, then with the Phoenix Suns, posted his diet on his Facebook page. He's "sensitive to milk," so he starts his day with almond or rice milk on his gluten-free cereal, and stays hydrated with plain water, whole-fruit smoothies, and green tea. So what's Nash doing on a Body by Milk poster, sporting a milk mustache as he makes a pass?

What do you think?

- When you see celebrity endorsements, what—if any—assumptions do you make? Even if you recognize that the celebrities shown may not actually use the products they promote, are you comfortable with these kinds of ads being aimed at kids? Why or why not?

- Typical milk alternatives have at least as much calcium per glass as cow's milk, along with vitamins A, D, and B$_{12}$. They're also free of saturated fat and cholesterol, and soymilk is high in protein. Do posters showing athletes with a milk mustache mislead kids into believing that cow's milk is the only beverage that can help them grow "big and strong"?

- On his Facebook page, Nash is clearly trying to share what he's learned about healthful eating. Do you feel that celebrity athletes have an ethical responsibility to promote health and fitness?

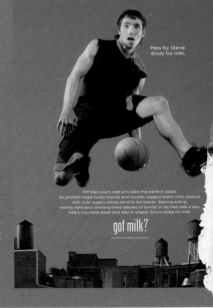

Pass by Steve.
Body by milk.

Off the court, milk provides the perfect assist. Its protein helps build muscle and studies suggest teens who choose milk over sugary drinks tend to be leaner. Staying active, eating right and drinking three glasses of lowfat or fat free milk a day helps you look great and stay in shape. Score three for milk.

got milk?

PHYSICAL ACTIVITY FOR FITNESS & HEALTH

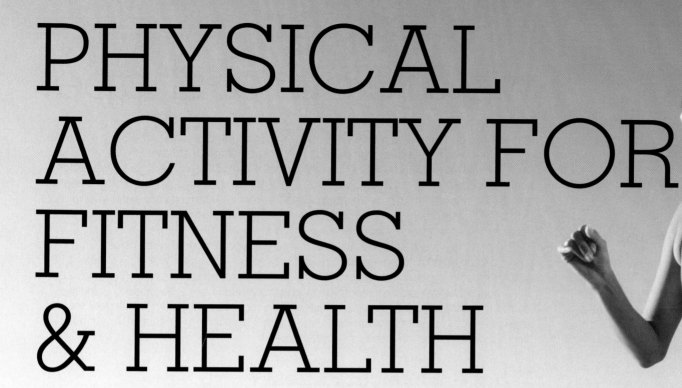

People who are physically active for about **7 hours** a week have a **40%** lower risk of dying early than those who are active for less than 30 minutes a week.[i]

Young adults 18 to 30 years old with low cardiovascular fitness levels are **two to three** times more likely to develop **diabetes** in 20 years than those who are fit.[ii]

In a recent study, women who performed one year of **strength training** significantly improved their ability to maintain **mental focus** and **resolve conflicts**.[iii]

Learning Objectives

IDENTIFY the five components of health-related physical fitness.

EXPLAIN the health benefits of physical activity.

IDENTIFY the principles of fitness training.

CONSIDER different types of physical activity for your fitness plan.

ASSESS how much physical activity you need.

DISCUSS how to exercise safely.

DESIGN an effective, personalized fitness program.

As a society, we are out of shape.

Many of our daily activities no longer require significant physical effort, and busy schedules cut into our time for exercise—an especially critical problem for students, who often see their physical activity levels decline in college. Even when we do have time for recreation, hours that could be spent getting exercise or playing sports are instead too often spent in the car, in front of the TV, or on the computer. The result: Americans are experiencing more long-term health problems, such as overweight and obesity, diabetes, cardiovascular disease, and even reduced mental health.

The good news is that in recent years the percentage of people in the United States who report getting at least some regular physical activity has grown somewhat, with about 47% of those 18 years old or older meeting guidelines for cardiorespiratory activity, about 24% meeting guidelines for strength-training activity, and about 20% meeting guidelines related to flexibility.[1] And if given the chance to be more active, our bodies thrive. Even small changes in physical activity levels can make a significant difference in your fitness and health, both in school now and in the years ahead.

What Is Physical Fitness?

Most of us equate fitness with appearance. We assume that those of us with trim builds are more fit, while those of us with flabby triceps are less fit. But physical fitness is not that simplistic. **Physical fitness** is the ability to perform moderate to vigorous levels of activity, and to respond to physical demands without excessive fatigue. Physical fitness can be built up through physical activity or exercise. **Physical activity** is bodily movement that substantially increases energy expenditure. Taking the stairs instead of the elevator, or biking to class instead of driving, count as types of physical activity. **Exercise** is physical activity that is carried out in a planned and structured format. Any type of activity will provide health benefits, but optimal physical fitness can only be achieved through regular exercise. Team sports, brisk walks, and working out at the gym all count as exercise.

There are two types of physical fitness: **skills-related fitness** and **health-related fitness.** In this chapter, we will focus on health-related fitness. The five key components of health-related fitness are cardiorespiratory fitness, muscular strength, muscular endurance, flexibility, and body composition.

Cardiorespiratory Fitness

Put together "cardio" for heart and "respiratory" for breath, and you've got a good idea of what this component of fitness covers. **Cardiorespiratory fitness** refers to the ability of your heart and lungs to effectively deliver oxygen to your muscles during prolonged physical activity. Experts agree that cardiorespiratory fitness should be the foundation upon which all the other areas of fitness are built. It is the component that is the best indicator of overall physical fitness, and in addition helps lower your risk of chronic disease and premature death.[2] In fact, the American Heart Association believes that cardiorespiratory fitness is one of the most important factors in overall health, and poor cardiorespiratory

physical fitness The ability to perform moderate to vigorous levels of activity and to respond to physical demands without excessive fatigue.

physical activity Bodily movement that substantially increases energy expenditure.

exercise A type of physical activity that is planned and structured.

skills-related fitness The capacity to perform specific physical skills related to a sport or other physically demanding activity.

health-related fitness The ability to perform activities of daily living with vigor.

cardiorespiratory fitness The ability of your heart and lungs to effectively deliver oxygen to your muscles during prolonged physical activity.

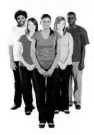

DIVERSITY & HEALTH

Men, Women, and Building Muscle

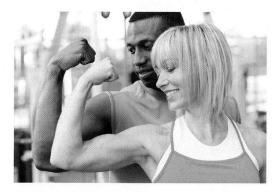

Men's and women's bodies react differently to resistance training.

All of us can benefit from resistance and strength training. But between men and women, lifting weights will often yield different results. Men are more likely to see increased muscle bulk, while women may notice less bulk even while seeing increased muscle strength and tone.

Many factors, including your diet, body type, and genetics, play a role in how your body responds to pumping iron. But your sex is a key differentiator, largely because of hormones. Certain hormones, such as testosterone and androgens, are linked to muscle growth. Because men's bodies make more of these particular hormones, their muscles are more likely to increase in size under a resistance-training program.

Differences in muscle size don't equal a difference in the benefits of strength training, however. Both men and women achieve valuable fitness and health gains from regular resistance workouts, including protection for our bones as we age. In women, for example, one study found a connection between muscle mass and bone health at locations where women are prone to fractures later in life, such as the hip.[1]

Critical-Thinking Questions

1. Have you noticed differences in the workouts that men and women prefer? What do you think are the causes of these differences?
2. What are some common stereotypes about men, women, and working out?
3. How might these stereotypes be detrimental to a person's overall level of fitness?

Reference: 1. "Skeletal Muscle Mass Is Associated with Bone Geometry and Microstructure and Serum Insulin-Like Growth Factor Binding Protein-2 Levels in Adult Women and Men," by N. Lebrasseur, S. Achenbach, L. Melton, 3rd, S. Amin, & S. Khosla, 2012, *Journal of Bone and Mineral Research, 10* (21), 59–69.

fitness is one of the strongest predictors of future risk for cardiovascular disease and other health problems—stronger, in fact, than other traditional risk factors like hypertension, smoking, obesity, elevated blood lipid levels, and type 2 diabetes.[3] You can boost your cardiorespiratory fitness by any continuous, rhythmic exercise that works your large muscle groups and increases your heart rate, such as brisk walking, swimming, or cycling.

Muscular Strength

Muscular strength is the maximum force your muscles can apply in a single effort of lifting, pushing, or pressing. Building stronger muscles will help keep your skeleton properly aligned, aid balance, protect your back, boost your athletic performance, and increase your metabolic rate. Building muscular strength also results in much higher bone mineral density and stronger bones.[4] You can build muscular strength by performing strength training exercises using machines, free weights, resistance bands, or simply the weight of your own body (as in push-ups, for example).

Muscular Endurance

Muscular endurance is the capacity of your muscles to repeatedly exert force, or to maintain force, over a period of time without tiring. Muscular endurance is measured in two ways: *static muscular endurance,* or how long you can hold a force that is motionless, and *dynamic muscular endurance,* or how long you can sustain a force in motion. A sustained sit-up, where you contract your abdominal muscles and do not move until they fatigue, is an example of static muscle endurance. Repeated sit-ups, done until you can't contract your abdominals any more, rely on dynamic muscle endurance. Muscular endurance is important for posture and for performing extended activities. Muscular endurance can be improved by gradually increasing the duration that your muscles work in each bout of strength exercises, such as slowly increasing the number of push-ups you perform during exercise.

Flexibility

Flexibility refers to the ability of your joints to move through their full ranges of motion, such as how far you can bend your trunk from side to side or how far you can bend forward from the hips toward your toes. Flexibility does not only pertain to the movement of muscle, but also depends on connective tissues such as your ligaments and tendons. Benefits of flexibility include the relief of muscle tension, reduction of joint pain, reduction of back pain, and improved posture. Flexibility can be improved through stretching exercises and activities such as yoga, Pilates, and tai chi.

Body Composition

Body composition refers to the relative proportions of fat tissue and lean tissue (such as muscle and connective tissues) in your body. A low ratio of fat to lean tissue is optimal. As we'll discuss in Chapter 6, many of us carry more body fat than is healthful. Excessive body fat, especially in the abdominal area, increases the risk of three of the four leading causes of death in the United States: heart

muscular strength The maximum force your muscles can apply in a single maximum effort of lifting, pushing, or pressing.

muscular endurance The capacity of muscles to repeatedly exert force, or to maintain a force, over a period of time.

flexibility The ability of joints to move through their full ranges of motion.

body composition The relative proportions of the body's lean tissue and fat tissue.

disease, cancer, and stroke. It is also related to other serious conditions, including osteoarthritis, diabetes, hypertension (high blood pressure), and sleep apnea. Research indicates that even if you are healthy in other ways, having too much body fat will still negatively impact your health.[5] Body composition affects your level of fitness, but the reverse is also true—as you become more physically fit, your body composition will usually improve.

What Are the Benefits of Physical Activity?

Physical activity is one of the best things you can do for yourself. It benefits every aspect of your health, at every stage of your life. Some of these benefits are purely physical, such as a stronger heart and healthier lungs. But physical activity can also put you in a better mood and help you to manage stress. As you age it will help postpone physical decline and many of the diseases that can reduce quality of life in your later years.

Figure 5.1 summarizes the major benefits of physical activity; we'll discuss each one next.

Stronger Heart and Lungs

As the organs that pump your blood and deliver oxygen throughout your body, your heart, lungs, and entire circulatory system literally keep you going. By increasing your body's demand for oxygen, physical activity helps keep these systems strong and efficient, even as you age. Physical activity also appears to help stabilize the parts of your brain that control the function of these vital systems.[6]

Participating in physical activity and exercise can cut your risk of cardiovascular disease in half through its positive effect on several

Reduces risk of heart disease, strengthens heart, reduces risk of high blood pressure

Increases lung efficiency and capacity

Reduces risk of type 2 diabetes

Reduces risk of colorectal, breast, and ovarian cancers

Strengthens immune system

Strengthens bones

Reduces risk of bone, muscle, and joint injuries

Promotes healthful body composition and weight management

Benefits psychological health and stress management

FIGURE 5.1 Health Benefits of Physical Activity.

major risk factors: It lowers LDL (bad) cholesterol, raises HDL (good) cholesterol, helps prevent or control diabetes, and helps you lose excess weight.[7] In addition, because physical activity keeps your blood vessels healthier, it lowers your risk of high blood pressure.

The stronger your heart and lungs, the longer you're likely to live. One study followed more than 20,000 men who weren't overweight, but had differing levels of cardiorespiratory fitness.[8] The researchers found that just being thin isn't enough to protect your health—fitness is also key. In the eight-year-long study, thin men with low rates of cardiorespiratory fitness were twice as likely to die from any cause as thin men with higher rates of cardiorespiratory fitness.

Management and Prevention of Type 2 Diabetes

Exercise can control your blood glucose level and blood pressure, help you lose weight and maintain weight loss, and improve your body's ability to use insulin, all of which help control or prevent type 2 diabetes. If you have type 2 diabetes, any daily physical activity is helpful. If you are at risk for the disease, even as little as 30 minutes of exercise a day five days a week can help lower your risk.[9] When combined with a healthful diet, exercise proves more powerful than prescription medication in lowering type 2 diabetes risk. A federal health study of people at high risk for diabetes showed that daily exercise and a healthful diet lowered risk by 58%, compared with a 31% reduction in risk for a common prescription diabetes drug.[9,10,11]

Reduced Risk of Some Cancers

Inactivity is one of the most significant risk factors for cancer that you can control. Physical activity lowers the long-term risks of developing colorectal cancer in men and women and breast and ovarian cancers in women.[12,13] One long-term study of more than 110,000 women found that those who performed at least five hours of moderate to strenuous exercise a week cut their risk of breast cancer by at least half.[14] Activity appears to help in part by controlling weight, a risk factor for certain cancers. It may also help by regulating certain hormones which are factors in some types of cancers and by encouraging your body to process and remove substances—including potential toxins that might cause cancer—more quickly.

Increased Immune Function

Do you want to lower your risk of getting sick during the next cold and flu season? Physical activity can help you fend off common illnesses by boosting your immune system. In one study, 60–90% of active individuals felt that they experienced fewer colds than their nonactive counterparts.[15] Scientists still aren't entirely sure how physical activity helps build immunity, but exercise's role in flushing impurities from the body, along with regulating hormones related to immune function, may play a part.[16]

Stronger Bones

Physical activity builds and protects your bones.[17] Weight-bearing exercise such as walking, running, or lifting weights makes your bones denser and stronger. Non–weight-bearing exercise, such as swimming, is healthful in other ways but does not strengthen bones. Bone strength helps protect your skeleton from injury, so it is important for everyone, but it is especially important for those at risk for **osteoporosis,** a serious condition that mostly

osteoporosis A condition in which reduced bone mineral density causes the bones to become weak and brittle.

affects older adults, in which reduced bone mineral density causes the bones to become weak and brittle. Although many college-aged students don't think they need to worry about osteoporosis, bone density peaks during early adulthood, so this is precisely the time to build the bone strength that could prevent the disease's onset later.

Reduced Risk of Injury

The stronger bones, muscles, tendons, and ligaments that result from physical activity can help protect you from injury. A strong back, for example, is much less likely to get strained and sore the next time you lift boxes while moving to a new dorm or apartment. Strong muscles can help you keep your balance and avoid falls, and strong joint-supporting muscles can help reduce the risk of a variety of injuries including sprains, tendinitis, runner's knee, and shin splints.

Healthful Weight Management

Physical activity helps you lose and control weight in more ways than one. Not only does it burn calories, but it also boosts your metabolism, so your body uses more calories. This boost in metabolism occurs both during and after workouts. Consistent exercise can slowly lower your overall percentage of body fat and help build and maintain muscle, whereas if you try to lose weight by dieting alone, you risk burning muscle mass along with body fat. Having more muscle also increases your metabolism and helps you maintain your weight long-term.

Benefits to Psychological Health, Stress Management, and Sleep

When people say they work out to "blow off steam," they are describing the effect physical activity has on their stress levels. Physical activity reduces stress and anxiety, and also helps boost concentration. These benefits appear to hold true no matter what type of physical activity you enjoy.

Certain studies have shown that exercise can be just as effective in relieving depression as antidepressant medication.[18] And the latest research concludes that exercise can prevent depression in the first place.[19] Any type of physical activity is considered helpful, but in one study of college women with signs of depression, vigorous-intensity exercise classes led to the most significant decrease in symptoms.[20]

In addition, active lifestyles may help you be more focused during the day and more tranquil at night. Physical activity may be associated with higher levels of alertness and mental ability, including the ability to learn and achieve academically.[5, 21] Cardiorespiratory fitness, in particular, can promote academic achievement and job productivity.[3] A physically active lifestyle may also be beneficial when bedtime rolls around—a daily routine that includes at least moderate levels of exercise has been associated with improved sleep quality.[22]

Principles of Fitness Training

You'll receive the greatest health benefits if you approach your exercise routine in a systematic way. In order to design an effective fitness program, you should first understand the basic principles of fitness training: *overload, specificity, reversibility,* and *individuality*.

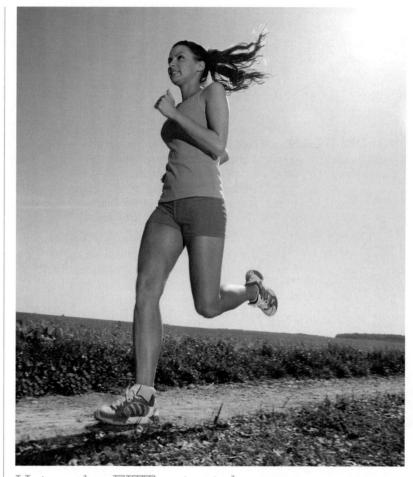

Using the FITT principle will help you achieve progressive overload.

Overload

Whatever your fitness capabilities, improving means pushing yourself to the next level. The **overload** principle requires that you increase the stress placed on your body, creating a greater demand than your body is accustomed to meeting. This forces your body to adapt and become more fit. In other words, you improve by exercising beyond your comfort zone.

For overload to work effectively, new stresses should be steady and gradual. This requires **progressive overload,** or increasing the demands on your body gradually and safely over time to avoid injury. You can achieve progressive overload safely by modifying and personalizing one or more of the exercise variables collectively known as **FITT,** which stands for:

- **Frequency,** or the number of times you engage in a particular physical activity each week.
- **Intensity** refers to the level of effort at which you exercise. For cardiorespiratory fitness, intensity is usually measured in terms of how fast you get your heart beating (your heart rate). For muscular strength and endurance training, intensity depends on the amount of resistance and number of repetitions. For flexibility, intensity is measured by the depth of the stretch.

overload Increasing the stress placed on your body through exercise, which results in an improved fitness level.

progressive overload Gradually overloading the body over time in order to avoid injury.

FITT Exercise variables that can be modified in order to accomplish progressive overload: frequency, intensity, time, and type.

Cardiorespiratory Fitness

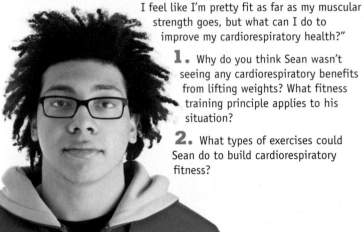

"HI, I'M SEAN. I've been lifting weights for the past two years. I've gained about 12 pounds of muscle since I started lifting, yet I get tired very easily doing any cardiorespiratory exercises like jogging. I feel like I'm pretty fit as far as my muscular strength goes, but what can I do to improve my cardiorespiratory health?"

1. Why do you think Sean wasn't seeing any cardiorespiratory benefits from lifting weights? What fitness training principle applies to his situation?

2. What types of exercises could Sean do to build cardiorespiratory fitness?

- **Time** (duration), or the amount of time you spend on a particular exercise.
- **Type,** or the sorts of exercise you choose to engage in.

Exercise type is closely linked to the principle of specificity, which we'll look at next. (To see the FITT principle applied to various types of workouts, see **Table 5.1**.)

Specificity

The **specificity** principle means that in order to improve a specific component of fitness, you must perform exercises designed to address that component in a deliberate, targeted way. Many exercises will improve some components of fitness but not others. Cycling, for example, is great for cardiorespiratory fitness, but doesn't build upper body strength or increase your flexibility. You should take into account the principle of specificity when deciding which activities you choose to perform.

Reversibility

Your personal level of fitness can easily go up—or down. The **reversibility** principle states that your fitness level will decline if you don't maintain your physical activity. Fitness declines can happen quickly, sometimes in as little as 10 days.[23] Therefore, it is important to maintain a consistent exercise routine to avoid reversing your fitness gains. Even if you can't take on a new round of progressive overload and increased physical stress at a particular time, maintaining your current workout will help keep your level of fitness from declining.

Individuality

The principle of **individuality** means that you will respond to the demands you place on your body in your own unique way. We each react differently to specific exercises, with some people gaining more benefit from a particular exercise than others. Identifying the exercises best suited to you is a key part of designing an effective fitness program. Whatever your individual needs and responses, however, one overarching principle applies to all of us: We can all benefit from exercise.

What Types of Physical Activity Should You Consider?

Any type of regular, sustained physical activity is beneficial, especially if you have been inactive for a while. However, in order to increase your overall health and fitness, you should look into activities that increase your cardiorespiratory fitness, muscular strength and endurance, and flexibility.

specificity The principle that a fitness component is improved only by exercises that address that specific component.

reversibility The principle that fitness levels decline when the demand placed on the body is decreased.

individuality The principle that individuals will respond to fitness training in their own unique ways.

TABLE 5.1 The FITT Principle in Action

FITT Dimensions	Cardiorespiratory Exercise	Strength Training	Flexibility
Frequency	Three to five times per week	Two to three times per week	At least two to three days per week, preferably more
Intensity	60–85% of personal maximum heart rate	Eight to 12 repetitions, or until the point of muscle fatigue	Tension (not pain), followed by feeling of release of tension
Time	At least 20 minutes or more (continuous)	As needed to work out safely	30 to 60 seconds
Type	Running, hiking, walking, swimming, rowing, stair climbing, vigorous dancing	Weight machines, free weights, resistance bands	Stretching

Source: Data from Physical Activity and Public Health: Updated Recommendation for Adults from the American College of Sports Medicine and the American Heart Association, by W. L. Haskell, I. M. Lee, R. R. Pate, K. E. Powell, S. N. Blair, B. A. Franklin, C. A. Macera ... A. Bauman, 2007, *Medicine & Science in Sports & Exercise, 39* (8), pp. 1423–1434.

Aerobic Exercise

You can build cardiorespiratory fitness through **aerobic exercise,** which is any prolonged physical activity that raises your heart rate and works the large muscle groups. Aerobic exercise makes your heart, lungs, and entire circulatory system stronger by requiring them to work harder to deliver adequate oxygen to your muscles.

Types of Aerobic Exercise

There are numerous forms of popular aerobic exercise, including:

- Running and jogging
- Hiking or brisk walking for extended periods of time
- Cycling and "spinning" (a structured workout on a stationary bicycle)
- Swimming
- Fast-paced running-based games, such as basketball or soccer
- Cardio classes, including aerobic dance videos and step aerobics training
- Vigorous martial arts, such as karate or cardio kickboxing

The types of aerobic exercise you choose, however, represent just one step toward improved fitness. As the FITT principle discussed earlier outlined, you'll also need to consider other factors—including just how hard you work out.

Intensity of Aerobic Exercise

Aerobic intensity is usually measured by heart rate because increased heart rate indicates that your cardiorespiratory system is working harder. In order to achieve the maximum cardiorespiratory benefit, you should aim to raise your heart rate so that it falls within your **target heart rate range.** For healthy adults who are not entirely sedentary or exceptionally active, the American College of Sports Medicine (ACSM) recommends a target heart rate range of anywhere from 64% to 91% of your maximum heart rate.[24] See the **Self-Assessment** on page 106 for how to determine these indicators.

Aerobic exercises are often categorized as lifestyle/light-intensity, moderate-intensity, or vigorous-intensity activities. According to the Centers for Disease Control and Prevention, light-intensity activity gets you moving but raises your heart rate to less than 50% of your maximum heart rate; moderate-intensity activities will raise your heart rate to 50–70% of your maximum heart rate; and vigorous-intensity activities raise your heart rate to 70–85% of your maximum heart rate.[25] **Table 5.2** shows the examples and benefits of these three categories of aerobic activities.

The best way to begin an aerobic exercise program is to start by performing exercises at intensities near the low end of your target heart rate range, or even lower if you have not exercised in a while. Start with a minimum of 10 minutes of activity at a time, more if you are able. Slowly increase the duration of your exercise by 5–10 minutes every 1–2 weeks for the first 4–6 weeks of your program.[24] After that, you can build fitness by gradually increasing the duration, frequency, or intensity of exercises.

> **aerobic exercise** Prolonged physical activity that raises the heart rate and works the large muscle groups.
>
> **target heart rate range** The heart rate range to aim for during exercise. A target heart rate range of 64–91% of your maximum heart rate is recommended.

TABLE 5.2 Physical Activity Intensities

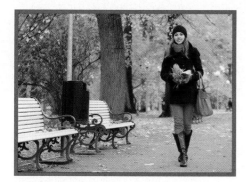

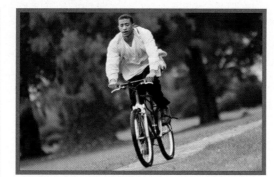

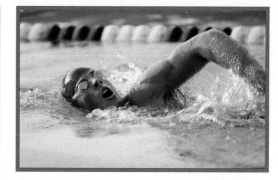

Activity Intensity Level: Lifestyle/light **Heart Rate Range:** Less than 50% maximum heart rate **Examples:** Light yard work and housework, leisurely walking, self-care and bathing, light stretching, light occupational activity **Health Benefits:** A moderate increase in health and wellness in those who are completely sedentary; reduced risk of some chronic diseases

Activity Intensity Level: Moderate **Heart Rate Range:** 50–70% maximum heart rate **Examples:** Walking 3–4.5 miles per hour on a level surface, resistance training, hiking, climbing stairs, dancing, doubles tennis, using a manual wheelchair, recreational swimming, water aerobics, moderate yard work and housework **Health Benefits:** Increased cardiorespiratory endurance, lower body fat levels, improved blood cholesterol and pressure, better blood sugar management, decreased risk of disease, increased overall physical fitness

Activity Intensity Level: Vigorous **Heart Rate Range:** 70–85% maximum heart rate **Examples:** Jogging, running, basketball, soccer, circuit training, backpacking, aerobic classes, competitive sports, swimming laps, martial arts, singles tennis, heavy yard work or housework, hard physical labor/construction, bicycling 10 miles per hour or faster up steep terrain **Health Benefits:** Increased overall physical fitness, decreased risk of disease, further improvements in overall strength and muscular endurance

Source: Adapted from *Physical Activity for Everyone: Target Heart Rate and Estimated Maximum Heart Rate,* from the Centers for Disease Control and Prevention website, 2009; and Hopson, Janet, Donatelle, Rebecca, and Littrell, Tanya, *Get Fit, Stay Well!,* Brief Ed., © 2012. Reprinted and Electronically reproduced by permission of Pearson Education, Inc., Upper Saddle River, New Jersey.

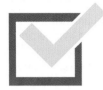

SELF-ASSESSMENT
Determining Your Maximum Heart Rate and Target Heart Rate Range

During aerobic exercise, the rate at which your heart is working lets you know if you are exercising effectively. You will gain the most cardiorespiratory benefit if you exercise within your target heart rate range.

Maximum Heart Rate

To start, you need to know your maximum heart rate. The American College of Sports Medicine (ACSM) has found the most accurate way to determine your maximum heart rate is through the following equation:[1]

$$206.9 - (0.67 \times age) = \text{maximum heart rate}$$

Step 1: _____ × 0.67 = _____
(your age)

Step 2: 206.9 − _____ = _____ = maximum heart rate
(answer from Step 1)

Target Heart Rate Range

You can narrow down the ACSM's target heart rate range of 64–91% of your maximum heart rate based on your current activity level.[2]

- If you perform only minimal physical activity right now, aim for a target heart rate of about 64–74% of your maximum heart rate. Use the following formulas to determine your target heart rate range:

Low end of target heart rate range: _____ × 0.64 = _____
(maximum heart rate)

High end of target heart rate range: _____ × 0.74 = _____
(maximum heart rate)

- If you perform sporadic physical activity right now, aim for a target heart rate of about 74–84% of your maximum heart rate. Use the following formulas to determine your target heart rate range:

Low end of target heart rate range: _____ × 0.74 = _____
(maximum heart rate)

High end of target heart rate range: _____ × 0.84 = _____
(maximum heart rate)

- If you perform regular physical activity right now, aim for a target heart rate of about 80–91% of your maximum heart rate. Use the following formulas to determine your target heart rate range:

Low end of target heart rate range: _____ × 0.80 = _____
(maximum heart rate)

High end of target heart rate range: _____ × 0.91 = _____
(maximum heart rate)

Measuring Your Heart Rate

While you exercise, take your pulse by placing your first two fingers (not your thumb) on the side of your neck next to your windpipe. Using a clock or watch, take your pulse for six seconds and then multiply that number by 10. The result will be your number of heartbeats per minute, which is your heart rate.

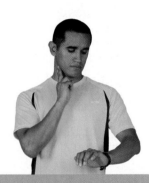

HOW TO INTERPRET YOUR SCORE

- Some cardiorespiratory equipment in gyms, such as stair climbers, offer real-time heart rate calculators. But you can easily track your heart rate using the measurement method above.
- If your heart rate is below your target heart rate range, increase your intensity until you are in your target range; if your heart rate is above your target heart rate range, reduce your intensity.

- There are several methods for calculating maximum heart rate and target heart rate ranges. The formula presented above is the ACSM's most accurate method; some organizations or online calculators may calculate your target heart rate range differently.

To complete this Self-Assessment online, visit MasteringHealth™

References: **1.** *ACSM's Guidelines for Exercise Testing and Prescription*, 8th ed., by the American College of Sports Medicine, 2010, p. 155. Baltimore, MD: Wolters Kluwer/Lippincott Williams & Wilkins. **2.** Ibid., pp. 166–167.

Always be sure to warm up before and cool down after an aerobic session, and to follow other safety precautions for exercise. See pages 115–120 for more about warming up, cooling down, and safety.

Incorporating Aerobic Exercise into Your Daily Life

Dedicated time for aerobic exercise is important, but doesn't hinge on time at the gym. Even engaging in activity for as little as 10 minutes can be an effective way to get more exercise into your life. Simple changes, such as doing some errands on foot instead of in the car, can quickly add up to significant aerobic exercise.

Even if you don't have time for a long walk, try breaking your time on foot into shorter stretches that fit into your daily routine. One study found that people who met physical activity guidelines but did so through bouts of exercise that lasted less than 10 minutes still saw some health improvements.[26] In another study of young men, 10 three-minute brisk walks per day were as effective at lowering resting blood pressure and levels of fats in the blood after meals as one longer walk.[27]

There are lots of other ways to get moving. Ride your bike instead of driving. Take the stairs. If you like being outside, try hiking, swimming,

or games like Ultimate Frisbee or soccer. If you prefer indoor exercise, consider an elliptical trainer, a Zumba class, or an aerobic workout DVD at home. It's easy to make aerobic exercise fun if you find activities that are so enjoyable that the time—and your workout—flies by.

Exercise for Muscular Strength and Endurance

Not all full-body exercises increase cardiorespiratory fitness. Short, intense activities, such as sprint running, sprint swimming, or heavy weight lifting, usually require more oxygen than the body can take in and deliver quickly. As a result, the muscles develop an oxygen deficit and you tire in a short amount of time. However, these **anaerobic exercises** increase your body's ability to deliver short bursts of energy and build muscular strength.

anaerobic exercise Short, intense exercise that causes an oxygen deficit in the muscles.

Many people think building muscle means increasing the amount of weight you can lift—in other words, building strength. But endurance is also an important component of muscular fitness. Strength allows you to lift that heavy box when you move to your next apartment, but muscular endurance will let you carry it all the way out to the moving truck.

In order to build muscle, the muscle must work against some form of resistance—this is called *resistance training* or *strength training*. There are several ways to create resistance that your muscles can work against: free weights (such as dumbbells or barbells), weight machines, resistance bands, or even using your own body weight. You can perform a variety of different exercises with free weights, resistance bands, and your own body weight, whereas weight machines are usually designed for only one or two specific exercises. Weight machines, however, promote correct movement and safe lifting and allow you to easily change the amount of resistance or pinpoint specific muscles.

Isometric versus Isotonic

You can do several different types of exercises while your muscles work against resistance. In **isometric exercise,** the muscle contracts but there is no visible movement. This is accomplished by working against some immovable form of resistance such as your body's own muscle (pressing the palms together) or a structural item (pushing against a door frame). It is most helpful to hold isometric contractions for 6–8 seconds and to perform each exercise 5–10 times. During **isotonic exercise,** muscle force is able to cause movement. The tension in the muscle remains unchanged, but the muscle length changes. Performing a biceps curl with a free weight, walking up stairs, and punching a punching bag are examples of isotonic exercises.

Repetitions and Sets

When developing your resistance training program, you should decide on the numbers of sets and repetitions that you will do for each exercise. **Repetitions** are the number of times you perform

the exercise continuously. **Sets** are separate groups of repetitions. The numbers of sets and repetitions to do depends on whether you are trying to build strength or endurance. Strength develops best when you do a few repetitions (approximately 8–12) with heavier weights or more resistance. Endurance develops best when you do more repetitions (approximately 15–25) with lighter weights or less resistance. Increase the amount of resistance once you can easily perform the desired number of repetitions.

Training Tips

When participating in a resistance training program, be sure to follow these guidelines:

- Use proper technique when performing weight-lifting exercises. See **Practical Strategies: Safe Weight Lifting** on page 110.
- Because resistance exercises are specific to the particular muscles they are designed for, be sure to include exercises for all the major muscle groups.
- Rest for 2–3 minutes between sets. If you are building muscular endurance you can slightly shorten the time between sets.[24]
- Vary your resistance training routine from time to time to lessen the risk of injury and keep your workouts from getting dull. Revisit your program as you get stronger. You may also need different levels or types of resistance training to preserve fitness and muscle mass as you get older.

Figure 5.2 on pages 108–109 shows examples of some simple resistance exercises you can perform.

Recovery

Once you've begun a resistance program, be sure to allow overloaded muscle at least 48 hours for repair and **recovery** before another exercise bout. However, because muscles begin to atrophy after about 96 hours, don't let too much time pass without another training session. If different muscle

isometric exercise Exercise where the muscle contracts but the body does not move.

isotonic exercise Exercise where the muscle contraction causes body movement.

repetitions The number of times you perform an exercise repeatedly.

sets Separate groups of repetitions.

recovery The period necessary for the body to recover from exercise demands and adapt to higher levels of fitness.

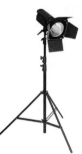

SPOTLIGHT

Core Concerns: Why You Should Strengthen Your Core

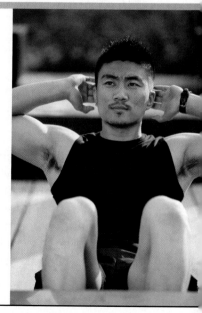

Your core muscles run the entire length of your torso, stabilizing the spine, pelvis, and shoulders. They also provide a solid foundation for movement of the arms and legs and make it possible for you to stand upright, move on two feet, balance, and shift movement in any direction. Standing upright and walking around on two feet is not easy on your body. A strong core distributes the stresses of bearing your weight and protects the back.

Weak core muscles can compromise the appropriate curvature of your spine, often resulting in low back pain and other injuries. The greatest benefit of core strength is increased functional fitness—the fitness that is essential to

both daily living and regular activities. Core strength can be built through exercises such as abdominal curls, planks, back extensions, Pilates, and any other exercises that work core muscles.

 Watch a video about core training at www.youtube.com/watch?v=Lj0q_L2U7EQ.

(a) Squat

Stand with feet shoulder-width apart, toes pointing forward, hips and shoulders aligned, abdominals pulled in. Bend your knees and lower until you have between a 45- and 90-degree angle. Keep your knees behind the front of your toes. Contract your abdominals while coming up.

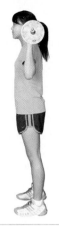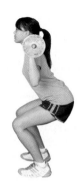

(b) Lunge

Stand with feet shoulder-width apart. As you step forward, keep your front knee in line with your ankle; make sure the front knee does not extend over your toes. Distribute your weight evenly between the front and back leg.

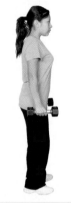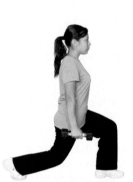

(c) Leg Abduction

Connect a resistance band to a stable object and loop around your outside leg. Stand with good posture and hold onto something stable. Slowly extend your leg out and return.

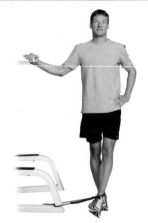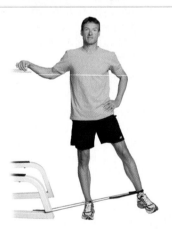

(d) Biceps Curl

Sit on a bench or chair with a dumbbell in each hand. Sit with good posture (ears and shoulders over hips and abdominals contracted) and your feet planted on the ground for balance. Lift one dumbbell up to your shoulder, turning your palm toward your shoulder as you lift. Slowly lower the dumbbell to the starting position as you lift the dumbbell in your other hand.

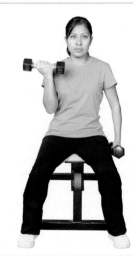

FIGURE 5.2 Simple Resistance Exercises. Be sure to perform exercises equally on both sides.

Source: Text from Hopson, Janet, Donatelle, Rebecca, and Littrell, Tanya, *Get Fit, Stay Well!* 2nd ed. © 2013, Fig. 5.8, pp. 127–139. Reprinted and Electronically reproduced by permission of Pearson Education, Inc., Upper Saddle River, New Jersey.

(e) Curl-Up

Lie on a mat with your arms by your sides, palms down, elbows straight, and fingers extended. Bend your knees at about 90-degrees. Curl your head and upper back upward, reaching your arms forward, then curl back down so that your upper back and shoulders touch the mat. During the entire curl-up, your feet and buttocks should stay on the mat.

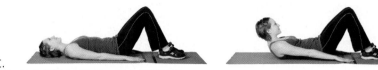
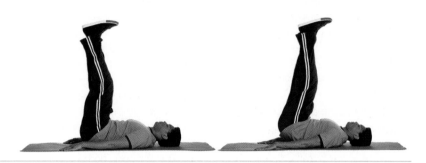

(f) Reverse Curl

 Lie on your back and place your hands near your hips. Lift your legs to 90-degrees from the floor. Your knees may be bent or straight. Contract your abdominals, pulling them in, while you lift your hips off the floor. Slowly return hips to the floor. Be careful not to rock back and forth.

(g) Back Extension

 Start lying on your stomach with your arms and legs extended, forehead on the mat. Lift and further extend your arms and legs using your back muscles. Hold for 3–5 seconds and slowly lower back down.

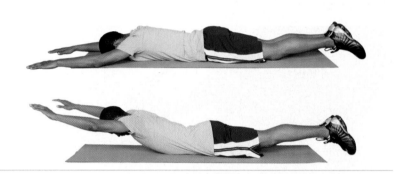

(h) Plank

 Support yourself in plank position (from the forearms or hands) by contracting your trunk muscles so that your neck, back, and hips are completely straight. Hold for 5–60 seconds, increasing time as you become stronger. Your forearms should be slightly wider than your shoulders.

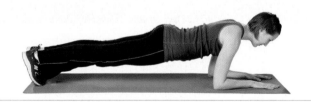

(i) Modified Push-Ups

 Support yourself in push-up position as shown by contracting your trunk muscles. Place hands slightly wider than your shoulders. Keep your neck, back, and hips completely straight; do not let your trunk sag in the middle or raise your hips. Slowly lower your body down toward the floor, being careful to keep a straight body position. Your elbows will press out and back as you lower to a 90-degree elbow joint. Press yourself back up to start position.

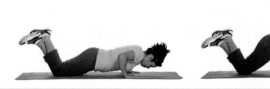

Practical Strategies

Safe Weight Lifting

- If you are just beginning to use weights, make an appointment with a fitness specialist who can teach you the proper techniques that reduce the risk of injury and maximize the benefits you receive.
- Always warm up before weight lifting.
- Take your time and lift mindfully.
- Breathe out as you lift the weight and in as you release the weight—don't hold your breath, it can cause dangerous increases in blood pressure.

- Focus on the muscle you're trying to work. Feel the effort in the muscle, not in the joint.
- Equally train opposing muscle groups, such as the lower back and abdomen or the biceps and triceps.
- Use only the amount of weights that your body can handle without having to cheat by using other muscles or momentum.
- When using free weights, always have a partner who can check your form and "spot" for you.

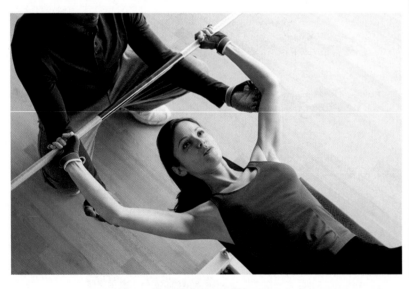

groups are worked on different days (for example, lower body versus upper body), it is acceptable to perform resistance exercise on consecutive days as long as each muscle group receives the recommended 48 hours of recovery time.

 Keep a log of your workouts so you can be sure to allow each muscle group adequate recovery time. Try these online logs: www.wellsphere .com, www.sparkpeople.com, **and** www.supertracker.usda.gov/ physicalactivitytracker.aspx.

Exercises for Improving Flexibility

There are two major types of flexibility. **Static flexibility** is the ability to reach and hold a stretch at one endpoint of a joint's range of motion. **Dynamic flexibility** is the ability to move quickly and fluidly through a joint's entire range of motion with little resistance. Static flexibility

determines whether a martial artist can reach her leg as high as her opponent's head, but it is dynamic flexibility that enables her to kick her leg that high in one fast, fluid motion. Flexibility can vary a lot among individuals, but everyone can increase flexibility through consistent stretching exercises.

Stretching

Stretching applies gentle, elongating force to both a muscle and its connective tissue. **Static stretching,** the most common form of stretching, involves a gradual stretch and then hold of the stretched position for a certain amount of time. Static stretching can be either active or passive. **Active stretching** is where you apply the force for the stretch. **Passive stretching,** on the other hand, is performed with a partner who gently applies the force to the stretch. Passive stretching may provide a more intense flexibility workout but also increases the risk of injury because you are not controlling the stretch yourself. **Ballistic stretching** focuses on the use of dynamic repetitive bouncing movements to stretch a muscle beyond its normal range of motion. If ballistic stretching is performed improperly, it can increase the risk of injury, so it is best for recreational exercisers to avoid this form of stretching.[28] **Dynamic stretching,** or slow movement stretching, incorporates movements performed in a controlled manner that mimic a specific sport or exercise and are often included during the warm-up or in preparation for a sports event. An example in soccer would be gently swinging a leg back and forth as if to kick an imaginary ball.

Flexibility varies for each joint, and flexibility exercises are specific to the joint they're designed for, so when creating a flexibility program, be sure to stretch all the major muscle and joint areas of the body (neck, shoulders, upper and lower back, pelvis, hips, and legs). Don't stretch cold muscles. Instead, warm up by walking or jogging or some other low-intensity activity for at least 5 minutes prior to stretching, or stretch at the end of your workout. The following tips will help you create your flexibility program:[29]

- Hold static stretches for 10–30 seconds.
- Perform two to four repetitions of each stretch, accumulating 60 seconds per stretch.
- Stretch at least 2–3 days per week.
- Stretch until your muscle feels tight or until you feel slight discomfort.
- Do not hold your breath while stretching. Try to relax and breathe deeply.
- Do not lock your joints while stretching.

static flexibility The ability to reach and hold a stretch at one endpoint of a joint's range of motion.

dynamic flexibility The ability to move quickly and fluidly through a joint's entire range of motion with little resistance.

static stretching Gradually lengthening a muscle to an elongated position and sustaining that position.

active stretching A type of static stretching where you gently apply force to your body to create a stretch.

passive stretching Stretching performed with a partner who increases the intensity of the stretch by gently applying pressure to your body as it stretches.

ballistic stretching Performing rhythmic bouncing movements in a stretch to increase the intensity of the stretch.

dynamic stretching A type of slow movement stretching in which activities from a workout or sport are mimicked in a controlled manner, often to help "warm up" for a game or event.

Holistic Flexibility Programs

In addition to regular stretching exercises, there are several other types of mind- and whole body–centered activities that increase flexibility. These types of activities are also sometimes referred to as *neuromotor exercise*, or workouts designed to improve balance and agility. Three of the most popular are yoga, Pilates, and tai chi:

- **Yoga** moves you through a set of carefully constructed poses designed to increase flexibility and strength. Yoga also addresses mood and thought, using techniques such as breathing exercises to reduce stress and anxiety.
- **Pilates** combines stretching and resistance exercises to create a sequence of precise, controlled movements that focuses on flexibility, joint mobility, and core strength. Because Pilates movements are so precise, it is recommended to begin Pilates in a group or private class.
- **Tai chi** is a Chinese practice designed to work the entire body gently through a series of quiet, fluid motions. The discipline also focuses on your energy, referred to in Chinese as "chi" (sometimes spelled "qi") or life force. The practice aims to keep a participant's body and chi in balance, requiring a focus on mood and thought.

Figure 5.3 on pages 112–113 shows simple flexibility exercises you can easily perform on your own as well.

>> Wherever you download apps, search for podcasts on topics like running, action sports, yoga, or activities in the great outdoors.

How Much Physical Activity Do You Need?

Creating a fitness program is more than determining what types of exercise to do; you'll also want to decide how often to be active so that you can move from overload to recovery and back again in an effective, consistent way.

Guidelines for Health Maintenance

The *Physical Activity Guidelines for Americans* from the U.S. Department of Health and Human Services recommends the following activity levels for the creation and maintenance of health-related fitness in healthy adults:[30]

- At least 2 hours and 30 minutes (150 minutes) of moderate-intensity aerobic activity each week

OR

- At least 1 hour and 15 minutes (75 minutes) of vigorous-intensity aerobic activity each week

OR

- An equivalent mix of moderate- and vigorous-intensity aerobic activity each week

AND

- Resistance exercise 2 days a week or more, for all major muscle groups, in sets of at least 8–12 repetitions

More detailed guidelines from the American College of Sports Medicine build on the government fitness recommendations, and include specific suggestions for flexibility and neuromotor exercise. **Table 5.3** and **Figure 5.4** on pages 114-115 summarize this set of exercise recommendations.

A good way to meet the aerobic guidelines is to perform 30 minutes of moderate-intensity activity 5 days a week. For greater health benefits, increase your weekly aerobic activity to 300 minutes (5 hours) of moderate-intensity activity or 150 minutes (2 hours and 30 minutes) of high-intensity activity.[30] If weight loss or maintenance of weight loss is one of your fitness goals, aim for at least 60–90 minutes of moderate-intensity physical activity a day.[31]

Avoid Sustained Sitting

Figure 5.4 includes a type of activity that should be minimized as much as possible: "sustained sitting," or sedentary behaviors. Sedentary behavior is typically defined as any behavior with exceedingly low energy expenditure. These behaviors include seated "couch potato activities" such as watching television, playing video games, and staring at computer screen. In one recent study, researchers found that the amount of leisure time spent sitting is linked to increased risk of death, even if you work out.[32] The researchers found that sitting six or more hours a day outside of work or class, compared to less than three hours, was significantly associated with a greater risk of death. Try to limit the overall quantity of daily sustained sitting, as well as to take frequent breaks to interrupt and intersperse sustained sitting by standing up and moving about briefly every 30 minutes.

Increase Your Level of Activity

The following tips can help you increase your activity levels and meet—or even go beyond—the physical activity recommendations.

If You Aren't Active Now

If you usually get little or no regular physical activity, start by doing what you can, and then look for ways to add more. If you tire easily, you can work out in as little as 10-minute intervals.[33] Below are a few easy ways you can add activity into your life:

- Park your car at the far end of the parking lot.
- Walk briskly or ride your bike to class.
- Begin an active new social hobby like tennis, yoga, or dance classes.
- Don't forget to include resistance and flexibility exercises at least two days per week.

If You Get Some Physical Activity Now

If you engage in some physical activity on a regular basis, focus on increasing your activity level:[33]

- Increase the intensity of your aerobic exercise by replacing moderate- with vigorous-intensity activities.
- Be active for longer; instead of walking for 30 minutes, try walking for 50 minutes.

> " *A good way to meet the aerobic guidelines is to perform 30 minutes of moderate-intensity activity 5 days a week.* "

(a) Neck Stretches

Head turn: Gently turn your head to look over one shoulder, keeping both of your shoulders down.
Head tilt: Keeping your chin level and your shoulders down, tilt your head to one side.

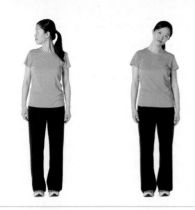

(b) Upper-Back Stretch

Reach your arms in front of you and clasp your hands while rounding your back and lowering your head.

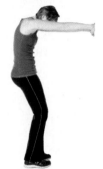

(c) Shoulder Stretch

Reach one arm across your chest and hold it above or below the elbow with the other hand.

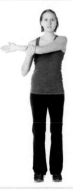

(d) Tricep Stretch

Lift your arm overhead, reaching the elbow toward the ceiling. Press the arm back from the front or reach your other arm over your head and gently pull the elbow toward your head.

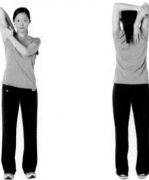

(e) Torso Twist

Sit with your legs straight out in front of you. Bend one knee and cross it over your other leg. Turn your body toward the bent knee and twist to look behind you. Place the opposite arm on the bent leg to gently press the stretch further.

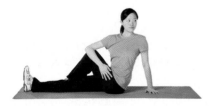

FIGURE 5.3 Simple Stretching Exercises. Be sure to perform exercises equally on both sides.

Source: Text from Hopson, Janet, Donatelle, Rebecca, and Littrell, Tanya, *Get Fit, Stay Well!* 2nd ed. © 2013, Fig. 6.3, pp. 169–174. Reprinted and Electronically reproduced by permission of Pearson Education, Inc., Upper Saddle River, New Jersey.

(f) Hip Stretch

While lying on your back, bend one knee and hip 90-degrees and keep the other leg straight. Slowly move the bent leg across your body toward the floor. Keep your arms wide and both shoulders down.

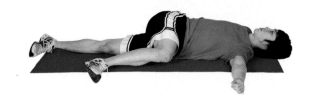

(g) Inner-Thigh Butterfly Stretch

Bring the bottoms of your feet together and pull your feet gently toward you. Actively contract your hip muscles to lower your knees closer to the ground.

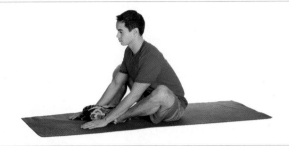

(h) Hip Flexor Stretch

Stand tall with one foot forward and one foot back in a lunge position. Lift up the heel of the back leg and press your hips forward.

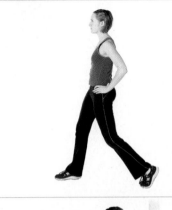

(i) Quadriceps Stretch

Grab your foot from behind and pull it back toward your rear until you feel a stretch in the front of your thighs. Maintain straight body alignment and keep your thighs parallel. Assist your balance by holding onto a stable object.

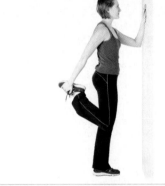

(j) Hamstrings Stretch

Sit with one leg extended and the other leg bent with the knee facing sideways. Keeping your back as straight as possible, lean your body forward, moving your chest closer to your extended leg. If you are moderately flexible, you can reach for and hold your foot but only if this does not cause pain.

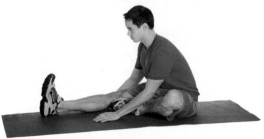

(k) Gluteal Stretch

Lie on your back with one leg bent and the foot on the floor. Place the ankle of the other leg on your thigh just above the knee (toward the hip). Lift both legs toward the chest and support them with your hands clasped behind your thigh.

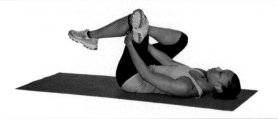

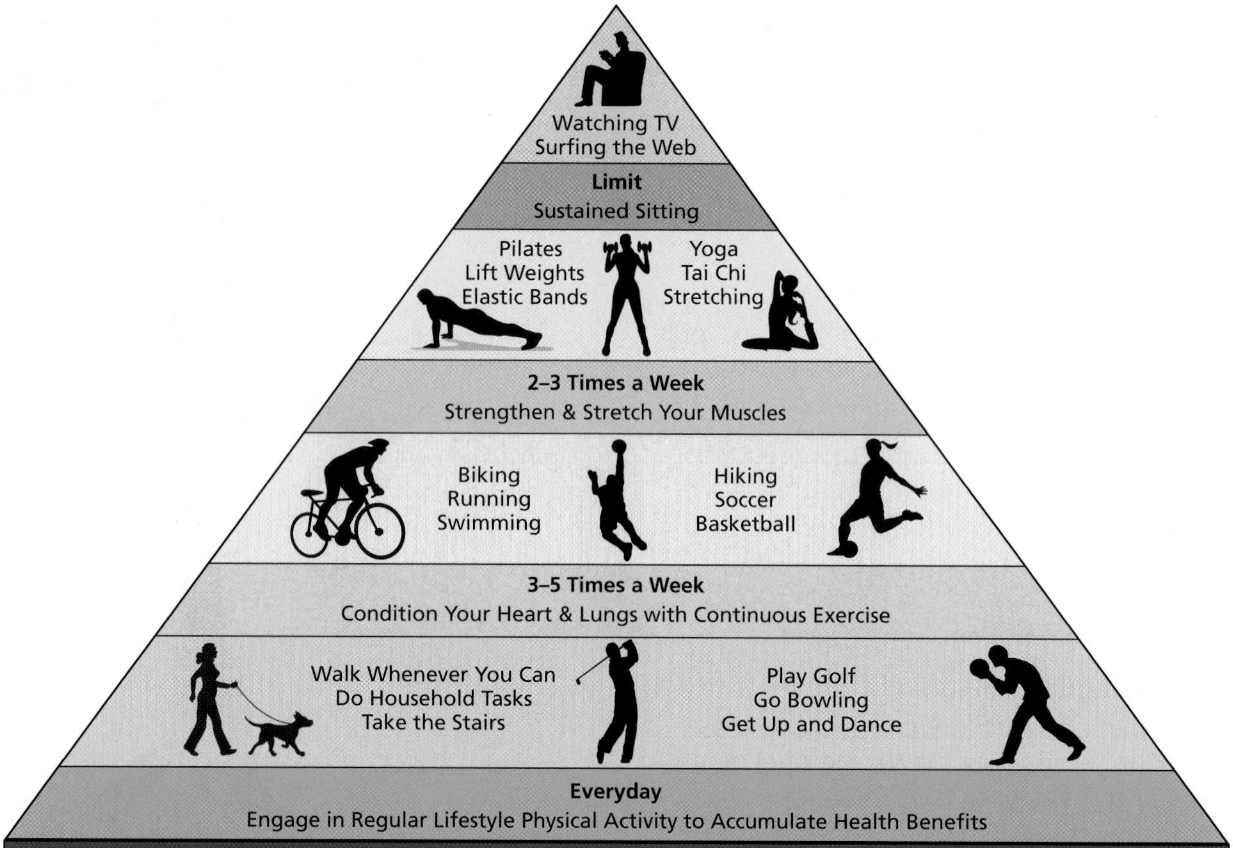

Watching TV
Surfing the Web
Limit
Sustained Sitting
Pilates
Lift Weights
Elastic Bands
Yoga
Tai Chi
Stretching
2–3 Times a Week
Strengthen & Stretch Your Muscles
Biking
Running
Swimming
Hiking
Soccer
Basketball
3–5 Times a Week
Condition Your Heart & Lungs with Continuous Exercise
Walk Whenever You Can
Do Household Tasks
Take the Stairs
Play Golf
Go Bowling
Get Up and Dance
Everyday
Engage in Regular Lifestyle Physical Activity to Accumulate Health Benefits

My Physical Activity & Exercise Pyramid

Lifestyle Physical Activity	Cardiorespiratory Exercise	Resistance, Flexibility, & Neuromotor Exercise	Sedentary Behavior
Engage in daily physical activity at home or work or by commute. Some activity is better than none. Engage in intermittent light- or moderate-intensity physical activity anytime, anywhere. Engage in ≥ 30 min. daily, preferably ≥10 min. at a time. Accumulate ≥150 min. per week. More min. = more health benefits.	Plan aerobic exercise that elevates your training heart rate to a moderate or vigorous intensity. Plan 5 moderate sessions of ≥ 30 min. or 3 vigorous sessions of ≥ 20 min. or a combination of both weekly. Plan sporting or recreational activities that involve moderate or vigorous bursts of aerobic activity with brief rest periods.	Strengthen major muscle groups. Perform 8 to 12 reps per set, do 2 to 4 sets per exercise. Stretch major muscle groups. Hold each stretch 10–30s, repeat to accumulate 60s. Select functional fitness exercises that simultaneously use multiple muscles and joints to improve strength, balance, and agility.	Too much sustained sitting is not the same as too little exercise or physical activity. Trim daily sustained sitting time to lessen the effects of sedentarism on metabolic health. Take frequent breaks to interrupt and intersperse sustained sitting. Stand up occasionally and move briefly every 30 minutes.

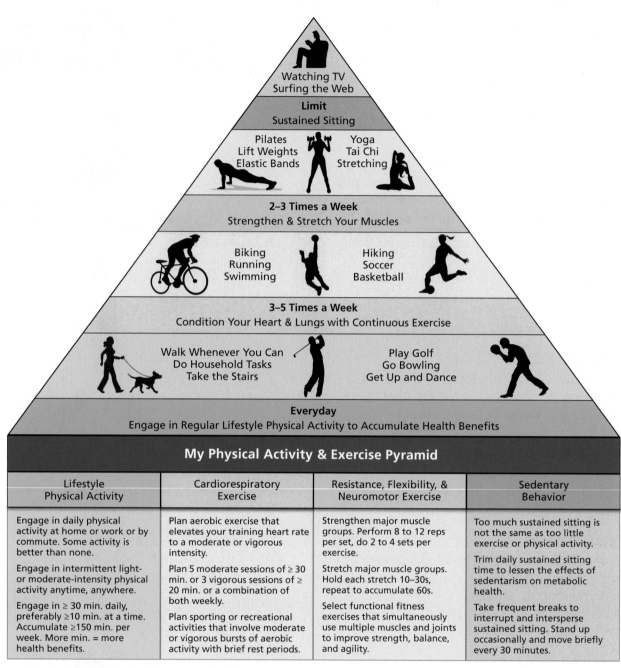

FIGURE 5.4 My Physical Activity and Exercise Pyramid. This pyramid summarizes the physical activity recommendations for adults.

Source: "My Physical Activity and Exercise Pyramid" by Dr. Jerome E. Kotecki, Ball State University. © 2012 by Jerome Kotecki. Reprinted with permission.

- Be active more often; if you work out two days a week, try building up to four days a week.
- If you already meet the minimum recommendations for activity, strive for the elevated recommendations of 300 minutes of moderate-intensity or 150 minutes of vigorous-intensity activity per week.

If You Are Overweight

Many people who are overweight or obese feel that they can't start an activity program, but that isn't true. To get started with an activity program, try the following:

- If your current weight puts stress on your joints, choose non–weight-bearing exercise. Swimming and water-based exercise classes can get you moving without stressing your joints.
- Remember that everyday activities, such as housework, walking the dog, or washing the car, can get you moving. Any activity that puts your body in motion helps. Try increasing your physical activity slightly each day.
- If you haven't worked out in a while, begin with light-intensity (40–50% of your maximum heart rate) aerobic activity that gets your whole body moving. This will provide health benefits, expend energy to help with weight loss, and set the foundation for progression to higher intensities.

TABLE 5.3 Exercise Guidelines from the ACSM

Exercise Type	ACSM Guidelines
Cardiorespiratory	Adults should get at least 150 minutes of moderate-intensity exercise per week or 75 minutes of vigorous-intensity exercise per week, or an equivalent mix of both.
	Exercise recommendations can be met through 30–60 minutes of moderate-intensity exercise (five days per week) or 20–60 minutes of vigorous-intensity exercise (three days per week), or an equivalent mix of both.
	One continuous session and multiple shorter sessions (of at least 10 minutes) are both acceptable to accumulate the desired amount of daily exercise.
	Gradual progression of exercise time, frequency, and intensity is recommended for best adherence and least injury risk.
	People unable to meet these minimums can still benefit from some activity.
Resistance	Adults should train each major muscle group two or three days each week using a variety of exercises and equipment.
	Two to four sets of each exercise will help adults improve strength and power.
	For each exercise, 8–12 repetitions improve strength and power, 10–15 repetitions improve strength in middle-aged and older persons starting exercise, and 15–20 repetitions improve muscular endurance.
	Adults should wait at least 48 hours between resistance training sessions.
	Very light or light intensity is best for older persons or previously sedentary adults starting exercise.
	A gradual progression of greater resistance, and/or more repetitions per set, and/or increasing frequency is recommended.
Flexibility	Adults should do flexibility exercises at least two or three days each week to improve range of motion.
	Each stretch should be held for 10–30 seconds to the point of tightness or slight discomfort.
	Repeat each stretch two to four times, accumulating 60 seconds per stretch.
	Static, dynamic, ballistic, and PNF stretches are all effective.
	Flexibility exercise is most effective when the muscle is warm. Try light aerobic activity or a hot bath to warm the muscles before stretching.
Neuromotor	Neuromotor exercise (sometimes called "functional fitness training") is recommended for two or three days per week.
	20–30 minutes per day is appropriate for neuromotor exercise.
	Exercises should involve motor skills (balance, agility, coordination, and gait), proprioceptive exercise training, and multifaceted activities (tai chi and yoga) to improve physical function and prevent falls in older adults.

Data from *Quantity and Quality of Exercise for Developing and Maintaining Cardiorespiratory, Musculoskeletal, and Neuromotor Fitness in Apparently Healthy Adults: Guidance for Prescribing Exercise,* by C. Garber, B. Blissmer, M. Deschenes, B. Franklin, M. Lamonte, I. Lee, D. Nieman, & D. Swain, 2011, *Medicine & Science in Sports & Exercise. 43* (7), pp. 1334–1359.

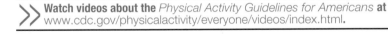

>> **Watch videos about the** *Physical Activity Guidelines for Americans* **at** www.cdc.gov/physicalactivity/everyone/videos/index.html**.**

Exercise Safe, Exercise Smart

Exercising safely is not difficult, if you keep a few basic guidelines in mind.

Get Medical Clearance

Before you begin any exercise program, make an appointment with a doctor to make sure you do not have any health conditions that should be taken into account before you begin an exercise program.

Warm Up and Cool Down

Before you start any moderate- to vigorous-intensity exercise, give yourself about 15 minutes to warm up. Warming up is not the same as stretching; effective warm-up involves gentle overall motion or a slowed-down version of the activity you are about to pursue, which increases your heart rate and blood flow to the muscles needed for exercise. When you are finished with your workout, give yourself another 15 minutes to cool down by performing slower and less intense movements, slowly returning your body to a less active state.

Get Training

Learning proper workout techniques from a qualified instructor will help prevent injury and increase your success at the activity. When you are choosing a trainer or fitness instructor, look for certifications from nonprofit organizations like the American College of Sports Medicine. Trainers and instructors should be knowledgeable in CPR and first aid; they should also undergo ongoing professional training on new techniques. Before settling on a fitness instructor, make sure that person makes you feel comfortable and provides helpful feedback to you during your workout.

Wear Suitable Clothes

Clothes made of lightweight, breathable fabrics such as 100% cotton will help keep you comfortable as you exercise and allow for full range of movement. Clothing marketed as moisture-wicking will pull sweat away from your body to increase comfort as well. Use sun protection and a hat if you will be outside, even if it is overcast. Wear a helmet, pads, and other protective gear when cycling, skateboarding, or participating in any other activities where a fall is possible. It's also important to wear the proper athletic shoes for the activity you are pursuing. See the **Consumer Corner** box on page 118 for more information on how to pick a proper shoe for exercise.

Eat Right

What food should you eat when you exercise? Consider these suggestions, adapted from the Mayo Clinic:[34]

- **Eat breakfast.** Your body needs fuel before exercise. If you plan to eat within an hour of your workout, reach for something lighter, such as whole grain cereal.
- **Need a snack before your workout?** Think small and healthful. Good options include fresh fruit, yogurt, and crackers with peanut butter.
- **After your workout, eat within two hours.** Smart snacks include yogurt and fruit, nuts, and string cheese and crackers. If it's time for a meal, be sure it includes protein, carbs, and fiber.

What About Protein?

Athletes and those who train like athletes have higher protein needs than the standard recommendation for Americans of 0.8 grams of protein per kilogram of body weight.[35] It is recommended that endurance athletes consume 1.2 to 1.4 grams of protein per kilogram of ideal weight each day. Strength athletes should consume slightly more, between 1.5 and 1.7 grams of protein per kilogram of ideal weight each day. In reality, however, most nonvegetarian Americans consume enough protein each day to meet even these higher protein needs.[36] Additionally, although adequate protein consumption is of great importance to athletes, more is not always better. The overconsumption of protein, in excess of 2 grams per kilogram per day, has not been proven to improve strength or performance.[35]

Stay Hydrated

Adequate water consumption is a critical part of any workout. Studies show that dehydration limits strength, power, and endurance.[37] It is most effective to keep drinking water before, during, and after exercise as opposed to gulping down water all at once at the end of your workout. If you find yourself feeling thirsty, fatigued, with weak muscles and a minor headache, you may need to rehydrate.

To stay hydrated, fitness specialists say that water is your best choice. If, however, activity is prolonged and performed at a high intensity level, you may consider commercial sports drinks. These beverages combine water with flavorings, sugars that provide energy, and *electrolytes,* salts that help your body function properly. For everyday workouts, however, sports drinks are often unnecessary. These beverages are often expensive, provide little essential nutrition, and contain unnecessary levels of sugar. If you prefer the taste of sports drinks to plain water but aren't performing vigorous-intensity, prolonged exercise, try mixing just a little sports drink, juice, or a few slices of lemon or lime into a bottle of water.

Prepare for Hot or Cold Weather

If you exercise outside, always check the weather report before you go out. In cold weather you need layered clothing that keeps you warm

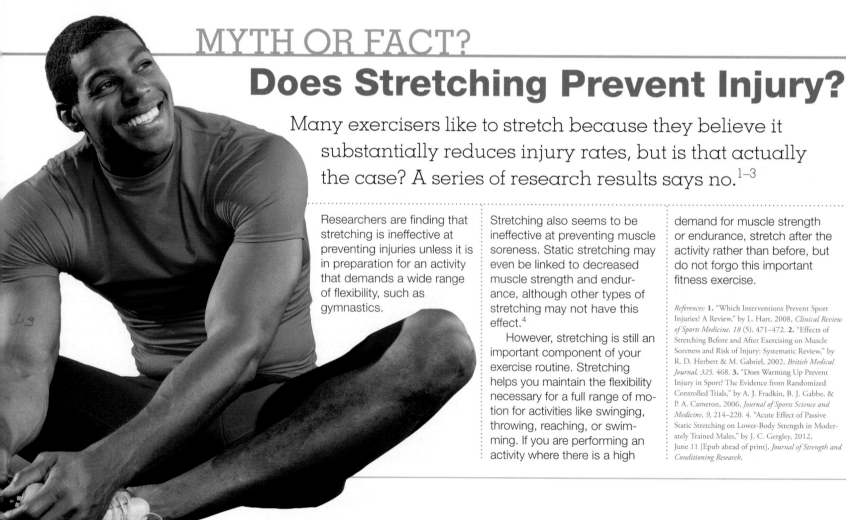

MYTH OR FACT?

Does Stretching Prevent Injury?

Many exercisers like to stretch because they believe it substantially reduces injury rates, but is that actually the case? A series of research results says no.[1–3]

Researchers are finding that stretching is ineffective at preventing injuries unless it is in preparation for an activity that demands a wide range of flexibility, such as gymnastics.

Stretching also seems to be ineffective at preventing muscle soreness. Static stretching may even be linked to decreased muscle strength and endurance, although other types of stretching may not have this effect.[4]

However, stretching is still an important component of your exercise routine. Stretching helps you maintain the flexibility necessary for a full range of motion for activities like swinging, throwing, reaching, or swimming. If you are performing an activity where there is a high

demand for muscle strength or endurance, stretch after the activity rather than before, but do not forgo this important fitness exercise.

References: **1.** "Which Interventions Prevent Sport Injuries? A Review," by L. Hart, 2008, *Clinical Review of Sports Medicine, 18* (5), 471–472. **2.** "Effects of Stretching Before and After Exercising on Muscle Soreness and Risk of Injury: Systematic Review," by R. D. Herbert & M. Gabriel, 2002, *British Medical Journal, 325,* 468. **3.** "Does Warming Up Prevent Injury in Sport? The Evidence from Randomized Controlled Trials," by A. J. Fradkin, B. J. Gabbe, & P. A. Cameron, 2006, *Journal of Sports Science and Medicine, 9,* 214–220. 4. "Acute Effect of Passive Static Stretching on Lower-Body Strength in Moderately Trained Males," by J. C. Gergley, 2012, June 11 [Epub ahead of print], *Journal of Strength and Conditioning Research.*

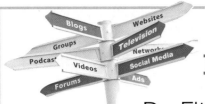

media and FITNESS

Do Fitness Apps Work?

When working out, more and more people bring a new piece of gear along with their towel and water bottle: their phone. In one recent survey of smartphone users, 38% of those who had downloaded a health-related app had included at least one fitness app in their selections.[1] But mobile apps are a relatively new part of fitness, and at least so far, appear to offer mixed results in improving your workout.

Apps can be fun, give you new workout suggestions, and provide connections to others with similar fitness goals and challenges. But not all are based on sound fitness science. In one key study, researchers found that many fitness apps aren't based on the scientific theories and guidelines proven to motivate real health behavior change.[2] One common shortcoming is the limited ability for users to customize an app to important personal factors such as height, weight, or age.[2] When choosing an app, consider those that allow you to personalize your experience.

Another study found that health-related apps with slightly higher costs (more than the popular $0.99 price for many apps) were more likely to be based on factors important to lasting behavior change.[3] In other words, it may be worth paying a little more for an app, to get help achieving long-term results. Fee-based apps that have received positive feedback for quality include C25K (Couch to 5k), iTreadmill, iFitness, and FitnessBuilder.

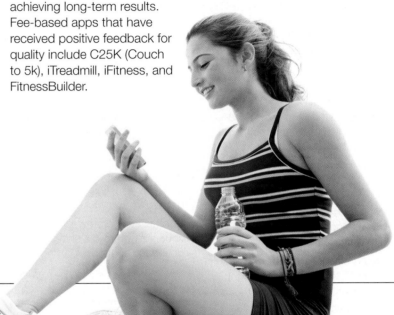

Critical-Thinking Questions

1. Have you used a fitness-related app to help with a workout? Why or why not?

2. What are some of the benefits of social connection and support in using fitness apps? What might be some of the drawbacks?

3. Based on what you've learned about behavior change, what are two or three important factors that would form the basis of a fitness app more likely to help you achieve long-term results?

References: 1. "Mobile Health 2012," by the Pew Internet and American Life Project, 2012, retrieved from http://www.pewinternet.org/Reports/2012/Mobile-Health.aspx. 2. "Apps of Steel: Are Exercise Apps Providing Consumers with Realistic Expectations? A Content Analysis of Exercise Apps for Presence of Behavior Change Theory," by L. Cowan, S. Van Wagenen, B. Brown, R. Hedin, Y. Seino-Stephan, P. Hall, & J. West, 2012, Health Education & Behavior, 1090198112452126. 3. "There's an App for That: Content Analysis of Paid Health and Fitness Apps," by J. West, C. Hall, C. Hanson, M. Barnes, C. Giraud-Carrier, & J. Barrett, 2012, Journal of Medical Internet Research, 14 (3), e72.

and wicks sweat away from your body, but lets you move at the same time. Wear a hat, because much of your body heat is lost through your head, and protect your fingers and toes from the cold. If you start shivering, stop your workout, add more layers of clothing, and head inside. Constant shivering is an early sign of **hypothermia,** a potentially fatal condition in which your core body temperature dips too low. If your core temperature isn't raised you will become uncoordinated, drowsy, and confused and will have difficulty speaking. If anyone you work out with develops these symptoms, he or she should be warmed up and taken to a hospital.

hypothermia A potentially fatal condition in which your core body temperature becomes too low.

heat exhaustion A mild form of heat-related illness that usually occurs as the result of exercising in hot weather without adequate hydration.

heatstroke A life-threatening heat-related illness that occurs when your core temperature rises above 105 degrees Fahrenheit.

If you are working out in the heat, try to exercise in early morning or evening, when the weather tends to be cooler and less humid. If you get too dehydrated in hot weather, you put yourself at risk for **heat exhaustion,** a mild form of heat-related illness. Symptoms of heat exhaustion include nausea, headache, fatigue, and faintness, and mean you need to slow down, drink water, and head for a cooler spot.

If your overheating worsens, you face the possibility of **heatstroke,** a potentially fatal condition. In heatstroke, your overheated core body temperature overwhelms your body's cooling capabilities,

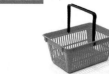

CONSUMER CORNER

Choosing Athletic Shoes

When shopping for athletic shoes it's important to choose shoes that are made for the particular activity you are participating in, because while athletic shoes look similar on the outside, each kind is constructed differently. The following tips will help you pick the best shoe:[1, 2]

- Always go to a store that specializes in athletic shoes to find the best selection and the most knowledgeable salespeople.

- Shop for shoes at the end of the day, when your feet are at their largest.

- Wear the type of socks you plan on wearing with the shoes, in order to get the best fit.

- Watch for width. If the sides of the heel, toes, or arch feel tight, it's not wide enough.

- If you have high arches, make sure to purchase a shoe or separate insoles with lots of arch support and cushioning.

- Purchase shoes made specifically for your sex. However, women with wide feet may consider trying men's or boy's shoes, which are made a bit larger throughout the heel.

- Bring your old shoes with you. Shoe professionals can give you tips based on the wear pattern on your old shoes.

- Try on both shoes, and walk, run, or perform the types of movements you will use the shoe for. The shoes should feel immediately comfortable, and your heel should fit snugly in each shoe and not slip as you walk.

- Don't assume you wear the same shoe size in athletic shoes as you do in regular shoes.

Running shoes should be replaced every 300–500 miles, cross-training shoes after 5–7 months, and aerobic shoes after 100–120 hours of use.[2, 3] If your shoes are wearing through, it's time to replace them regardless of how long you've had them.

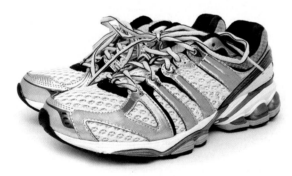

This interactive graphic can help you select the best walking shoes:
www.mayoclinic.com/health/medical/FS00001.

References: 1. "Walking Shoes: Features and Fit That Keep You Moving," by the Mayo Clinic, 2009, retrieved from http://www.mayoclinic.com/health/walking/HQ00885_D. 2. "Smart Shopping for Athletic Shoes," by K. A. Laux, 2009, retrieved from http://www.livestrong.com/article/353-smart-shopping-athletic-shoes. 3. "Selecting Workout Shoes: Proper Sports Shoes Can Increase Pleasure and Reduce Pain," by C. Christian, 2007, retrieved from http://fitness.suite101.com/article.cfm/selecting_workout_shoes.

causing dry, hot skin and rapid heart rate. Brain damage and death can follow. If you experience any of the symptoms, you need rest, a cooler location, ice packs applied to your body, especially your armpits and groin area, and lots of cool fluids to drink immediately. Outdoor sports that require heavy pads, such as football, make it tough for your body

to regulate its temperature effectively on hot days and put you at higher risk for heatstroke. If you participate in gear-heavy sports that leave you feeling overheated, such as football, talk to your coach about taking steps to make everyone cooler.

Start Slow and Watch Out for Red Flags

It's important to start slowly when you begin an exercise program, in order to avoid injuries. If you experience any of the following symptoms while exercising, stop immediately, no matter your level of fitness. Talk with your doctor or campus health service about any of these symptoms:

- Pain, tightness, or pressure in your chest, neck, arm, or shoulder
- Dizziness or nausea
- Cold sweats
- Severe muscle cramps
- Extreme shortness of breath
- Pain in your joints, feet, ankles, or legs

Care for Injuries

Injuries occasionally do happen when exercising. Common complaints include contusions (bruises), joint sprains, muscle strains, shin splints, and tendinitis. These injuries most often cause pain, swelling, or skin discoloration.

Another common complaint during exercise is **cramps.** These severe muscle contractions are your body's way of making you take a break. If you get a cramp, stop your activity. Drink some water and massage or apply pressure to the cramped muscle. You can also try taking a few deep breaths to give your body—and your cramped muscles—extra oxygen.

Minor injuries to the muscles and joints should be treated with the RICE protocol: rest, ice, compression, and elevation. The first step is to rest the injured area; stop exercising as soon as you feel pain. Second, ice the injured area for no more than 20 minutes at a time intermittently for the first 24–48 hours. The cold of the ice helps to decrease the swelling. After 48 hours you can apply a heating pad to the area, which improves blood flow and promotes healing. Third, compress the area with an elastic bandage, both to hold the ice in place and to decrease the swelling. Finally, if you can elevate the injured area above your heart, do so. It will minimize swelling and discomfort.

Be Wary of Performance-Enhancing Drugs

Prominent athletes, including well-known Olympic athletes, cyclists, and players in Major League Baseball, have made headlines after investigators discovered their use of performance-enhancing drugs. But use of these substances isn't confined to the top tiers of sports. According to health estimates, up to three million Americans have used performance-enhancing drugs, including an estimated 4.7% of males and 1.2% of females.[38] In a national survey, about 40% of high school seniors described these substances as "fairly easy" or "very easy" to get.[39] Some performance-enhancing drugs carry dangerous side effects, and a few are even illegal for use or sale in the United States. Common types of performance-enhancing drugs include:

- **Anabolic steroids.** Synthetic derivatives of the male hormone testosterone, anabolic

cramp An involuntary contracted muscle that does not relax, resulting in localized intense pain.

When you want to boost your **fitness level,** how you get started can make you stronger—or leave you sidelined. To pursue fitness in a healthy way:

CHOOSE THIS.

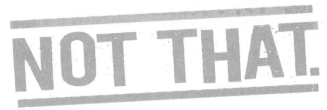

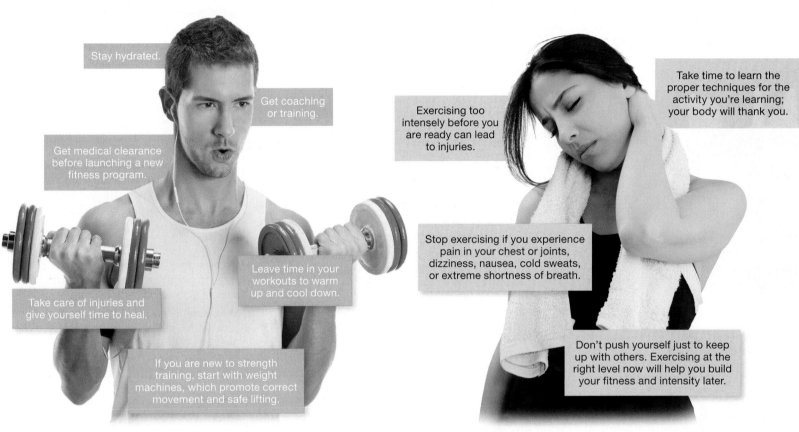

Stay hydrated.

Get coaching or training.

Get medical clearance before launching a new fitness program.

Take care of injuries and give yourself time to heal.

Leave time in your workouts to warm up and cool down.

If you are new to strength training, start with weight machines, which promote correct movement and safe lifting.

Exercising too intensely before you are ready can lead to injuries.

Take time to learn the proper techniques for the activity you're learning; your body will thank you.

Stop exercising if you experience pain in your chest or joints, dizziness, nausea, cold sweats, or extreme shortness of breath.

Don't push yourself just to keep up with others. Exercising at the right level now will help you build your fitness and intensity later.

Slow and Steady:

Assess your current level of fitness realistically, and build from there. You can start with as little as 10 minutes at a time.

Fast and Furious:

Don't let a desire for ideal athleticism push you into overly ambitious patterns that can leave you injured.

---

steroids can encourage muscle growth and build lean body tissue. It is illegal to use anabolic steroids to improve athletic performance, and they pose serious health risks, including liver cancer, fluid retention, high blood pressure, and severe acne. Men who use anabolic steroids may see their testicles shrink and their sperm counts drop. In women, steroid use can cause cessation of the menstrual cycle, growth of facial and body hair, and deepening of the voice. Anabolic steroids can also lead to dangerous psychological side effects, including aggression, extreme mood swings, rage, and even violent behavior.

- **Creatine.** Creatine is a substance naturally produced by the body and stored in skeletal muscles. Creatine is thought to help muscles during short, high-intensity activity, but research on creatine has been inconclusive. Taking creatine may cause dehydration, reduced blood volume, and produce imbalances in blood chemistry. Federal health officials warn that creatine should only be used under a doctor's care.[40]

- **Human growth hormone.** Also known as HGH, human growth hormone is a naturally occurring compound made by the body to fuel cell growth and regeneration. Its use as an athletic supplement has been widespread because HGH is difficult to detect during drug testing. Scientists warn that the long-term effects of using HGH are unknown, and researchers have found no significant athletic benefits tied to use of the hormone. Use of HGH in athletes, for example, did not improve strength and actually appeared to worsen athletic performance. HGH users also experienced more soft tissue swelling and fatigue.[41]

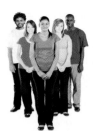

DIVERSITY & HEALTH

Safe Exercise for Special Populations

Exercise can do everyone good. If you have health concerns, the key is to modify your fitness program to reduce risk and maximize the benefits you receive. The following measures can help you have a safe and effective workout.

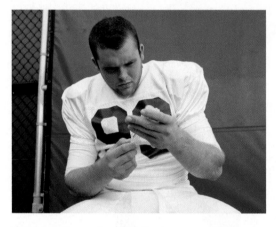

This college football player with diabetes is preparing an insulin injection for himself.

Asthma

- If prescribed, use pre-exercise asthma inhalers before beginning exercise.
- Extend your warm-up and cool-down to help your lungs prepare for and recover from exercise.
- Check for environmental irritants that could promote an asthma attack, such as a recently mowed lawn, high pollen counts, or high levels of air pollution, and consider exercising indoors at those times. If exercising in cold weather, cover your mouth and nose with a scarf or mask.
- Try swimming. The warm, moist environment is soothing, and swimming helps build cardio-respiratory endurance.
- If you begin to cough, wheeze, have difficulty breathing, or have tightness in your chest, halt exercise and use your inhaler or other pre-scribed medication.

Pregnancy

- Avoid contact sports or activities that may cause trauma or a fall. Walking and swimming are great low-impact options, but you can also dance, run, or hike.

- You can still perform resistance exercises. Focus on muscular endurance exercises rather than strengthening exercises.
- Halt exercise if you experience vaginal bleeding, dizziness, headache, chest pain, calf pain or swelling, pre-term labor, or decreased fetal movement.
- After the first trimester, avoid exercises in which you lie on your back; they can reduce blood flow to the uterus.

Diabetes

- Monitor your blood glucose before and after exercise, especially when beginning or modifying your exercise program.
- Wear a diabetes ID bracelet during exercise.
- Carry a snack if you will be active for a few hours.
- If you begin to feel shaky, anxious, or suddenly begin to sweat more, halt exercise and consume a fast-acting carbohydrate.
- Make sure to wear well-fitting shoes and check your feet for blisters or sores before and after exercise.

- **Androstenedione.** A steroid precursor that is thought to enhance athletic performance and boost testosterone, androstenedione has been linked to many high-profile controversies among professional athletes. Androstenedione is illegal for sale or use in the United States, and its side effects include breast development and impotence in men, abnormal periods and facial hair in women, and liver disease and blood clots.
- **Ephedra.** Typically used to boost energy and promote weight loss, ephedra has such serious adverse effects that the U.S. Food and Drug Administration has banned its sale. Research has not shown ephedra to be effective in boosting energy or athletic performance, and its side effects include high blood pressure, irregular heartbeat, stroke, gastrointestinal distress, and psychological problems.[42]

Change Yourself, Change Your World

Improved fitness is as much a public health goal as it is a personal one. Some of the factors that contribute to one's level of fitness reflect individual choice—whether to drive or cycle, watch TV or go outside, spend time online or spend time at the gym. But the communities in which we live also play a key role. Getting fit starts with you, but

through the choices you make, you also have the potential to help improve the lives of others.

Personal Choices

In the busy life of a student, scheduling regular exercise may seem daunting. But if you set goals, find activities you enjoy, and periodically reassess your progress, you'll be able to stay motivated, have fun, and enjoy the benefits of fitness.

Set Realistic Goals

One of the most important aspects of a fitness program is working at an intensity and rate that makes sense for you as you are. It is important to realistically assess your current fitness level in order to set fitness goals that are appropriate. Fitness goals can be based on a specific activity-related improvement you want to make, such as cycling 40% farther than you currently can; a health-related goal you may have, such as reducing your blood pressure; or a social or lifestyle desire, like preparing for a backpacking trip with your friends. Make sure your goals are easily measurable, so you can clearly tell when you've met one. If you don't make a particular goal you have set, don't get discouraged. Take that chance to reevaluate your goal and possibly break it down into smaller sub-goals.

>> **Take this self-assessment for a quick idea of how fit you are:**
www.nhs.uk/Tools/Pages/Fitness.aspx.

Find Activities You Enjoy

To exercise on a regular basis, focus on physical activities you naturally enjoy. Ask yourself which of those activities will help you reach the fitness goals you have set for yourself, which ones you are most likely to stick with, and which ones you can afford. Don't be afraid to mix it up—a wide range of activities can bring you all the benefits of fitness and will stave off boredom. If you can only afford to take tennis lessons twice a month, combine that with free aerobics classes at school and resistance exercises you can perform at home.

Schedule Time

One key to sticking with exercise is to schedule in exercise as you would a job or a class. If you have a set time devoted to exercise, you will be more likely to stick with it. See Step 3 of the **Choosing to Change Worksheet** at the end of this chapter for a schedule where you can plan activity.

Team Up!

Find a friend or family member with similar fitness goals and make plans to work out together regularly. You'll not only enjoy the company and extra motivation to stay on track, but may achieve greater health benefits. One study found that people with regular workout partners, especially workout partners who'd received a significant amount of fitness training and coaching, lost more weight compared with those who trained alone.[43]

Overcome Obstacles

You can probably come up with a long list of reasons for why you do not exercise regularly. Here are some common obstacles and solutions for overcoming them:

- **I don't have time.** Remember that only 30 minutes of moderate exercise a day can improve or maintain your fitness and that amount can be broken down into 10-minute sessions. Substituting exercise for TV or computer time is a good place to start. If you don't have time for the gym, exercise at home. If you have children, actively play with them. Some gyms also offer free or inexpensive child care.

- **I don't know how.** If you don't know how to play a particular sport, take a class. Consider working with a personal trainer, who will build your skills with lots of one-on-one attention. Many campus wellness centers offer low-cost personal training and classes.

- **I don't like the gym.** If working out on the machines isn't your thing, try alternative exercises, like rock climbing, Ultimate Frisbee, or video games designed for fitness, like the Wii Fit™.

- **I'm embarrassed about how I look.** If you aren't ready to hit the campus pool in a bathing suit, start with activities where you'll be comfortable in sweat pants and a T-shirt. Also, seek out exercise environments in which you feel comfortable (for example, a women-only fitness center).

- **I don't have the money.** If you can't afford a gym membership, choose exercises that require no more than a good pair of shoes, such as walking or running. Or, purchase low-cost equipment like exercise bands, exercise balls, or dumbbells. Your campus or community recreation center may have free or low-cost gyms or classes.

Assess Your Progress

Every four to six weeks, get motivated by assessing how far you've come. Look back on all the exercise you've done, think about the positive effects on how you feel or how fit you are becoming, and evaluate how close you are to the goals you set. At the beginning of an exercise program you may want to assess your progress even more often.

Adapting Exercise to My Needs

 "HI, I'M MOLLY. I have hip dysplasia so some of the movements that other people can do, I can't do as well. I don't have as good flexibility and mobility and sometimes when I run or I do other things for a long time, they hurt. So I've had to adapt the way that I exercise so that I can still get that activity, but do it in a way that doesn't hurt me. And one of those ways is that I swim. I'll do laps or go swimming with my friends and that is something that doesn't put pressure on my hips but it's still a great way to exercise. And I also like to ride my bike. I reach my target heart rate and it's something that I can do just as well as anyone else."

1. Do you have any needs—physical or otherwise—that you want to structure your exercise around? How will you go about doing that?

2. Exercising with friends and varying your exercise activities, as Molly does, can help you stay motivated. What else will help you stay motivated with your fitness program?

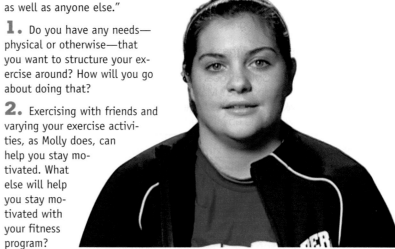

Campus Advocacy

All across the country, people are working to create communities that make physical activity an easier part of everyday life. Look around your campus to start or join the following types of projects:

- Walkability: Want to improve pedestrian ease and safety? Go to WalkingInfo.org (**www.walkinginfo.org/library/details.cfm?id=12**) for ideas on fixing problems.

- Bicycle safety: Across the country, bicycle clubs meet regularly to cycle local streets and advocate for community improvements that make cycling safer. Visit the League of American Bicyclists for tools that can help you be a bike safety advocate (**www.bikeleague.org/bfa/toolkit**). If your campus doesn't provide incentives for cyclists, such as reduced tuition or other fees for students who bring a bike rather than a car to campus, start advocating for them.

- Find fitness improvement projects in your community and share their stories to help inspire others and drive change.

>> **Watch videos of real students discussing physical activity and fitness at** MasteringHealth™

Learning Objectives

IDENTIFY important factors in body image and body weight.

DESCRIBE alarming trends in weight gain.

EXPLAIN the risks and costs of obesity.

IDENTIFY factors that contribute to weight gain.

EXPLAIN how to maintain a healthful weight.

COMPARE weight-management programs for overweight and obesity.

DESCRIBE common body image and eating disorders.

Excess body weight is one of our society's most serious health concerns—

so much so that the Centers for Disease Control and Prevention has declared obesity a national epidemic. An estimated 69.2% of American adults over age 20 are **overweight** or **obese**.[1] Among children and teenagers, an estimated 18% of those aged 6 to 11 years and 18.4% of those aged 12 to 19 years are obese.[1] The problem is also spreading globally: Between 2005 and 2015, the number of obese adults is estimated to grow from 400 million to 700 million worldwide, affecting those in both industrialized and developing nations.[2]

Amid this pressing public health concern, others face difficult issues at the other end of the weight spectrum. In the United States, nearly 2% of adults and over 5% of college students are underweight.[3,4] Some of these individuals may need nutritional or medical help in reaching a healthful weight, while others may be suffering from potentially dangerous eating disorders such as bulimia or anorexia nervosa.

Why should you care? Being overweight or underweight affects your life in a myriad of ways every day. Both conditions increase your risk of disease and, in more serious cases, early death. Moreover, your body weight influences your self-confidence and self-image, which in turn affects your relationships, goals, and activities—essentially all aspects of your life.

Body Image and Body Weight

When was the last time you looked at your body in a mirror and thought it could be more attractive? When did you last criticize yourself for your body shape or size? Did you use harsh terms that you'd never use to describe a friend? If you are like many of us, those self-criticisms come easily, and all too often.

The way you view, critique, and feel about your own body is called **body image**. Whether positive or negative, how you view your body can shape the way you feel, the way you treat yourself, and the way you eat—all of which have important health implications. Body image concerns affect males and females of all ages:

- Numerous studies have found that children absorb adult ideas about thinness and ideal body type, often from media images, and then use these ideas to judge themselves.[5]

overweight The condition of having a body weight that exceeds what is generally considered healthful for a particular height. A weight resulting in a BMI of 25 to 29.9.

obese A weight disorder in which excess accumulations of nonessential body fat result in increased risk of health problems. A weight resulting in a BMI of 30 or higher.

body image A person's perceptions, feelings, and critiques of his or her own body.

- Men often share women's self-criticisms of size and shape, although they may experience them more sharply at different points in their lives. One 20-year-long study found that men's dissatisfaction with their bodies went up with time and age. Women, while persistently displeased with their bodies, were often more critical when they were younger, and become more self-accepting as they grew older.[6]
- College is prime time for harsh self-judgment. In a study of college students, about 70% of female students and 35% of male students were dissatisfied with their bodies.[7] About 70% of female students considered themselves unattractive to the opposite sex, as did about 45% of male students.

 Beauty-product manufacturer Dove has created a series of videos called Real Beauty Sketches, which explore women's body images. Watch the videos here: http://realbeautysketches.dove.us.

Many Factors Influence Body Image

For the vast majority of us, external influences shape our body image. Every day we see hundreds of images of women who appear to be effortlessly fit and thin, and of men who seem to have been born buff. The opinions of friends and family also contribute to our perceptions of our bodies.

Girls and women are often under the most pressure to conform to societal ideals of the "beautiful body." Magazines and fashion-oriented websites geared toward young women are packed with images that associate extreme thinness with beauty, desirability, and success. Numerous research studies have linked viewing such images to the development of negative self-perceptions. In one study in which college women were shown either neutral images or "thin-ideal" images from magazines, exposure to the skinny imagery was directly linked to an increasingly negative view of one's own body, regardless of the person's actual size.[8] These external influences are not all-powerful, however: Other studies have shown that heightened media literacy, such as awareness that many media images have been digitally altered, can put societal influences in perspective and help to improve one's own body image.[9]

Defining a Healthful Body Weight

If media images and social pressures are poor guides for assessing one's weight, where should each of us look to determine our most healthful weight and shape? Some of the answers lie in numbers—measurements that indicate everything from weight to percentage of body fat. Others depend on more personal factors. We'll look at the numbers first.

Body Mass Index (BMI)

Body mass index, or **BMI**, is one of the most common methods for assessing weight, as well as for defining *overweight* and *obese*. A ratio between your height and your weight, BMI is one of several indicators used to predict risk factors for health problems later in life. To determine your own BMI, see **Figure 6.1** on page 129 and the **Self-Assessment** on page 130.

A BMI between 18.5 and 24.9 indicates a **healthful weight**. If your BMI falls below 18.5, you are considered **underweight**. A BMI of 25–29.9 indicates overweight, and a BMI of 30 or above is defined as obese. Generally, people with a BMI between 18.5 and 24.9 have few weight-related health risks. Risks increase as BMI falls below or rises

above this range, indicating that both underweight and overweight can impair health.[10]

BMI, however, is not always an accurate health indicator. Athletes with large amounts of lean muscle mass, for example, may have BMIs that classify them as overweight, even though they are at a healthful weight for their build. BMI also sometimes underestimates total body fat in older people who have lost muscle. In addition, one large recent scientific analysis of many weight-related studies found that, especially for older people, having a BMI that equaled being overweight—but not obese—lowered the risk of death compared with people of normal weight.[11] Based on such findings, many experts increasingly say that many factors, such as cholesterol levels or blood pressure, need to be considered alongside BMI, and that BMI should not be used as the sole indicator of weight-related health.

Body Measurements

Beyond BMI, other measurements used to predict weight-related health problems include *waist circumference* and *waist-to-hip ratio*. Waist circumference is an indicator of how much body fat you carry. If you carry fat mainly around your waist (so called *apple-shaped* fat patterning), you are more likely to develop health problems than if you carry fat mainly in your hips and thighs (also called *pear-shaped* fat patterning). This is true even if your BMI falls within the normal range. To find out how to accurately measure your own waist, see the **Self-Assessment** on page 130. In general, a waist measuring more than 35 inches in a

>> **You can skip the math and use these online calculators:** www.nhlbi.nih .gov/guidelines/obesity/BMI/bmicalc.htm **and** www.healthcalculators .org/calculators/waist_hip.asp.

body mass index (BMI) A numerical measurement, calculated from height and weight measurements, that provides an indicator of health risk categories.

healthful weight The weight at which health risks are lowest for an individual; usually a weight that will result in a BMI between 18.5 and 24.9.

underweight A weight resulting in a BMI below 18.5.

> " *Generally, people with a BMI between 18.5 and 24.9 have few weight-related health risks. Risks increase as BMI falls below or rises above this range, indicating that both underweight and overweight can impair health.*"

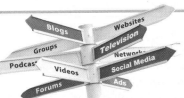

media and BODY IMAGE

Beauty in the Age of Photoshop: Seeing Shouldn't Be Believing

They surround you while you are standing in the grocery checkout aisle: magazine after magazine showing perfect-looking models and celebrities on the covers.

But how realistic are those photos? The truth is, the vast majority of them have been digitally altered—boosting a curve here, shaving off a few pounds there. The result, media critics say, is a distorted representation of "the perfect body" that encourages unhealthful body perceptions in the rest of us. What's more, showcasing such unrealistic physical "ideals" can produce the desire to achieve the unattainable. Studies have shown that such images can increase body dissatisfaction, concerns over weight, and risk for eating disorders in both women and men.[1, 2]

It's not always obvious where and how a photo has been changed. But every so often, original and retouched versions of the same photo appear in public. After singer Britney Spears held a fashion photo shoot, she allowed both the original and "after" images to be released, with the alterations (slimmer thighs, a smaller backside, and the removal of cellulite) easy to spot. Spears said she released the photos to demonstrate the intensity of the pressure on women—including celebrities such as her—to look perfect.[3]

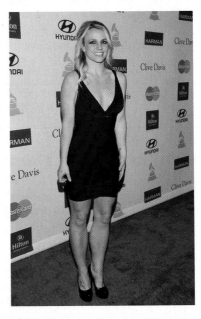

Britney Spears released "before" and "after" images from a recent photo shoot to highlight the effects of Photoshop.

Critical-Thinking Questions

1. When you see staged photos of fashion shoots, does it routinely occur to you that these images may have been altered?

2. What effects do you think altered photos have on your standards of ideal body size, and your body image? Even if you know an image is altered, do you think it still affects your idea of what beauty is?

3. What can you do to avoid comparing yourself unfavorably to images in magazines or advertisements? The next time you see a photo that looks a little too perfect, what will you tell yourself?

Want to see more examples of fake photos exposed? Visit Photoshop Disasters at www.psdisasters.com, **view the Dove Evolution video at** www.youtube.com/watch?v=iYhCn0jf46U, **and watch a** *New York Times* **video about Photoshop and media at** www.nytimes.com/video/opinion/1194838469575/op-ed-sex-lies-and-photoshop.html.

References: 1. "Influence of Mass Media on Body Image and Eating Disordered Attitudes and Behaviors in Females: A Review of Effects and Processes," by G. Lopez-Gulmera, M. P. Levine, D. Sanchez-Carracedo, & J. Facquet, 2010, *Media Psychology, 13,* pp. 387–416. 2. "Meta-Analyses of the Effects of Media Images on Men's Body-Image Concerns," by C. P. Barlett, C. L. Vowels, & D. A. Saucier, 2008, *Journal of Social and Clinical Psychology, 27,* pp. 279–310. 3. "Britney Spears Bravely Agrees to Release Un-Airbrushed Images of Herself Next to the Digitally Altered Versions," by the *Daily Mail Reporter,* April 13, 2010, retrieved from http://www.dailymail.co.uk/tvshowbiz/article-1265676/Britney-Spears-releases-airbrushed-images-digitally-altered-versions.html#axzz2KXR0eWXL.

---

woman or 40 inches in a man points to greater health risks. As waist circumference increases, disease risks increase.

Waist-to-hip ratio, determined by dividing your waist circumference by your hip circumference, also can be used to predict health risks. To find out how to measure and assess your waist-to-hip ratio, see the **Self-Assessment** on page 130.

Health-care professionals commonly use BMI and waist circumference measures because they are easy and inexpensive to perform. Together, these measures can be valuable in assessing some of a person's weight-related health risks, such as heart disease risk, and monitoring changes over time.[12]

		Underweight		Healthful weight						Overweight					Obese						Extreme obesity			
BMI	**17**	**18**	**18.5**	**19**	**20**	**21**	**22**	**23**	**24**	**25**	**26**	**27**	**28**	**29**	**30**	**31**	**32**	**33**	**34**	**35**	**36**	**37**	**39**	**≥40**
Height										**Weight in pounds**														
4'10"	81	86	89	91	96	100	105	110	115	119	124	129	134	138	143	148	153	158	162	167	172	177	186	191
4'11"	84	89	92	94	99	104	109	114	119	124	128	133	138	143	148	153	158	163	168	173	178	183	193	198
5'	87	92	95	97	102	107	112	118	123	128	133	138	143	148	153	158	163	158	174	179	184	189	199	204
5'1"	90	95	98	100	106	111	116	122	127	132	137	143	148	153	158	164	169	174	180	185	190	195	206	211
5'2"	93	98	101	104	109	115	120	126	131	136	142	147	153	158	164	169	175	180	186	191	196	202	213	218
5'3"	96	102	104	107	113	118	124	130	135	141	146	152	158	163	169	175	180	186	191	197	203	208	220	225
5'4"	99	105	108	110	116	122	128	134	140	145	151	157	163	169	174	180	186	192	197	204	209	215	227	232
5'5"	102	108	111	114	120	126	132	138	144	150	156	162	168	174	180	186	192	198	204	210	216	222	234	240
5'6"	105	112	115	118	124	130	136	142	148	155	161	167	173	179	186	192	198	204	210	216	223	229	241	247
5'7"	109	115	118	121	127	134	140	146	153	159	166	172	178	185	191	198	204	211	217	223	230	236	249	255
5'8"	112	118	122	125	131	138	144	151	158	164	171	177	184	190	197	203	210	216	223	230	236	243	256	262
5'9"	115	122	125	128	135	142	149	155	162	169	176	182	189	196	203	209	216	223	230	236	243	250	263	270
5'10"	119	126	129	132	139	146	153	160	167	174	181	188	195	202	209	216	222	229	236	243	250	257	271	278
5'11"	122	129	133	136	143	150	157	165	172	179	186	193	200	208	215	222	229	236	243	250	257	265	279	286
6'	125	133	136	140	147	154	162	169	177	184	191	199	206	213	221	228	235	242	250	258	265	272	287	294
6'1"	129	137	140	144	151	159	166	174	182	189	197	204	212	219	227	235	242	250	257	265	272	280	295	302
6'2"	132	140	144	148	155	163	171	179	186	194	202	210	218	225	233	241	249	256	264	272	280	287	303	311
6'3"	136	144	148	152	160	168	176	184	193	200	208	216	224	232	240	248	256	264	272	279	287	295	311	319
6'4"	140	148	152	156	164	172	180	189	197	205	213	221	230	238	246	254	263	271	279	287	295	304	320	328

FIGURE 6.1 Body Mass Index (BMI). BMI is often used to predict risk factors for health problems later in life. To determine your BMI, find your height and then scan across to find your weight. Then, scan up to find your BMI.

Personal Factors

Personal factors, such as your age, genetics, and body type should influence your assessment of your body weight. Consider the following questions:

- **What is a healthful *range* of weight for you?** There is no single ideal weight that is right for all of us. Identifying a healthful range of weight and accepting that it's normal for your weight to fluctuate within that range is a much more practical approach. The following section will discuss several methods for determining the range of weight that's most healthful for you.

- **What's your body composition?** Your *body composition,* or the percentage of fat compared to muscle and other tissues that we just discussed, matters more than the number on your bathroom scale. Although it varies with age, healthful amounts of total body fat range from 8% to 24% for adult men; adult women should have a body fat range between 21% and 35%.[13]

- **How old are you?** Most of us gain weight as we age. It's not realistic to expect that you will always weigh what you did in high school.

- **What's going on in your life?** Are you working a job while studying for finals and trying to write your senior thesis? Extremely busy

SELF-ASSESSMENT
Assessing Your Weight-Related Health Risks

To assess your health risks related to weight, use these three key measures: BMI, waist circumference, and waist-to-hip ratio.

Determine Your BMI

The formula for computing BMI is (your weight in pounds × 703)/your height (in.).[2]

Classification of Overweight and Obesity by BMI

	BMI	Obesity Class
Underweight	< 18.5	
Normal	18.5–24.9	
Overweight	25.0–29.9	
Obesity	30.0–34.9	I
	35.0–39.9	II
Extreme Obesity	≥ 40.0	III

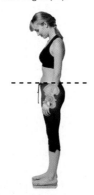

Measure Your Waist Circumference

1. Place a tape measure around your bare abdomen, just above your hip bones (see photo).

2. Be sure that the tape is snug, but not pushing into your skin.

3. Breathe out, and measure the girth of your abdomen.

Calculate Your Waist-to-Hip Ratio

1. Measure your waist as described.

2. Use the same technique to measure your hips at the widest part.

3. Divide your waist measurement by your hip measurement.

Waist-to-Hip Ratio and Associated Health Risk Levels

Classification	Men	Women
Lower Risk	< 0.90	< 0.80
Moderately High Risk	0.90–1.0	0.80–0.85
High Risk	> 1.0	> 0.85

HOW TO INTERPRET YOUR SCORE

- BMI: Calculate your BMI and check it against the BMI table. Underweight, overweight, obesity, and extreme obesity are all associated with increased health risks.
- Waist circumference: A waist measuring more than 35 inches in a woman or 40 inches in a man points to greater health risks.

- Waist-to-hip ratio: Calculate your waist-to-hip ratio and check it against the Waist-to-Hip Ratio table. This ratio is an indicator of where you carry your excess fat. A higher ratio can mean you carry excess fat in your abdomen; a lower ratio indicates you carry more fat in your lower body.

To complete this Self-Assessment online, visit Mastering Health™

---

periods in our lives often make it tougher to stay at the lower range of a healthy weight.

- **How does gender factor in?** As we discuss on page 134, men and women tend to gain and store weight in different ways.
- **What's your body type?** Some of us are naturally willowy, others stocky, and others curvy. Aim to look and feel like a healthy version of yourself, not someone else.

Alarming Trends in Body Weight

With two out of every three American adults qualifying as overweight or obese, weight concerns are a major personal and public health problem. But this wasn't always the case. Rates of overweight and obesity began trending upward in the late 1980s.

Weight Trends in the United States

Adult weight statistics by state show the spread of the obesity epidemic throughout the United States over the last two decades.[14]

- In 1990, no state taking part in a federal weight-tracking project had an obesity rate of 15% or more. Ten states had an obesity rate below 10%.
- By 2000, no state had a prevalence of obesity less than 10%. While 23 states had a prevalence of obesity of 20–24%, no state had a prevalence of 25% or higher.

- By 2011, every single state had an obesity rate of at least 20% or more, and 12 states had an obesity rate of 30% or more **(Figure 6.2)**.
- If these patterns continue, researchers predict that 42% of U.S. adults will qualify as obese by 2030.[15]

>> **A coproduction of HBO and the National Institutes of Health, the documentary _Weight of the Nation_ goes in-depth into America's obesity epidemic. Stream it for free at** http://theweightofthenation.hbo.com/films.

Weight Trends Around the World

Weight concerns are hardly confined to the United States. Globalization has spread Western eating and lifestyle habits—especially an affinity for high-fat, high-sugar foods and a decline in physical activity—worldwide. International health experts are now tackling overweight and obesity as global problems.

According to the World Health Organization, there are more than 1 billion overweight adults globally, and at least 400 million of them are obese. Obesity rates have grown threefold since 1980 in parts of Europe, the Middle East, the Pacific Islands, Australia, New Zealand, and China.[2]

As in the United States, an increase in chronic disease is following this rise in weight. Countries such as India and China, which once had

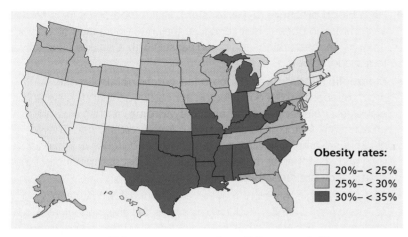

FIGURE 6.2 Obesity in the United States, 2011.

Data from *Adult Obesity Facts, Prevalence of Self-Reported Obesity Among U.S. Adults, BRFSS, 2011,* by the Centers for Disease Control and Prevention, retrieved from http://www.cdc.gov/obesity/data/adult.html#Prevalence.

Obesity rates:
- 20%– < 25%
- 25%– < 30%
- 30%– < 35%

relatively low rates of heart disease and diabetes, are already seeing significant increases in these conditions. In 2010, heart disease emerged as the top cause of death and disability worldwide; just 20 years earlier, it was the fourth-leading cause.[16] In an especially cruel twist, problems of weight and malnutrition often coexist in some developing countries, with richer residents seeing rapid weight gains even as some of their fellow citizens suffer from a lack of adequate nutrition.

Weight Trends on Campus

When you started college, you likely heard warnings about gaining 15 pounds your first year. Most students, it turns out, don't bulk up quite that much so quickly. But avoiding early weight gain can be a challenge.

Most first-year students do gain some weight once they start college—usually about 7 to 8 pounds.[17] More importantly, this weight often doesn't disappear once the first year is over. Instead, many students gain a few more pounds every year of college. In one study that tracked a group of male and female students over their four years in college, about 70% gained weight (almost 12 pounds on average) between freshman year and graduation, and the percentage qualifying as overweight or obese climbed from 18% to 31%.[18] Male students experienced weight gain more often—about 35% of them qualified as overweight, compared with about 20% of female students. In another survey, about 50% of college students said they were trying to lose weight.[19]

What's the big culprit behind campus weight gain? While excess calories clearly contribute, a decline in physical activity also appears to be a major factor. Female students, for example, often find that their level of physical activity drops substantially in college.[20, 21] For all students, larger amounts of time spent watching television and smaller amounts of physical activity have been closely linked with excess weight.[18]

The problem is compounded by the fact that more students are starting college at heavier weights than ever before. Almost 17% of American children and adolescents between the ages of 2 and 19 are obese, compared with a teen obesity rate of 5% in 1970.[22] For many, these problems start during early childhood, with 9.7% of infants and toddlers qualifying as overweight.[22] Overweight children are far more likely to carry extra pounds into adulthood.[10]

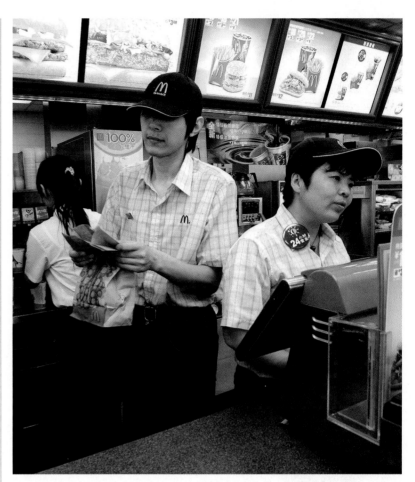

As developing countries adopt more Westernized diets, their rates of overweight and obesity are increasing.

Risks and Costs of Obesity

You could be tempted to think: How bad can a few extra pounds be, when so many people you know carry some? But just because weight concerns are common doesn't make them any less serious.

Health Risks

Being overweight or obese is associated with many health problems, including:[23, 24]

- **Type 2 diabetes.** Type 2 diabetes is strongly associated with increased body weight. More than 85% of people with type 2 diabetes are overweight or obese.[24] Excess fat makes your cells resistant to insulin, a hormone that allows glucose to be transported out of the bloodstream and into cells. When *insulin resistance* develops, glucose stays in the bloodstream, leaving cells depleted of energy and causing damage to blood vessels throughout the body.

- **Abnormal levels of blood lipids.** Obesity is associated with low blood levels of HDL cholesterol ("good" cholesterol) and high levels of LDL cholesterol ("bad" cholesterol) and triglycerides. Over time, abnormal blood lipids can contribute to *atherosclerosis*—an accumulation of deposits on the lining of blood vessels that narrows them and impedes blood flow. Atherosclerosis puts a person at risk for coronary heart disease and stroke. With increasing weight, there is a 9–18% increase in the prevalence of abnormal blood lipids.[25]

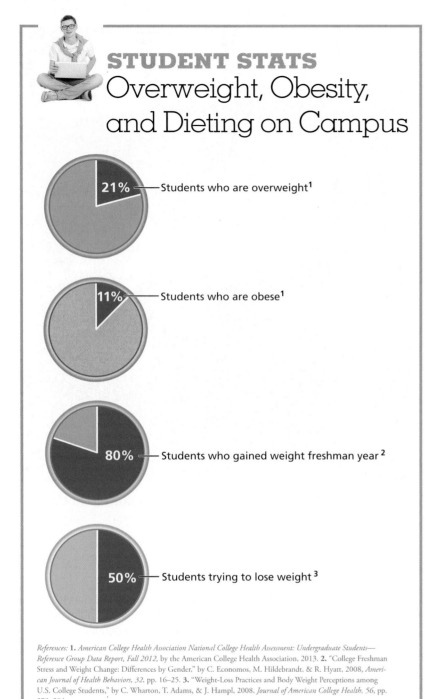

STUDENT STATS
Overweight, Obesity, and Dieting on Campus

21% ——— Students who are overweight[1]

11% ——— Students who are obese[1]

80% ——— Students who gained weight freshman year[2]

50% ——— Students trying to lose weight[3]

References: **1.** *American College Health Association National College Health Assessment: Undergraduate Students—Reference Group Data Report, Fall 2012,* by the American College Health Association. 2013. **2.** "College Freshman Stress and Weight Change: Differences by Gender," by C. Economos, M. Hildebrandt, & R. Hyatt. 2008, *American Journal of Health Behaviors, 32,* pp. 16–25. **3.** "Weight-Loss Practices and Body Weight Perceptions among U.S. College Students," by C. Wharton, T. Adams, & J. Hampl. 2008, *Journal of American College Health, 56,* pp. 579–584.

- **Coronary heart disease (also called coronary artery disease).** This disease results from atherosclerosis in arteries that supply the heart. The narrowed arteries reduce the amount of blood that flows to the heart. Diminished blood flow to the heart can cause chest pain (angina). Complete blockage can lead to a heart attack.
- **Stroke.** Atherosclerosis occurs in arteries throughout the body, including those that feed the brain. A stroke occurs when an artery supplying a region of the brain either becomes completely blocked or ruptures. In either case, brain tissue in that region is deprived of blood, and the functions controlled by it cease. Being obese raises your risk for having a stroke.

- **High blood pressure (hypertension).** High blood pressure is twice as common in obese adults because they have increased blood volume, higher heart rates, and blood vessels with a reduced capacity to transport blood.
- **Metabolic syndrome and increased cardiometabolic risk.** A group of obesity-related risk factors for cardiovascular disease and diabetes is referred to as **metabolic syndrome**, and an expanded group of risk factors is referred to as *cardiometabolic risk*. They include, for example, a waist measurement of 40 inches or more for men and 35 inches or more for women. (We discuss metabolic syndrome and cardiometabolic risk in Chapter 12.)
- **Cancer.** Being overweight may increase your risk for developing several types of cancer, including colon, rectal, esophageal, and kidney cancers. Excess weight is also linked to uterine and postmenopausal breast cancer in women and prostate cancer in men.
- **Osteoarthritis.** This joint disorder most often affects the knees, hips, and lower back. Excess weight places extra pressure on these joints and wears away the cartilage that protects them, resulting in joint pain and stiffness. For every two-pound increase in weight, the risk for developing arthritis increases 9% to 13%.
- **Sleep apnea.** Sleep apnea causes a person to stop breathing for short periods during sleep. A person who has sleep apnea may suffer from daytime sleepiness, difficulty concentrating, and even heart failure. The risk for sleep apnea is higher for people who are overweight.
- **Gallbladder disease.** The gallbladder is a small sac that stores bile from the liver and secretes it into the small intestine to break apart dietary fats. Gallbladder disease includes inflammation or infection as well as the formation of gallstones (solid clusters formed mostly of cholesterol). Overweight people may produce excessive cholesterol and/or may have an enlarged gallbladder that may not work properly.
- **Fatty liver disease.** The level of stored fat often increases in the livers of overweight and obese people. When fat builds up in liver cells it can cause injury and inflammation leading to severe liver damage, cirrhosis (scar tissue that blocks proper blood flow to the liver), or even liver failure.
- **Fertility problems.** Approximately 10% of women of childbearing age experience polycystic ovary syndrome (PCOS), which is the most common cause of female infertility.[26] Many women with PCOS are overweight or obese.
- **Pregnancy complications.** Pregnant women who are overweight or obese raise their risk of pregnancy complications for both themselves and their child. These women are more likely to develop insulin resistance, high blood glucose, and high blood pressure. The risks associated with surgery, anesthesia, and blood loss also are increased in obese pregnant women.

Excess weight is also linked to physical discomfort, social and emotional troubles, and (in the case of obesity) lower overall life expectancy. A long-term study conducted by Oxford University found that life expectancy of severely obese individuals may be

metabolic syndrome A group of obesity-related factors that increase the risk of cardiovascular disease and diabetes, including large waistline, high triglycerides, low HDL cholesterol, high blood pressure, and high fasting blood glucose.

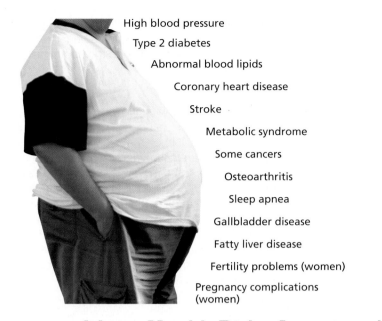

High blood pressure

Type 2 diabetes

Abnormal blood lipids

Coronary heart disease

Stroke

Metabolic syndrome

Some cancers

Osteoarthritis

Sleep apnea

Gallbladder disease

Fatty liver disease

Fertility problems (women)

Pregnancy complications (women)

FIGURE 6.3 Major Health Risks Associated with Overweight and Obesity.

reduced by 3 to 10 years.[27] **Figure 6.3** summarizes some of the major health risks associated with overweight and obesity.

Financial Burden of Obesity

Recently, a national group of financial experts took a close look at obesity. Their findings were staggering. They estimated that over-weight and obesity cost the United States and Canada about $300 billion a year in health-care costs and lost productivity, with $270 billion of that total belonging to the United States.[28] Another study found that some states spend up to $15 billion a year on obesity-related health care, with a significant portion of that cost paid for by the public.[29]

The individual costs are high as well—especially for women. In a study of the personal costs of obesity, researchers found that it costs an obese woman about $4,870 more per year to live in the United States compared with a woman of healthy weight, and it costs an obese man about $2,646 more per year than a healthy-weight man.[30] Some of these costs are medical, such as for doctor's visits and medi-cations. Others are work-related, pertaining to wages and missed work days. And some are personal, such as for transportation and life insur-ance premiums.

Factors That Contribute to Weight Gain

Many of us watch the number on the bathroom scale rise or fall be-cause of a simple concept: **energy balance**. The calories in the foods and beverages you consume are a form of "energy in." Your body uses this energy to perform all of its activities, from breathing and circulation to studying and exercising. Think of these activities as "energy out." If, over time, the calories you consume match the calories you expend, then you are in energy balance and your weight will not change. If you take in fewer calories than you use, you'll lose weight. Take in more calories than you use, and you'll gain weight **(Figure 6.4)**.

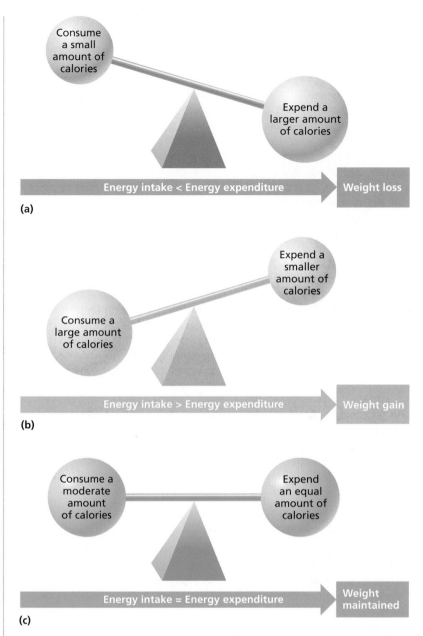

(a) Energy intake < Energy expenditure → Weight loss

Consume a small amount of calories / Expend a larger amount of calories

(b) Energy intake > Energy expenditure → Weight gain

Consume a large amount of calories / Expend a smaller amount of calories

(c) Energy intake = Energy expenditure → Weight maintained

Consume a moderate amount of calories / Expend an equal amount of calories

FIGURE 6.4 Energy Balance. Energy balance is attained when the calories you consume equal the calories you expend.

Source: Thompson, Janice. and Melinda Manore, *Nutrition: An Applied Approach*, 2nd ed., © 2009, p. 448. Reprinted and Electronically reproduced by permission of Pearson Education, Inc., Upper Saddle River, New Jersey.

But while excess weight ultimately results from an energy intake in excess of energy used, many factors influence how that equation plays out in each of us. We discuss these factors next, starting with those that are less controllable.

Biology and Genetics

Why does it seem as if some people can eat whatever they want all day long and not gain a pound, while others who monitor every mouthful just keep watching the scale go up? This is partly due to

energy balance The state achieved when energy consumed from food is equal to energy expended, maintaining body weight.

misperceptions; for instance, some people fail to count snacks that add up during the day. But it also occurs because factors unique to us as individuals affect our energy needs.

Differences in Basal Metabolism

About two-thirds of the energy a person needs each day goes toward *basal metabolism*—that is, the body's maintenance of basic physiological processes (like keeping vital organs functioning) when at complete digestive, physical, and emotional rest. The remainder of energy a person uses is for food digestion, adjusting to environmental changes such as temperature, stress, and engaging in physical activity.

The rate at which basal metabolism occurs in an individual is his or her **basal metabolic rate (BMR)**. A similar measure of energy output, called *resting metabolic rate* (RMR), is measured when a person is awake and resting quietly. BMR and RMR may vary greatly from person to person and may vary for the same person with a change in circumstance or physical condition. In general, BMR and RMR are highest in people who are growing (children, adolescents, pregnant women), are tall (greater surface area = more heat loss = more calories burned), and have more lean body mass (physically fit people and males).

Regular physical activity can build your muscles, a component of your lean body mass. If you increase your physical activity from light to moderate or heavy, you will burn more energy through exercise while increasing your BMR; together these factors can contribute greatly to weight loss.

Age

As people age, they tend to become less active and lose muscle mass. Because of this, BMR declines about 2% for each decade.[31] This reduced energy expenditure in turn reduces calorie needs. However, older adults who remain active can avoid gaining weight as they age. Aerobics, strength training, and flexibility exercises are all recommended.

Sex and Gender Differences

Men and women each have unique factors that contribute to weight gain. Men may be more likely than women to consume high-calorie diets in response to social expectations. "Real men," according to the stereotype, eat ribs, not salad. In one study of college students, male students were less interested in making careful food choices. Some male students in the survey said more healthful eating was a female concern, not something men would focus on.[32] However, preventing weight gain is just as important in men as in women, if not more so. Men are more likely to store fat in their abdomens, which, as discussed earlier, confers greater health risks, such as heart disease.[33, 34]

Women, on the other hand, have unique health considerations that increase their risk of excess weight. Female hormones play an important role in fat storage.[35] Women's bodies need adequate fat for the production of female reproductive hormones, and women naturally keep body fat stores in reserve for pregnancy and breast-feeding. As evidence of that, it is not uncommon for women with inadequate body fat to cease menstruating. Because women tend to have a higher percentage of body fat than men, and body fat burns less energy than lean tissue, women, on average, need fewer calories than men do.

Life cycle factors also affect women's weight more drastically than men's. While pregnancy leads to necessary weight gain, many women find that the extra pounds are difficult to lose afterward. Additionally, between puberty and menopause, women are more likely to store body fat in their hips and thighs, but after menopause, fat storage patterns begin to more closely resemble men's, with fat storage shifting to the abdominal area, increasing the risk of conditions such as heart disease.

basal metabolic rate (BMR) The rate at which the body expends energy for only the basic functioning of vital organs.

Genetics

Overweight and obesity often run in families. If one or both of your parents are overweight or obese, your chances of being overweight increase. To be sure, some of this influence may be due more to habits than genes. Families tend to share eating and exercise patterns (whether the habits are healthful or unhealthful). However, studies have shown that genes, too, can affect the tendency to gain weight, how much fat a person stores, and where he or she carries excess weight. Scientists are studying specific genes, such as a certain variation of a gene that is related to fat mass and obesity, known as FTO. FTO appears to increase a person's risk of obesity by 30% to 70%, depending on the specific variety of FTO and how many copies of that obesity-linked variation a person carries.[36]

Race and Ethnicity

Overweight and obesity disproportionately affect certain racial and ethnic groups. Overweight and obesity are problems for:[37, 38]

- 76.7% of African Americans.
- 72.2% of Native Americans/Alaskan Natives.
- 78.8% of Hispanic Americans.
- 66.7% of Caucasian Americans.
- 42.1% of Asian Americans.
- 64.9% of other racial or ethnic groups.

The reasons for these disparities are complex. Factors may include cultural differences in diet and exercise, socioeconomic differences in patterns of food consumption, inequalities in access to nutritious food, and inequalities in access to education about nutrition and fitness. Other influences may arise from genetic differences. For more detail, see the **Diversity & Health** box for a discussion of theories behind one particular gene—dubbed the "thrifty gene"—that may affect weight-gain tendencies among people of different ancestries.

The disparities occur in more than just body weight. One study of *central obesity*, or excessive fat concentrated in the abdomen, found that while levels of abdominal fat have increased for Caucasian Americans, African Americans, and Mexican Americans since 1900, African American women have seen the largest shifts.[39] If patterns of central obesity increases continue, the researchers estimate that by 2020, about 71% of African American women would qualify as having central obesity and would be likely to face the increased health risks it confers.

Health History

Certain health issues or medications may trigger weight gain. In some cases, weight gain may reflect hormonal imbalances triggered by an underactive thyroid. In this condition, called hypothyroidism, the thyroid gland fails to make enough thyroid hormone, leading to a variety of symptoms, including excess weight, fatigue, and being more sensitive to cold. If you have concerns about your thyroid, your doctor can check your thyroid hormone levels with a simple blood test.

Individual Behaviors

Although factors such as biology and genetics are an important consideration in an individual's weight, they cannot alone explain the dramatic surge in weight gain seen worldwide in recent decades. Personal choices related to diet and physical activity clearly have had a major effect.

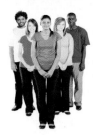

Overweight, Obesity, Ancestry, and the "Thrifty Gene"

While the reasons behind disproportionate rates of obesity among certain racial and ethnic groups are complex, researchers speculate that an ancient factor may be at work among some populations in our modern environment: a gene intended to prevent starvation.

This theory, centered around the idea of a "thrifty gene," is based on the fact that

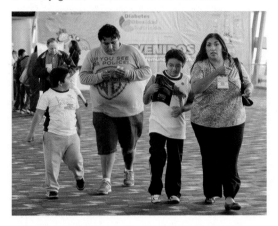

Does a "thrifty gene" promote weight gain in Native Americans, Latinos, and other groups?

for thousands of years, certain populations, such as the native populations of the Americas, relied on hunting, fishing, and gathering for their food.[1] Access to food was seasonal and cyclical, swinging between times of plenty and times when food was scarce. To compensate, these populations developed a gene that allowed them to store fat easily when food was plentiful so as to prevent starvation later. Fast-forward to today, however, and the same gene overcompensates, encouraging fat storage even though the food supply is more reliable, encouraging weight gain and obesity among contemporary populations such as modern-day Native Americans, who have high rates of obesity and diabetes. Latinos, whose ancestors often include Native American peoples, may also be affected.

Although this theory is still under study, geneticists have identified a particular gene called PPARγ as one likely "thrifty gene."[2] This gene affects energy metabolism and fat storage, and a particular variant of the gene linked to an increased risk for obesity and type 2 diabetes has been found in some Native Americans strongly affected by weight concerns.[3] Further research will help determine if this gene variant is often found in other populations, and over

time may help provide strategies for how to better address the effects of this ancient gene in today's society.

Critical-Thinking Questions

1. While populations who might carry a "thrifty gene" have high rates of type 2 diabetes, this condition is common among Americans of many backgrounds. What are other factors driving the increase in type 2 diabetes? What can you do to reduce your own risks?

2. Do weight-related genetic predispositions, such as the "thrifty gene," mean that a person is guaranteed to be overweight?

3. How can you better understand any genetic predispositions toward certain weight-management issues you may have? What can you do to factor these predispositions into your own weight-management plan?

References: **1.** "The Pima Indians: Obesity and Diabetes," by the National Institute of Diabetes and Digestive and Kidney Diseases (date not provided), retrieved from http://diabetes.niddk.nih.gov/dm/pubs/pima/obesity/obesity.htm. **2.** "PPARγ, the Ultimate Thrifty Gene," by J. Auwerx, 1999, *Diabetologia, 42*, pp. 1033–1049. **3.** "A Functional Variant in the Peroxisome Proliferator-Activated Receptor Gamma2 Promoter Is Associated with Predictors of Obesity and Type 2 Diabetes in Pima Indians," by Y. Muller, C. Bogardus, B. Beamer, A. Shulinder, & L. Baier, 2003, *Diabetes, 52*, pp. 1864–1871.

Increased Calorie Consumption

The average American today consumes about 570 more calories per day than in 1977.[40] Many of these increased calories are in the form of fats and sugar: In 2005, total added fats and oils available for consumption in the U.S. diet reached 86 pounds per person, compared with 53 pounds per person in 1970, and total sugars and sweeteners reached 142 pounds per person, compared with about 120 pounds.[41] Our diets are especially high in saturated fats (fried foods, fatty meats, cheeses), added sugars (especially in soft drinks, many breakfast cereals, and desserts), and refined grains (pasta, white bread, flour tortillas).

Large portion sizes and dining away from home also increase calorie intake. Across the board, portion sizes have ballooned. Servings of fast foods and soft drinks, for example, often are two to five times larger now than when they were introduced.[42] For example, in 1954, a serving of McDonald's French fries weighed 2.4 ounces and contained 210 calories. By 2013 the fries had reached 5 ounces and 500 calories.[42, 43]

>> **Take the Portion Distortion Quiz to see how increasing portion sizes piles on the calories at** www.nhlbi.nih.gov/health/public/heart/obesity/wecan/portion/index.htm

Lack of Physical Activity

Fewer than one in three Americans gets the recommended minimum of 30 minutes of moderate activity a day, most days of the week. In fact, one-third of Americans over the age of 18 do not engage in any leisure-time physical activity at all, and that percentage climbs steadily with age.[44] About 25% of those between the ages of 18 and 24 get no leisure-time physical activity, and among those 65 or older, that number jumps to 49%.[45]

Many people now earn their living while sitting for hours. In 1860, the average workweek was 70 hours of heavy physical labor, compared with 40 hours of sedentary work today. The least physically active groups are older adolescents and adults over 60 years old who spend about 60% of their waking time in sedentary pursuits.[45] According to the Nielsen Company's "Cross Platform Report" (measuring television, computer, and cell phone usage), during 2011, Americans watched about five hours of video per day on average.[46]

Coupled with the fact that Americans typically spend almost an hour a day commuting to and from work, little time is left in the day for physical activity.[47] With less physical activity, lean body mass decreases and fat takes its place.

Losing Weight

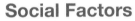

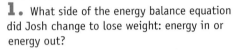

"HI. MY NAME IS JOSH. As a teenager, I often struggled with my weight. When I was 14 or 15 I was overweight, and I felt really down about myself and had low self-esteem. So, in an effort to lose weight and to get more healthy, I started looking for activities that I enjoyed and I found basketball and I found running. And through these activities, I started gradually losing weight, and I stuck to it. And so, if I could suggest anything for losing weight, I'd say find an activity that you like and which you can motivate yourself to do."

1. What side of the energy balance equation did Josh change to lose weight: energy in or energy out?

2. Do you think it really matters that Josh likes the activities he's doing, or will any activity work to lose weight?

3. What activities do you like that you could use to lose weight?

STUDENT STORY

Social Factors

Although most people seem to appreciate the importance of a healthful diet and regular physical activity, many social factors in our everyday lives encourage behaviors that run counter to healthful weight management:

- Long work and school days, combined with commuting, leave many people little time for staying healthy. One study of commuting patterns found that time spent commuting detracted directly from time spent sleeping and being physically active.[48] Another study of college students found that those with a drive time of 16 minutes or more were 64% more likely to be overweight or obese.[49]

- Most of us are stressed, and some people reach for food as comfort. One study found that the stresses of everyday life often trigger the urge to eat, with many people favoring less healthful food options.[50]

- The fast food so many of us go for could be more aptly named "fat food." Most popular fast food choices are stuffed with calories and saturated fat.[51]

While these social factors affect all aspects of American society, they play an especially acute role for those facing the greatest economic challenges. In what researchers sometimes call the "food insecurity-obesity paradox," individuals and families of lower socioeconomic status are often at the greatest risk for obesity. A complex web of factors appears to underlie this paradox, including limited ability to access and purchase healthful foods, fewer opportunities for physical activity, and high levels of stress. Also influential are cycles of food deprivation and overeating, in which lack of food at some points leads to overeating and weight gain at others.[52] Many nutrition experts now push for food assistance programs that provide healthy nutrition choices and promote physical activity, rather than simply providing adequate calories.[53]

Physical Factors

Look at the built environment, and you'll likely see examples of how we have literally helped construct the obesity epidemic. Health experts now describe many of our built areas as "obesogenic environments," meaning that they are spaces that promote obesity. Here are just a few examples:

- Many neighborhoods lack sidewalks, resulting in more driving and less walking. Protected bike routes are rare in many communities.

- In some neighborhoods, supermarkets are scarce, leaving residents to rely on smaller stores that rarely carry healthful choices such as fresh fruits and vegetables. In many such neighborhoods, fast food is often the most available restaurant option.

- Many of us don't have ready access to gyms or other opportunities for physical activity and recreation. Paradoxically, those of us at the greatest risk for obesity often have the least access. One group of researchers found that when they built a playground and a walking path in a lower-income neighborhood, the proportion of residents observed being active increased significantly, indicating that even relatively simple improvements to the built environment can carry important benefits.[54]

Public Policy

Laws, regulations, and federally sponsored promotional programs around food also affect our nutritional environment, perhaps not always for the better. While public health officials now pour substantial money and attention into understanding and addressing the obesity epidemic, critics argue that other agencies create policies that make obesity more likely, sometimes by promoting the consumption of foods higher in fat and calories over those that are less calorie dense. According to one group's research, more than 60% of recent agricultural subsidies have directly and indirectly supported meat and dairy production, while less than 1% have gone to fruits and vegetables.[55]

Change Yourself, Change Your World

For most people, the key to healthful weight management lies in the ability to ensure that less energy is coming in and more energy is going out. This requires consistent work. Losing weight doesn't have to mean depriving yourself. But it does mean eating wisely and changing your lifestyle to be as physically active as possible.

Some of us practice successful weight management on our own. But many of us benefit from some support, whether that help comes from a friend, a trainer, a counselor, a formal program, or even a doctor.

Personal Choices

Did you grab a snack before sitting down to study this chapter? If so, what did you choose? Seemingly small decisions about what and how much you eat can affect successful weight management. The **Practical Strategies** box on page 140 lists several helpful choices to try.

Can Dieting Work?

Hunger is the physiological sensation caused by a lack of food. Hunger is triggered in our brains, as a response to signals sent by the digestive tract and hormones circulating in our blood. Hunger is different from **appetite**, the psychological

hunger The physiological sensation caused by the lack of food.

appetite The psychological response to the sight, smell, thought, or taste of food that prompts or postpones eating.

response to the sight, smell, thought, or taste of food that prompts or postpones eating. Appetite can prove helpful, stimulating you to eat before you get too hungry. It can also prove harmful, steering you toward too much food or toward tempting but unhealthful food choices. When we've eaten and relieved or prevented hunger, a feeling called **satiety** helps turn off the desire to eat more.

Given that both hunger and appetite compel us to eat, can dieting work? Weight-loss diets can be helpful for some people, especially those who like the support of a structured plan or program. However, dieting is a slow, steady process. You can't achieve healthful or permanent weight loss by starving yourself for a week. Diets also work best if they are accompanied by regular exercise. To keep the weight off, successful dieters must work to make their new eating and exercise habits into a way of life that they can sustain long term.

Millions of Americans follow weight-loss diets (**Table 6.1 on pages 138-139**). In a year-long study that compared four popular diets—Atkins, Ornish, The Zone, and Weight Watchers—roughly half the participants lost an average of 7 pounds and improved some of their health indicators, such as heart disease risk.[56] But in a pattern familiar to many dieters, the other half of the study's participants dropped out.

Three common dieting approaches are low-calorie diets, low-fat diets, and low-carbohydrate diets.

Low-Calorie Diets. Cutting 500 to 1,000 calories a day typically leads to a loss of 1 or 2 pounds a week. **Figure 6.5** shows a healthful way to reduce the calories in a daily diet.

But a low-calorie diet is rarely a simple matter of food math. Without a healthful eating plan in place, abruptly restricting one's daily calorie intake below recommended levels can be dangerous and deprive you of the energy you need for daily activities. You may find yourself withholding calories all day, only to lunge for a double cheeseburger at night.

>> *Frontline: Diet Wars* investigates popular diets and America's obesity problem. View this program online at www.pbs.org/wgbh/pages/frontline/shows/diet.

Low-Fat Diets. Diets that focus on reducing daily fat intake are also common. Most aim to cut the dieter's total fat intake to about 25% of calories or less. Some of these diets are vegetarian, others vegan, and others allow lean meats, poultry, and fish. Long-term weight loss is a challenge with low-fat diets, because dieters find them difficult to follow and to maintain. That said, we can all benefit from following these general fat intake guidelines:

- Cut *trans* fats from your diet. *Trans* fats are created when manufacturers add hydrogen to vegetable oil—a process called hydrogenation. Consumption of *trans* fats reduces your "good cholesterol" (HDL) and raises your "bad cholesterol" (LDL), thereby increasing your risk of cardiovascular disease. Prepackaged snack and dessert foods (crackers, chips, cookies, cakes, pies, etc.) were once the largest sources of *trans* fat in our diet, although in recent years, due to the

satiety Physical fullness; the state in which there is no longer the desire to eat.

Higher-Calorie Diet (about 3,300 calories/day)	Lower-Calorie Diet (about 1,700 calories/day)
Breakfast: 1½ C. Fruit Loops cereal 1 C. 2% milk 1 C. orange juice 2 slices white toast 1 Tbsp. butter (on toast) 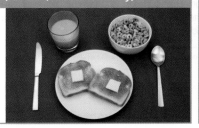	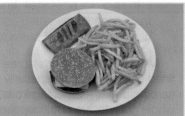 **Breakfast:** 1½ C. Cheerios cereal 1 C. skim milk ½ fresh pink grapefruit
Lunch: McDonald's Big Mac hamburger French fries, extra-large 3 Tbsp. ketchup Apple pie	**Lunch:** Subway cold cut trio 6-inch sandwich Granola bar, hard, with chocolate chips (24 g) 1 fresh medium apple
Dinner: 4½ oz. ground beef (80% lean, crumbled), cooked 2 medium taco shells 2 oz. Cheddar cheese 2 Tbsp. sour cream 4 Tbsp. store-bought salsa 1 C. shredded lettuce ½ C. refried beans 6 Oreos 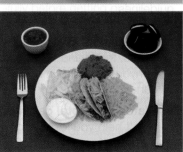	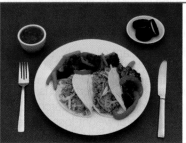 **Dinner:** 5 oz. ground turkey, cooked 2 soft corn tortillas 3 oz. low-fat Cheddar cheese 4 Tbsp. store-bought salsa 1 C. shredded lettuce 1 C. cooked mixed veggies 3 Oreos

FIGURE 6.5 How to Cut Calories While Maintaining a Balanced Diet.
The meals on the right show healthful alternatives to the higher-calorie meals on the left.

Source: Thompson, Janice, and Melinda Manore. *Nutrition: An Applied Approach.* 2nd ed., © 2009, p. 464. Reprinted and Electronically reproduced by permission of Pearson Education, Inc., Upper Saddle River, New Jersey.

Practical Strategies

Cutting Calories, Not Nutrition

You can reduce the total number of calories you eat while boosting your intake of healthful nutrients by following these basic guidelines:

- **Shop smart.** Never shop on an empty stomach! You'll make wiser purchases if you're not particularly hungry. Also, avoid buying high-calorie foods that you'll have difficulty eating in moderate amounts. And don't be fooled by "low-fat" foods. They may be just as high in calories as the regular versions, because manufacturers often make up for the fat with added carbohydrates.

- **Track your food intake.** Use a free online tracker, like the MyPlate SuperTracker (www.supertracker.usda.gov) or www.sparkpeople.com, to calculate the calories you are consuming and compare them with your MyPlate calorie intake recommendations.

- **Practice portion control.** Match the amount of food on your plate to your desired servings and calorie intake level. Try gauging the higher-calorie foods you tend to choose (such as red meats, fats, and sweets), cutting their portion sizes in half, and replacing the rest with lower-calorie options.

- **Fill your plate!** Low-calorie meals do not have to be skimpy. If you fill most of your plate with legumes and other vegetables alongside smaller portions of foods higher in calories, you can still have an ample, nutritious meal without busting your calorie count for the day.

- **Choose healthful fats.** Nuts, seeds, and most plant oils are excellent sources of healthful unsaturated fats. Salmon and other fish are good sources of essential fatty acids.

- **Eat whole foods as close to their natural state as possible.** Highly processed foods are more likely to contain empty calories. If you reach for an apple instead of a cup of sweetened applesauce, for example, you will avoid the calories that were added during the manufacturing process. You will also be consuming more fiber, which helps you feel full longer.

- **Don't skip meals.** This will only leave you overwhelmingly hungry later on. If you're often too rushed to eat breakfast, fix yourself a peanut butter and banana sandwich on whole grain bread before you go to bed, and grab it on your way out the door the next morning.

- **Avoid drastic measures.** Cutting your calorie intake in half may help you lose a few pounds for a week or two, but it's a losing strategy. That's because your BMR drops right along with your calorie cutting. At the same time, your feelings of hunger and deprivation make you crave food even more strongly. Sustained weight loss requires steady, gradual lifestyle change. Aiming to lose 10% of your body weight over a six-month period is a reasonable goal.

- **Drink water instead of sugary drinks filled with calories.** Approximately 20% of our total calorie consumption comes from what we drink.[1] Juices, "vitamin waters," soft drinks, and energy drinks are all extra sources of calories. If plain water gets a little dull, opt for sparkling water flavored with a wedge of lemon, or make yourself a spritzer by adding a dash of juice to a glass of sparkling water.

- **Use artificial sweeteners in moderation.** Artificial sweeteners are low- or no-calorie sugar substitutes. Artificial sweeteners containing aspartame (for example, Equal and NutraSweet) have been studied extensively, and while many studies have found them to be safe in moderation, newer research indicates that these sweeteners may actually affect blood sugar levels and increase diabetes risk.[2, 3] However, people with phenylketonuria (PKU) should avoid aspartame because it contains phenylalanine, which their bodies cannot process.

- **Change one habit at a time.** Instead of trying to overhaul all of your eating habits at once, choose one meal or snack and make small changes little by little. At lunch, for example, opt for fruit instead of dessert. Give that new habit some time to "stick" before trying another change.

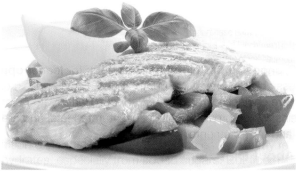

References: **1.** "Effects of Soft Drink Consumption on Nutrition and Health: A Systematic Review and Meta-Analysis," by L. R. Vartanian, M. B. Schwartz, & K. D. Brownell, April 2007, *American Journal of Public Health. 97*, pp. 667–675. **2.** "Aspartame: Review of Safety," by Harriett H. Butchko, 2002, *Regulatory Toxicology and Pharmacology, 35*, pp. S1–S93, 200. **3.** "Consumption of Artificially and Sugar-Sweetened Beverages and Incident Type 2 Diabetes in the Etude Epidemiologique aupres des Femmes de la Mutuelle Generale de l'Education Nationale-European Prospective Investigation into Cancer and Nutrition Cohort," by G. Fagherazzi, A. Vilier, D. Saes Sartorelli, M. Lajous, B. Balkau, & F. Clavel-Chapelon, January 30, 2013, *American Journal of Clinical Nutrition.* (Epub ahead of print.)

- From December 2008 to May 2009, the FDA recalled over 70 weight-loss supplements because they were found to illegally contain prescription-drug ingredients.

- Even though the FDA prohibited the sale of weight-loss supplements containing the ingredient ephedra more than a decade ago, pills claiming to contain ephedra still appear for sale on the Internet. The ingredient has been linked to thousands of cases of side effects that include tremors, insomnia, heart palpitations, and increased risk of heart attack and stroke.[65]

>> **Visit *Medline Plus* for reliable information about drugs and supplements at** www.nlm.nih.gov/medlineplus/druginformation.html.

Only one pill has received full clearance from the FDA for sale as an over-the-counter weight-loss medication. Alli, a lower dose of the prescription weight-loss medication orlistat, was released to the public in 2007. The drug works by causing your body to excrete some of the fat that passes through your digestive tract, and is intended to help you lose about 5% of your body weight over time. But side effects, such as digestive discomfort and gas with oily spotting, can be unpleasant. Alli is also expensive, costing about $50 for a one-month supply of the pills.

Get Physically Active

Physical activity does more than burn off calories and reduce body fat. While a particularly strenuous workout might leave you reaching for a snack, regular exercise over time appears to help reduce feelings of hunger and mediate appetite.[66] It also builds muscle, which burns more calories than fat tissue. Choose an activity you like. If you make exercise fun, weight loss will be more enjoyable!

Keep in mind the basic exercise guidelines we discussed in Chapter 5. If you are trying to maintain weight loss or lose weight, aim for 60–90 minutes each day. At least two to three times a week, some of that exercise should focus on building muscle. If you have time for nothing else, try to build a little more walking into your routine each day. It can make a significant difference over the long term.

>> **There are lots of free online programs that can track your diet and physical activity, such as** www.supertracker.usda.gov, www.sparkpeople.com, **and** www.fitday.com.

Finding Help

If you've tried to lose weight, you may have discovered how difficult it can be to do it on your own. There are people and organizations that can give you support.

Start by visiting your campus health and fitness centers. Many offer a variety of services and programs related to achieving a healthy weight. If you are a student, these services are often less expensive than you'll find elsewhere.

You can also consider joining a community-based or commercial weight-loss program. Nonprofit groups such as Overeaters Anonymous or TOPS (Take Off Pounds Sensibly) provide supportive help in understanding and rethinking emotional responses to food, and are either free or relatively low cost. Commercial groups, such as Weight Watchers or Jenny Craig, are also readily available, although at a higher price. Some base their weight-loss plans around purchasing prepared meals from the program, which can get expensive, especially on a student budget.

When deciding whether any weight-loss program is right for you, federal health experts suggest looking for these elements:[67]

- Healthy eating plans that reduce calories but do not forbid specific foods.
- Tips to increase moderate-intensity physical activity.
- Tips on healthy habits that also keep your cultural needs in mind, such as lower-fat versions of your favorite foods.
- Slow and steady weight loss. Depending on your starting weight, experts recommend losing weight at a rate of 1/2 to 2 pounds per week.
- Medical care if you are planning to lose weight by following a special formula diet, such as a very low-calorie diet (a program that requires careful monitoring from a doctor).
- A plan to keep the weight off after you have lost it.

>> **If you're interested in joining a commercial weight-loss program or trying a new product, the Federal Trade Commission has resources to help you assess them:** www.consumer.ftc.gov/topics/weight-loss-fitness.

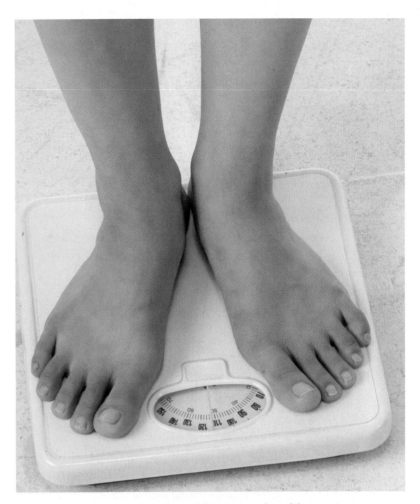

Talking to someone at your campus health center or joining a weight-loss program can be a first step to losing weight.

Clinical Options for Obesity

In 2012, almost 5% of college students described themselves as "very overweight."[4] Because obesity is a significant health risk, your doctor may recommend medical treatment if your BMI is 30 or higher. Options range from psychotherapy to prescription drugs to weight-loss surgery.

Psychotherapy. Psychotherapy can be a vital component of both weight-loss and weight-management programs. This is especially true for people who turn to food to reduce stress or assuage depression. Others may have significant body image issues that are most effectively addressed with the help of a therapist. Psychologists have found that both individual and group therapy can be helpful in treating obesity and related issues such as shame or a distorted view of one's own body.[68]

Prescription Drugs. Prescription weight-loss medications include those approved by the U.S. Food and Drug Administration (FDA) for short-term use in weight loss, including diethylpropion, phendimetrazine, and phentermine, and one approved for long-term use, orlistat. Each has side effects ranging from increased blood pressure, sleepiness, nervousness, dizziness, and headaches to cramping and

When you want to lose some weight, you can reach your goal healthfully, or set yourself up for frustration. To drop pounds in a healthy way:

CHOOSE THIS.

NOT THAT.

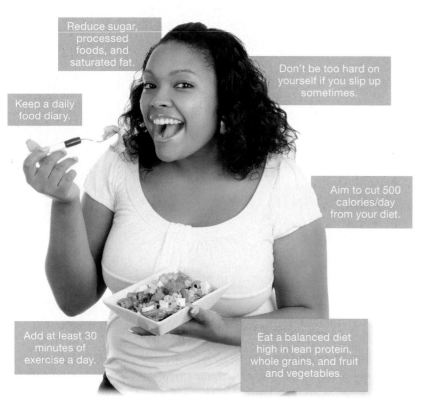

Reduce sugar, processed foods, and saturated fat.

Don't be too hard on yourself if you slip up sometimes.

Keep a daily food diary.

Aim to cut 500 calories/day from your diet.

Add at least 30 minutes of exercise a day.

Eat a balanced diet high in lean protein, whole grains, and fruit and vegetables.

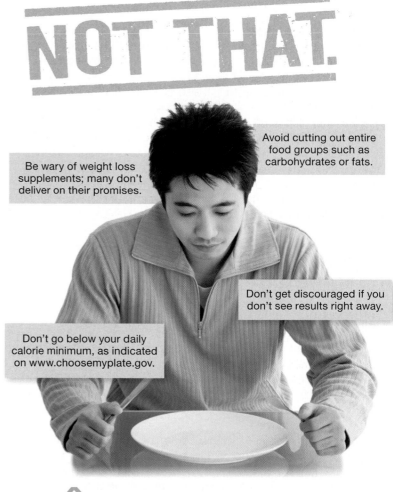

Avoid cutting out entire food groups such as carbohydrates or fats.

Be wary of weight loss supplements; many don't deliver on their promises.

Don't get discouraged if you don't see results right away.

Don't go below your daily calorie minimum, as indicated on www.choosemyplate.gov.

A Pound or Two Each Week:

When you want to lose weight, you want the pounds gone NOW. But a slower, steadier pace will be more manageable and bring longer-lasting results.

Crash Diet:

Trendy diets may sound like a path to getting skinny fast, but they are often not balanced and will leave you feeling depleted. They also don't help keep weight off later.

---

explosive diarrhea. They are typically prescribed only for obesity, not more moderate cases of weight management.

These drugs help patients shed only a small percentage of body weight, and only when combined with changes in diet and exercise. They are usually prescribed to obese patients who are experiencing health problems due to their weight, and only for short periods of time. In 2010, the FDA required a new safety warning label for orlistat to alert patients that a few people using the drug had suffered severe liver injury, and to watch for symptoms of liver trouble, such as yellow eyes or skin, when taking the drug.[69]

Surgery. A growing number of obese people—about 200,000 each year in the United States alone—are opting for surgery to alter the sizes of their stomachs and reduce the amount of food they can ingest.[70] This type of surgery, called **bariatric surgery**, comprises

several different types of procedures. One subset of procedures, known as *gastric banding*, involves partitioning off part of the stomach with a removable band. The other subset, *gastric bypass*, involves permanently reducing the size of the stomach. After either type of procedure, the reshaped stomach can only hold a limited amount of food—sometimes as little as an ounce—resulting in greatly reduced calorie intake. In more extreme types of surgery, other portions of the digestive tract are also altered to limit calorie absorption.

Weight-loss surgery may be increasingly common, but it's

bariatric surgery Weight-loss surgery using various procedures to modify the stomach or other sections of the gastrointestinal tract in order to reduce calorie intake or absorption.

not for everyone. Doctors only recommend weight-loss surgical procedures for people who:

- Have a BMI of 40 or more. That usually means you are about 100 pounds or more overweight.
- Have a lower BMI (between 35 and 40) but also have a dangerous obesity-related health condition, such as heart disease, type 2 diabetes, severe joint pain, or high cholesterol.
- Have tried and failed to lose weight other ways.
- Fully understand the risks, and realize that the surgery is just one step in making dramatic, long-term lifestyle changes to lose weight and keep it off. Weight-loss surgery doesn't give you the freedom to gorge on burgers and chocolate afterward. It's part of a lifetime commitment to weight management.

In early 2011, the FDA also approved the use of a relatively less invasive weight-loss procedure, called LAP-BAND, in those with a BMI of 30 or higher who have at least one obesity-related condition.

Some patients see significant weight loss and other health improvements after undergoing these procedures, such as a significant reduction in blood glucose. But others eventually gain back the weight they lost, find they can no longer absorb certain nutrients properly, or experience chronic diarrhea or vomiting or other problems. Also, any major surgery involving an obese patient carries an unusually high risk for complications such as infection and the formation of blood clots. Overall, about 1 in 200 patients dies within 90 days following the surgery.[71]

What If You Want to Gain Weight?

If you want or need to gain weight for optimal health, you should consume more calories than you expend. Consider the following approaches:

- Boost your calories, but in healthful ways. Piling the cheese on your pizza isn't a good way to gain weight. Instead, reach for a diverse mix of foods, including 100% fruit juices, nuts and seeds, dried fruits, peanut butter, hummus, and energy bars. Keep a supply of nut-based trail mix with you as a snack. **Table 6.2** lists a healthful 3,000-calorie-per-day diet that can be used to gain weight.
- Eat smaller meals more frequently throughout the day. If you don't have much of an appetite, try eating four or five smaller meals throughout the day, rather than two or three big ones.
- Add calories to your favorite meals. If you enjoy salad, for example, choose an olive oil dressing instead of a fat-free version. Add in some protein as well, such as diced chicken, cheese, avocado, or tofu.

>> Take a small step toward achieving your target weight. Visit http://people .bu.edu/salge/52_small_steps/weight_loss/index.html **for 52 tips on eating better, getting more active, and tracking your progress toward your goals.**

- Get regular exercise to build both appetite and muscle. Participate in activities such as weight lifting to increase muscle mass and swimming to improve cardiovascular fitness.

How Do You Maintain a Healthful Weight?

Reaching or being at a healthful weight is only one piece of the puzzle. Once you've achieved your target weight, you have to maintain it.

TABLE 6.2 Healthful Weight Gain: A Sample 3,000-Calorie Diet

Meal	Food
Breakfast	1 cup Grape Nuts 2 cup 2% milk 1 cup cranberry juice
Snack	6 Tbsp. raisins 1 cup orange juice
Lunch	8 oz. 2% milk 3 oz. tuna 2 tsp. mayonnaise 1 bun Lettuce, tomatoes, sprouts 2 oz. chips/snack food 1 cup whole baby carrots
Snack	Met-Rx fudge brownie bar 1 cup orange juice
Dinner	5 oz. chicken 1 cup instant mashed potatoes with 1/3 cup 2% dry milk powder 1 cup 2% milk 1 Tbsp. *trans* fat–free margarine 1 cup green beans Lettuce salad with vegetables 2 Tbsp. salad dressing
Snack	16 oz. water 16 animal crackers

Long-term weight management doesn't have to mean endless days of dull meals or counting calories. Instead, look at your food habits, your level of physical activity, and your feelings about eating, and choose options that make it easy and fun to keep your weight in balance. Keep in mind:

- **Your healthful weight is a range, not a fixed number.** If you find your weight creeping up, reduce your calorie intake a bit and exercise a little more. A flexible approach lets you manage your weight and still enjoy your life.
- **Find reasons to be active.** Often, we make excuses for not exercising. Try turning that habit around. Leave your car at the far end of the parking lot and walk. Turn off your laptop or TV for a couple of hours and join an intramural sports team instead. Look for part-time work that requires being on your feet, not sitting at a desk.
- **When choosing physical activity, aim for consistency over intensity.** A half-hour brisk walk every day will do more for you in the long run than a 2-hour intense workout done only on Saturdays. In one study of college students, those with four or more low-intensity workouts a week were twice as likely to have healthful BMIs.
- **Snack smarter.** Replace higher-calorie snacks such as chips and energy bars with fruits and vegetables. If you crave something more substantial, reach for whole grains or nuts. Store snacks in cupboards rather than leaving them lying around in plain sight.
- **Don't be too hard on yourself.** If you have a few high-calorie days, don't tell yourself that you've blown your diet. Instead, follow up with a few days of lower-calorie choices.

Helping a Friend

The motto of weight-loss support group Overeaters Anonymous is, "I put my hand in yours, and together we can do what we could never do alone." And social support doesn't have to be face to face. An analysis of 500,000 users of the calorie-tracking app MyFitnessPal revealed that the more friends users had, the more weight they lost.[72] If you want to help a friend shed pounds for good, try the following:

- Find fun in something other than food. Go to the movies, catch a game, or work out.
- Don't coach—join in! Instead of suggesting your friend walk more often, arrange to walk to class together in the morning rather than drive.
- Let the slip-ups pass. If your friend couldn't pass up a doughnut today, calling attention to the fact might only generate guilt and resentment. Instead, suggest your friend join you for an after-class workout.

Campus Advocacy

College doesn't have to mean scary food in the dining hall and worrying about the "freshman 15." Get involved to help bring healthier options to your school.

For inspiration, check out the Real Food Challenge (**www.realfood-challenge.org**), a network of students working to bring better options to campuses. This group, which has chapters at about 300 colleges and universities so far, aims to "shift $1 billion of annual college food purchases away from industrial agriculture towards local, sustainable, and fair sources." That's an ambitious goal, but the group provides support and training for campus chapters, and also has ways to start smaller, such as getting just one real food item into the menu at your dining hall. If your school doesn't have a chapter, start one, and if it does, get involved. Groups such as these show that students don't have to be at the mercy of the campus food service.

Maybe you make most of your own meals. If so, consider starting a cooking club with like-minded friends, where you share the planning, shopping, cooking—and mealtime.

If your campus doesn't offer safe walking and biking options, work with other students to lobby the administration and make these changes happen. In addition to working toward a healthful campus environment, it's also essential to avoid judging others because of weight. Many colleges and universities now offer courses in so-called "Fat Studies," which prompt students to research issues such as how weight is perceived in different countries, and what our media obsession with thinness reveals about our values as a society. Or check out NAAFA, the National Association to Advance Fat Acceptance at **www.naafaonline.com.**

Body Image and Eating Disorders

Have you ever thought about the fact that ads for junk foods like chips or cheeseburgers are funding videos and programs featuring actors so thin they look like they've never had a bite of either? For some people, contradictions like this contribute to the development of a distorted view of their body, or a dangerous relationship with food.[73]

Body Image Disorders

While many of us have concerns about our bodies and our appearance from time to time, some people experience worries about body image to such a strong degree that their thoughts and perceptions interfere with their happiness and daily life.

Body Dysmorphic Disorder

In **body dysmorphic disorder**, a person can't stop thinking about a perceived flaw with his or her appearance, even though the flaw is typically minor or imagined. Though this disorder can apply to any physical feature, it often centers on weight and body shape, and often starts during the teen years. Men and women experience the disorder in equal numbers.[74]

This condition can have serious effects, including depression, anxiety, social isolation, eating disorders, seeking out unnecessary cosmetic procedures or surgeries, and even suicidal thoughts. Treatment often centers on psychotherapy, although in some cases, antidepressant medications may also be recommended.

Social Physique Anxiety

Many of us get a little uncomfortable at the thought of appearing before others in shorts or a bathing suit, but for those with **social physique anxiety**, this concern is amplified to a degree that makes them extremely nervous and fearful of having their bodies judged by others. Psychologists have developed a 12-point scale to help understand the severity of this disorder, with people at the higher end of the scale more likely to experience consequences such as social isolation or extreme self-criticism.[75] While males and females may both experience this disorder, women and girls are more likely to have higher levels of social physique anxiety and lower levels of physical self-esteem than males.[76]

If you know someone who might have one of these body image disorders, encourage him or her to seek professional help. Your campus health center is often a good place to start.

Eating Disorders

Sometimes people let negative body image or other psychological factors steer them toward unhealthful eating behaviors. When these behaviors produce drastic weight changes and put health

body dysmorphic disorder Mental disorder characterized by obsessive thoughts about a perceived flaw in appearance.

social physique anxiety Mental disorder characterized by extreme fear of having one's body judged by others.

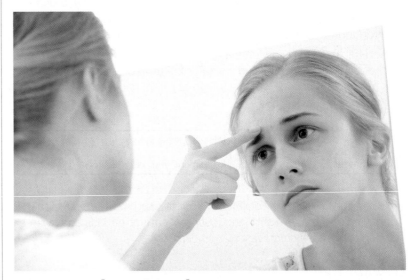

Being overly critical of your body can interfere with your happiness.

and even life at risk, they are called **eating disorders**. Teenage girls are most at risk for eating disorders, especially if they are preoccupied with being thin, experience social or family pressure to be thin, come from more affluent families, and have tendencies toward extreme self-control and perfectionism. But young men and athletes under pressure to adhere to a particular body shape are also vulnerable. According to national estimates, about 2.7% of 13- to 18-year-olds, including 3.8% of girls and 1.5% of boys, suffer from an eating disorder.[77]

Three dangerous eating disorders are anorexia nervosa, bulimia nervosa, and binge eating disorder. Other eating and weight-related behaviors, while not yet classified by medical experts as full-blown eating disorders, can also have serious health effects; these include night-eating syndrome and the female athlete triad.

Anorexia Nervosa

People with **anorexia nervosa** see food as an enemy that must be controlled. They eat as little as possible, often setting up elaborate rituals and practices to control food intake. They have an extremely unhealthful body image, seeing themselves as fat even when they are dangerously underweight. In the United States, experts estimate that about 0.6% of the population suffers from anorexia, including about 0.9% of women and 0.3% of men.[78] About 0.3% of teenagers develop the condition.[79]

Although the exact cause of anorexia nervosa is unknown, a variety of factors play a role in many cases. Psychological factors, such as a tendency toward obsessive-compulsive personality traits, may make it more possible for some people to focus intently on their weight and forgo food even when hungry. Environmental factors, such as the body image concerns and media influences discussed earlier, often play a part.

Signs and symptoms of anorexia nervosa include:

- An intense fear of gaining weight or being overweight.
- A highly distorted body image that continues to see fat where none exists.
- A refusal to maintain a normal body weight.
- A refusal to eat, or eating patterns that tightly restrict food intake.

Anorexia nervosa is classified as a serious mental disorder. Starvation leads to wasting: A body deprived of calories will begin to break down the proteins in muscle and other body tissues to use for energy. This can cause serious and sometimes irreparable damage throughout the body, especially to the heart muscle, and can prompt sudden death. People suffering from anorexia nervosa are 18 times more likely to die early than people in the same age group in the general population.[80] Other physical consequences of anorexia nervosa are illustrated in **Figure 6.6**.

Treatment for the disorder is key, although experts estimate that only about 34% of those with the disorder receive care.[81] The good news, though, is that once treatment is accessed, most patients do respond. In one survey of teenagers diagnosed with anorexia, more than 65% followed their treatment plan closely, and the vast majority showed healthful, positive outcomes in the years following their care.[82] The type and duration of treatment varies according to the severity of the illness. Patients with less severe cases often receive a blend of treatment and support services, such as

Brain and Nerves
Can't think right, fear of gaining weight, sad, moody, irritable, bad memory, fainting, changes in brain chemistry

Hair
Hair thins and gets brittle

Heart
Low blood pressure, slow heart rate, fluttering of the heart, palpitations, heart failure

Blood
Anemia and other blood problems

Muscles, Joints, and Bones
Weak muscles, swollen joints, bone loss, fractures, osteoporosis

Kidneys
Kidney stones, kidney failure

Body Fluids
Low potassium, magnesium, and sodium

Intestines
Constipation, bloating

Hormones
Periods stop, growth problems, trouble getting pregnant. If pregnant, higher risk for miscarriage, having a C-section baby with low birth weight, and postpartum depression.

Skin
Bruise easily, dry skin, growth of fine hair all over body, get cold easily, yellow skin, nails get brittle

FIGURE 6.6 Major Physical and Health Effects Associated with Anorexia.

Source: Adapted from *Anorexia nervosa Fact Sheet,* from the U.S. Department of Health and Human Services Womenshealth website, 2009.

psychiatric care, medications, and nutritional counseling in outpatient settings that allow them to continue to live at home. Patients with more severe cases, especially those whose life is at risk, may receive treatment in the hospital, where patient care, including nutritional support in the form of supervised feedings, can be more closely monitored.[83]

During and after treatment for anorexia nervosa, support from family and friends is key. Many treatment plans include family therapy to help loved ones find new ways to support the patient and each other, and avoid prior patterns of behavior that may have contributed to the condition. Patients also benefit from finding new ways to manage stress and reduce anxiety, helping themselves acquire a more healthful body image and relationship with food. Patients are also helped by disengaging from "pro-anorexia" websites and online forums where those with untreated anorexia nervosa discuss how they sustain their disorder or hide it from friends and family. To help, several large blogging and social media platforms recently announced that they would start removing posts and websites that could promote anorexia and other eating disorders.[84]

Bulimia Nervosa

This disorder is marked by an ongoing cycle of seeking large amounts of food and then trying to

eating disorders A group of mental disorders, including anorexia nervosa, bulimia nervosa, and binge eating disorder, that is characterized by physiological and psychological disturbances in appetite or food intake.

anorexia nervosa Mental disorder characterized by extremely low body weight, body image distortion, severe calorie restriction, and an obsessive fear of gaining weight.

get rid of the calories consumed. People who have **bulimia nervosa** have elaborate food rituals that typically start with **binge eating**, the consumption of a large amount of food in a short amount of time. After a binge, bulimics then try to remove these calories from their bodies by **purging** through self-induced vomiting, heavy laxative use, fasting, or excessive exercise.

An estimated 0.3% of American adults develop bulimia nervosa in any given year, including about 1.5% of women and 0.5% of men.[85] About 0.9% of teenagers develop the condition.[78] Unlike anorexia nervosa, those suffering from bulimia nervosa often maintain a healthy or normal weight, but as in anorexia nervosa, bulimics are often intensely anxious about gaining weight and extremely critical of their own bodies. Many conduct bulimic behavior in secret, sometimes as often as several times each day.[86]

Bulimia nervosa carries serious health risks, including dental problems such as cavities and tooth enamel erosion, dehydration from vomiting and other forms of forced purging, stomach problems such as ulcers and even stomach rupture, and cardiac risks including irregular heartbeat and heart failure. Signs of bulimia nervosa include:

- Regular binge eating episodes, at a rate of at least two per week for several months
- Binges followed by purging, strict dieting, or excessive exercise to prevent weight gain
- Using self-induced vomiting or laxatives as part of purging
- An obsession with weight and body shape

As with anorexia nervosa, treatment for bulimia nervosa can be extremely effective. Bulimia treatments usually focus on a combination of medical, psychiatric, and psychosocial care tailored to the needs of the individual patient. Some patients also benefit from antidepressant medications such as fluoxetine (Prozac), which is the only prescription drug approved by the FDA as a treatment for bulimia. These medications help some patients reduce depression and anxiety, as well as reduce binge-purge behavior and the chance of relapse.[87]

Binge Eating Disorder

Binge eaters may periodically consume thousands of calories in a matter of hours, do little to burn off those calories afterward, and then repeat a session of binge eating within a few days. As more binges lead to weight gain, many binge eaters say they begin to feel depressed, worried, and concerned about their ability to control their appetite. Those feelings lead many binge eaters to eat in private or try to hide their eating from others. About 2.8% of U.S. adults, including 3.5% of women and 2% of men, suffer from binge eating disorder.[88] About 1.6% of teenagers develop the condition.[78]

Signs of binge eating disorder include:

- Eating large amounts of food in a relatively short period of time, whether you are hungry or not, at least twice a week.
- Eating until you feel overly full.
- Eating large amounts of food alone.
- Choosing to consume particular personal "comfort foods," such as certain types of cookies, ice cream, or other foods you find especially pleasurable, during these concentrated sessions of heavy eating.

---

bulimia nervosa Mental disorder characterized by episodes of binge eating followed by a purge behavior such as vomiting, laxative abuse, or extreme exercise.

binge eating The rapid consumption of an excessive amount of food.

purging Behaviors, such as vomiting, laxative abuse, or overexercising, intended to reduce the calories absorbed by the body.

disordered eating A range of unhealthful eating behaviors used to deal with emotional issues that does not warrant a diagnosis of a specific eating disorder.

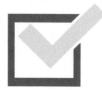
Treatment options for binge eating disorder are similar to those used to treat bulimia nervosa, and may include nutritional counseling, behavior therapy, and antidepressant medication.

Other Unhealthful Eating Behaviors

There are other unhealthful eating behaviors that do not qualify as full-blown eating disorders but still have serious effects on weight, mental health, and well-being. These behaviors are classified as **disordered eating**, a range of unhealthful eating habits in which food is used primarily to deal with emotional issues. Disordered eating is common on college campuses—in one study, about 17% of students said they had experienced some kind of disordered eating.[89]

Night-Eating Syndrome

While it's common for many of us to occasionally visit the fridge after dinner, some people suffer from a regular pattern of night-time eating, disrupted sleep, and mood disorders that can add up to depression and weight gain. Those with night-eating syndrome often skip breakfast and eat little during the first part of the day. Then, beginning in the evening, food intake increases dramatically, often focusing on starchy or sugary foods. People with this syndrome may eat before going to bed, and then wake up several times during the night for more food.

This syndrome isn't yet fully understood. Researchers suspect that a range of sleep and health difficulties may play a role, leading the body to seek food in an effort to better produce and regulate sleep-related hormones. Estimates of its prevalence vary widely—while experts estimate that about 1.5% of the general population suffers from the condition, a study of a group of college students found that about 5.7% experienced some form of the disorder.[90, 91] Night-eating syndrome can be difficult to treat, but is sometimes addressed with hormonal supplements such as melatonin or antidepressant medications.[88]

Female Athlete Triad

This multifaceted disorder is more prevalent in female athletes participating in sports that require a lower body weight, such as gymnastics, diving, or distance running. Women and girls with this syndrome experience a trio of disorders: disordered eating (focusing on weight control and calorie restriction), amenorrhea (irregular or absent menstrual period), and osteoporosis (low bone density).[92] The combination of disordered eating and frequent high-intensity exercise leaves the body with inadequate energy to maintain fat stores and reproductive functioning. Low blood levels of the female reproductive hormone estrogen lead to cessation of menstrual periods, and loss of bone density. This in turn increases the athlete's risk for fractures. Depending on the athlete's age, the loss of bone density may be irreversible, resulting in a lifelong increased risk for fractures. Because this disorder is difficult to treat, medical experts stress prevention, urging coaches, friends, and parents of female athletes to avoid excessive focus on an athlete's weight, watch for signs of the triad, and seek professional help if they suspect the disorder is present.[93]

Getting Help for a Body Image or Eating Disorder

If you struggle with a negative body image or unhealthful eating behaviors, seek support and treatment from trained professionals. Many people who experience eating disorders and disordered eating also get a great deal of help from guided support groups. In these groups, you'll not only receive help in shifting your self-perceptions and habits, but get valuable advice from others who've been in your shoes. If you have a serious eating disorder, you may first need medical treatment to stabilize your body and stop your health from deteriorating.

If you think someone you know has an unhealthful eating or weight-control behavior:

- Locate support and treatment resources on campus or in your community.
- Once you know where to find help, have a compassionate, open conversation with the person you are concerned about. Try to listen and talk about your worries, rather than accuse or blame.
- Try not to talk with your friend or loved one about dieting, body size, or weight. Instead, focus on behaviors that worry you and how they might be unhealthful.
- Offer to direct the person to the treatment resources you've found, and offer to go along for support if desired.
- Know that one conversation may not go far. Keep trying. If you let your friend or loved one know that you are concerned, that person will know where to turn when he or she is ready to seek help.

Personal Choices: Develop a More Positive Body Image

While energy balance—calories in versus calories burned—is important, it's also critical to understand how you view your body and your health. Here are a few strategies for building a more positive body image to help yourself achieve and maintain a healthy weight and shape:

- Accept yourself for who you are. Beauty comes in many shapes and sizes.
- Pay attention to your fitness rather than your appearance. Build healthy habits that benefit both your mind and your body.
- Be kind to yourself. No one can look their healthiest or eat wisely all the time. Accept your setbacks as temporary obstacles, not personal failures.

Eating Disorders

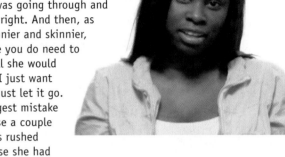

"HI, MY NAME IS VIEGE. My freshman year in college I had a friend named Lisa, who suffered from an eating disorder. She would always starve herself to try to look like other people or starve herself to get a guy. To be honest with you, I really didn't take it seriously. I just told her that it's just a phase she was going through and everything will be all right. And then, as I saw her getting skinnier and skinnier, I was like, hey, maybe you do need to get some help. And all she would say is, I'm not crazy. I just want to be beautiful. So I just let it go. And that was the biggest mistake I've ever made because a couple months later, Lisa was rushed to the hospital because she had something wrong with her heart.

So, if you do have a friend that's struggling with eating disorders, you should probably talk to them. You may not think of it as serious but it can be, even if they're young."

1. What do you think was wrong with Viege's friend's heart? What could have caused her to be hospitalized?

2. Do you think it's common for people to take eating disorders seriously? What would prompt you to talk to a friend about a possible eating disorder? Do you think it's your place to convince a friend to get help?

> **"** *Remember that your worth is not defined by your appearance, and your health is not defined by the number on the scale."*

- Know that the beauty and fitness industries are businesses designed to make money, not be health-care providers. Take corporate and mass media beauty and fitness advice with a large grain of salt.
- Remember that your worth is not defined by your appearance, and your health is not defined by the number on the scale.

>> **Watch videos of real students discussing weight management and body image at MasteringHealth™**

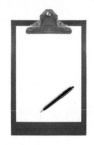

Choosing to Change Worksheet

To complete this worksheet online, visit MasteringHealth™

What can you do to manage your weight? What is an appropriate goal for weight management? Follow the steps below to develop a weight-management plan.

Directions: Fill in your stage of behavior change in Step 1 and complete the rest of the Worksheet with your stage of change in mind.

Step 1: *Your Stage of Behavior Change.* Please check one of the following statements that best describes your readiness to manage your weight.

_____ I do not intend to change my body weight in the next six months. (Precontemplation)

_____ I might change my body weight in the next six months. (Contemplation)

_____ I am prepared to change my body weight in the next month. (Preparation)

_____ I have been changing my body weight for less than six months. (Action)

_____ I have been changing my body weight for more than six months. (Maintenance)

Step 2: *Creating a Weight-Management Plan*

1. What does your BMI and waist-to-hip ratio tell you about the effect of your weight on your health? How do you feel about your weight when you look in the mirror? Do you want to maintain your current weight? Gain weight? Lose weight? By how many pounds? Write down exactly what you want to accomplish with your weight-management plan.

BMI and waist-to-hip ratio: _____

Effect on health: _____

Weight-management goal: _____

_____

2. Given your current stage of behavior change, what can you do next to accomplish your weight-management goal? Which side of the energy balance equation do you want to change: energy in or energy out? You can also modify both. Include a realistic timeline for your next step and list a reward for yourself once you have accomplished your next step.

Next step: _____

_____

Timeline: _____

Reward: _____

3. Consider that a healthful prescription for weight loss is cutting 500 to 1,000 calories a day, through reduced calorie intake or increased exercise. This typically leads to a weight loss of 1 or 2 pounds a week. To gain weight, you would add a similar amount of calories daily. Now, consider the weight-management techniques introduced in this chapter. Which techniques can you try to better manage your weight? Keep in mind that you should not cut calories below your recommended MyPlate levels that you can find at **www.choosemyplate.gov.**

_____

_____

_____

4. If you want to simply maintain your current weight, what will you do to ensure that your energy expenditure meets the energy you consume? Think about extended amounts of time when you might consistently consume more food (such as holiday breaks), or where you might be less active than usual (such as during finals). What steps can you take during those times to make sure you stay in energy balance?

_____

_____

_____

Step 3: _Promoting a Healthful Body Image._

1. What are your current feelings about your body? When you think about your body, are you usually thinking about how it looks? How it feels? What it does for you? Write down your general thoughts.

_____

_____

_____

2. What do you like about your body? Write down _at least_ three things.

_____

_____

_____

3. Are there factors that lead you to think negatively about your body (for example, images you see in the media, the opinions of friends or family, the presence of scars or injury, etc.)? If so, how could you combat those factors and improve your body image?

_____

_____

_____

Chapter Summary

MasteringHealth™

Build your knowledge—and health!—in the Study Area of **MasteringHealth**™ with a variety of study tools.

- Your weight affects your health, not just your appearance. Many of us, however, become preoccupied with body image when thinking about our weight.

- BMI, together with other factors such as waist circumference and waist-to-hip ratio, can help indicate whether your weight will increase your risk for certain health conditions and diseases.

- Overweight and obesity are serious and common health problems, not just in the United States, but around the world.

- Excess body weight is a critical issue for college students. Decline in physical activity is often a major contributor to college weight gain.

- Health risks of excess weight include high blood pressure, type 2 diabetes, abnormal blood fats, coronary heart disease, stroke, cancer, osteoarthritis, sleep apnea, gallbladder disease, fatty liver disease, and fertility and pregnancy complications.

- Your weight is shaped by your energy balance, physical activity, basic energy needs, age, genes, gender, and environment. Ultimately, excess weight results from an imbalance of calories consumed and calories used.

- To truly understand your weight and its effects on your health, you need to know your body composition, blood chemistry, and other factors, not just how much you weigh.

- Reaching a healthful lower weight requires consistent, long-term work on both eating habits and increasing physical activity. Short-term diets are often of limited help. Diet aids can be expensive, may not work, and may even be harmful.

- Medical options, including prescription drugs and bariatric surgery, may be beneficial for people who are extremely obese.

- To gain weight, boost your calories in healthful ways by eating nutritious foods like nuts, juices, peanut butter, and energy bars. Also, eat more often and get exercise to stimulate your appetite.

- Maintaining a healthful weight is most effective when you establish and consistently follow eating and exercise habits you enjoy, and use them to keep your weight within a healthful range.
- Societal contradictions that encourage weight gain while glorifying thinness lead many of us to have negative views of our own bodies. These body image issues contribute to disordered eating and eating disorders.
- Eating disorders are complicated psychiatric conditions that are affected by family, social dynamics, and feelings of self-worth. Eating disorders that carry significant health risks include anorexia nervosa, bulimia nervosa, and binge eating disorder.

- Disordered eating behaviors, while not qualifying as psychiatric disorders, are also unhealthful. These include night-eating syndrome and the female athlete triad.
- While eating disorders and disordered eating can significantly harm a person's health, or even lead to death in some cases, the good news is that treatments are available, and are often effective. If you know someone who you think might have an eating-related disorder, help them find resources on campus for support and treatment.

GET CONNECTED

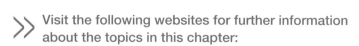

Visit the following websites for further information about the topics in this chapter:

- American College of Sports Medicine Exercise Guidelines
  www.acsm.org
- Academy of Nutrition and Dietetics
  www.eatright.org
- Centers for Disease Control and Prevention: Overweight and Obesity
  www.cdc.gov/obesity/index.html
- National Institute of Mental Health: Eating Disorders
  www.nimh.nih.gov/health/publications/eating-disorders/index.shtml
- USDA Nutritional Database
  http://ndb.nal.usda.gov
- World Health Organization: Obesity
  www.who.int/topics/obesity/en

MOBILE TIPS!

Scan this QR code with your mobile device to access additional weight-management and body image tips. Or, via your mobile device, go to **http://chmobile.pearsoncmg.com** and navigate to Chapter 6.

- FitDay (free online weight-loss journal)
  www.fitday.com

Website links are subject to change. To access updated web links, please visit MasteringHealth™

TEST YOUR KNOWLEDGE

1. Which of the following conditions is NOT related to being overweight?
   a. polycystic ovary syndrome
   b. high blood pressure
   c. fatty liver disease
   d. low LDL levels

2. What percentage of 18- to 24-year-olds engage in no leisure-time physical activity?
   a. 75%
   b. 50%
   c. 25%
   d. 10%

3. When most students start college, how many pounds do they gain?
   a. 1 to 4
   b. 7 to 8
   c. 9 to 12
   d. 13 to 16

4. What is the healthful weight range for someone who is 5 feet 11 inches tall?
   a. 133 to 172 pounds
   b. 140 to 171 pounds
   c. 149 to 183 pounds
   d. 164 to 196 pounds

5. What is BMI?
   a. a ratio between your height and your weight, used to help assess health risks
   b. a measurement of how much fat you have
   c. a measurement of how much muscle you have
   d. a 100% reliable indicator of how healthy you are

6. What is the best approach to weight loss?
   a. Eat more protein and drink more water.
   b. Take in fewer calories and exercise more.
   c. Avoid foods containing carbohydrates.
   d. Take in more energy and eat less fat.

7. What term best describes our response to the sight, smell, thought, or taste of food?
a. satiety
b. craving
c. hunger
d. appetite

8. In order to maintain weight loss, you should
a. eat as little as possible.
b. stop working out; it makes you hungry.
c. never allow yourself to have a high-calorie day.
d. focus on eating fruits and vegetables.

9. Which of the following statements about body image is true?
a. In body dysmorphic disorder, a person focuses on a perceived physical flaw.
b. Among college students, about 10% of males and 35% of females are dissatisfied with their body.
c. Men and boys are more likely to have higher levels of social physique anxiety than women and girls.
d. Women become less self-accepting of their bodies with age.

10. The risk for fractures is increased in women with
a. bulimia nervosa.
b. night-eating syndrome.
c. the female athlete triad.
d. compulsive overeating.

Get Critical

What happened

The fashion world revolves around women's appearance, but top Chanel designer Karl Lagerfeld may have taken his opinion a little too far when he decided to comment on the physique of rising singing star Adele when he told a reporter "She is a little too fat, but she has a beautiful face and a divine voice."[1]

Adele's many fans responded angrily, wondering why Lagerfeld would use the body size standards of his industry to critique others who never saunter down a runway. But no one hit back more eloquently than Adele herself, saying "I've never wanted to look like models on the cover of magazines. I represent the majority of women and I'm very proud of that."[2] Lagerfeld later apologized.[3]

What do you think?

- Does the entertainment industry support people of different physiques and sizes? If so, how? If not, why doesn't it?
- What effects do you think the body size standards favored by the fashion industry have on your standards of ideal body size, and your body image? Even if you know a model has had to severely restrict her eating to get down to runway size, do you think it still affects your idea of what beauty is?
- What could the worlds of fashion and entertainment do to represent people with many different body types?

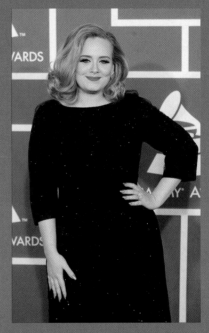

References: **1.** "Karl Lagerfeld on Adele, the Greek Crisis and M.I.A.'s Middle Finger (Updated)," by *Metro World News*, February 8, 2012, retrieved from http://www.metro.us/newyork/life/article/1089980--karl-lagerfeld-on-adele-the-greek-crisis-and-m-i-a-s-middle-finger. **2.** "All About Adele" by Joey Bartolomeo, from *People*, February 20, 2012, Volume 77(8). **3.** "EXCLUSIVE: Karl Lagerfeld: 'Adele, I Am Your Biggest Admirer'," by K. Hunt, February 8, 2012, retrieved from http://www.metro.us/newyork/entertainment/2012/02/08/exclusive-karl-lagerfeld-adele-i-am-your-biggest-admirer/.

DRUG USE AND ABUSE

More than **22 million** Americans age 12 and up currently use **illicit drugs**.[i]

The number of **drug overdose deaths** has climbed steadily every year for the past decade.[ii]

College students tend to **vastly overestimate** how many of their **peers** use illicit drugs.[iii]

7

DISCUSS the characteristics of addiction.

IDENTIFY four common behavioral addictions.

COMPARE the prevalence of drug use among college students and in the general population.

DISCUSS the physical and psychological effects of initial and chronic drug use.

IDENTIFY commonly abused drugs, describing their mechanisms, effects, and health risks.

DISCUSS three drug-prevention strategies used throughout the United States.

LIST community, campus-based, and clinical options for treatment of drug abuse.

DESCRIBE personal strategies for overcoming addictions and drug abuse.

Rock star checks into rehab!

Actor's spending out of control! When addiction or abuse involves a celebrity, you hear about it. But what about the untold stories—the more than 38,000 drug-overdose deaths in the United States each year, the 5% of female college students who have experienced a drug-related forcible sexual assault, the 22.5 million Americans who use illicit drugs, or the 2 million Americans whose lives are ruined by addiction to gambling?[1-4] Chances are, you've witnessed one or more of these stories among your own family members or friends—or maybe the untold story is your own.

Even if your life hasn't been directly touched by addiction, you share the costs. These include the economic burden of increased health care, social services, and law enforcement as well as the costs of broken families and ravaged communities.

What can you do about addictions and drug abuse? Change starts with knowledge—about the nature of addictions, how to avoid them, how to recover, and how to help a friend. Start here.

An Overview of Addiction

From time to time, we all do things for fun even though we know they might cause us trouble in the long term: We cut classes, eat that extra slice of pizza, or buy those concert tickets that we "really can't afford." Such behavior is normal—and reflects the power of the pleasure centers in our brains. But some people repeatedly engage in problematic behaviors that have long since stopped providing any real pleasure. In short, they develop an addiction.

What Is Addiction?

The American Society of Addiction Medicine defines **addiction** as a chronic disease of brain reward, motivation, memory, and related circuitry. Dysfunction in these brain circuits is characterized by the pursuit of reward and/or relief by substance abuse or other destructive behavior.[5]

Perhaps the most fundamental characteristic of addiction is craving.[5] The person experiences an uncontrollable compulsion to engage in the behavior, and seeks it out even in the face of significant negative consequences, such as poor grades, loss of relationships or employment, violence, or arrest. Although these negative consequences are entirely clear to others, the addict has a diminished capacity to recognize them. Denial of both the negative consequences and the addiction itself is common.[5]

Another characteristic of addiction is loss of pleasure. Although the person originally may have engaged in the activity for pleasurable recreation, he or she now derives very little satisfaction from it. Instead, the addict's motivation becomes an increasingly powerful compulsion to relieve the physical discomfort and emotional anguish experienced when abstaining. As a result, the person experiences an escalating loss of control over the act and comes to feel increasingly controlled by it.[5] At the same time, the person has an increased sensitivity to stressors as well as increased anxiety and emotional pain.

Without treatment, addiction is progressive; that is, the behavior becomes more frequent and/or severe.[5] Recovery is often preceded by one or more cycles in which the person abstains from the behavior, then relapses; however, with treatment, full recovery from addiction is possible.

How can you tell if you or someone you care about has an addiction? The nearby **Practical Strategies** box lists the signs to look for.

addiction A chronic, progressive disease of brain reward, motivation, memory, and related circuitry characterized by uncontrollable craving for a substance or behavior despite both negative consequences and diminishment or loss of pleasure associated with the activity.

Practical Strategies

Warning Signs of Addiction

How can you tell if you or someone you care about has an addiction? Look for the following signs:

- **Craving.** Does the person seem compelled to engage in a particular behavior, such as gambling or doing drugs and getting high?
- **Loss of control.** Does the person seem to be engaging in the behavior less because of the pleasure it brings and more because he or she can't stop?
- **Negative consequences.** Is the behavior becoming increasingly reckless, such as failing to study because of drug use, then skipping class, then missing exams? Does the person continue the destructive behavior despite serious negative consequences such as academic failure, financial ruin, injury or illness, arrest, or loss of relationships with others?
- **Denial.** Does the person fail to recognize or acknowledge that the addiction is causing problems?

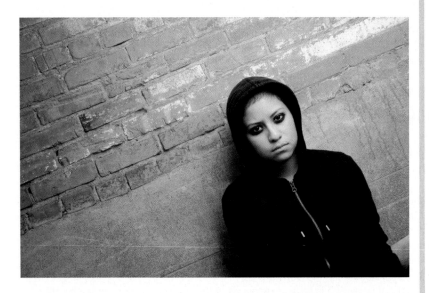

What Are Some Behavioral Addictions?

The American Psychiatric Association (APA) recognizes a category of diagnoses called **behavioral addictions** that can be applied to patients who are addicted not to a substance, but rather to an activity such as gambling.[6] The rationale for this category is that the patient's subjective experience, the brain networks involved, the progression of the disorder, and the effective treatment are equivalent to those for substance addictions. Let's look at a few of the most common behavioral addictions.

Pathological Gambling

About 85% of adults in the United States have gambled at least once in their life.[4] For most of us, a night at the casino doesn't pose a problem.

> **behavioral addiction** A form of addiction involving a compulsion to engage in an activity such as gambling, sex, or shopping rather than a compulsion to use a substance.

However, for an estimated 2 million people in the United States, roughly 1% of adults, gambling is an addiction.[4] Although gambling is illegal for anyone under age 21 in many states, most addicted gamblers get their start in high school, and young adults are especially vulnerable. Studies estimate that 6% of American college students have a serious gambling problem that can result in psychological difficulties, unmanageable debt, and failing grades.[7]

The APA considers a gambling habit *pathological* (harmful) when players experience destructive traits such as:

- Being preoccupied with thoughts and plans related to gambling
- Needing to gamble with increasing amounts of money in order to achieve the desired excitement
- Feeling restless or irritable when attempting to cut back or stop gambling, or being unable to do so
- Using gambling to escape feelings of helplessness, guilt, anxiety, or depression

Other telltale signs include lying to friends and family to hide the extent of the problem and borrowing from others or stealing to finance the habit.

Hypersexual Disorder

A variety of sources estimate that between 3% and 5% of the U.S. population could meet the criteria for sexual addiction, which the APA refers to as *hypersexual disorder*.[8] Characteristics include recurrent and intense sexual fantasies, urges, and behavior that consume excessive time and cannot be controlled, despite negative consequences such as sexually transmitted infections, unintended pregnancy, broken relationships, and financial problems. The person typically gains little satisfaction from sexual activity and in fact may experience feelings of deep guilt and shame.

Compulsive Spending

Compulsive spending (also referred to as compulsive buying or shopping) is thought to affect more than 1 in 20 U.S. adults.[9] Most are young and have incomes below $50,000. When a compulsive spender buys something, the act triggers the release of chemicals in the brain that cause a rush of euphoria. Compulsive spenders are also more likely than ordinary shoppers to experience uncontrollable buying binges, make senseless and impulsive purchases, and feel depressed after shopping.[9]

Addiction to Technology

A recent study in Europe and the United States suggests that about 1.5% to 8.2% of regular Internet users become addicted; that is, their Internet use interferes with their academic success, work, relationships, hours of sleep, or exercising.[10] Moreover, the addict turns to Internet use to alter his or her mood, especially to escape from depression or anxiety.

Another use of technology that's increasingly getting media attention is "addiction" to texting. Undoubtedly, Americans love to text: We send or receive about 5 billion text messages per day.[11] Many of these messages are sent by people of college age; a national survey found that 18% of adults aged 18 to 24 send more than 200 text messages a day.[12] Does this level of texting constitute an addiction? Those who say it does point to brain scans showing that the same areas of the brain light up when people text and when they use mind-altering drugs. Moreover, many people continue to text excessively despite serious negative consequences—including damage to the tendons in their hands. Other addiction experts say that, although frequent texting is a bad habit, before we can classify it as an addiction, more research is needed.

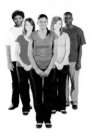

Drug Use Through the Lenses of Sex, Race, Age, and Geography

A recent national survey of drug use in the United States revealed the following information.

Overall

- About 9% of the U.S. population (an estimated 22.5 million individuals aged 12 or older) currently use illicit drugs. The most commonly used illicit drug is marijuana (18.1%), followed by prescription drugs used nonmedically (6.1%).

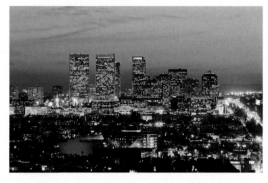

Rates of drug use are higher in metropolitan areas than in rural areas.

Sex

- 11.1% of males use illicit drugs, compared with 6.5% of females. Males are much more likely than females to use marijuana (9.3% of males, compared with 4.9% of females). Males also have slightly higher rates of use of prescription drugs for nonmedical purposes, hallucinogens, and cocaine.

Age

- The age group with the highest percentage of past-month illicit drug use is young adults aged 18 to 20 (23.8% in 2011). Adults aged 21 to 25 show the second highest percentage (19.9%), followed by teens aged 16 to 17 (17.2%).

Race

- Mixed-race individuals reported the highest rates of illicit drug use (13.5%), followed by Native Americans (13.4%), African Americans (10%), Caucasians (8.7%), Hispanics (8.4%), and Asian Americans (3.8%).

Geography

- Rates of illicit drug use are highest in the West (10.5%), followed by the Northeast (9.2%), Midwest (8.5%), and the South (7.5%). Illicit drug use is higher in densely populated areas. For instance, 9.2% of the population in large metropolitan counties use illicit drugs, compared with 5.7% in completely rural counties.

Critical-Thinking Questions

1. Are you surprised that the percentage of males using illicit drugs is almost 75% higher than the percentage for females? What factors can you think of that might account for this difference?

2. In Chapter 1, you learned about poverty as a determinant of health. How might poverty play a role in some of the statistics you see here?

3. How might access to illicit drugs influence these statistics?

Data from *Results from the 2011 National Survey on Drug Use and Health: Summary of National Findings*, NSDUH Series H-44, HHS Publication No. (SMA) 12-4713, by the Substance Abuse and Mental Health Services Administration, U.S. Department of Health and Human Services, 2012.

>> View the complete results of the 2011 national survey on drug use and health at www.samhsa.gov/data/NSDUH/2k11Results/NSDUHresults2011.htm.

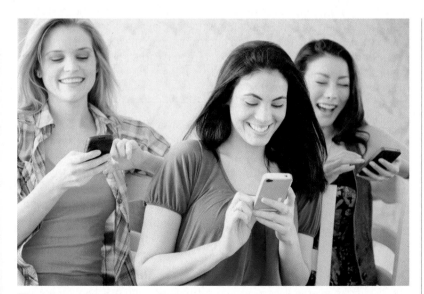

Technology addictions are becoming a concern in this gadget-friendly age.

Patterns of Drug Use

Do you use drugs? Many of us quickly say no, but the answer to this question is not simple. A **drug** is any chemical that is taken in order to alter the body physically or mentally for a non-nutritional purpose. Drugs that alter feelings, mood, perception, or psychological functioning are considered **psychoactive.** Although you may not realize it, you might routinely use one or more psychoactive drugs. If you drink caffeinated beverages or take certain pain relievers, sleeping pills, or allergy medicines, you are using psychoactive drugs. Of course, some are much more harmful than others: There is a big difference between having a daily cup of coffee and being addicted to cocaine.

In 2011, about 8.7% of Americans age 12 and older used **illicit drugs**; that is, drugs that are regulated by the

> **drug** A chemical substance that alters the body physically or mentally for a non-nutritional purpose.
>
> **psychoactive** Capable of altering feelings, mood, perceptions, or psychological functioning.
>
> **illicit drugs** Drugs regulated by the U.S. Drug Enforcement Agency as unlawful substances, including prescription medications used unlawfully.

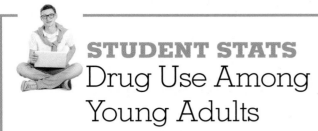

STUDENT STATS
Drug Use Among Young Adults

Three times as many young adults (age 18–25) use marijuana as any other drug

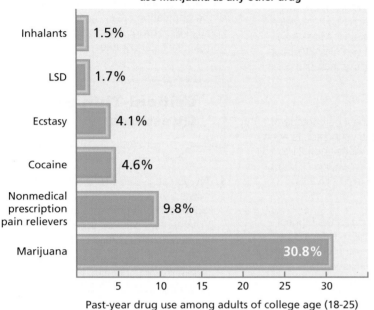

Inhalants	1.5%
LSD	1.7%
Ecstasy	4.1%
Cocaine	4.6%
Nonmedical prescription pain relievers	9.8%
Marijuana	30.8%

Past-year drug use among adults of college age (18-25)

Data from *Results from the 2011 National Survey on Drug Use and Health: Summary of National Findings* (NSDUH Series H-44, HHS Publication No. [SMA] 12-4713), Table 8.5: Past-Year Prevalence Estimates Among Young Adults, by the Substance Abuse and Mental Health Services Administration, 2012, Rockville, MD. http://www.samhsa.gov/data/NSDUH/2k11Results/NSDUHresults2011.htm.

U.S. Drug Enforcement Agency (DEA) as unlawful substances, including prescription medications used unlawfully.[3,13]

The rate of illicit drug use among people who are unemployed and among people who did not graduate from high school is more than double that of people with full-time jobs and college graduates.[3] The **Diversity & Health** box on page 155 examines other differences in patterns of illicit drug use among various demographic groups.

In 2011, 22% of full-time college students aged 18 to 22 reported using illicit drugs during the previous month.[3] This rate closely reflects drug use prevalence in this age group in general.

❝ *Although you may not realize it, you might routinely use one or more psychoactive drugs.*❞

Which illicit drugs do young adults most commonly use? To compare, check out the nearby **Student Stats** graph.

Interestingly, college students tend to vastly overestimate the percentage of their peers who use drugs. For example, in a national survey conducted in 2012, students reported believing that over 80% of their peers use marijuana, when only 15.3% of students reported actually using it.[14] The number of students who report using illicit drugs other than marijuana was even lower—12.7%. So as you read on in this chapter, it's important to bear in mind that *not everyone is using drugs*—far from it.

>> **View a video of young adults telling personal stories about their drug addictions at** http://pact360.org/programs/youth360.

How the Body Responds to Drugs

By definition, all psychoactive drugs intoxicate the brain, producing characteristic physical, psychological, and behavioral changes. Before we explore the chemistry behind these changes, let's define some terms.

Drug Misuse and Abuse

Drug misuse is the inappropriate use of a legal drug, either for a reason for which it was not medically intended, or by a person without a prescription. Using your roommate's amoxicillin because you think you have a sinus infection is an example of drug misuse.

In contrast, **drug abuse** is the use (most often the excessive use) of any legal or illegal drug in a way that is detrimental to your health. If, for example, you take prescription painkillers to get high or use street amphetamines to lose weight, you are abusing drugs. All drug use involves some level of health risks; however, the risks are significantly increased if you misuse or abuse drugs.

Initial Effects on the Brain

People self-administer drugs in a variety of ways, from ingestion to inhalation (**Table 7.1**). But no matter how they get into the body, once they enter the bloodstream, drugs chemically tap into and interfere with the brain's communication system, altering how nerve cells send, receive, and process information. The most addictive substances trigger a rush of the neurotransmitter *dopamine*. Dopamine is the brain's "feel good" chemical and causes feelings of pleasure and satisfaction. When the brain is overstimulated chemically, users experience a sense of euphoria that primes their bodies to repeat the stimulation. Eventually the brain adapts to the drug by producing less of its own neurotransmitters. As a result, when the drug is no longer externally supplied, users may feel "flat" or depressed, uninterested in things that used to bring them pleasure.

Effects of Chronic Use

Prolonged or repeated use of chemical substances can actually alter the brain's structure and how it works. The body can eventually develop **tolerance,** meaning that the brain has grown so

drug misuse The inappropriate use of a legal drug, either for a reason for which it was not medically intended, or by a person without a prescription.

drug abuse The use (most often the excessive use) of any legal or illegal drug in a way that is detrimental to your health.

tolerance Reduced sensitivity to a drug so that increased amounts are needed to achieve the usual effect.

TABLE 7.1 Common Methods of Drug Administration

Method	Description	Typical Drugs
Ingestion	Swallowing a drug and absorbing it through the digestive system	Alcoholic beverages, pills, LSD
Injection	Using a syringe to inject a drug directly into the skin, muscle, or bloodstream	Cocaine, methamphetamine, heroin
Inhalation	Breathing a drug into the lungs through the mouth or nostrils (snorting or smoking)	Marijuana, tobacco, cocaine (crack), inhalants such as paint thinner or glue
Mucosal absorption	Absorbing a drug through the mucous membranes	Chewing tobacco (absorbed through the membranes in the mouth); snorted cocaine (absorbed through the membranes in the nose)
Topical administration	Applying a drug directly onto a body surface, like the skin	Nicotine patch

accustomed to the drug that more of the drug is required to achieve the effect that a smaller amount used to have. Tolerance may also cause users to need to keep using a drug just to feel "normal."

This cycle of drug use and tolerance feeds drug addiction. Like other forms of addiction, drug addiction is a complex condition characterized by uncontrollable craving and use—despite negative consequences. In the past, people believed that drug addiction was due to moral failure, laziness, or lack of willpower. Today, addiction to drugs is typically described in terms of **dependence,** which has both psychological and physical roots.

Psychological dependence ("psychological addiction") means a mental attachment to a drug—the belief that a drug is needed to relieve stress, anxiety, or other feelings of mental discomfort. With *physical dependence*, the body requires the regular use of a substance in order to function. A physically dependent person also develops tolerance; therefore, larger and larger doses are needed to achieve a high, or even feel normal. Both psychological dependence and physical dependence are characterized by intense cravings for the drug.

The APA defines *substance dependence* as a pattern of substance use that leads to "significant impairment or distress" and that is characterized by at least three or more of the following within a one-year period:[15]

- The development of tolerance to the substance
- Using the substance in larger quantities or over a longer period than intended
- Inability to cut down or control one's use of the substance
- Spending an inordinate amount of time on activities aimed at obtaining the substance, using it, or recovering from its effects
- Sacrificing important social, occupational, or recreational activities due to the substance use
- Continuing use of the substance despite knowledge that the substance has either caused or is exacerbating a physical or psychological problem

dependence The state of being mentally attached to and/or physically needing a drug.

withdrawal The process in which, and symptoms that develop when, a person stops using a drug.

toxicity The dosage level at which a drug becomes poisonous to the body.

- The experience of withdrawal symptoms. **Withdrawal** refers to the process and experience of ceasing to take a drug that has created a physical dependence. Withdrawal can make some drugs extremely difficult to quit. Effects include craving, headaches, nausea, and vomiting.

How Drugs Leave the Body

Both the extent and the duration of a drug's effect on the body depend on several factors, from body size to ethnicity. For example, a heavyset person will be less affected by the same dose of the same drug as a slender person, and Caucasians generally clear psychoactive drugs from the body more quickly than do Asian Americans. Moreover, drugs differ in their *distribution half-life,* the amount of time it takes a drug to move from the bloodstream to body tissues such as muscle and fat. The liver is responsible for metabolizing (breaking down) all kinds of toxins, from pesticide residues and pollutants to psychoactive drugs, into chemicals that can be excreted by the bowels in stool and by the kidneys in urine. Some substances can also be eliminated through exhaled breath, sweat, saliva, or in the breast milk of nursing mothers.

A drug's physiological effect on the body can also be affected when two or more drugs are combined. In *additive interactions,* the effect of one drug is combined with the effect of another. In *antagonistic interactions,* the effect of one drug is diminished when combined with another drug. The dosage level at which the drug becomes poisonous to the body and can cause temporary or permanent damage is referred to as its **toxicity.**

Commonly Abused Drugs

As noted earlier, illicit drug use includes unlawful use of prescription drugs, which is a growing problem in the United States. The following section discusses these and other commonly abused drugs.

Prescription and Over-the-Counter Medications

Taken as directed, medications can restore and improve health and boost quality of life, but all carry risks, including unwanted side effects. These risks increase when medications are not taken properly. The four most common types of misuse are:

- Taking the incorrect dose
- Taking the medicine at the wrong time
- Forgetting to take a dose
- Failing to take all the medicine

These behaviors can retard healing, promote the development of complications, or, in the case of antibiotics, lead to the reproduction of so-called super germs that are resistant to the drug.

In addition to these problems of misuse, public health and law enforcement authorities are becoming increasingly concerned by America's outright abuse of prescription drugs, which is now considered the fastest growing drug problem in the United States.[16] A national survey conducted by the American College Health Association found that almost 13% of college students reported using prescription drugs that were not prescribed to them.[14]

Abuse of Prescription Opioids

In 2011, more than 1.8 million Americans reported abusing prescription pain medications in the past year.[3] The most commonly abused are prescription *narcotics* (from the Greek word meaning

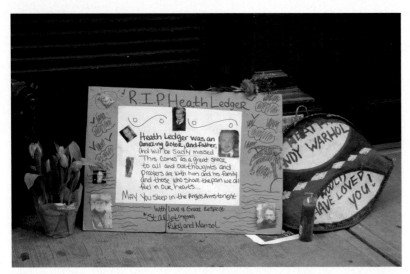

Misusing prescription drugs—especially more than one—is dangerous. A lethal combination of prescription drugs caused the death of actor Heath Ledger.

"numbing"), pain relievers that were originally derived from opium, a milky fluid found in the unripe seedpods of the opium poppy. Today, most narcotics are synthetic versions called **opioids.** They include morphine, which is often given to patients before or after surgery to alleviate severe pain, and codeine, which is used for milder analgesia (pain relief) or severe coughs. Other prescription opioids include hydrocodone (Vicodin) and oxycodone (marketed under the brand names OxyContin, Percodan, and Percocet). Heroin, a nonprescription opioid, is discussed later in this chapter.

Narcotics attach to special receptors on body cells and block the transmission of pain signals to the brain. When taken as directed, they can manage pain effectively; however, common side effects are nausea and constipation, and in too large a dose, they can cause respiratory depression, coma, and death. In fact, abuse of prescription narcotics is implicated in hundreds of thousands of emergency department visits annually in the United States and is now the primary cause of overdose deaths, including more than 16,000 in 2010.[1,17]

Other Prescription Drug Abuse

The second most commonly abused class of prescription drugs are stimulants, including drugs traditionally prescribed for attention deficit hyperactivity disorder (ADHD) such as Ritalin and Adderall. In 2011, 670,000 Americans abused prescription stimulants.[3] The average age at which this abuse began was 22, and the problem is increasing on campus. (See the **Special Feature: Are "Study Drugs" Smart—and Safe?**)

Other commonly abused prescription drugs include sedatives, antidepressants, and erectile dysfunction drugs. Again, many prescription drugs, including opioids and stimulants, have a high potential for addiction. And prescription drug abuse—especially when it involves combinations of drugs—can be fatal.

>> **View a PBS Newshour segment on the increasing misuse and abuse of prescription drugs at** http://video.pbs.org/video/2365004668/.

Over-the-Counter (OTC) Drugs

Over-the-counter (OTC) drugs are medications available for purchase without a prescription. OTC drugs include aspirin, allergy pills, and cough or cold medications. There are now more than 700 OTC products available that contain ingredients that were available only by prescription three decades ago—some at greater dosage strength.[18]

OTC drugs pose many of the same challenges as prescription drugs. They are not meant to be taken in higher doses or for longer periods than is indicated on the label. If symptoms do not go away after a few days of using an OTC drug, it is time to see your health-care provider. Some OTC medications can interact with other medicines, herbal supplements, foods, or alcohol. Some OTC drugs are hazardous for people with certain medical conditions, such as asthma. Pregnant women should always check with a doctor before taking any OTC drug.

The U.S. Food and Drug Administration (FDA) cautions against the misuse of several common OTC pain relievers.[19] For example, taking too much acetaminophen (a common pain-relief drug, sold as Tylenol among other brand names) can lead to serious liver damage. If ingested with alcohol—as little as three drinks per day—the risk of liver damage increases. The OTC anti-inflammatory drug ibuprofen also has serious adverse effects if taken to excess or if taken with alcohol. These include diarrhea, nausea, and vomiting, ulcers, internal bleeding, and kidney damage.

Cough and cold formulations can also be dangerous, especially when given to children. The FDA has withdrawn some of these medications for children younger than age 2 and advises that caregivers always consult the child's pediatrician before using OTC remedies.[20]

Marijuana

Although Colorado and Washington states allow its recreational use, **marijuana** is still classified as an illicit drug and is in fact the most commonly used illicit drug in the United States.[3] According to the most recent National Survey on Drug Use and Health, 18.1 million Americans reported using marijuana in the past 30 days, representing about 7% of the population over the age of 12.[3]

Marijuana (the plant *Cannabis sativa*) grows wild and is farmed in many parts of the world. "Pot"—a dry, shredded mix of flowers, stems, seeds, and leaves of the plant—is usually rolled and smoked as a cigarette (a "joint"), or by using a water pipe (a "bong") that passes the smoke through water to cool it. It is also sometimes mixed in food such as brownies, or brewed as a tea.

Short-Term Effects

Over the years, marijuana growers have bred the plant to contain increasingly higher percentages of its psychoactive ingredient, THC (tetrahydrocannabinol). When a person inhales THC in marijuana smoke, it takes just a few minutes to move from the lungs to the bloodstream to the brain. Ingesting marijuana from food is slower. In the brain, THC binds to cannabinoid receptors, initiating a series of cellular reactions that ultimately result in a surge of dopamine that causes users to experience a high. The heart beats faster (in some users, double the normal rate); the bronchi (large air passages in the lungs) become enlarged; and blood vessels in the eyes expand, reddening the whites of the eye. Other manifestations include dry mouth ("cotton mouth"), hunger, and sleepiness.

Some users report that the drug makes them feel relaxed and that time seems to slow, whereas others feel euphoric,

opioids Drugs derived from opium or synthetic drugs that have similar sleep-inducing, pain-reducing effects.

marijuana The most commonly used illegal drug in the United States; derived from the plant *Cannabis sativa.*

Are "Study Drugs" Smart—
—and Safe?

In recent years, there has been an increase in college students' misuse of prescription stimulants, such as Adderall, Ritalin, and Concerta, which are intended for the treatment of attention deficit hyperactivity disorder (ADHD). Evidence from a variety of surveys suggests that between 6% and 34% of college students have used a prescription stimulant (PS) without a valid prescription.[1, 2]

The drugs work by increasing blood flow and levels of neurotransmitters in a region of the brain involved in decision-making and impulse regulation. Users believe that the drugs help keep them alert and focused for extended periods, allowing them to finish academic papers and study longer for exams. But does PS use translate into academic success?

It would seem logical that drugs that improve attention and concentration should also promote learning and academic achievement. But studies have found a correlation between PS use and improvement in rote memory, not complex memory, which is more likely to be required for college exams.[3] Moreover, because the drugs cause students to think more narrowly, they can stifle creativity—thinking outside the box. So students may be better able to process data but less able to make meaningful connections.

In addition, in a variety of types of academic skills, modest improvements with PS use were mainly limited to subjects who had lower levels of ability to begin with, indicating that the drug is more effective at correcting deficits than "enhancing performance."[3] Or to put it another way, smart, creative students don't need to misuse PS and derive little benefit from doing so.

Interestingly, the placebo effect may contribute to students' perceptions of PS use improving their performance. In one study, subjective feelings of

being stimulated were produced solely by *expecting* to receive a PS.[3]

Whereas the academic benefits of PS misuse are small, the academic risks are significant. First, these drugs are controlled substances; thus, their unauthorized use—including use without a prescription—is a violation of most campus drug policies (not to mention a federal crime). Corrective actions may range from requiring participation in drug treatment to suspension or dismissal. Second, PS misuse is cheating. Duke University in North Carolina, for example, prohibits the non-medical use of prescription stimulants for any academic purposes. Such use has been added to the university's formal definition of cheating.[3]

PS misuse also poses significant health risks.[2, 3] Large doses can lead to psychosis, seizures, and an increased or erratic heart rate that can result in heart attack, stroke, and sudden death. Even at

small doses, the drugs almost universally disrupt normal sleep patterns and cause nervousness, headaches, decreased appetite, and fever. Many of the drugs have "a high potential for abuse" and are highly addictive: In addition to craving, withdrawal symptoms can include exhaustion, depression, anxiety, insomnia, and thoughts of suicide.

Cases of suicide among students using prescription stimulants are increasingly in the news. In early 2014, for example, hearings will begin in a medical-malpractice lawsuit against Harvard University, which was filed by the parents of student John Edwards. A sophomore, Edwards committed suicide six months after a clinical nurse specialist at the campus health services center prescribed Adderall following a single consultation. Edwards' parents contend their son never had ADHD.[4]

As a result of such cases, dozens of colleges are tightening the rules under which their health services staff are allowed to prescribe medicine for ADHD. Moreover, many are requiring students to sign contracts in which they promise to visit a mental health professional monthly, to submit to regular blood testing, and to not share or sell the pills.[5]

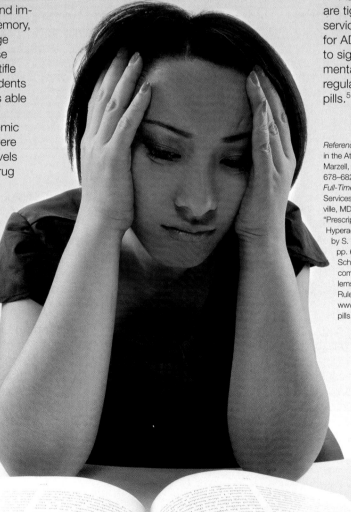

References: **1.** "Judging Cheaters: Is Substance Misuse Viewed Similarly in the Athletic and Academic Domains?" by T. Dodge, K. J. Williams, M. Marzell, & R. Turrisi, 2012, *Psychology of Addictive Behaviors, 26*(3), pp. 678–682. **2.** *The NSDUH Report: Nonmedical Use of Adderall® Among Full-Time College Students,* by the Substance Abuse and Mental Health Services Administration, Office of Applied Studies, April 7, 2009, Rockville, MD. http://www.samhsa.gov/data/2k9/adderall/adderall.htm. **3.** "Prescription Stimulants in Individuals with and Without Attention Deficit Hyperactivity Disorder: Misuse, Cognitive Impact, and Adverse Effects," by S. E. Lakhan & A. Kirchgessner, 2012, *Brain and Behavior, 2*(5), pp. 661–677. **4.** "Harvard Student's Suicide as Case Study," by A. Schwartz, May 3, 2013, *The New York Times,* http://www.nytimes.com/2013/05/01/us/harvard-suit-highlights-adhd-medication-problems.html?src=recg. **5.** "Attention-Deficit Drugs Face New Campus Rules," by A. Schwartz, April 30, 2013, *The New York Times,* http://www.nytimes.com/2013/05/01/us/colleges-tackle-illicit-use-of-adhd-pills.html?ref=us.

Tainted Drugs

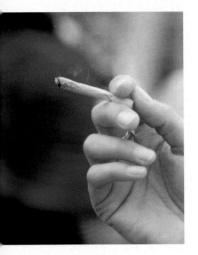

"HI, I'M ANDREA.* One Halloween, me and my friends were at a party and we got a call saying we had to pick up my friend's boyfriend. So we picked him up, and he had marijuana on him, which he offered to us. We smoked it, thinking it's her boyfriend, so it must be okay. Well, it ended up being laced with PCP and it was one of the worst things I've ever gone through. The day after that, when I woke up, I could not stop jittering. My chest felt like it was going to explode. It was a really bad experience and ultimately made me give up marijuana for good."

1. Was there any way Andrea could have known that the marijuana was laced with another drug?

2. If a friend offered you marijuana, how would you respond?

*Name changed at student's request.

Can lead to addiction

Increases risk of chronic cough, bronchitis

Increases risk of schizophrenia in vulnerable individuals

May increase risk of anxiety and depression

Impairs attention, memory, and learning

FIGURE 7.1 Long-Term Effects of Marijuana Use. Smoking marijuana can cause health problems throughout the body.

---

with colors and sounds seeming more intense. Physicians in 18 states can prescribe marijuana for medical use. Patients report that, although it does not relieve pain, it helps them tolerate it.

Other short-term effects are less pleasant. They include impaired coordination; confusion; difficulty thinking, solving problems, learning, and remembering; and reduced reaction time. These effects can last for days or weeks in chronic users.[21] Moreover, because marijuana raises the heart rate, the risk for a heart attack in the hour after its use increases more than fourfold.[21] Finally, THC has a well-documented effect of making users get "the munchies" (feel hungry), and weight gain is not uncommon with frequent use.

Long-Term Effects

Chronic marijuana use can have serious effects on mental and physical health **(Figure 7.1)**. Indeed, opponents of medical marijuana use often cite these adverse effects in explaining their opposition.

A number of studies have shown an association between chronic use and increased rates of anxiety, depression, psychosis, and personality disturbances; however, it is not clear whether marijuana use causes these disorders, exacerbates them, or reflects an attempt to self-medicate symptoms already present.[21] Long-term attention, learning, and memory have all been shown to be impaired in heavy, chronic marijuana users.

Marijuana smoke contains more cancer-causing chemicals than tobacco smoke and is similarly irritating to lung tissues. Thus, people who smoke marijuana can end up with many of the same respiratory problems associated with tobacco smokers, including daily cough and phlegm production and

stimulants A class of drugs that stimulate the central nervous system, causing acceleration of mental and physical processes in the body.

caffeine A widely used stimulant found in coffee, tea, soft drinks, chocolate, and some medicines.

lung infections. Frequent and/or long-term marijuana use may also increase a man's risk of developing the most aggressive type of testicular cancer.[21, 22]

Increasingly, research is finding that marijuana can be a hard habit to kick. Addiction develops in about 9% of all users, but in 25–50% of daily users.[21]

>> **For more information on the health effects of marijuana, visit** www.drugabuse.gov/publications/drugfacts/marijuana.

Stimulants

Stimulants are a class of drugs that stimulate the function of the central nervous system, resulting in increased heart rate, blood pressure, and alertness. Commonly referred to as "uppers," stimulants also elevate mood. Legal stimulants include nicotine, caffeine, and prescription stimulants lawfully used. Illegal stimulants include cocaine, amphetamines, methamphetamine, and "bath salts" as well as prescription stimulants used nonmedically.

Caffeine

Caffeine is a white crystalline powder that, in its pure form, tastes very bitter. However, as a component in coffee, tea, soft drinks, energy drinks, and chocolate, it is the most popular psychoactive drug in the world. **Table 7.2** lists the caffeine content in some common foods and beverages, and it is also found in some prescription and OTC medications, including some headache remedies.

TABLE 7.2 Caffeine Content of Selected Foods and Beverages

Food/Beverage/Pill	Caffeine (milligrams)
Generic brewed coffee, 8 oz.	95–200
NoDoz, maximum strength, 1 tablet	200
Excedrin, extra strength, 2 tablets	130
Rockstar, 8 oz.	79–80
Red Bull, 8.4 oz.	76–80
Restaurant-style espresso, 1 oz.	40–75
Black tea, 8 oz.	14–61
Mountain Dew, 12 oz.	46–55
Coca-Cola Classic, 12 oz.	30–35
Generic decaffeinated brewed coffee, 8 oz.	2–12
Arizona iced tea, lemon flavored, 8 oz.	11
Hershey's kisses, 9 pieces	9

Source: Data from Caffeine Content for Coffee, Tea, Soda and More, by the Mayo Clinic, 2012.

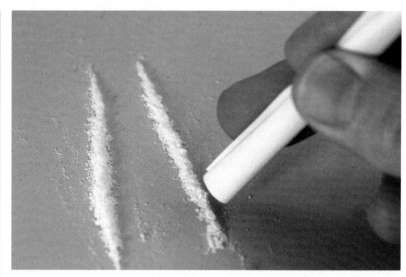

Cocaine use can result in heart damage, stroke, and sudden death.

The effects of caffeine start in less than an hour after consumption. As the drug stimulates the body's central nervous system, users feel more alert and energetic. Heart rate and blood pressure increase, and both concentration and athletic performance can improve. However, although most people can safely drink two to four cups of coffee a day, excessive caffeine consumption can cause restlessness, anxiety, dehydration, and irritability. Caffeine can also trigger headaches and insomnia and lead to abnormal heart rhythms. Pregnant women who drink a cup and a half of coffee a day may double their risk of having a miscarriage.[23]

Caffeine is physically addictive, and regular users can suffer withdrawal symptoms if they suddenly go "cold turkey." Withdrawal usually lasts for 2 to 9 days and may include headaches, anxiety, fatigue, drowsiness, and depression.

Cocaine

Cocaine is derived from South American coca leaves, which people have ingested for thousands of years. "Coke" refers to cocaine in its fine white powder form. It is inhaled (snorted) or dissolved in water and injected intravenously. *Freebase cocaine* is a rocklike crystal that is heated so that its vapors can be smoked (inhaled). It is also known as "crack," which refers to the crackling sound that freebase makes when heated.

Cocaine is a strong central nervous system stimulant that triggers the release of dopamine. Almost immediately, its use causes a rush of euphoria. These effects typically disappear within a few minutes or a few hours. To continue the euphoria, users must continue taking the drug.

Taken in small amounts, cocaine usually makes the user feel energetic and mentally alert. It can also temporarily reduce appetite. Whereas some people find it helps them perform simple physical and mental tasks more quickly, others experience confusion. Paranoia is also common.

Some of cocaine's more common side effects include increased heart rate, blood pressure, and respiration, chest pain, blurred vision, fever, and muscle spasms. Less commonly, cocaine use can cause abnormal heart rhythms, heart damage, strokes, abdominal pain and nausea, seizures, coma, and death.

Continued use of cocaine commonly leads to tolerance. Repeated snorting of cocaine can lead to nosebleeds, a reduced sense of smell, and a chronically runny nose. Injection can trigger allergic reactions and put users at risk for blood-borne diseases such as HIV and hepatitis. Another hazard of the powder is that dealers often dilute it with cornstarch, talcum powder, or sugar, or with other stimulants such as amphetamines.

Mixing cocaine and alcohol is especially dangerous. Taken together, the two drugs are converted by the body into cocaethylene, which is more toxic than either drug alone, and can cause death.

>> **Learn more about cocaine abuse at** www.drugabuse.gov/publications/research-reports/cocaine-abuse-addiction.

Amphetamines

Amphetamines exert their stimulant effects by increasing the concentration of neurotransmitters in different regions of the brain. This increases the user's sense of alertness, decreases appetite and the need for sleep, and enhances physical performance. Amphetamines also induce feelings of well-being and euphoria.

Both the effects and the risks of amphetamines resemble those of cocaine. Even healthy young adults have suffered heart attacks after using them. Addiction is especially common with amphetamines because their effect causes users to take them again and again to avoid the "down" they begin to feel as soon as the drug wears off.

cocaine A potent and addictive stimulant derived from leaves of the coca shrub.

amphetamines Central nervous system stimulants that are chemically similar to the natural stimulants adrenaline and noradrenaline.

Amphetamines are legally classified as Schedule II drugs, meaning that they have a high potential for abuse and addiction, but also have a recognized medical use. They are found in the prescription drugs for ADHD mentioned earlier as well as in drugs used for certain rare sleep disorders and for chronic fatigue syndrome.

Methamphetamine

The highly addictive **methamphetamine** is a chemical similar to amphetamines, but it is much more potent, longer lasting, and more harmful to the central nervous system. Methamphetamine is prescribed medically for ADHD and extreme obesity; however, because of its high potential for abuse, it is legal only by a one-time, nonrefillable prescription. Most methamphetamine that is sold on the street is made by small illegal labs from household materials. It can be ingested, injected, smoked, or snorted. "Crystal meth" refers to methamphetamine in its clear, chunky crystal form.

>> View "before" and "after" images of people who became addicted to methamphetamine at www.facesofmeth.us/main.htm.

Short-Term Effects. Like amphetamines, methamphetamine exerts its effects by causing the brain to flood with neurotransmitters. However, its added "methyl" group allows it to cross into the brain more efficiently and to degrade more slowly. Even small amounts of methamphetamine can cause a rapid or irregular heartbeat, boost blood pressure, and reduce appetite. Other side effects include irritability, anxiety, insomnia, confusion, and tremors. Users quickly develop tolerance, needing more of the drug to get the same high. But increasing the dose can cause convulsions, cardiovascular collapse, and death.

Long-Term Effects. Chronic methamphetamine use may alter areas of the brain associated with emotion and memory, which could account for many of the emotional and cognitive problems that have been observed in abusers.[24] It may also result in aggressiveness, anorexia, hallucinations, and a paranoia that sometimes causes homicidal or suicidal thoughts. Some users hallucinate that bugs are crawling all over them and therefore scratch themselves repeatedly.

Over time, some methamphetamine users begin to develop what is known as "meth mouth"—severely stained teeth that appear to be rotting away or falling out. Methamphetamine can also damage tissues and blood vessels, promote acne, and slow down the healing of sores. Open sores, in fact, are a hallmark of methamphetamine use **(Figure 7.2)**.

Despite such serious side effects, users often find themselves hooked by intense craving for the drug. The addiction is very difficult to treat.

Bath Salts

The term **bath salts** refers to drugs containing one or more chemicals related to the stimulant cathinone.[25] They are typically sold in small packets marketed as bath salts, plant food, or jewelry cleaner. Users ingest, inhale, or inject them.

The stimulant effect of these drugs is said to be as much as 10 times more potent than that of cocaine, but they also induce hallucinations. Together, the combination can produce extreme agitation, panic attacks, paranoia, delirium, suicidal thoughts, and violent behavior. Moreover, heart attack, stroke, seizures, and kidney failure have been reported following use. Criminal assaults and emergency department visits are not uncommon consequences

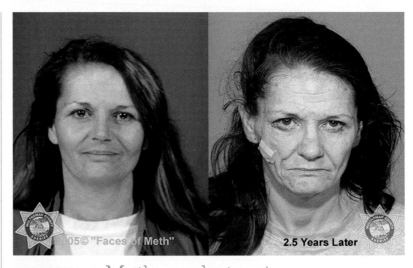

FIGURE 7.2 Methamphetamine.
Methamphetamine use can take a dramatic physical toll.

of use, and numerous deaths have been reported. Moreover, the drugs produce intense cravings and are highly addictive.[25]

Hallucinogens

Hallucinogens are so named because, in addition to altering perceptions, thoughts, and mood, they cause hallucinations. That is, people who use hallucinogenic drugs often report seeing "real" things and hearing "real" sounds that others know do not exist. Some hallucinogens come from plants, like the button-shaped top of the mescal cactus that produces mescaline, and certain types of mushrooms. But other, manufactured hallucinogens can be more potent.

LSD

LSD (lysergic acid diethylamide) is one of the strongest mood-altering chemicals. Commonly known as "acid," it is derived from lysergic acid, which is found in a fungus called *ergot,* which grows on rye and other grains. Its hallucinogenic effects were discovered in 1943 when the scientist who first synthesized it accidentally swallowed some. LSD "trips" were promoted in the 1960s as a means of enhancing creativity or experiencing spiritual insight, and the fad emerged again among teens in the 1990s.

The effects of LSD are unpredictable, varying according to the amount taken, the user's personality, and the surroundings in which the drug is used. First effects are often felt within 30 to 90 minutes as the user moves from one emotion to another or feels several emotions simultaneously. A heavy dose can cause delusions and visual hallucinations. Physical changes include dilated pupils; increased body temperature, heart rate, and blood pressure; sweating; sleeplessness; and tremors.

LSD is not addictive, but some users grow tolerant. Sometimes LSD users have "bad trips" that are extremely disturbing, or experience "flashbacks," meaning they relive parts of a previous LSD experience long after the drug has worn off. Flashbacks may occur a few days or even a few years after actual use.

methamphetamine A highly addictive and dangerous stimulant that is chemically similar to amphetamine, but more potent and harmful.

bath salts Any of a group of drugs containing a synthetic compound similar to cathinone, an amphetamine-like stimulant.

hallucinogens Drugs that alter perception and are capable of causing auditory and visual hallucinations.

LSD (lysergic acid diethylamide) A powerful hallucinogen manufactured from lysergic acid, a substance found in a fungus that grows on rye and other grains.

PCP

The street names for **PCP (phencyclidine)** include "angel dust," "killer weed," "embalming fluid," and "rocket fuel." As these names suggest, the drug can have volatile and even fatal effects. Originally developed in the 1950s as an anesthetic, its medical use was discontinued because of its adverse effects, and, today, street PCP comes from illegal labs. Users typically apply it to a smokable, leafy material such as mint or marijuana. Many people take in PCP unknowingly when someone else adds it to marijuana, LSD, or methamphetamine.

PCP is a **dissociative drug,** meaning it produces feelings of detachment from a person's surroundings. Whereas some users say PCP gives them the perception of strength and invulnerability, others have very bad reactions, including confusion, agitation, and delirium. No one knows why reactions vary so much. Other effects can include shallow breathing, flushing, sweating, numbness of the extremities, and poor muscular coordination.

At high doses, the effects can range from nausea and vomiting to blurred vision, seizures, coma, and death. PCP is known for triggering violent behavior in people, and suicides have been associated with PCP. Some symptoms, such as memory loss, difficulties with speech, and depression, can last for up to a year after taking PCP.

Psilocybin (Magic Mushrooms)

Psilocybin, also known as "magic mushrooms," is a hallucinogen present in certain mushrooms grown in South America, Mexico, and parts of the United States. The mushrooms are often brewed as a tea or eaten with foods that mask their bitter flavor.

Within 20 minutes of ingestion, users begin to notice changes, usually hallucinations and an inability to separate fantasy from reality. Panic attacks can also occur. The effects usually fade away after 6 hours. Psilocybin is not known to be addictive, and there seem to be no withdrawal effects. But serious risks include the onset of psychosis in susceptible users, and poisoning if another, deadlier mushroom (of which there are many) has been confused with the psilocybin mushroom.

"Club Drugs"

The National Institute on Drug Abuse uses the term **club drugs** to refer to methamphetamine, LSD, and several other psychoactive substances that tend to be used at bars, nightclubs, and parties.[26] A few of these are discussed here.

MDMA (Ecstasy)

Methylenedioxymethamphetamine (MDMA), commonly known as ecstasy, is a synthetic drug chemically similar to methamphetamine. It was used by 4.1% of young adults in 2011.[3] Ecstasy comes in tablets, often colorful round pills imprinted with smiley faces, peace signs, or hearts. It is also known as "E," "X," and "XTC."

Typically, an ingested tablet takes about 15 minutes to enter the bloodstream and reach the brain. Its positive effects can include feelings of self-confidence, peacefulness, empathy, and increased energy. About 45 minutes later, the user feels the peak of the high, which can last for 3 to 6 hours.

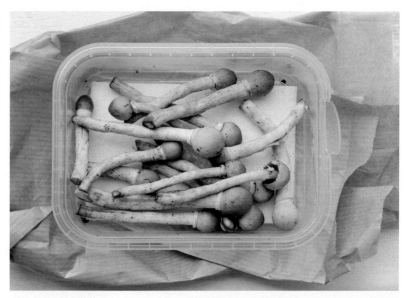

Psilocybin, also called "magic mushrooms," induces hallucinations and can cause psychosis in some users.

>> View a segment about the dangers of Molly, a new formulation of MDMA www.today.com/video/today/52904627#52904627.

PCP (phencyclidine) A dangerous synthetic hallucinogen that reduces and distorts sensory input and can unpredictably cause both euphoria and dysphoria.

dissociative drug A medication that distorts perceptions of sight and sound and produces feelings of detachment from the environment and self.

psilocybin A hallucinogenic substance obtained from certain types of mushrooms that are indigenous to tropical regions of South America.

club drugs Illicit substances, including MDMA (ecstasy), GHB, and many others that are commonly used at nightclubs and parties.

methylenedioxymethamphetamine (MDMA) A synthetic drug, commonly called "ecstasy," that works as both a stimulant and a hallucinogen.

GHB (gamma-hydroxybutyric acid) A central nervous system depressant known as a "date rape drug" because of its use to impair potential victims of sexual assault.

Ecstasy's negative effects are similar to those of stimulants.[27] These include confusion, anxiety, and paranoia. More distinctly physical effects can include nausea, blurred vision, chills, sweating, muscle tension, rapid eye movement, involuntary teeth clenching, faintness, and increases in heart rate and blood pressure. Because the stimulant effects enable users to dance for long periods, some have suffered dehydration and heatstroke. Heatstroke can lead to kidney, liver, or cardiovascular failure, and if left untreated is nearly always fatal.

Regular use can cause depression, anxiety, insomnia, and memory problems that last for up to a few weeks. Studies have shown that some regular users of MDMA have significant memory loss and attention deficits.[27]

"Date Rape Drugs"

Less commonly used club drugs include GHB and Rohypnol, both of which are referred to as "date rape drugs" because perpetrators commonly slip them into drinks in order to make victims drowsy or unconscious. The Drug-Induced Rape Prevention and Punishment Act of 1996 increased the federal penalties for using any controlled substance to aid in a sexual assault.

GHB (gamma-hydroxybutyric acid) is used for its euphoric effects and for the perception of increased libido and sociability. High doses are associated with seizures, respiratory distress, and comas. GHB is addictive, and users who try to kick the habit often experience insomnia, anxiety, tremors, and sweating.

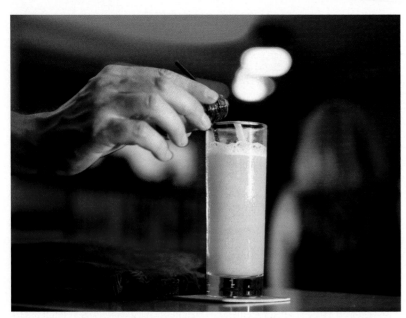

Date rape drugs, such as GHB or Rohypnol, can be slipped into drinks when you're not looking.

Rohypnol is a sedative and can cause drowsiness, visual disturbances, dizziness, and confusion. It can also cause partial amnesia, rendering users unable to remember certain events that they experienced while under the influence of the drug, including sexual assault.

Inhalants

Psychoactive **inhalants** include more than 1,000 common household items, such as paint, glue, and felt-tip markers, which people sniff in order to get high. In 2011, 1.5% of young adults reported abusing an inhalant in the past year.[3]

Types of Inhalants

Common household chemicals are commonly used as inhalants.[28] These include:

- Solvents (liquids in which chemicals are dissolved) such as paint thinners or removers, gasoline, and glue
- Aerosols (a suspension of liquid or solid particles in a gas) such as spray paints, hair spray, vegetable oil sprays, and aerosol computer cleaning products
- Gases such as refrigerant gases, ether, chloroform, or nitrous oxide ("laughing gas")
- Nitrites (chemical compounds that include the element nitrogen), such as room fragrance sprays, leather cleaners, or "liquid aroma" products

Effects of Inhalants

Inhalants typically cause a feeling of intoxication similar to that of alcohol, usually for just a few minutes.[28] By repeated sniffing, users extend the high for several hours. At first, inhalants make people feel slightly stimulated. After repeated inhalations, they can feel less inhibited but also less in control.

Health risks vary by type of inhalant but include permanent hearing loss, bone marrow damage, and brain damage.[28] Butane, propane, and the chemicals in aerosols have all been linked to what is known as "sudden sniffing death"—fatal heart failure within minutes of repeated inhalations. Some young users also cover their heads with a paper or plastic bag to inhale a higher concentration of chemical. This can cause suffocation.

Chronic abuse of solvents specifically can cause severe damage to the liver and kidneys.

Depressants

Depressants (also known as "downers") include alcohol, barbiturates, and benzodiazepines. All are substances that depress the central nervous system and slow the brain's activity. The effect is a drowsy or calm feeling that can reduce feelings of anxiety or pain, and help induce sleep. Misuse of depressants can result in addiction, health problems, and even death.

Barbiturates and Benzodiazepines

Barbiturates are a type of central nervous system depressant typically prescribed to induce sleep and reduce anxiety. Barbiturate sedation can range from mild and short term to severe and long term (inducing coma). The drugs were extremely popular in the early 20th century, but because of their side effects, potential for abuse, and safety concerns, fewer than 10% of current depressant prescriptions in the United States are for barbiturates.

Benzodiazepines are commonly prescribed to induce sleep, relieve anxiety and panic attacks, and help prevent seizures. They were first marketed in the 1960s and, because they're considered safer and less addictive than barbiturates, have become the depressant of choice in many medical practices. More than a dozen benzodiazepines are approved for use in the United States, including lorazepam (Ativan), alprazolam (Xanax), and diazepam (Valium).

Effects

In a small dose, depressants reduce inhibition, induce calmness and muscle relaxation, and impair judgment. An excessive dose can cause slurred speech and loss of motor coordination. Very high doses can lead to respiratory depression, coma, and death. Veterinarians routinely use barbiturates to euthanize animals, and 1 in 10 humans who overdose on barbiturates do not survive.[29]

Depressants are not usually prescribed for long-term use, which can result in memory loss, irritability, amnesia, hostility, and disturbing dreams. Long-term users can develop tolerance and physical dependence, and withdrawal can be dangerous. Because depressants work by slowing the brain's activity, abruptly ending long-term use can cause the brain to race out of control. Insomnia and anxiety—the same symptoms that may have prompted a person to use these drugs in the first place—are common. More severe withdrawal can include fever, delirium, seizures, and cardiovascular collapse. Anyone who is dependent on depressants should seek medical treatment before giving them up. Hospitalization may be required.

rohypnol A powerful sedative known as a "date rape drug" because of its use to impair potential victims of sexual assault.

inhalants Chemical vapors that, when inhaled, produce mind-altering effects.

depressants Substances that depress the activity of the central nervous system and include barbiturates, benzodiazepines, and alcohol.

barbiturates Types of central nervous system depressants often prescribed to induce sleep.

benzodiazepines Medications commonly prescribed to treat anxiety and panic attacks.

Heroin

Earlier we discussed the growing epidemic of prescription opioid abuse. The most abused nonprescription opiate is **heroin,** a fast-acting, highly addictive, illicit drug. Heroin is typically sold as a white or brown powder, or as a sticky black substance known as "black tar heroin." Known on the street as "smack," "H," and "junk," heroin is usually injected directly into a vein, although it can also be smoked. About 280,000 people in the United States report past-month heroin abuse.[3]

Heroin is particularly addictive because it crosses into the brain quickly, producing an intense "rush" of pleasure accompanied by a sensation of heaviness. Withdrawal symptoms may begin within a few hours, and include drug craving, restlessness, muscle and bone pain, diarrhea, and vomiting. Although these symptoms typically subside after about a week, they persist in some people for many months. Nearly a quarter of people who use heroin become dependent.[30]

Table 7.3 provides a summary of commonly abused drugs, their intoxication effects, and the health risks of using them.

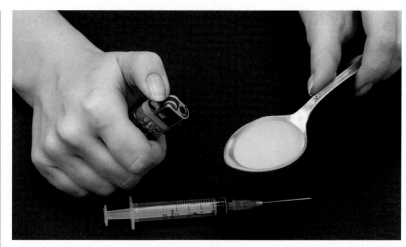

Heroin users can develop collapsed veins, infections, and liver disease.

Prevention Strategies: Do They Work?

The aim of prevention programs is to reduce the factors that contribute to drug abuse while simultaneously promoting protective factors. Parental involvement, for example, is a known protective factor: Communicating the risks of drug abuse to children and teens cuts their risk of engaging in the behavior in half.[31] When valid substance abuse prevention programs are properly implemented, they can be effective.[32]

The following prevention strategies are in use throughout the United States:

- Public awareness campaigns. The federal government has spent millions of dollars on public awareness campaigns meant to discourage drug use. Although the effectiveness of these campaigns is the subject of some debate, the National Institute on Drug Abuse reports that rates of abuse do go down when perceptions of harm go up, and that typically happens with public awareness campaigns. Moreover, two research studies have found that youths who reported exposure to a public awareness campaign on the risks of marijuana were less likely to begin use.[33]

- Drug testing. In an effort to discourage people from using drugs—and to catch those who do—some schools, athletics organizations, the U.S. military, and many workplaces conduct *random drug testing.* The process usually involves taking a urine sample and testing for traces of common drugs.

heroin An illicit, highly addictive opioid.

TABLE 7.3 Commonly Abused Drugs

Category	Representative Drugs	Method of Administration	Intoxication Effects and Health Risks
Cannabis	Marijuana (street names: pot, dope, weed, grass, joint, reefer)	Inhaled or ingested	Effects: Psychoactive agent THC causes a sense of euphoria. Heart rate increases, bronchi enlarge, blood vessels expand.
			Risks: Addiction, impaired cognition, lung damage, increased cancer risk
Stimulants	Cocaine (street names: crack, rock, blow, C, coke, snow)	Inhaled or injected	Effects: Derived from coca leaves, this drug first produces feelings of increased energy and euphoria. Heart rate and blood pressure increase, appetite drops.
			Risks: Addiction, irritability, anxiety, paranoid or violent behavior, damage to heart, brain, and other vital organs
	Amphetamines (street names: speed, uppers, crank)	Inhaled, ingested, injected	Effects: This large, varied group of synthetic drugs improves mood and alertness. Heart rate and blood pressure increase.
			Risks: Addiction, restlessness, appetite suppression, hallucinations, erratic or violent behavior
	Methamphetamines (street names: meth, crystal, ice, glass, tina) *Shown at left*	Inhaled, ingested, injected	Effects: A common form of amphetamine, this highly addictive drug quickly produces a sense of euphoria followed by a dramatic drop in emotion and energy as the drug wears off.
			Risks: Addiction, appetite suppression, dental damage, brain damage, psychosis, paranoia, aggression

(continued)

TABLE 7.3 Commonly Abused Drugs (continued)

Category	Representative Drugs	Method of Administration	Intoxication Effects and Health Risks
Hallucinogens 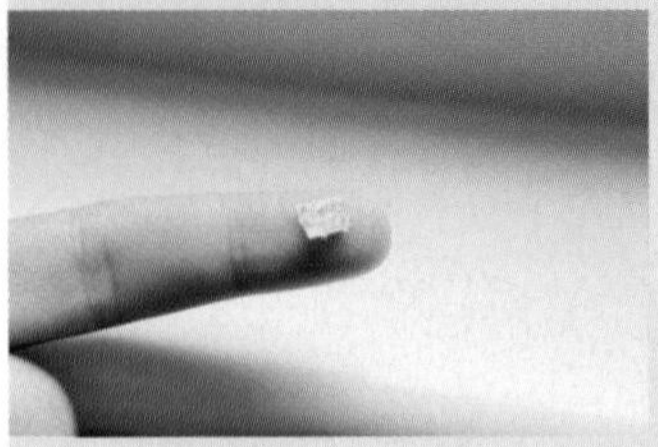	LSD (street names: acid, blotter) *Shown at left*	Ingested	Effects: Effective even at very low doses, this drug is known for producing powerful hallucinations. Other effects include nausea, increased heart rate, tremors, and headaches. Risks: Shortened attention span, miscarriage and pre-term labor in pregnant women, paranoia, disordered thinking
	PCP (street name: angel dust)	Inhaled, ingested, injected	Effects: This synthetic drug can lead to both euphoria and extreme unhappiness and can also produce hallucinations. Risks: Slurred speech, poor coordination, loss of sensitivity to pain, nausea, vomiting, violent behavior, coma, and even death
	Psilocybin (street names: shrooms, magic mushrooms)	Ingested	Effects: This group of mushrooms, if ingested, has effects similar to those of LSD. Effects last for up to 6 hours. Risks: Paranoia, disordered thinking, nausea, erratic behavior
Club Drugs 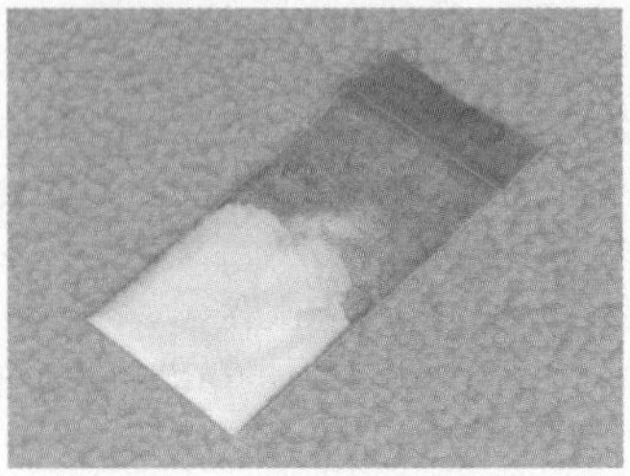	MDMA (street names: ecstasy, E, X, XTC, Molly)	Ingested	Effects: This synthetic drug creates feelings of warmth and friendliness and also increases heart rate and blood pressure. Risks: Hallucinations, brain damage, disordered thinking, disturbed sleep. Extremely dangerous if mixed with alcohol
	GHB (street name: G)	Ingested	Effects: This is a central nervous system depressant that disrupts memory and can lead to unconsciousness. Risks: Temporary amnesia, nausea, vomiting, seizures, memory loss, hallucinations, coma
	Rohypnol (street name: roofies)	Ingested	Effects: This drug is a powerful tranquilizer that slows physical and mental responses and is the best known of the so-called date rape drugs. Risks: Temporary amnesia, slowed physical and mental reactions, semi-consciousness, unconsciousness
Inhalants 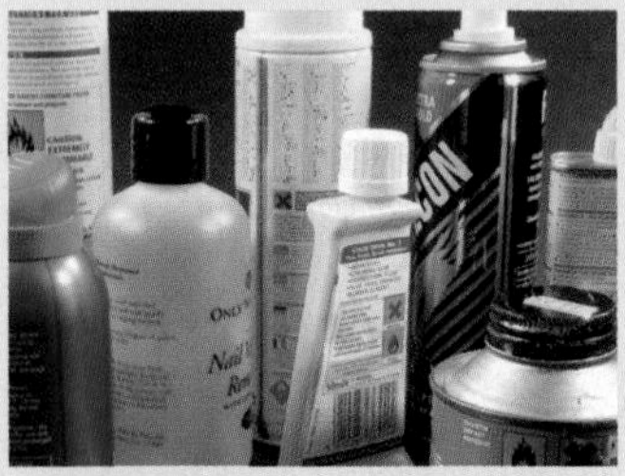	Solvents (e.g., paint thinner), aerosols (e.g., spray paint), gases (e.g., nitrous oxide), nitrites (e.g., leather cleaner)	Inhaled	Effects: Found in ordinary household products, these substances can produce a feeling of being "high" or drunk. Risks: Dizziness, impaired speech, impaired physical coordination, vomiting, hallucinations, loss of consciousness, death
Depressants 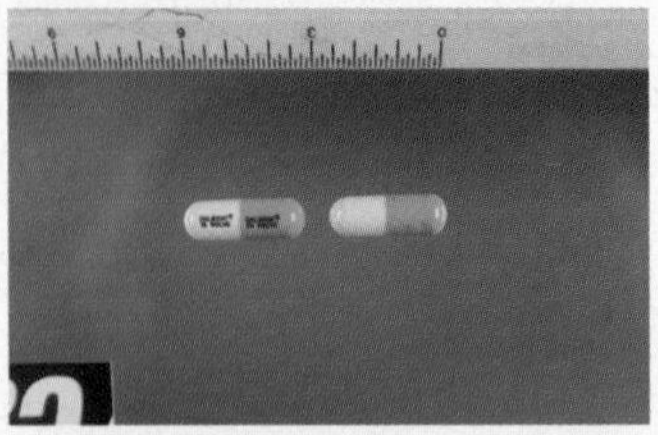	Barbiturates (street names: barbs, downers)	Ingested or injected	Effects: This group of drugs slows the functions of the central nervous system and is legally prescribed for anxiety and insomnia. Risks: Slowed pulse and breathing, slurred speech, impaired memory, addiction, sleep problems, impaired coordination
	Benzodiazepines (street names: downers, benzos) *Shown at left*	Ingested or injected	Effects: This group of depressants functions as tranquilizers and includes common medications such as Valium. Risks: Drowsiness, dizziness, loss of libido, confusion, depression; less addictive than barbiturates
Opioids 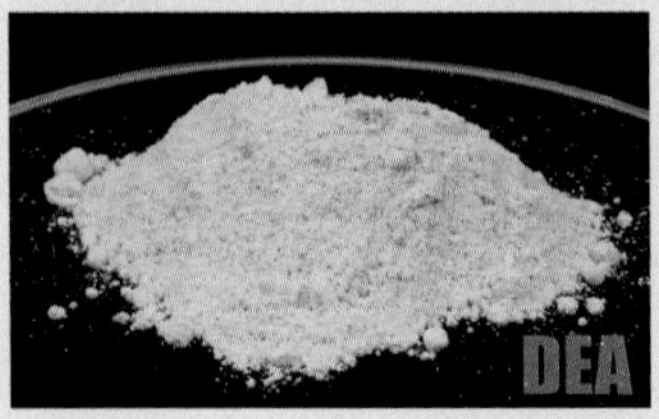	Heroin (street names: smack, H, brown sugar, junk, horse) *Shown at left*	Injected or inhaled	Effects: This opioid produces a feeling of drowsiness, dreaminess, and euphoria and can also lead to dramatic mood swings. Risks: Addiction, cardiovascular damage, respiratory illnesses, internal infections, death
	Prescription opioids (street names: Oxy, Captain Cody)	Ingested	Effects: This group of drugs produces feelings of sleepiness, dreaminess, and a reduced sensitivity to pain. Risks: Addiction, dangerous interactions with other drugs, nausea, vomiting, lack of physical coordination

The Occupational Safety and Health Administration (OSHA) recommends a strategy in which companies that perform random drug testing also offer employees drug education and assistance programs.[34]

- Federal policies. In 2010, the Obama administration announced a new National Drug Control Strategy to reduce drug use. Some of its key initiatives include increased public awareness campaigns, increased monitoring of prescription drugs, including narcotics, increased availability of drug treatment programs, and increased law enforcement.[35]

Getting Help for a Drug Problem

Historically, drug abuse in the United States was seen as more of a moral problem than as a public health problem. The legacy of that stance is that arrest and punishment took precedence over placing drug users into treatment programs. However, courts now often try to strike a balance between punishment and the goal of recovery. And, of course, many people enter drug treatment without ever coming into contact with the legal system. Unfortunately, in 2011, more than 19 million Americans needed treatment for substance abuse but did not receive it. Of those who sought treatment but did not receive it, the number one reason reported was lack of health insurance and inability to afford treatment without it.[3]

Campus and Community-Based Options

So-called **12-step programs,** such as Narcotics Anonymous (NA), are free of charge and help many people struggling with substance abuse. Men and women come together to share their problems with drugs and their strategies for drug-free living as well as to support others. The 12 steps take addicts through a process of self-growth, such as asking them to admit they have no control over their addiction and to make amends to all the people they have harmed. NA members have an average of nine years drug free.[36]

Your campus health services center may offer assistance for students struggling with substance abuse. These services may include drug treatment, weekly support group meetings, substance-free housing, and opportunities to participate in community service projects. These services can be highly effective: Records from one Midwestern college show that, of an average of 60 students per year served in the previous decade, only 8 per year relapsed.[37]

 View personal stories of hope and recovery from drug addiction at www.youtube.com/youarenotalone.

Clinical Options

The long-term goal of clinical drug treatment programs is, of course, to get people off harmful drugs for good. Many outpatient programs are available, but residential treatment is often necessary for persistent and severe addictions. In residential programs, the patient lives at the treatment center and away from old habits and social circles for weeks or months at a time.

Programs typically move through stages, beginning with *detoxification,* a process by which the person is therapeutically supported (with medications and other interventions) while the body clears itself of the drug and its byproducts and undergoes the withdrawal stage. This is followed by treatment, which may also include medications as well as psychotherapy.

Coping with Addiction

 "HI, I'M ANA. I come from a background of alcoholism and addiction in my family. I've also struggled with it myself ever since I was 14. My dad was never around, and when he was around he struggled with addiction. I grew up thinking that was normal, despite what was taught at school. About a year ago, I heard about AA, Alcoholics Anonymous, and NA, Narcotics Anonymous, and I've been with the program for a year. My dad's also with the program and it's been great to have each other for support.

I used to drink a lot—binge drink with my friends—because that's what everybody did. And being around party drugs, designer drugs, was really kinda hard, just seeing everyone else use them, you really fall into the peer pressure of it all.

Now I definitely don't hang out with the same crowd. My friends and I were each others' crutches and pulled each other down. So, not being around those kind of people has really helped me a lot because I'm not around drugs or alcohol anymore, so I don't have the temptation there. I don't have the drugs to turn to.

AA and NA have helped because they're about getting over the fear of being judged and speaking about it. Often times we feel like we're going to be ostracized from society if we admit—or we admit to our parents—that we have a problem with addiction. But it's just really important to speak out about it and ask for help, especially at such a young age before all the other problems develop."

1. What factors put Ana at increased risk for addiction?

2. Ana talks about the fear of being judged for having an addiction. Why else might someone avoid admitting that she or he has an addiction? What types of things might cause someone to finally admit an addiction?

3. Ana mentions other problems that could develop due to addictions. What do you think she means? What types of problems does addiction cause in people's lives?

Medications commonly used for opiate addiction include methadone and buprenorphine, which act on the same receptors as heroin and morphine, suppressing withdrawal symptoms and relieving cravings. All medications help patients disengage from drug seeking and become more receptive to behavioral treatments.[38]

Recovery from addiction is often more complicated for a **polyabuser**—a person who abuses multiple drugs, often including alcohol. Polyabuse is commonly a factor in drug overdose incidents and deaths; in fact, a significant majority of emergency department visits for drug overdose in the United

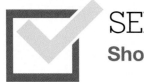

SELF-ASSESSMENT
Should You Seek Drug Treatment?

Answer Yes or No to the following 20 questions.

1. Have you used drugs other than those required for medical reasons?
2. Have you abused prescription drugs?
3. Do you abuse more than one drug at a time?
4. Do you use drugs more than once a week?
5. Have you tried to stop using drugs and were not able to do so?
6. Have you had blackouts or flashbacks as a result of drug use?
7. Do you ever feel bad or guilty about your drug use?
8. Does your spouse or parents ever complain about your involvement with drugs?
9. Has drug abuse created problems between you and your spouse or your parents?
10. Have you lost friends because of your use of drugs?
11. Have you neglected your family because of your use of drugs?
12. Have you been in trouble at work because of your use of drugs?
13. Have you lost a job because of drug abuse?
14. Have you gotten into fights when under the influence of drugs?
15. Have you engaged in illegal activities in order to obtain drugs?
16. Have you been arrested for possession of illegal drugs?
17. Have you ever experienced withdrawal symptoms (felt sick) when you stopped taking drugs?
18. Have you had medical problems as a result of your drug use, such as memory loss, hepatitis, convulsions, bleeding, etc.?
19. Have you gone to anyone for help for a drug problem?
20. Have you been involved in a treatment program especially related to drug use?

HOW TO INTERPRET YOUR SCORE
The more "Yes" answers you gave, the more likely it is that you should seek treatment for your drug use.

To complete this Self-Assessment online, visit MasteringHealth™

Source: DAST-20 Drug Abuse Screening Test, reproduced by permission of Dr. Harvey A. Skinner. © Copyright 1982 by Harvey A. Skinner, PhD and the Centre for Addiction and Mental Health, Toronto, Canada. Reprinted by permission.

States involve polyabuse.[39] The behavior is particularly dangerous because of the collective toxicity of the drugs.

Should you seek drug treatment? Find out by completing the **Self-Assessment** above.

Change Yourself, Change Your World

If you currently abuse drugs—or find yourself strongly tempted to do so—seek help now. If instead you're concerned about peer pressure, academic stress, or other issues pulling you toward drug abuse in the future, then your best strategy may be to think about yourself as your own personal advocate. Just as you surely have been advised to "think before you drink," health experts encourage you to consider all of the ramifications before you light up or shoot up. Do you understand the short- and long-term health risks involved in the use of this drug? Is a temporary high worth the risk of addiction and other health problems, family and relationship conflict, academic problems, financial trouble—maybe even arrest—or death?

Personal Choices

By now you're familiar with the process of behavior change. But overcoming drug abuse can be more challenging than other types of behavior change because of the chemical effects that psychoactive drugs have on your brain. Employing the strategies discussed here can help.

Value Your Values

What are your values? Health, independence, financial security, achievement, caring relationships, honesty, integrity . . .? What about your goals? Do you want to be accepted into medical school, get a job in high tech, or land a role on Broadway? Challenging yourself to identify how your choices about drugs reflect and support—or deny and derail—your values and goals can be an enlightening exercise.

The next step is identifying what specific steps you need to take to live in closer alignment with your values and to achieve your goals.

Make Some Trade-Offs

If you're tempted to abuse drugs, or to continue to abuse them, you may believe that they'll provide a quick fix for whatever might be troubling you. Although it's true that, for a few minutes or hours, you'll escape, what about those short- and long-term consequences? Make a better trade-off. **Endorphins** are your body's own "feel-good" chemicals. When they bind to opiate receptors in the brain, they increase pleasure and decrease pain. There are many healthful ways to prompt your brain to produce this "natural high," including exercise, meditation, creative writing, volunteer work, and spending time with people you love. Many people find that challenging themselves to overcome fears—by performing, for instance, or public speaking, or rock climbing—boosts their endorphins.

Another important trade-off you might have to make is in your circle of friends. Tell them in unambiguous language that you're drug free. True friends will not only accept, but respect your decision. Those who ridicule you about it, or try to talk you out of it, still deserve your care and concern, but not your time. Let them know you have no hard feelings but won't be able to hang out with them anymore. Recognize your vulnerable times—for instance, Friday and Saturday nights—and schedule some drug-free activities in advance to make sure your calendar is filled. That way, you can honestly say, "Sorry, I'm busy," if someone asks you to a party where drugs will be available.

Build a Healthier Lifestyle

If you're in recovery, the experience will go more smoothly if you take care of yourself. Although withdrawal often disturbs sleep patterns, go to bed at a reasonable hour and try to get 7 to 8 hours of sleep. If your mind races, try repeating a positive affirmation or sending loving thoughts to any friends who you know are struggling with abuse and addiction, too.

endorphins Hormones that act as neurotransmitters and bind to opiate receptors, stimulating pleasure and relieving pain.

Don't ignore your diet. Depending on the drug you used, you may have lost significant weight. Yet withdrawal from certain drugs can promote gastrointestinal problems such as diarrhea, vomiting, and nausea, just at a time when you need nutrients, including fluids, to support your recovery. Guidelines from the National Institutes of Health recommend that you:[40]

- Stick to regular mealtimes.
- Eat a diet that is relatively low in fat and has adequate protein and complex carbohydrates (including plenty of vegetables and whole grains).
- Take a multivitamin-mineral supplement.
- Eat nutritious snacks.
- Don't mistake hunger or thirst for a drug craving. If a craving hits, eat a healthy meal or snack, or drink a glass of water, milk, or 100% juice.

Finally, exercise. The endorphins released during vigorous physical activity will help decrease cravings and elevate your mood.

Ask for Help

If you're trying to quit, but a craving hits you in the middle of the night, who is the one person you know you could call on for help? Maybe it's your mom or dad, maybe a close sibling or your best friend . . . or maybe a member of your 12-step program or support group. Whoever it is, tell that person what you're going through and ask him or her to be "on call" for you. And remember, you don't have to "tough it out"—medications and clinical counseling are a phone call away. The Substance Abuse and Mental Health Services Administration's nationwide treatment referral help line is available 24 hours a day at 1-800-662-HELP.

 You can also locate treatment centers in your area by clicking on the map at http://findtreatment.samhsa.gov.

Deal with Relapse

More than half of patients in drug treatment experience relapse.[32] Often, relapse occurs during times of stress. But some people are tempted to abuse again when they are well into their recovery, feeling healthy and strong. At these times, people can begin to feel nostalgic for their "early days" of drug use, when they felt they were in control. They may believe that they can return to this casual level of use, not realizing that the chemical changes prompted by their addiction don't make this possible.[41,42]

Experts stress that "falling off the wagon" does not mean treatment doesn't work or that a user will never be free of the drug. Relapse can, however, be extremely demoralizing. It is better to look at relapse not as a failure, but as practice. As with every challenge in life, you may need to try several times before finally getting something right.

intervention A technique used by family and friends of an addict to encourage the addict to seek help for a drug problem.

Helping a Friend

As drug dependence progresses, it commonly changes brain functioning significantly enough that users do not realize they have a problem or that it is interfering with their lives. In such cases, friends and family may stage what is called an **intervention,** an organized attempt to encourage a loved one to get professional help. Interventions usually involve direct, face-to-face demonstrations of love, support, and encouragement to enter treatment. Before you consider an intervention, meet with a substance abuse counselor for guidance and for information about available treatment options.

 An excellent resource for helping a loved one with a drug addiction is **The Partnership at** www.drugfree.org.

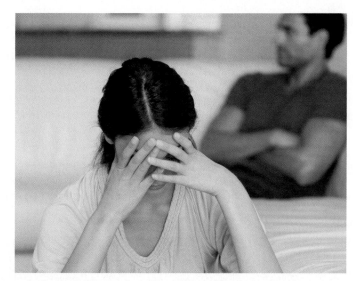

Don't be afraid to talk to someone if you're suffering with addiction.

Campus Advocacy

How can you promote a campus environment where drug abuse and addiction are recognized as serious health problems? Here are some ways to get involved:

- Recognize that, every time you say no to drugs, you're challenging the idea that drug use is normal. Still, it's hard to "just say no," especially if you value fitting in. So be ready with "a line"; for instance: "No thanks, I've got a paper due tomorrow." Or, "I'm working on a health challenge right now, and that would only make it worse." Or try humor: "Sorry, but I need to preserve all the brain cells I have!"
- Spread the word. Although information alone usually isn't enough to stop drug abuse, when combined with other prevention and treatment efforts, it does make a difference, especially when the information comes from peers. For instance, let's say you know that a friend is abusing a prescription drug but mistakenly thinks that, because it was prescribed for a family member, it's safe and legal. Take the opportunity to ask some questions: *Do you know about the health risks of using this drug? Do you know that what you're doing is illegal?* Let your friend know you're concerned and offer to help.
- Get your message out online. Use your social networking sites to raise awareness, and send short articles about the consequences of student drug abuse to your school's online newspaper.
- Visit the office of your dean of students or your student government association and lobby for chem-free housing and campus-sponsored activities. Join drug-free organizations on campus, and attend their activities. If a club you belong to doesn't have a drug-abuse policy, suggest that the members establish one.
- Volunteer to become a peer mentor. Many colleges have peer mentoring associations (PMAs) whose volunteers help their peers overcome substance abuse and other challenges.

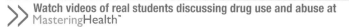 Watch videos of real students discussing drug use and abuse at MasteringHealth™

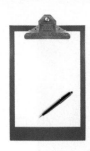

Choosing to Change Worksheet

To complete this worksheet online, visit MasteringHealth™

Although you may not realize it, you might routinely use one or more psychoactive drugs. If you drink caffeinated beverages like coffee, tea, cola, or energy drinks, or drink alcohol or smoke cigarettes, or take pain relievers, sleeping pills, or allergy medicine, you are using a psychoactive drug. Monitor your drug use for a week.

Part I. Keep a Drug Diary
List the drugs you consumed daily over the course of a week. Did you drink coffee? List the number of cups. How about energy drinks or caffeinated sodas? Tea? Did you smoke cigarettes? How many? Drink alcohol? Did you take prescription medications? Over-the-counter medications? Also make note of your stress level and mood at the time you used the drug.

Example:

Day	Substance	Amount	Drug	What Did it Do for You?	Stress Level 1 = low stress 2 = moderate stress 3 = high stress	Mood (angry, happy, depressed, bored, frustrated, etc.)
1	Coffee	3 cups	Caffeine	Helped me wake up	3	Frustrated

Your Turn:

Day	Substance	Amount	Drug	What Did it Do for You?	Stress Level 1 = low stress 2 = moderate stress 3 = high stress	Mood (angry, happy, depressed, bored, frustrated, etc.)
1						
2						
3						
4						
5						
6						
7						

Review and Reflect on Your Drug Diary

1. Were you surprised about anything from your drug diary? _____ If yes, what surprised you?

_____

2. Did you notice any patterns in your use of drugs? _____ If yes, what patterns were apparent?

_____

3. Are you using any drugs as a coping mechanism to deal with your stress levels or moods? _____ If yes, which drugs?

_____

4. Looking at your drug diary, are there any substances you would like to reduce or eliminate?

_____

Part II: Reducing or Eliminating Drug Use
Directions: Fill out your stage of change in Step 1 and complete the remaining steps depending on which one applies to your stage of change.

Step 1: *Your Stage of Behavior Change.* Please check one of the statements on the next page that best describes your readiness when it comes to reducing or eliminating the drug listed in question 4, above.

_____I do not intend to eliminate or reduce use of this drug in the next six months. (Precontemplation)

_____I might eliminate or reduce the use of this drug in the next six months. (Contemplation)

_____I am prepared to eliminate or reduce the use of this drug in the next month. (Preparation)

_____I eliminated or reduced use of this drug less than six months ago. (Action)

_____I have eliminated or reduced use of this drug for more than six months and want to maintain it. (Maintenance)

Step 2: *Precontemplation, Contemplation, and Preparation Stages.* Write down a healthier behavior you could replace your drug use with. If you are in the Preparation stage, create a SMART goal for your behavior change.

_____

_____

_____

Tell someone what you plan to do. Being accountable to others motivates you and also offers you the support and encouragement of others. Who did you tell?

_____

Step 3: *Action and Maintenance Stages.* Track your progress. For 3 days after you start reducing or eliminating your drug use, keep track of the results. Evaluate your progress and explain whether or not you intend to modify your plan.

_____

_____

_____

If you still have trouble cutting back on your drug use, see a health professional for help. Reread pages 167–168 of the chapter for information on where to find professional help. List the professional resources that will help you achieve your goal:

_____

_____

Step 4: *I Don't Use Drugs But Am Concerned About Someone Who Does.* Ask yourself the following questions about your friend or loved one's drug use.

1. Are you concerned with the amount of drugs your friend or loved one uses?   Yes   No

2. Does trying to talk about your friend or loved one's drug or alcohol use cause a fight?   Yes   No

3. Do you worry about how much money and time your friend or loved one devotes to alcohol or drugs?   Yes   No

4. Do you make excuses or lie to cover up your friend or loved one's behavior when he or she using?   Yes   No

5. Has he or she ever hurt or embarrassed you because he or she was drunk or high?   Yes   No

6. Does his or her behavior when he or she is drinking or using ever scare you or make you nervous?   Yes   No

7. Have you ever thought of calling the police on your friend or loved one while he or she is drunk or high?   Yes   No

8. Does his or her using make you feel stressed out?   Yes   No

9. Are you forced to take on his or her responsibilities because he or she is drunk, high, or hung over?   Yes   No

Source: Adapted from *Concerned About Someone?* by the National Council on Alcoholism and Drug Dependence, Inc. (NCADD). Available at http://www.ncadd.org/index.php/for-youth/concerned-about-someone. Reprinted with permission from NCADD. www.ncadd.org.

If you answered "Yes" to any of the nine questions, you may want to talk to your friend or loved one right away. Also, reread pages 167–168 for information on professional resources that may help and reread the information on page 169 about how to help a friend with addiction.

Chapter Summary

- *Addiction* is a chronic disease of brain reward, motivation, memory, and related circuitry. One of its most fundamental characteristics is craving.

- Two recognized behavioral addictions are pathological gambling and hypersexual disorder. Some psychologists recognize other behavioral addictions, such as compulsive spending and addiction to technology.

- As a group, college students greatly overestimate how many of their peers are using illicit drugs. Self-reported marijuana use is below 16%.

- *Drug misuse* is the inappropriate use of a legal drug. *Drug abuse* is the use of any drug that results in harm to your health.

- Chemicals called neurotransmitters—including dopamine and others—facilitate the transport of messages throughout the nervous system. Psychoactive drugs typically trigger a surge of these chemicals, resulting in a sense of euphoria.

- The body develops tolerance to many illicit drugs, so progressively larger amounts are needed to achieve an effect. Psychological dependence is a mental attachment to a drug. Physical dependence occurs when the body requires the regular use of a drug in order to function. Withdrawal from a drug provokes a variety of challenging symptoms, from nausea and vomiting to insomnia and panic attacks.

- Commonly abused drugs include prescription and over-the-counter medications, marijuana, stimulants (e.g., caffeine, cocaine, amphetamines, and methamphetamine), hallucinogens (e.g., LSD, PCP, and psilocybin), "club drugs" (e.g., MDMA, GHB, and Rohypnol), inhalants, depressants (e.g., barbiturates and benzodiazepines), and opioids, including certain prescription pain relievers and heroin.

- Prevention efforts, including public awareness campaigns, can be effective, especially when combined with treatment.

- Most people who need drug treatment do not receive it. Community-based programs such as Narcotics Anonymous can help. A growing number of colleges are offering on-campus support services and "communities" for students attempting to overcome substance abuse.

- Clinical drug treatment includes walk-in clinics and on-site residential programs, both of which may offer medications and counseling.

- In attempting behavior change for drug abuse or addiction, you may need to commit to several trade-offs—in the way you attempt to manage your mood, the people you hang out with, and the activities you engage in. It also helps to practice good sleep habits, eat a nourishing diet, get exercise, and talk to a friend.

- An intervention is an organized attempt by an individual, family, or other group to encourage a loved one to get professional help.

GET CONNECTED

>> Visit the following websites for further information about the topics in this chapter:

- The Science of Addiction
  www.drugabuse.gov/publications/science-addiction
- Drugs of Abuse Information
  www.drugabuse.gov/drugs-abuse
- Narcotics Anonymous
  www.na.org
- National Center on Addiction and Substance Abuse at Columbia University
  www.casacolumbia.org

MOBILE TIPS!

Scan this QR code with your mobile device to access additional tips about avoiding drug misuse or abuse. Or, via your mobile device, go to **http://chmobile.pearsoncmg.com** and navigate to Chapter 7.

Website links are subject to change. To access updated web links, please visit MasteringHealth™

TEST YOUR KNOWLEDGE

1. One of the most fundamental characteristics of addiction is
   a. recognition that the behavior is causing significant harm.
   b. intense craving.
   c. sleep disturbances.
   d. euphoria.

2. Which of the following is a behavioral addiction?
   a. gambling
   b. hypersexual disorder
   c. addiction to video games
   d. addiction to texting

3. The rate of drug abuse among full-time college students is
   a. significantly higher than the rate among college-age adults in general.
   b. significantly lower than the rate among college-age adults in general.
   c. about the same as the rate among college-age adults in general.
   d. somewhat higher than most college students believe it is.

4. A person who must use more of a drug to experience an effect that a smaller dose used to produce has developed
   a. tolerance.
   b. psychological dependence.
   c. hypersensitivity to the drug.
   d. signs of withdrawal.

5. Which of the following is responsible for the greatest percentage of overdose deaths?
   a. heroin
   b. cocaine
   c. methamphetamine
   d. prescription narcotics

6. Adderall is grouped within the same class of drugs as
   a. methamphetamine.
   b. barbiturates.
   c. LSD.
   d. Oxycontin.

7. Impaired memory is a potential adverse effect of use of
   a. marijuana.
   b. methamphetamine.
   c. MDMA.
   d. all of these drugs.

8. The Occupational Safety and Health Administration recommends which of the following drug-abuse prevention strategies?
   a. mandatory random drug testing for all American workers
   b. termination of employees who test positive for drug abuse
   c. federal tax incentives for companies that perform regular random drug testing
   d. employee drug education and assistance programs for companies that perform random drug testing

9. Which of the following statements about drug treatment options is true?
   a. Membership fees for participation in Narcotics Anonymous are usually covered by health insurance providers.
   b. The most common reason people give for not entering treatment for drug abuse is lack of health insurance coverage and an inability to pay out-of-pocket.
   c. Community support groups and outpatient therapy are usually effective treatment options even for people with persistent and severe addictions.
   d. All are true.

10. The return to drug abuse after a period of conscious drug abstinence is called
    a. persistence.
    b. remediation.
    c. relapse.
    d. codependency.

Get Critical

What happened

On November 8, 2011, the parents of aspiring medical student Richard Fee found their son's body in his apartment in Norfolk, Virginia. He had committed suicide. Fee had been severely addicted to Adderall, a potent amphetamine commonly prescribed for attention deficit hyperactivity disorder (ADHD).

Fee had never shown any signs of ADHD from kindergarten through high school. But then, as an undergraduate, he'd started taking Adderall to help him finish papers and cram for exams. No one knows who supplied it. After graduation, while studying for his medical school entrance exams, he visited a psychiatric clinic. There, he filled out a short questionnaire and got a prescription for an amphetamine similar to Adderall.

Fee failed to get into medical school, moved back home, and consulted a local psychiatrist who prescribed a fast-acting form of Adderall. He began exhibiting insomnia and paranoia, then became violent. After an arrest for assault, he consulted a new psychiatrist, who prescribed more Adderall. Fee became suicidal and was hospitalized in the summer of 2011. After his release, his psychiatrist refused another prescription. Two weeks after Fee took his last dose of Adderall, he hanged himself.

After Fee's death, a close friend recalled, "He had it in his mind that because it came from a doctor, it was okay."[1]

What do you think?

- Fee's parents repeatedly begged their son's psychiatrists to stop the prescriptions for Adderall. Were Fee's physicians in any way responsible for their patient's death?

- Richard Fee received a prescription for amphetamines, a controlled substance, after filling out a short questionnaire. A recent study found that ADHD assessment tools are incapable of distinguishing between patients with ADHD and people who are faking. If no reliable ADHD diagnostic tool exists, should psychiatrists be allowed to prescribe a treatment with a high potential for addiction?

- Selling or giving away even one Adderall pill is a federal crime. So is buying or accepting. Do you see this behavior among your peers? Do you participate? If so, are you concerned about the health and legal risks? Why or why not?

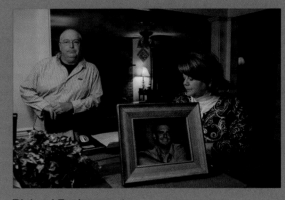

Richard Fee's parents.

Reference: 1. "Drowned in a Stream of Prescriptions," by A. Schwartz, February 2, 2013, *The New York Times.*

ALCOHOL AND TOBACCO USE AND ABUSE

Alcohol is a factor in about **60%** of fatal burn **injuries**, drownings, and homicides; **50%** of severe trauma injuries and sexual assaults; and **40%** of fatal motor vehicle **crashes**, suicides, and fatal falls.[i]

Over 24% of U.S. college students have never had a **drink** at all.[ii]

1 out of every **5 deaths** in the United States is caused by a **smoking-related** illness.[iii]

Secondhand smoke, laden with **toxic chemicals**, is responsible for **almost 50,000** smoking-related **deaths** each year.[iii]

8

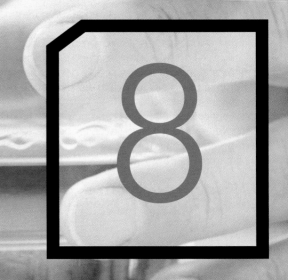

Learning Objectives

DISCUSS the prevalence of alcohol use in the United States.

IDENTIFY the components of alcohol.

DESCRIBE how the body absorbs and metabolizes alcohol.

DESCRIBE the short-term and long-term health effects of alcohol use.

EXPLAIN how alcohol affects behavior.

RECOGNIZE the types and signs of alcohol abuse.

OUTLINE strategies for preventing alcohol abuse and for treating alcoholism.

DISCUSS the prevalence of tobacco use in the United States.

IDENTIFY the components of tobacco and cigarettes.

IDENTIFY the short-term and long-term health effects of tobacco use.

IDENTIFY a range of tobacco products.

OUTLINE strategies for quitting smoking.

UNDERSTAND how to promote a smoke-free environment on campus.

There will be many times in college when you are exposed to two of the most popular drugs

in the United States: alcohol and tobacco. Both are easily accessible on college campuses, and students often feel pressure to try them. Although experimenting with these drugs may seem like a harmless rite of passage, their use can carry serious consequences. Just one drunken night can result in a fatal vehicle accident or make you vulnerable to sexual assault. Alcohol and tobacco are also both highly addictive. Many alcoholics trace the roots of their alcoholism to their college years, and smoking is notoriously hard to quit. The long-term health consequences of heavy drinking and smoking can be devastating and include diseases like cirrhosis (scarring of the liver), cancer, and heart disease.

Students tend to underestimate how easy it is to develop a drinking or smoking problem and how difficult it is to overcome one. By setting limits—or by abstaining from alcohol and tobacco altogether—you can reduce the likelihood that these addictive drugs might one day control you.

Alcohol Use in the United States

According to national surveys, slightly more than half the adults in the United States drink alcohol—about 133.4 million people.[1] Among men, about 57% report being current drinkers compared to 47% of women. However, among those aged 12 to 17, the percentages of male and female drinkers are very similar (both about 13–14%). Among Caucasian adults of either sex, about 57% drink alcohol—a higher percentage than reported by any other racial or ethnic group.[1] See the **Diversity & Health** box on page 176 for a more detailed snapshot of drinking in the United States.

The 1984 Federal Uniform Drinking Age Act (FUDAA) financially penalizes any state that fails to prohibit the purchase or public possession of any alcoholic beverage by a person under 21. Because all states ultimately complied, the act effectively raised the national minimum legal drinking age to 21. Research shows that the FUDAA has had positive effects on health and safety, primarily in decreasing traffic crashes and fatalities, suicide, and decreased consumption by those under age 21.[2, 3, 4, 5]

Alcohol Use and Binge Drinking on Campus

An estimated 76% of college students nationwide have tried alcohol, and 39% report **binge drinking**.[1,6] Binge drinking, or *heavy episodic drinking*, is defined by the National Institute on Alcohol Abuse and Alcoholism as a pattern of drinking alcohol that results in a blood alcohol concentration (BAC) of 0.08% or above (we will discuss BAC in more detail shortly).[7] For a typical adult,

> **binge drinking** A pattern of drinking alcohol that results in a blood alcohol concentration of 0.08 or above (about five or more alcoholic drinks within 2 hours for men, or four or more alcoholic drinks within 2 hours for women).

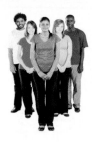

Alcohol Use Through the Lenses of Sex, Race/Ethnicity, Age, Education, and Geography

Although alcohol use and abuse cuts across all demographic groups, some groups show heavier patterns of drinking than others. A recent national survey conducted by the Substance Abuse and Mental Health Services Administration revealed the following patterns.

Overall

- Among people aged 12 or older, 51.8% reported being current drinkers: about 133.4 million people.
- Among people aged 12 or older, 6.2% reported heavy drinking (having five or more drinks on one occasion, on at least 5 days over the course of the previous month).

Sex

- Of males aged 12 or older, 56.8% reported being current drinkers, compared to 47.1% of females in the same age group.

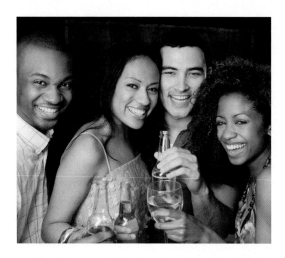

- Among those aged 12 to 17, there was no difference between male and female drinkers: 13.3% of males in this age group were current drinkers compared to 13.3% of females.

Race/Ethnicity

- Among Caucasians, 56.8% report being current drinkers, the highest rate of any racial/ethnic group.
- Among mixed-race individuals, 46.9% report being current drinkers.
- Among Native Americans, 44.7% report being current drinkers.
- Among Hispanics, 42.5% report being current drinkers.
- Among African Americans, 42.1% report being current drinkers.
- Among Asian Americans, 40% report being current drinkers.
- Rates of binge drinking (defined in this survey as having five or more drinks on at least one occasion over the previous month) were highest among Native Americans (24.3%), Caucasians (23.9%), Hispanics (23.4%), African Americans (19.4%), those of mixed race (18.6%), and Asian Americans (11.6%).

Age

- Among individuals aged 21–25, 69.7% reported being current drinkers, the highest rate of any age group.

Education

- Among individuals aged 26 and older, the rates of binge drinking or heavy drinking were lower

among college graduates than among those who had attended some college but not yet obtained a degree. For binge drinking, 21.8% of college graduates reported engaging in that behavior, compared to 26.7% of non-college graduates. For heavy drinking, 5.4% of college graduates reported doing so, compared to 7.9% of non-college graduates.

Geography

- The rates of alcohol use are lower in the South (46.7%) than in the Northeast (57.1%), Midwest (53.9%), or the West (50.7%).

Critical-Thinking Questions

1. These figures on drinking include people as young as 12 years old. What, if any, drinking did you notice among your peers in high school? How is it different from what you are experiencing in college?

2. What are some of the possible reasons behind varying rates of alcohol use in different parts of the country?

3. Why do you think drinking rates are the same for both sexes as teens, but diverge as people get older?

Data from *Results from the 2011 National Survey on Drug Use and Health: National Findings,* from the Substance Abuse and Mental Health Services Administration website, 2012.

this corresponds to consuming five or more drinks (for men), or four or more drinks (for women), in about 2 hours. Note that some organizations define binge drinking even more narrowly, that is, as equivalent to consuming four or more drinks (for men) and three or more drinks (for women) within 2 hours.

The incidence of binge drinking is highest among young adults aged 18 to 24, whether they are in college, the military, or the workforce. In fact, the highest prevalence of alcohol dependence occurs in this age group.[7] Studies indicate that 12th graders heading to college are consistently less likely than their non–college-bound counterparts to report

binge drinking.[8] However, once at college, these same students report more binge drinking than their peers who entered the workforce.

Binge drinking is arguably the most significant health risk behavior among college students today. If you consider the consequences—and just how widespread binge drinking is—it is easy to see why. Alcohol is a factor in about 60% of fatal burn injuries, drownings, and homicides; 50% of severe trauma injuries and sexual assaults; and 40% of fatal motor vehicle crashes, suicides, and fatal falls.[9] Additionally, binge drinking can lead to drunk driving, violence, vandalism, risky sex, forced sex, and poor academic performance.[10] Binge drinkers not only place themselves in harm's way, but also raise risks for those around them. Those who live with or near heavy drinkers are exposed to more property damage, fights, and noise disturbances than those who do not.[11] Non-drinking students also report experiencing verbal abuse, drunk driving, and harassment of minority and international students at the hands of peers who have had too much to drink.[12] Of even more concern is the fact that each year, more than 696,000 students between the ages of 18 and 24 are assaulted by another student who has been drinking, and more than 97,000 students between the ages of 18 and 24 are victims of alcohol-related sexual assault or date rape.[13]

Although college students of all types may binge drink, it is most common in athletes, sports fans, fraternity and sorority members, and extremely social students. Women and minorities, and religious, married, and older students tend to drink less.[14] The **Student Stats** feature provides a snapshot of overall drinking patterns on campus, based on a recent nationwide survey of college students.

>> Listen to a Centers for Disease Control podcast on the dangers of binge drinking at www2c.cdc.gov/podcasts/player.asp?f=11157.

Why Students Drink

Students cite many different reasons for reaching for a drink. Researchers have classified the motivations into four different categories: coping (to avoid problems), conformity (to gain peer acceptance), enhancement (to induce a positive mood), and social (to make parties and outings more enjoyable).[15]

Peer pressure is often a major factor. When students are frequently offered alcoholic beverages at parties or goaded into consuming multiple drinks at a time by their friends, they may come to think that heavy drinking is normal behavior. Aware of the impact of social norms on students' drinking behaviors, alcohol abuse prevention experts try to counter student perceptions of their peers' drinking behaviors with the fact that the overwhelming majority of students drink responsibly. In fact, in a recent national survey, 13.6% of U.S. college students who had tried alcohol reported that they had not had a single alcoholic beverage within the past 30 days, and 24.4% of college students in this survey reported that they had never tried alcohol at all.[6]

Parents are also a major influence on the drinking patterns of college students. Parents who allow their children to drink alcohol in high school are not protecting their children from abusing alcohol when they leave the home for college. On the contrary, students whose parents allowed alcohol consumption in high school were significantly more at risk for alcohol misuse and its consequences in college.[16] Meanwhile, parental disapproval of drinking in high school does seem to have a protective effect against alcohol misuse in college.[16]

>> Is your drinking pattern risky? Assess yourself at http://rethinkingdrinking.niaaa.nih.gov/IsYourDrinkingPatternRisky/WhatsYourPattern.asp.

The Makeup of Alcohol

Alcohol is a chemical substance that is toxic to the body. The key ingredient in every can of beer, glass of wine, and shot of tequila is **ethyl alcohol,** or **ethanol**. This intoxicating substance

ethyl alcohol (ethanol) The intoxicating ingredient in beer, wine, and distilled liquor.

proof value A measurement of alcoholic strength, corresponding to twice the alcohol percentage (13% alcohol equals 26 proof).

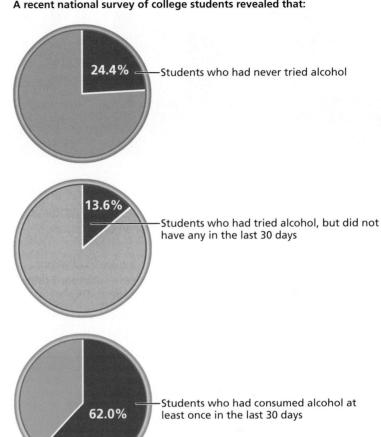

is produced through a process called *fermentation,* in which natural sugars are converted into alcohol and carbon dioxide with the help of yeast. To produce beer and wine, manufacturers add other ingredients, such as water, that dilute the drinks. To create hard liquor, they put the ethyl alcohol through another process, known as *distillation.* Distillation involves heating and then cooling the fermented liquid so that it ends up with a higher alcoholic concentration than before. These stronger beverages are often referred to by their **proof value,** a measure of their ethyl alcohol content. A proof is double the actual alcohol percentage—for example, 100-proof bourbon contains 50% alcohol by volume. Many red wines have an alcohol percentage of around 13%, or a proof value of 26.

>> For more information on what constitutes a "standard drink," visit http://pubs.niaaa.nih.gov/publications/Practitioner/pocketguide/pocket_guide2.htm.

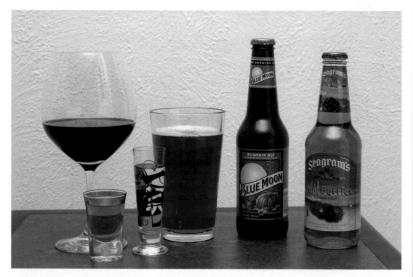

FIGURE 8.1 "Standard" Serving Sizes.
A 5-ounce glass of wine, a 1.5-ounce shot of liquor, and a 12-ounce can of beer are all "standard" servings containing about the same amount of alcohol: 14 grams (½ ounce).

Because different beverages have such varying levels of alcohol, a "standard" serving size also varies by drink type. A **standard drink** contains about 14 grams (or ½ ounce) of pure alcohol. That is the equivalent of a 12-ounce can of beer, or 8 to 9 ounces of malt liquor. A 5-ounce glass of table wine is considered standard, as is 1.5 ounces of 80-proof liquor—roughly one shot glass **(Figure 8.1)**. Although these amounts may seem intuitive enough, researchers at the University of California at Berkeley found that when people were asked to serve themselves a standard drink at home, they poured considerably more alcohol than they should have.[17]

How the Body Absorbs and Metabolizes Alcohol

When you consume an alcoholic beverage, the alcohol passes from your stomach and small intestine into your bloodstream, a process known as **absorption.** The alcohol then travels to your liver, where it is broken down by enzymes in a process known as **metabolism (Figure 8.2)**. (A small amount of alcohol is metabolized in the stomach as well, but 80% of alcohol metabolism takes place in the liver.) One enzyme in particular, *alcohol dehydrogenase*

standard drink A drink containing about 14 grams pure alcohol (one 12-oz. can of beer, one 5-oz. glass of wine, or 1.5 oz. of 80-proof liquor).

absorption The process by which alcohol passes from the stomach or small intestine into the bloodstream.

metabolism The breakdown of food and beverages in the body to transform them into energy.

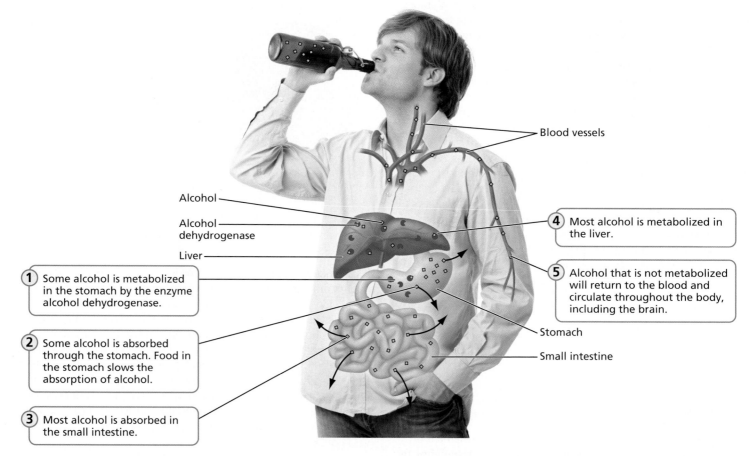

1 Some alcohol is metabolized in the stomach by the enzyme alcohol dehydrogenase.

2 Some alcohol is absorbed through the stomach. Food in the stomach slows the absorption of alcohol.

3 Most alcohol is absorbed in the small intestine.

4 Most alcohol is metabolized in the liver.

5 Alcohol that is not metabolized will return to the blood and circulate throughout the body, including the brain.

Blood vessels
Alcohol
Alcohol dehydrogenase
Liver
Stomach
Small intestine

FIGURE 8.2 Alcohol Absorption and Metabolism. Alcohol is absorbed into the bloodstream through the stomach and small intestine. Metabolism takes place in the stomach and in the liver.

Source: Adapted from Blake, Joan Salge. *Nutrition and You.* 2nd ed., ©2012. Reprinted and electronically reproduced by permission of Pearson Education, Inc., Upper Saddle River, New Jersey.

(ADH), converts alcohol into a byproduct called *acetaldehyde.* The acetaldehyde is then quickly transformed into acetate by other enzymes and is eventually metabolized to carbon dioxide and water. Some alcohol, however, is not metabolized by the body, and is excreted in urine, sweat, and breath. It can be detected in breath and urine tests that gauge blood alcohol levels.

The liver can metabolize only a small amount of alcohol at a time, roughly one standard drink per hour, although metabolism varies among individuals. Alcohol that is not immediately metabolized by the liver continues to circulate in the bloodstream to other parts of the body, including the brain. If a person consumes alcohol at a faster rate than the liver can break it down, the person will become intoxicated.

Blood Alcohol Concentration

The amount of alcohol contained in a person's blood is known as **blood alcohol concentration (BAC)**. BAC is measured in grams of alcohol per deciliter of blood and is usually expressed in percentage terms. Having a BAC of 0.08% means that a person has 8 parts alcohol per 10,000 parts blood in the body. Also referred to as *blood alcohol level,* BAC can be affected by several factors, including:

- **How much and how quickly you drink.** Binge drinking causes a large amount of alcohol to enter your body in a very short period. Because your body cannot process alcohol at a fast pace, this results in a higher BAC.

- **What you drink.** All drinks are not created equal. The water in beer and wine acts as a buffer for alcohol so that people feel the effects of these beverages a little less than if they had downed a straight shot of hard liquor. Champagne, on the other hand, contains carbon dioxide, which increases the rate of alcohol absorption and causes a more rapid intoxication. Mixers can also make a big difference. Water and fruit juices mixed with alcohol may slow the absorption and intoxication process, whereas soda and other carbonated beverages speed it up. The temperature of the alcohol also affects absorption with a hot toddy moving into the bloodstream more quickly than a frosty margarita.

- **Your sex.** Women are more vulnerable to alcohol than men and will have a higher BAC after drinking the same amount of alcohol. This occurs for several reasons. First, women typically are smaller and consequently have less blood volume than men. They also have a higher percentage of body fat. Because alcohol is not easily stored in fat, it will enter the bloodstream more quickly in women. Men have significantly more muscle and consequently have a higher percentage of water in their bodies. The added water helps dilute the alcohol men consume. Women absorb about 30% more alcohol into the bloodstream than men do. This is primarily because women produce less alcohol dehydrogenase, the enzyme responsible for the breakdown of alcohol in the stomach. **Figure 8.3** shows how BAC levels differ between men and women of similar weights.

- **Your age.** Research indicates that as people age, they become more sensitive to alcohol's effects.[18] The same amount of alcohol can have a greater effect on an older person than on a younger one.

- **Your weight.** The less you weigh, the less blood and water you have in your body to dilute alcohol. As a result, a lighter person will have a higher BAC than a heavier person who drinks the same amount.

- **Your physical condition.** People who are fatigued or stressed out tend to be more affected by moderate amounts of alcohol.

- **Your food intake.** Eating a meal before drinking, especially one high in protein and fat, helps slow the absorption of alcohol into the bloodstream. Conversely, drinking on an empty stomach speeds absorption. BAC rises more rapidly when you have not eaten because there is no food in your stomach in which to dilute the alcohol.

- **Medications.** Aspirin and other medications, including many sold over the counter, prevent the enzyme ADH from breaking down alcohol. This causes alcohol to accumulate in the blood faster (resulting in a higher BAC) and have longer lasting effects. Women on birth control pills process alcohol more slowly than other women, and remain drunk longer.

>> **Use this calculator to estimate your blood alcohol concentration:** www.ou.edu/oupd/bac.htm.

blood alcohol concentration (BAC)
The amount of alcohol present in blood, measured in grams of alcohol per deciliter of blood.

For Women

Drinks per hour	Body weight in pounds					
	100	120	140	160	180	200
1	0.05	0.04	0.03	0.03	0.03	0.02
2	0.09	0.08	0.07	0.06	0.05	0.05
3	0.14	0.11	0.10	0.09	0.08	0.07
4	0.18	0.15	0.13	0.11	0.10	0.09
5	0.23	0.19	0.16	0.14	0.13	0.11
6	0.27	0.23	0.19	0.17	0.15	0.14
7	0.32	0.27	0.23	0.20	0.18	0.16
8	0.36	0.30	0.26	0.23	0.20	0.18
9	0.41	0.34	0.29	0.26	0.23	0.20
10	0.45	0.38	0.32	0.28	0.25	0.23

For Men

Drinks per hour	Body weight in pounds					
	100	120	140	160	180	200
1	0.04	0.03	0.03	0.02	0.02	0.02
2	0.08	0.06	0.05	0.05	0.04	0.04
3	0.11	0.09	0.08	0.07	0.06	0.06
4	0.15	0.12	0.11	0.09	0.08	0.08
5	0.19	0.16	0.13	0.12	0.11	0.09
6	0.23	0.19	0.16	0.14	0.13	0.11
7	0.26	0.22	0.19	0.16	0.15	0.13
8	0.30	0.25	0.21	0.19	0.17	0.15
9	0.34	0.28	0.24	0.21	0.19	0.17
10	0.38	0.31	0.27	0.23	0.21	0.19

FIGURE 8.3 Blood Alcohol Concentration (BAC) Tables. The orange areas indicate legal intoxication.

Source: Adapted from "Alcohol Impairment Charts," by Pennsylvania Liquor Control Board's Bureau of Alcohol Education, published by the Pennsylvania Liquor Control Board, with data gathered from The National Clearinghouse for Alcohol and Drug Information, Substance Abuse, and Mental Health Services Administration. Adapted with permission.

Intoxication

In the most basic sense, **alcohol intoxication** is just another term for being drunk. In a legal sense, it means having a BAC of 0.08% or greater. Intoxication levels vary, but generally a person weighing 150 pounds can expect the following symptoms:[19]

- At a BAC of 0.03% (after about one drink), you feel relaxed and slightly exhilarated.
- At a BAC of 0.06% (after two drinks), you feel warm and relaxed as well as experience decreased fine-motor skills.
- At a BAC of 0.09% (after three drinks), you notice a slowed reaction time, poor muscle control, slurred speech, and wobbly legs.
- At a BAC of 0.12% (after four drinks), you have clouded judgment, a loss of self-restraint, and an impaired ability to reason and make logical decisions.
- At a BAC of 0.15% (after five drinks), you have blurred vision, unclear speech, an unsteady gait, and impaired coordination.
- At a BAC of 0.18% (after six drinks), you find it difficult to stay awake.
- At a BAC of 0.30% (after 10 to 12 drinks), you are in a stupor or deep sleep.
- At a BAC of 0.50%, you are in a deep coma and in danger of death.

The Effects of Alcohol on the Body

Excess alcohol consumption negatively affects the health of the drinker on many different levels **(Figure 8.4)**. Not only do heavy drinkers put themselves at a higher risk of accidental injury and violence, they also increase their risks of developing lasting neurological problems and serious diseases, such as cancer, heart disease, and liver disease.

Immediate Effects of Alcohol on the Body

Within moments of ingestion, alcohol begins to cause changes in the body. As mentioned, as BAC increases, the drinker will experience symptoms such as lightheadedness, relaxation, loss of inhibition, compromised motor coordination, slowed reaction times, slurred speech, dulled senses (i.e., less acute vision, hearing, smelling, and taste), and clouded judgment. Other short-term effects of alcohol use include:

- **Dehydration.** Alcohol is a diuretic, triggering more frequent urination. This can lead to dehydration and an electrolyte imbalance. Symptoms of mild to moderate dehydration include thirst, weakness, dryness of mucous membranes, dizziness, and lightheadedness.
- **Gastrointestinal problems.** Alcohol irritates the stomach and intestines, causing inflammation and indigestion. This is especially true when a person drinks a beverage with an alcohol concentration greater than 15%.[20]
- **Sleep disturbances.** Although alcohol has sedative effects that can make people feel sleepy, it actually tends to *disrupt* sleep and throw off the biological rhythms of the body. As a result, alcohol-induced sleep is often shorter in duration and poorer in quality. In addition, alcohol relaxes the throat muscles, facilitating snoring.
- **Alterations in the metabolic state of the liver and other organs.** These changes result in low blood sugar levels.

The effect many drinkers fear most, however, is a **hangover,** which begins within several hours after drinking has stopped and can last for up to 24 hours. A hangover is the constellation of unpleasant physical and mental symptoms that accompany a bout of heavy drinking. They include fatigue, headache, increased sensitivity to light and sound, redness of the eyes, dry mouth, muscle aches, thirst, vomiting, diarrhea, dizziness, vertigo, depression, and irritability.

Researchers believe that key contributors to hangovers are compounds found in alcoholic beverages known as *congeners*.[21] Congeners contribute to the taste, smell, and appearance of alcoholic drinks, but the body metabolizes them very slowly, and they are more toxic than ethanol. Research has shown that beverages containing a large number of congeners, such as whiskey,

alcohol intoxication The state of physical and/or mental impairment brought on by excessive alcohol consumption (in legal terms, a BAC of 0.08% or greater).

hangover Alcohol withdrawal symptoms, including headache and nausea, caused by an earlier bout of heavy drinking.

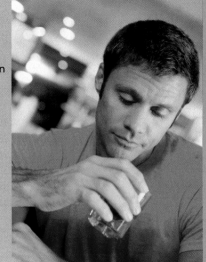

Short-term effects:
- Lightheadedness
- Relaxation
- Loss of inhibition
- Compromised motor coordination
- Slowed reaction times
- Slurred speech
- Dulled senses (i.e., less acute vision, hearing, smelling, taste)
- Clouded judgment
- Dehydration
- Digestive problems
- Sleep disturbance
- Low blood sugar levels due to alterations in metabolism
- Hangover
- Memory loss
- Alcohol poisoning
- Drug-drug interactions

Long-term effects:
- Increased risk of cancer
- Increased risk of cardiovascular disease
- Increased risk of liver disease (fatty liver disease, hepatitis, cirrhosis)
- Neurological problems
- Tolerance and addiction
- Fetal alcohol syndrome in infants (if alcohol is consumed during pregnancy)

FIGURE 8.4 Short- and Long-Term Health Effects of Alcohol Use.

brandy, and red wine, cause greater hangover effects than beverages composed of more pure ethanol, such as gin and vodka.[22]

Alcohol Poisoning

Every year, dozens of students from universities and colleges across the country die from **alcohol poisoning** as a result of a dangerously high level of alcohol consumption and the toxic byproducts that result when alcohol is metabolized by the body. When the body absorbs too much alcohol, it can depress the central nervous system, slowing breathing, heart rate, and the gag reflex that is needed to prevent choking. Inebriated students can lose consciousness, choke on their own vomit, and die from asphyxiation. In addition, victims can experience *hypothermia* (low body temperature) and *hypoglycemia* (too little blood sugar), which can lead to seizures. Vomiting can also cause seizures, resulting in permanent brain damage.

Signs of alcohol poisoning include mental confusion, vomiting, seizures, slow or irregular breathing, low body temperature, and skin that is pale or bluish in color. If a

alcohol poisoning Dangerously high level of alcohol consumption, resulting in depression of the central nervous system, slowed breathing and heart rate, and compromised gag reflex.

person cannot be roused, that is another indication that emergency medical care is needed.

Alcohol poisoning should be taken as seriously as any other kind of poisoning. Giving a grossly intoxicated person a cup of coffee or a cold shower will not help. Neither will having him or her sleep or "walk it off." A person's blood alcohol concentration can continue to rise even while

> " *A person's blood alcohol concentration can continue to rise even while he or she is passed out. It is dangerous to assume the person will be fine if left alone to sleep.*"

MYTH OR FACT?

Can Coffee Cure a Hangover?

A hangover is the body's reaction to being poisoned with too much alcohol. Excessive drinking traumatizes the central nervous system, resulting in headaches, dizziness, nausea, dehydration, and even a weakened immune system.

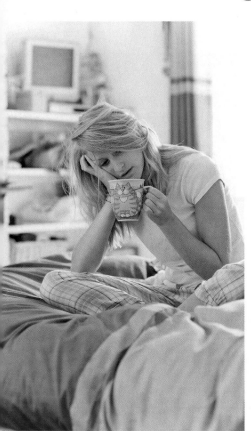

Alcohol is a diuretic and consequently increases urination, which leads to dehydration. Coffee is not an effective hangover cure because the caffeine in it causes even more dehydration—and could actually make your hangover worse! The morning after, stick to water for rehydration. Sports drinks might also be a good choice because they will both counter dehydration and replace lost electrolytes.

While we're at it, let's look at other supposed hangover "cures":

- Can a Bloody Mary (vodka and spiced tomato juice) cure a hangover? No. Drinking additional alcohol the morning after may *postpone* the symptoms of a hangover but cannot prevent them.

- Will eating before you go to bed help alleviate your hangover symptoms the next day? No. In order for food to have any impact, it needs to be in your stomach *while* you are drinking, when it can slow the absorption of alcohol and reduce your level of intoxication.

- What about taking over-the-counter painkillers before going to bed? No. These painkillers peak in about 4 hours,

so unfortunately, the effect of a bedtime dose will be gone by morning. Also, note that taking acetaminophen (e.g., Tylenol) immediately after drinking can be downright dangerous. Alcohol disrupts how the liver processes acetaminophen, which can lead to liver inflammation and permanent damage.

What's the only surefire way to avoid a hangover? Don't drink to excess in the first place.

he or she is passed out. It is dangerous to assume the person will be fine if left alone to sleep. If you encounter someone who you suspect may have alcohol poisoning, call 911 immediately if the person:

- Is unconscious and you can't rouse him or her even by shaking.
- Has consumed other drugs.
- Is experiencing seizures.
- Is injured.
- Has a respiration rate of fewer than 8 breaths per minute.
- Is experiencing shallow or irregular breathing (10 seconds or more between breaths).

Long-Term Effects of Alcohol on the Body

It is difficult to find a part of the body that alcohol does not damage if it is abused for long periods. Chronic, heavy use of alcohol has been linked to cancer, heart disease, liver problems, neurological ailments, and stomach disorders.

Cancer

Study after study has linked cancer and excessive alcohol use.[23] Cancers of the liver, breast, esophagus, mouth, larynx, and throat have all been associated with chronic drinking patterns.[23] Among women assessed in one important study, breast cancer was responsible for the majority of alcohol-related cancer deaths, whereas among men, cancers of the esophagus and upper airway were especially notable.[23] Drinkers who consumed more than 20 grams of alcohol (about 1.5 drinks) per day made up more than one-quarter of all alcohol-related cancer deaths.[23]

Certain populations may be more at risk for certain alcohol-related cancers. Scientists have known that approximately 36% of East Asians (Japanese, Chinese, and Koreans) experience a facial flushing response to alcohol.[24] This flush occurs because of an inherited deficiency in an enzyme that helps metabolize alcohol, aldehyde dehydrogenase 2 (ALDH2). There is accumulating evidence that ALDH2-deficient people are at much higher risk of esophageal cancer from alcohol consumption than those with fully active ALDH2.

Cardiovascular Disease

Although there is some evidence that *moderate* alcohol use may lower the risk of some types of heart disease (see **Spotlight: Can Alcohol Have Health Benefits?**), excessive chronic alcohol use can raise the blood levels of triglycerides, a type of fat. It can also lead to high blood pressure, heart failure, and, in some chronic drinkers, stroke. Excessive use of alcohol can also have a direct toxic effect on the heart muscle cells, causing *cardiomyopathy.* Cardiomyopathy is a serious disease in which the heart muscle becomes inflamed and weakened. As a result, it cannot pump blood efficiently. The lack of blood flow affects all parts of the body, resulting in damage to multiple tissues and organ systems.

Liver Disease

Alcohol can cause three kinds of liver disease:

- **Fatty liver.** A buildup of fat cells in the liver that can cause abdominal discomfort.
- **Alcoholic hepatitis.** Also called inflammation of the liver. About a third of heavy drinkers will develop alcoholic hepatitis, which causes progressive liver damage and is marked by nausea, vomiting, fever, and jaundice.
- **Alcoholic cirrhosis.** The most serious type of alcohol-related liver disease. An estimated 48.2% of the 31,500 deaths from cirrhosis each year are alcohol-related, according to a national study.[25] With cirrhosis, normal liver tissue is replaced with scar tissue, causing life-threatening damage.

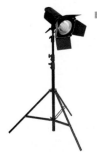

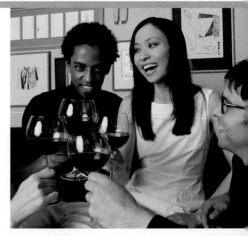

SPOTLIGHT

Can Alcohol Have Health Benefits?

Can a drink a day actually help keep you healthier? Although some studies have said yes, the science is far from conclusive.

There is some evidence that people who regularly consume *small* amounts of alcohol may have a decreased risk of coronary heart disease, high blood pressure, and stroke compared with people who do not drink at all.[1] Other studies have shown that moderate drinkers (defined as people who regularly have 1–2 drinks per day) have the lowest mortality rate, whereas heavy drinkers have the highest, and teetotalers (those who don't drink) and light drinkers have rates that fall somewhere in the middle.[2]

However, another analysis looked broadly at studies supporting the health benefits of alcohol in heart disease and found fundamental problems with almost all of them, raising questions about how accurate the health claims for alcohol might truly be.[3] Women should also be aware that alcohol use, even moderate use, has been linked to an increased risk of breast cancer.[4] Among young people in particular, alcohol use is associated with *increased* risk of premature death from accidents or injuries. College students should not take up drinking or drink more frequently with the goal of improving their health.

References: **1.** "Association of Alcohol Consumption with Selected Cardiovascular Disease Outcomes: A Systematic Review and Meta-Analysis," by P. Ronksley, S. Brien, B. Turner, K. Mukamal, & W. Ghali, 2011, *British Medical Journal, 342,* p. d671. doi: 10.1136/bmj.d671. **2.** "The Health Benefits of Moderate Drinking Revisited: Alcohol Use and Self-Reported Health Status" by M. T. French & S. K. Zavala, 2007, *American Journal of Health Promotion, 21*(6), pp. 484–491. **3.** "Health Benefits of Moderate Alcohol Consumption: How Good Is the Science?" by T. Stockwell, A. Greer, K. Fillmore, T. Chikritzhs, & K. Zeisser, 2012, *British Medical Journal, 2012,* p. 344, e2276. **4.** "Moderate Alcohol Intake and Cancer Incidence in Women" by N. E. Allen, V. Beral, D. Casabonne, S. W. Kan, G. K. Reeves, A. Brown, & J. J. Green, 2009, *Journal of the National Cancer Institute, 101*(5), pp. 296–305.

Neurological Effects

Alcohol can cause severe and possibly lasting brain damage in people under age 21, according to the American Medical Association. The brain grows and changes during adolescence and into the college years and alcohol can negatively affect two brain areas involved in learning and behavior. Moderate drinking impairs learning and memory far more in youth than adults with adolescents only needing to drink half as much to suffer the same negative brain effects.[26]

Alcohol and Pregnancy

A pregnant woman is not only "eating for two," she is also "drinking for two." The ingestion of high levels of alcohol during the first trimester of a pregnancy can cause a miscarriage. Alcohol that is ingested at other points in the pregnancy can lead to health problems and even brain damage in the fetus. Scientists coined the term **fetal alcohol syndrome** more than three decades ago to describe a pattern of birth defects that appeared in the children of mothers who drank while pregnant. The telltale signs of the condition include facial abnormalities, retarded growth, and permanent intellectual and behavioral problems.

Today, drinking while pregnant is recognized as the leading cause of birth defects, developmental disabilities, and mental retardation. The prevalence of fetal alcohol syndrome is estimated to be between 0.5 and 2 for every 1,000 births, and approximately 40,000 newborns are affected by an alcohol-related disorder each year.[27] Despite the known risks, an estimated 9.4% of pregnant women reported consuming alcohol while pregnant in a recent national survey.[28]

The highest risk is to babies whose mothers are heavy drinkers, but scientists are unsure whether there is any safe level of alcohol use during pregnancy. In 2005, the U.S. Surgeon General issued an advisory to pregnant women urging them to abstain from alcohol altogether. Stating that it is "in the child's best interest for a pregnant woman to simply not drink alcohol," Dr. Richard Carmona said studies also indicate babies can be affected by alcohol just after conception, before a woman even knows she is pregnant. For that reason, the federal government has begun recommending that women who may possibly be pregnant avoid alcohol.

The Effects of Alcohol on Behavior

Alcohol does not just have physical effects on the body—it is also associated with poor decision making and risky behavior. Among the most serious risks associated with alcohol use are drunk driving and alcohol-related sexual activity.

Drinking and Driving

In 2011, 9,878 people died in alcohol-related car crashes in the United States—about 27 deaths every day on our roadways, or about 1 every 53 minutes. Weekends were about twice as deadly in terms of drinking and driving—about 31% of drivers in fatal crashes on weekends were alcohol-impaired, compared to about 15% on weekdays.[29]

College students are disproportionately affected by drunk driving. One study found that more than 1,825 students aged 18 to 24 died from alcohol-related car crashes and unintentional injuries in a single year.[13] More than one-fourth of college students in the United States have driven under the influence of alcohol.[13]

> **fetal alcohol syndrome** A pattern of mental and physical birth defects found in some children of mothers who drank excessively during pregnancy.

Negative Effects from Drinking

"HI, I'M COURTNEY. Out of my friends, most of us drink. There have been a lot of negative effects from drinking. This year alone, one of my sorority sisters fell and broke her hand. Another one has fallen and chipped a tooth. A lot of us spend way too much money when we go out. There's lots of negative effects.

A lot of people drink because it loosens them up to be able to socially interact. But I would tell someone who doesn't want to drink to definitely join organizations on campus. There are a lot of things that you can do to meet other people that have nothing to do with drinking."

1. Courtney lists injuries and financial impacts as negative effects from drinking. What other negative effects can you think of?

2. What factors make Courtney vulnerable to high-risk drinking?

How does alcohol affect driving skills? The following are only some of the common impairments:

- **Judgment.** Alcohol reduces reason and caution, so you're more likely to take risks, from speeding to failing to stop at a light that's changing to red. Research has shown that as few as one or two drinks can impair mental and motor skills necessary for safe driving.[19]

- **Vision and hearing.** Alcohol reduces the acuity of hearing and vision, including depth perception, which helps you relate the position of your vehicle to others on the road.

- **Reaction time.** Impairments in focusing your attention, understanding your situation, and coordinating your response all contribute to significantly slowed reaction time.

Having a BAC of 0.08% or greater will qualify you for a DWI arrest in all 50 states if you are 21 years of age or older. Under zero-tolerance laws, it is illegal to have any alcohol in your system if you are underage and driving a vehicle. In practice, many states have a cutoff of 0.02% to allow for consumption of minute amounts of alcohol—for instance in cough syrups or wine sipped in religious services. Still, teenagers who are caught operating a motor vehicle after having even half a drink could be charged in civil or criminal courts with a DWI or similar charge and, if convicted, could have their license suspended—in some states for one year or until they reach age 21, whichever is longer.

>> The Mothers Against Drunk Driving (MADD) website includes statistics on drunk driving, victim services, and opportunities to help eliminate drunk driving: www.madd.org. To see personal stories about the devastating harm caused by drunk driving, go to MADD's collection of videos at www.youtube.com/watch?v=LrG-jHdupw0.

Practical Strategies

Accidents or injuries resulting from alcohol-related behavior are all too common on college campuses. The following guidelines can help keep you safe.

- **Don't drink to get drunk.** Alcohol-related risks increase dramatically with intoxication, so if you drink, drink moderately. Eat before you start consuming any alcohol, and keep eating while you drink. During the evening, take breaks between drinks by alternating alcoholic beverages with non-alcoholic ones. Avoid drinking games that can cause you to drink alcohol more quickly than your body can handle.

- **Pair-up with a friend.** If you are drinking away from home, don't do it alone. Always pair-up with a friend and make a pact to stick together.

- **Make arrangements for getting home safely.** If you are heading to a drinking event, arrange for a sober driver or contact a cab company ahead of time. Most colleges have "safe ride" systems that provide safe late night transportation services from popular night spots.

- **Don't accept drinks from strangers.** While at a party, club, or bar, don't give anyone the opportunity to slip drugs like Rohypnol or GHB into your drink. Never put your drink down. If your drink is out of sight, even for a few minutes, don't finish it. Get yourself a new one. Don't accept an open drink from anyone. If you order a drink in a bar, make sure you watch the bartender open the bottle or mix your drink.

- **Know the signs of alcohol poisoning.** Be prepared so that you can help a friend if the situation arises. If the person is unconscious, cannot be roused, has consumed other drugs, is experiencing seizures, is injured, and/or is exhibiting shallow or irregular breathing, call 911 immediately. Remember that other signs of alcohol poisoning include mental confusion, vomiting, low body temperature, and skin that is pale or bluish in color.

Although penalties vary by state, a first conviction for DWI may result in jail time, a fine ranging from several hundred to several thousand dollars, and/or community service. The offender's driver's license will be suspended for a period, and he or she will be required to enroll in an alcohol rehabilitation program. In some states, a DWI conviction—even if a first offense—may remain on the person's criminal record for life. A second offense may involve mandatory prison time and a much higher fine. In addition, in at least 22 states, repeat offenders must have their cars outfitted with an ignition-interlock system, which detects alcohol use and prevents people from starting their vehicle if they have been drinking.[30]

Alcohol and Sexual Activity

Engaging in sexual intercourse while inebriated can be just as dangerous as riding in a speeding car after the driver has had a few too many drinks. In one study, 21.3% of college students reported participating in unplanned sexual activities after having too much to drink.[31] Drinking may also make it less likely that partners use protection while having sex under the influence, possibly exposing themselves to sexually transmitted diseases, such as AIDS or hepatitis B, as well as unplanned pregnancy.

For women, the risks can be even greater. Heavy drinking increases the odds that a woman will become a victim of violence or rape. One survey of college students between the ages of 18 and 24 years old found that in a single year, about 97,000 were victims of alcohol-related sexual assault or date rape.[13]

Alcohol and Other Problems

Students who engage in heavy drinking also increase their risks of other problems. One of the most common consequences of high-risk drinking among college students is difficulty keeping up with academic responsibilities. In one survey, 25% of college students said they had missed class, fallen behind, flunked exams, or received lower grades as a result of their drinking.[32] Alcohol use is also closely associated with depression and can increase the risk that a depressed person will attempt suicide. Alcohol intoxication increases suicide risk up to 90 times, as compared with abstinence.[33]

A common refrain on vintage T-shirts states, "I don't have a drinking problem. I drink, I get drunk. I fall down. No problem!" Health experts, however, are not laughing. One study found that in a single year, more than one million college students were injured or assaulted in drinking-related incidents.[13]

Alcohol Abuse

Excessive drinking is a pervasive problem in American society. In the United States, 17.6 million adults meet the criteria for either alcohol abuse or alcohol dependence.[34] **Alcohol abuse** refers to drinking that gets in the way of work, school, or home life and causes interpersonal, social, or legal problems. **Alcoholism**, technically known as **alcohol dependence**, is problem drinking taken a step further—alcoholics do not just enjoy drinks, they crave them and experience withdrawal symptoms whenever they stop drinking.

Alcoholism

Alcoholism is defined as exhibiting at least three of the following symptoms during a one-year period:

- **Tolerance.** Needing to drink more and more alcohol to get drunk.

- **Withdrawal symptoms.** Having a physical dependence on alcohol to the extent that nausea, sweating, shakiness, tremors, seizures, and anxiety are experienced after stopping drinking.

- **Loss of control.** Drinking more or longer than intended.

- **Desire or an inability to quit.** Having a persistent

alcohol abuse Drinking alcohol to excess, either regularly or on individual occasions, resulting in disruption of work, school, or home life and causing interpersonal, social, or legal problems.

alcoholism (alcohol dependence) A physical dependence on alcohol to the extent that stopping drinking brings on withdrawal symptoms.

desire to cut down on drinking or attempting unsuccessfully to do so.

- **Overwhelming time commitment.** Spending an excessive amount of time buying alcohol, drinking it, and recovering from its effects.
- **Interference with life.** Experiencing a reduction in social, recreational, or work activities due to alcohol use.
- **Continued use.** Drinking despite the knowledge that it is causing physical or psychological problems.

Risk Factors for Alcoholism

Genetic, physiological, psychological, and social factors all play a role in determining a person's susceptibility to alcoholism. To what extent each factor influences a person's susceptibility depends on the individual. The risk of alcoholism is higher for people who have a parent who abused alcohol, for instance, but not all children of alcoholics become alcoholics themselves. Other factors that increase a person's risk for abusing alcohol include low self-esteem, impulsiveness, a need for approval, peer pressure, poverty, and being a victim of physical or sexual abuse. Individuals who are under a great deal of chronic stress are also vulnerable. They may turn to alcohol to cope with their problems and try to make themselves feel better, a potentially destructive behavior that is called **self-medicating**.

The age at which a person begins drinking can also raise his or her risk for alcohol abuse. People who begin drinking as teenagers are more likely to develop problems with alcohol. Gender is another risk factor; statistics show that men are much more likely to become dependent on alcohol than women are.[1]

No matter what the cause, once people begin abusing alcohol, the problem often perpetuates itself. Heavy drinking can deplete or increase the levels of some chemicals in the body, causing it to crave or need alcohol to feel good again. Some people keep drinking simply to avoid the uncomfortable withdrawal symptoms.

Common Profiles of Alcoholics

Alcoholism knows no demographic boundaries. It can affect men and women of any race, class, age, and social group. That said, researchers have identified five types of alcoholics that are the most prevalent in our society.

- **The young adult subtype.** Usually alcoholics by their 21st birthday, these young adult drinkers typically do not abuse other drugs and are free of mental disorders. They usually lack a family history of alcoholism and rarely seek help for their drinking problem. They may drink less often than other alcoholics but tend to binge drink when they do. They account for 31.5% of alcoholics in the United States.[35]
- **The young antisocial subtype.** These drinkers start at an earlier age than the young adult subtype and tend to come from families suffering from alcoholism. About half could be considered antisocial, and many have major depression, bipolar disorder, or anxiety problems. They are more likely to smoke cigarettes and marijuana as well as use cocaine. They account for 21% of all alcoholics.[35]
- **The functional subtype.** Typically middle-aged, well-educated, and smokers, these drinkers have stable jobs, good incomes, and families. About one-third have a family history of alcoholism, and about one-fourth have had

a major bout of depression. They make up 19.5% of the alcoholic population.[35]

- **The intermediate familial subtype.** These middle-aged drinkers tend to have alcoholic parents. About half have been depressed. Most smoke cigarettes, and nearly one in five have had problems with cocaine and marijuana use. They account for 19% of alcoholics.[35]
- **The chronic severe subtype.** Chronic severe drinkers typically start drinking early in life—and develop alcohol problems at a young age, too. They tend to be middle-aged, antisocial, and prone to psychiatric disorders, including depression. They exhibit high rates of smoking, marijuana use, and cocaine dependence. Although they account for only 9% of U.S. alcoholics, about two-thirds of chronic severe drinkers seek help for their drinking problems, making them the most prevalent type of alcoholic in treatment.[35]

Although 22 is the average age when alcohol dependence begins, the onset varies from the mid-teens to middle age.[36]

Are you at risk for developing alcoholism or alcohol abuse? Take the **Self-Assessment** on page 186.

Getting Help for a Drinking Problem

Few people who abuse alcohol acknowledge that they have a drinking problem. Fewer still seek treatment or counseling for it. It can take a major health problem, accident, or hitting "rock bottom" to motivate a problem drinker to change his or her behavior. Even when drinkers decide that they want to quit, they may not know how to do so on their own. An estimated 21.6 million people in the United States need treatment for an alcohol use problem (about 8.4% of the population aged 12 or older), but only 2.3 million receive treatment at a specialized facility.[1]

Treatment Options

Advances in alcoholism treatment in recent years have provided more choices than ever for patients and health professionals. They include:

- **Medications.** Newer medications (naltrexone, topiramate, and acamprosate) can make it easier to quit drinking by offsetting changes in the brain caused by alcoholism and reducing the craving for alcohol. They don't make you sick if you drink, unlike an older medication (disulfiram). None of these medications are addictive. They can also be combined with support groups or alcohol counseling.
- **Alcohol counseling or "talk therapy."** There are several counseling approaches that are about equally effective—12 step, cognitive-behavioral, motivational enhancement, or a combination of these. Getting help in itself appears to be more important than the particular approach used, as long as it offers empathy, avoids heavy confrontation, strengthens motivation, and provides concrete ways to change drinking behavior. These programs usually focus on abstinence from alcohol. They may offer individual or group therapy, connect patients with alcoholism support groups, provide informational lectures, or lead activity therapy sessions. Specialized counseling may focus on the individual or family and may involve months of sessions or just occasional appearances. Short, one-on-one counseling sessions known as "brief interventions" have been increasing in popularity in recent years. Unlike traditional alcoholism treatments that emphasize complete abstinence from alcohol, interventions encourage sensible drinking at healthy levels. They require minimal follow-up and can be very effective.[37]

self-medicating Using alcohol or drugs to cope with sadness, grief, pain, or mental health problems.

SELF-ASSESSMENT
Alcohol Use Disorders Identification Test (AUDIT)

Is the way or amount you drink harming your health? Should you cut down on your drinking? Taking the following Self-Assessment will help you answer these questions.

Please mark the answer that is correct for you.

1. How often do you have a drink containing alcohol?
   ☐ Never ☐ Monthly or less ☐ 2 to 4 times a month
   ☐ 2 to 3 times per week ☐ 4 or more times per week

2. How many drinks containing alcohol do you have on a typical day when you are drinking?
   ☐ 1 or 2 ☐ 3 or 4 ☐ 5 or 6 ☐ 7 to 9 ☐ 10 or more

3. How often do you have six or more drinks on one occasion?
   ☐ Never ☐ Less than monthly ☐ Monthly ☐ 2 to 3 times per week
   ☐ 4 or more times a week

4. How often during the last year have you found that you were not able to stop drinking once you had started?
   ☐ Never ☐ Less than monthly ☐ Monthly ☐ 2 to 3 times per week
   ☐ 4 or more times a week

5. How often during the last year have you failed to do what was normally expected from you because of drinking?
   ☐ Never ☐ Less than monthly ☐ Monthly ☐ 2 to 3 times per week
   ☐ 4 or more times a week

6. How often during the last year have you needed a first drink in the morning to get yourself going after a heavy drinking session?
   ☐ Never ☐ Less than monthly ☐ Monthly ☐ 2 to 3 times per week
   ☐ 4 or more times a week

7. How often during the last year have you had a feeling of guilt or remorse after drinking?
   ☐ Never ☐ Less than monthly ☐ Monthly ☐ 2 to 4 times per week
   ☐ 4 or more times a week

8. How often during the last year have you been unable to remember what happened the night before because you had been drinking?
   ☐ Never ☐ Less than monthly ☐ Monthly ☐ 2 to 3 times per week
   ☐ 4 or more times a week

9. Have you or someone else been injured as a result of your drinking?
   ☐ No ☐ Yes, but not in the last year ☐ Yes, during the last year

10. Has a relative or friend, or doctor or other health worker, been concerned about your drinking or suggested you cut down?
    ☐ No ☐ Yes, but not in the last year ☐ Yes, during the last year

HOW TO INTERPRET YOUR SCORE

The Alcohol Use Disorders Identification Test (AUDIT) can detect alcohol problems experienced in the last year. Questions 1–8 are scored as 0, 1, 2, 3, or 4 points from first to last option. Questions 9 and 10 are scored 0, 2, or 4 only. A score of 8 or above on the AUDIT generally indicates harmful or hazardous drinking.

To complete this Self-Assessment online, visit MasteringHealth™

Source: The Alcohol Use Disorders Identification Test: Interview Version from AUDIT Manual, box 4, p. 17, World Health Organization, Division of Mental Health and Prevention of Substance Abuse. Copyright ©2001 by World Health Organization. Reprinted with permission.

- **Self-help groups.** Mutual help organizations include the 12-step program Alcoholics Anonymous. People in these groups attend general meetings and support each other by sharing advice and their personal experiences with alcohol abuse and recovery.

- **Intensive treatment programs.** These include 14- to 28-day residential programs that typically employ a 12-step approach combined with individual and group therapy in a strictly scheduled abstinence environment. They also include longer-term (three- to four-month) programs and halfway houses that offer life skill and job training as well as treatment for substance dependence and mental health problems.

>> **Looking for an alcohol treatment center? Visit** http://findtreatment.samhsa.gov, **which allows you to search for a treatment program near you.**

>> **This site provides self-help strategies for cutting back on or quitting drinking:** http://rethinkingdrinking.niaaa.nih.gov/Support/ChooseYourApproach.asp.

Dealing with Relapse

Once an alcoholic has decided to curb or stop drinking altogether, he or she must confront the possibility of *relapse*. **Relapse**—resuming the behavior of drinking to excess, or "falling off the wagon"— is experienced by up to 90% of drinkers when they first try to quit.[38] With hard work and commitment, however, it can be overcome. Research from the National Institute on Alcohol Abuse and Alcoholism reveals that 20 years after the onset of alcohol dependence, about three-fourths of individuals were fully recovered.[36] Even more surprising, more than half of these individuals were able to drink at low levels without showing symptoms of alcohol dependence.[36] That said, many alcoholics find that abstinence is ultimately the only way to keep alcohol use from disrupting their lives.

Beating any addiction requires both patience and practice. The body has to be weaned off a substance it has been dependent on, and the mind has to give up a long-time emotional crutch. Recovering alcoholics often have to change their social patterns and entire lifestyle. If you relapse while trying to quit drinking, don't give up. Learn from what happened and decide what to do next.

relapse Returning to drinking after a period of sobriety.

Change Yourself, Change Your World

Reducing alcohol-related risks happens one drink at a time. Some simple choices can help you keep your drinking under control, reduce your risk of becoming a victim of others' drinking, and help your peers make more healthful choices, too.

Personal Choices

If your drinking is getting out of hand, what can you do to take control? Step one: Make sure you haven't given someone else—for instance, your peer group—the power to control your decisions about drinking. Check out the **Special Feature** box on page 188 for tips on resisting peer pressure. In addition, here are other personal choices you can make to cut down on your drinking and reduce your risks.

Start by respecting your limits. Remember that your liver can break down the amount of alcohol in just one standard drink per hour, on average. So if you're at a party, try to stay within that limit:[39]

- **Pace and space.** Sip slowly. Make every other drink totally alcohol free.
- **Include food.** Don't drink on an empty stomach.
- **Shuffle things up.** Don't just drink. Get out on the dance floor, join the group watching a movie, or talk with friends outside.

What if you're planning to attend a club or off-campus party, and you've heard ahead of time that alcohol will be there? Offer to be the designated driver, or take a cab. If at all possible, attend the party with a trusted friend. Make a pact with each other not to engage in high-risk drinking, and help each other stick to it.

Another potentially life-saving precaution is to avoid consuming alcohol during swimming, boating, or other water activities. Alcohol is involved in over 60% of fatal drownings.[9] Moreover, the American Boating Association reports that alcohol is involved in 31% of boating fatalities.[40]

Also avoid using other potentially dangerous machinery and equipment if you've been drinking. The truth is, when you're intoxicated, anything from a candle flame to a flight of stairs could become a life-threatening hazard.

Helping a Friend

What if you suspect that someone you care about is engaging in high-risk drinking? Trust your feelings. Confronting your friend now might save his or her academic career, health, or life. Here are some guidelines from the University of Texas at Dallas for talking to your friend about getting help for his or her high-risk drinking:[41]

- **Be informed.** Know before your talk where help is available, just in case he or she is ready to seek it.
- **Use "I" statements.** Say things like, "I'm afraid you'll get kicked out," or "I worry that you'll be charged with a DWI, or even worse—that you'll get killed . . . or kill somebody else." Pointing the finger or using the word "you" too much, as in "You've got to change," will only back your friend into a corner.
- **Don't judge and don't interrupt.** If your friend starts talking about the problem, don't break in. Sometimes just talking can lead to a huge revelation.
- **Don't expect your friend to seek help after just one discussion.** It's difficult to predict how any individual person will react when confronted with his or her drinking problem. But it's still important to begin the process.

Campus Advocacy

Students nationwide are helping to reduce high-risk drinking on their campuses. If you'd like to get involved, two national programs that may be active on your campus—and looking for student volunteers—include the following:

- **The BACCHUS Network.** Since 1975, the mission of the BACCHUS Network has been to actively promote student leadership on health and safety issues such as alcohol abuse. One of its goals is to train a network of peer educators who in turn empower other students. For information on starting a chapter or getting involved on your campus, visit **www.bacchusnetwork.org**.
- **Students Against Destructive Decisions.** Founded in Massachusetts in response to the impaired driving deaths of local teens, SADD's original mission was to help young people say "No" to drinking and driving. Today, its broader mission is to provide students with the best prevention tools to deal with issues of underage drinking, other drug use, impaired driving, and other destructive decisions.[42] To get involved, check out **www.sadd.org**.

Smoking in the United States

Each year, 443,000 people in the United States die prematurely because of smoking-related illnesses.[43,44] That translates to 1 of every 5 deaths in the United States. Tobacco use is the leading cause of preventable death in the United States, with one study finding that it causes more deaths each year than other significant, preventable health problems such as obesity, physical inactivity, or high blood pressure.[45] Although smoking rates have dropped in recent years, approximately 57 million Americans aged 12 or older—about 22% of the population—remain smokers.[1]

The **Diversity & Health** box on page 191 provides a closer look at the prevalence of smoking among different demographic groups.

Smoking on Campus

Of all tobacco users, the age group with the highest rate of use is people between 18 and 25 years old with a total of 39.5% of people in that age range using tobacco.[45] About 29.3% of college students have tried smoking cigarettes at least once, although only 13.2% report smoking in the previous 30 days, and just 3.9% report smoking daily.[6] If you thought the rates of smoking on your campus were higher, you're not alone: The **Student Stats** box examines actual versus perceived use of cigarettes among college students.

Why Do Some Students Smoke?

It would be difficult to find a student who has not heard that smoking can kill you. Why, then, do some students smoke? There are as many different factors and reasons as there are individuals.

> ❝ *Make sure you haven't given someone else—for instance, your peer group—the power to control your decisions about drinking.*❞

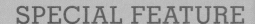

Peer Pressure: Resisting the Pitch

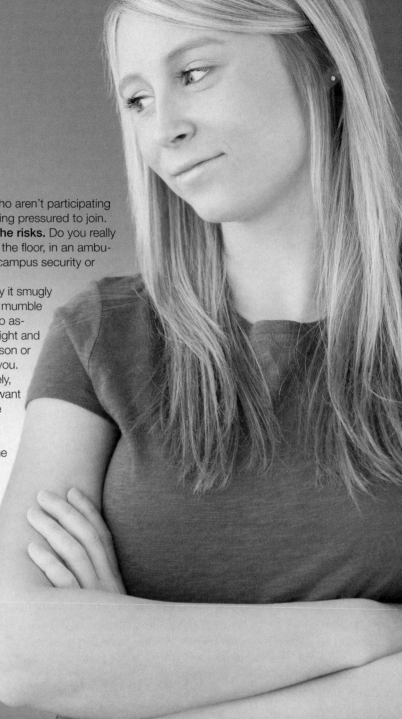

When was the last time you did something against your better judgment? Maybe last Saturday night? Did you give in to peer pressure and do something you really did not want to do? How can you stand your ground next time?

The National Institute on Alcohol Abuse and Alcoholism identifies a few of the most common reasons people give in to peer pressure.[1] Do any of these sound familiar?

- Desire to be liked, to be popular, and to not lose friends

- Desire to appear sophisticated, hip, cool, one of the "in" crowd

- Fear of being rejected, put down, teased, or ridiculed

- Worry about hurting a friend's feelings

- Uncertainty about what you really want

- Unawareness of how to get out of a bad situation

If you find yourself giving in to peer pressure for any of these reasons—or others—realize that although such feelings may be uncomfortable, they can motivate you to change. Here's how:[1]

Take a reality check. A friend may say to you, "Everybody else is okay with it. Why aren't you?" But how many students are really going to that pregame party, or mixing shots with their beer, or taking part in the drinking game in the lounge? If necessary, broaden your view: Remind yourself of students you like to hang out with who don't engage in high-risk drinking, and who aren't participating in the behavior you're being pressured to join.

Remind yourself of the risks. Do you really want to end the night on the floor, in an ambulance, or sobering up in campus security or the city jail?

Just say no. Don't say it smugly or aggressively, but don't mumble or apologize either. Say no assertively, standing up straight and looking directly at the person or group who is pressuring you. Speaking firmly and politely, and state that you don't want to join the behavior. Make it clear that this is your choice, but don't offer to explain your reasons. If the challenge continues, try countering: Repeat that you don't want to participate, and point out that real friends respect one another's choices.

Walk away. If necessary, be prepared to walk away from the situation.

Reference: 1. "Peer Pressure," by the National Institute on Alcohol Abuse and Alcoholism, 2010, retrieved from http://www.thecoolspot.gov/pressures.asp.

Genetics. Substantial evidence from a number of twin and adoption studies suggests that persistent smoking is significantly influenced by hereditary factors.[46] In addition, molecular studies suggest that genetic variations account for at least some of the susceptibility to become addicted to **nicotine**, the key psychoactive and addictive ingredient in tobacco.[47] Still, no specific genes have been reliably identified, and many researchers emphasize that persistent smoking and addiction to nicotine develop as a result of complex genetic–environmental interactions.[48]

Family and Peer Exposure. One environmental factor is family exposure. Research shows that if children have a parent who smokes, they are at significant risk of becoming smokers themselves, and that risk goes up further if both parents smoke.[49] Moreover, students whose friends smoke may begin smoking so that they can maintain acceptance from their peer group, or may begin smoking simply because they are more often in environments in which smoking is the norm. In one study, nonsmoking young adults who frequented bars, clubs, and similar establishments where smoking was unrestricted were at significantly higher risk for becoming smokers themselves.[50]

Age at Initiating Smoking. The younger people are when they start smoking, the more likely they are to become adult smokers. Research findings conclude that approximately 90% of adults who are regular smokers began at or before age 19.[51]

Psychosocial Factors. Stress is certainly a factor in tobacco use. Schoolwork, family tensions, and complicated social relationships with classmates have all been cited as reasons why students smoke.

Young people experiencing interpersonal stress may rebel by experimenting with substances that their parents—and other authority figures in their lives—would not approve of. The fact that smoking is "bad" can actually make it more appealing to a teen wishing to challenge authority. In addition, some teens curious to experiment with a variety of recreational drugs may begin with smoking.

Behind such experimentation, there's often a failure to appreciate the real risks of tobacco use. Young adults sometimes have poor decision-making and risk-judging skills, leading them to believe they're invulnerable to harm. In one study, adolescents who had the lowest appreciation for the long-term health risks of smoking were more than three times as likely to start smoking as adolescents with the highest appreciation of the risks.[52] In another study, Florida community college students who smoked rated the health risks of smoking to be less significant than did their nonsmoking peers. Moreover, the smokers viewed their personal risk as lower than the risk to other smokers.[53]

Desire to Lose Weight. For decades, public health researchers have speculated that concerns about body weight were important factors in initiation of tobacco use among adolescents, particularly females. A recent study supports this theory. It found that, in general, females who perceived themselves to be overweight in grades 8 and 11 were more likely to be smokers as young adults.[54] Although it is true that nicotine can suppress appetite, taking up smoking to lose weight is one of the worst decisions anyone can make. The damage to health caused by smoking far outweighs any benefits in weight management.

Role of Media and Advertising. Media and advertising, including films, music videos, and expensive promotional campaigns, play a significant part in glamorizing smoking and making

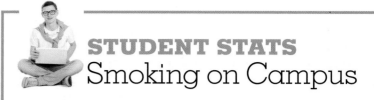

STUDENT STATS
Smoking on Campus

Students often greatly overestimate how many of their peers regularly smoke cigarettes.

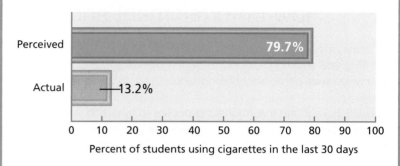

Perceived — 79.7%

Actual — 13.2%

Percent of students using cigarettes in the last 30 days

Data from *ACHA-NCHA II: UNDERGRADUATE STUDENTS—Reference Group Executive Summary Fall 2012*, by the American College Health Association, 2013.

it acceptable. Characters in movies are commonly shown smoking, for example, even though the majority of Americans don't share the habit. Overall, the total weight of evidence from multiple types of studies worldwide demonstrates not just an association, but a causal relationship, between tobacco promotion and increased tobacco use.[55]

For a deeper look at how entertainment and ads contribute to smoking and alcohol use, see the **Media and Alcohol and Tobacco Use** box on page 190.

What's in a Cigarette?

Smoking cigarettes is by far the most common form of tobacco use. A typical cigarette in the United States contains 50% shredded tobacco leaf, 30% reconstituted tobacco (made from other parts of the tobacco plant, such as the stem), and 20% expanded tobacco (tobacco that has been "puffed up" like popcorn and functions as "filler").[56] It also contains nearly 600 additives with a wide range of functions. Cocoa, licorice, and vanilla, for example, are among the additives that help hide the harsh taste of tobacco. Meanwhile, ammonia—a chemical commonly used for household cleaning—boosts the delivery of *nicotine* (the key psychoactive ingredient in tobacco) into the lungs and bloodstream.

When a cigarette is lit and smoked, it releases approximately 4,000 chemicals, more than 60 of which are **carcinogenic,** meaning they cause cancer. These carcinogens include arsenic (a poison), formaldehyde (used in embalming fluid), polonium-210 (a radioactive substance), and **tar.** Tar is a sticky, thick brown residue that forms when tobacco is burned and its chemical particles condense. Other harmful chemicals in cigarette smoke include hydrogen cyanide, benzene (found in gasoline), and **carbon monoxide,** an especially dangerous gas that inhibits the delivery of oxygen to the body's vital organs.

nicotine An alkaloid derived from the tobacco plant that is responsible for smoking's psychoactive and addictive effects.

carcinogenic Cancer-causing.

tar A sticky, thick brown residue that forms when tobacco is burned and its chemical particles condense.

carbon monoxide A gas that inhibits the delivery of oxygen to the body's vital organs.

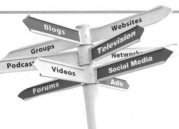

media and ALCOHOL AND TOBACCO USE

How Entertainment and Ads Drive Drinking and Smoking

The media play a crucial role in shaping perceptions and habits related to drinking and smoking. Unfortunately, the message that's usually portrayed to viewers is that alcohol or tobacco use is fun, sophisticated, or cool.

Studies have found that frequent exposure to television and video portrayals of alcohol consumption as desirable can trigger new or increased drinking, with one study noting that "alcohol advertising and promotion increases the likelihood that adolescents will start to use alcohol, and to drink more if they are already using alcohol."[1] Take, for example, a period in our recent history: the 1990s. During that time, increases in alcohol use were linked by researchers to a decline in public service announcements cautioning against alcohol use and a corresponding increase in pro-use messages from the entertainment industry. In 1997, for example, alcohol appeared in 93% of the 200 most popular movie rentals, and the same year, the alcohol industry spent more than $1 billion on television, radio, print, and outdoor advertising.[2]

If you think the amount spent on alcohol advertising is high, the tobacco industry leaves it in the dust. The major cigarette manufacturers spend more than $27.2 million *every day* to promote their products in the United States, and many of their efforts directly reach young adults.[3] Those efforts are also often apparently successful in both popularizing and triggering smoking—one large research analysis found that "nonsmoking adolescents who were more aware of tobacco advertising or receptive to it, were more likely to have experimented with cigarettes or become smokers" later.[4]

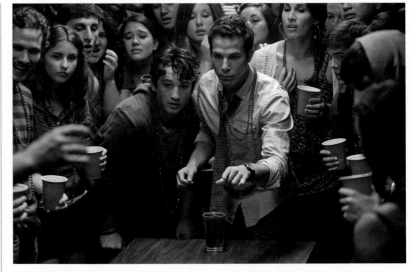

Movies that depict tobacco use or excessive drinking can promote those behaviors.

The depiction of smoking is pervasive in films, occurring in three-quarters or more of contemporary box-office hits.[5] Perhaps no form of media is more powerful in influencing smoking initiation: A 2008 report from the National Cancer Institute reached "the government's strongest conclusion to date" that smoking in films encourages smoking in youth.[5]

Critical-Thinking Questions

1. How often do you see ads and images glamorizing alcohol use as compared to ads or messages about its health risks, such as drunk driving?

2. How often are the depictions of smoking you see on film realistic in terms of everyday hassles (bad breath, smelly clothes) and health risks?

3. Why do you think smoking is so commonly shown in movies when the majority of the U.S. population doesn't smoke?

References: **1.** "Impact of Alcohol Advertising and Media Exposure on Adolescent Alcohol Use: A Systematic Review of Longitudinal Studies," by P. Anderson, A. Bruijn, K. Angus, R. Gordon, & G. Hastings, 2009, *Alcohol & Alcoholism, 44*(3), pp. 229–243. **2.** "Substance Abuse: The Nation's Number One Health Problem," by U.S. Department of Justice, 2001, OJJDP Fact Sheet, #17, retrieved from https://www.ncjrs.gov/pdffiles1/ojjdp/fs200117.pdf. **3.** "Cigarette Report for 2007 and 2008," by the U.S. Federal Trade Commission, 2011, retrieved from http://www.ftc.gov/os/2011/07/110729cigarettereport.pdf. **4.** "Impact of Tobacco Advertising and Promotion on Increasing Adolescent Smoking Behaviours," by C. Lovato, A. Watts, & L. Stead, 2011, *The Cochrane Collaboration*, Issue 10. Art. No.: CD003439. doi: 10.1002/14651858. **5.** "The Role of the Media in Promoting and Reducing Tobacco Use. NCI Tobacco Control Monograph Series," by the National Cancer Institute, 2008, retrieved from http://cancercontrol.cancer.gov/tcrb/monographs/19/docs/M19ExecutiveSummary.pdf.

>> **View video clips about the effects of tobacco advertising and more at** www.tobaccofree.org/clips.htm.

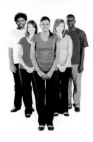

Tobacco Use Through the Lenses of Sex, Race/Ethnicity, Age, Education, and Geography

A recent national survey conducted by the Substance Abuse and Mental Health Services Administration revealed the following:

Overall

- An estimated 26.5% of those aged 12 or older (about 68.2 million people) use a tobacco

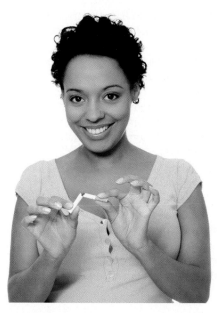

Smoking rates are highest among those aged 18–25.

product; 22.1% smoke cigarettes, 5.0% smoke cigars, and 3.2% use smokeless tobacco.

Sex

- Men are more likely to use a tobacco product than women. Of males aged 12 or older, 32.3% use a tobacco product compared to 22.1% of females.
- However, among those aged 12 to 17, there is not much difference in the rate of smoking in males (8.2%) versus females (7.3%).

Race/Ethnicity

- Among Native Americans, 43.0% report current tobacco use, the highest of any racial/ethnic group.
- Among people of mixed-race background, 36.1% use tobacco.
- Among Caucasians, 28.6% use tobacco.
- Among African Americans, 26.2% use tobacco.
- Among Hispanics, 20.4% use tobacco.
- Among Asian Americans, 13.0% use tobacco.

Age

- People aged 18–25 report a higher rate of current tobacco use (39.5%) than any other age group.

Education

- Adults with college degrees are less likely to use tobacco than those with less education.

Geography

- Rates of smoking are higher in the South (23.2%) and Midwest (24.2%) than in the West (18.1%) and Northeast (22.2%).

Critical-Thinking Questions

1. Why do you think people between the ages of 18 and 25 have the highest rate of tobacco use of any age group?

2. What are some of the possible reasons behind varying rates of tobacco use in different parts of the country?

3. Why do you think smoking rates are similar for both sexes as teens, but diverge as people get older?

Data from *Results from the 2011 National Survey on Drug Use and Health: National Findings* from the Substance Abuse and Mental Health Services Administration website 2012.

 Learn more about the chemicals found in cigarette smoke at www.lung.org/stop-smoking/about-smoking/facts-figures/whats-in-a-cigarette.html.

 See how nicotine works in the brain to create addiction at www.youtube.com/watch?v=5ewwzazHfq4.

Effects of Smoking on Health

Smoking harms nearly every organ of the body, including the lungs, kidneys, bladder, heart, pancreas, stomach, and esophagus. It weakens the immune system and shortens life expectancy. Adults who smoke have a life expectancy over 10 years shorter than those who don't smoke.[57] About half of long-term smokers will die because of their habit, according to the American Cancer Society.[58]

Short-Term Health Effects

From the moment a person takes the first puff of a cigarette, physiological changes take place in the body. Within 8 seconds of entering the body, nicotine is absorbed by the lungs and quickly moved into the bloodstream, where it is circulated throughout the brain. There, it triggers the release of large amounts of **dopamine**, a neurotransmitter that stimulates feelings of pleasure. Once smokers develop a tolerance to nicotine, they need more and more of it to achieve the same effects they experienced when they first began smoking. Eventually, smokers need to keep smoking just to feel "normal," as the body becomes addicted to nicotine. Stopping smoking can

dopamine A neurotransmitter that stimulates feelings of pleasure.

cause withdrawal symptoms such as cravings, irritability, insomnia, head-ache, inability to concentrate, and dry mouth.

Other short-term health effects of smoking include:

- **Increased heart rate and blood pressure.** Nicotine causes the heart to beat faster. It also raises blood pressure.
- **Shortness of breath and reduction in stamina.** The carbon monoxide in cigarette smoke binds to a protein in red blood cells, disrupting these cells' ability to effectively deliver oxygen to the rest of the body.
- **Coughing.** Cigarette smoke damages the respiratory passageways, increasing the production of mucus and triggering the need to cough.
- **Heightened alertness.**
- **Decreased skin temperature.** Nicotine constricts blood vessels, resulting in less blood flow to the skin (reducing its temperature) and to the legs and feet.
- **Increased blood sugar.**
- **Dulled sense of smell and taste.**
- **Bad breath.**
- **Smelling like smoke.**
- **Decreased urine production.**
- **Risks to a developing fetus.**

Long-Term Health Effects

Cigarette smoking is so harmful that the Surgeon General has called it "the leading preventable cause of disease and deaths in the United States." It raises the risk of cancer and cardiovascular disease and contributes to a host of other negative health effects.

Cancer

In the United States, smoking is responsible for 90% of lung cancer deaths in men and nearly 80% in women.[56] Smoking is also associated with cancers of the kidney, bladder, pancreas, stomach, esophagus, mouth, throat, larynx, cervix, and blood. A smoker's risk of developing these cancers increases with the number of cigarettes and the number of years they smoke. The risk, however, does begin to drop over time in those who are able to quit for good.

The risk of developing cancer is not insignificant. The odds of getting lung cancer are more than 23 times higher among men who smoke cigarettes than men who do not.[56] Women who smoke are 13 times more likely to develop the disease than women who do not.[59]

Cardiovascular Disease

Smoking is a key risk factor for three major types of cardiovascular disease:

- **Coronary heart disease.** The leading cause of death in the United States, coronary heart disease often stems from the development of *atherosclerosis*, a progressive hardening of the coronary arteries. Smoking contributes to the development of atherosclerosis, which can result in a heart attack. Indeed, you are four times more likely to die of coronary heart disease if you smoke.[56]
- **Stroke.** A stroke occurs when a blood vessel carrying oxygen and nutrients to the brain either bursts or is blocked by a clot. When that

happens, part of the brain cannot get the blood and oxygen it needs and starts to die. It can cause speech problems, vision problems, memory loss, and paralysis on one side of the body. It can also be fatal. Cigarette smoking doubles a person's odds of having a stroke. The risk, however, steadily decreases after quitting smoking with former smokers having roughly the same stroke risk as nonsmokers do 5 to 15 years after quitting.[56]

- **Abdominal aortic aneurysm.** An aortic aneurysm is a dangerously weakened and bulging area in the aorta, the major blood vessel that supplies blood to the body. A ruptured aortic aneurysm can cause life-threatening bleeding. Smoking is clearly associated with the condition. Several studies show that the risk of death from abdominal aortic aneurysm more than quadruples in smokers and doubles in former smokers.[56]

Respiratory Disease

Smoking damages the airways and alveoli of the lungs and can lead to **chronic obstructive pulmonary disease (COPD),** a category of diseases that includes emphysema, chronic bronchitis, and asthma.

In **emphysema,** the walls of the lungs' air sacs lose their elasticity and are destroyed. It becomes difficult for the lungs to transfer oxygen to the bloodstream, causing shortness of breath. Emphysema sufferers often have trouble performing simple physical activities such as shopping or climbing the stairs. As the disease progresses, many emphysema patients must rely on an oxygen tank to help them breathe.

Chronic bronchitis is an inflammation of the main airways in the lungs that continues for at least three months. Symptoms include a chronic cough that produces mucus, shortness of breath, wheezing, and frequent respiratory infections.

Asthma is a chronic pulmonary disease in which the air passages become inflamed. The inflammation causes a narrowing of the airways, making breathing very difficult. Asthma symptoms include wheezing, coughing, shortness of breath, and chest tightness.

In 2012, COPD was the third leading cause of death in the United States.[60] Smoking is considered the "primary causative factor" in 80% of COPD deaths.[61]

Other Health Effects

Aside from the increased risks for cancer, cardiovascular disease, and respiratory disease, smoking can have additional health consequences:

- Erectile dysfunction in men.
- Loss of bone density in women following menopause.
- Periodontitis, a gum infection that can lead to tooth loss.
- Increased risk of developing cataracts, a leading cause of blindness.
- Decreased fertility in women.
- Premature aging and wrinkling of skin.
- Stained teeth.

Figure 8.5 summarizes the short- and long-term health effects of smoking.

Smoking and Pregnancy

When a pregnant woman smokes, so does her unborn baby. The nicotine, carbon monoxide, benzene, and other cancer-causing chemicals that enter her bloodstream are passed on to her fetus.

chronic obstructive pulmonary disease (COPD) A category of diseases that includes emphysema, chronic bronchitis, and asthma.

emphysema A chronic disease in which the air sacs in the lung become damaged, making breathing difficult.

chronic bronchitis Inflammation of the main airways in the lungs that continues for at least three months.

asthma A chronic pulmonary disease in which the air passages become inflamed, making breathing difficult.

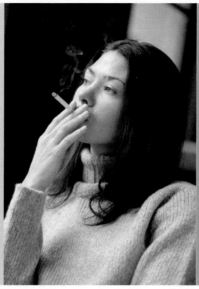

Short-term effects:
- Increased heart rate
- Increased blood pressure
- Shortness of breath
- Reduction in stamina
- Coughing
- Heightened alertness
- Decreased skin temperature
- Increased blood glucose
- Dulled sense of smell and taste
- Bad breath
- Smelling like smoke
- Health risks to developing fetus

Long-term effects:
- Greatly increased risk of cancer
- Greatly increased risk of cardiovascular disease
- Reduced lung function
- Periodontal disease
- Increased risk of gastroesophageal reflux
- Increased risk of peptic ulcers
- Reduced liver function
- Increased risk of type 2 diabetes
- Erectile dysfunction
- Decreased fertility
- Loss of bone density
- Vision impairment
- Premature aging and wrinkling of skin
- Stained teeth
- Nicotine addiction

FIGURE 8.5 Short- and Long-Term Health Effects of Smoking.

Nicotine also reduces the amount of oxygen that reaches the fetus, negatively affecting its growth.

Smoking while pregnant is like gambling—with the baby's life. Babies born to women who smoke are two to three times more likely to die of *sudden infant death syndrome* than babies born to women who did not smoke.[62] They also have 30% higher odds of being born prematurely and are more likely to weigh less than 5.5 pounds when they are born, increasing their risk for illness or death.[62] Smoking during pregnancy has also been linked to miscarriages and stillbirths. Up to 5% of infant deaths would be prevented if women did not smoke during their pregnancy.[63]

Secondhand Smoke

Secondhand smoke is a mixture of **sidestream smoke**—the smoke emanating from the burning end of a cigarette or pipe—and **mainstream smoke**, which is exhaled from the lungs of smokers. Also called **environmental tobacco smoke,** it contains more than 250 chemicals known to be toxic or capable of causing cancer, including arsenic, ammonia, formaldehyde, and benzene.[64]

The smoke that nonsmokers are exposed to actually has higher concentrations of some harmful chemicals than the smoke inhaled by the smoker, according to the American Lung Association. This is because sidestream smoke is not filtered through a cigarette filter or a smoker's lungs. As a result, secondhand smoke has at least twice the amount of nicotine and tar as mainstream smoke. It also has five times the amount of carbon monoxide and has higher levels of ammonia and cadmium (chemicals found in glass cleaner and batteries, respectively).

Millions of people in the United States are essentially *passive smokers:* people who breathe in secondhand smoke from their environment. In national surveys, 43% of passive smokers have been found to have detectable levels of *cotinine*—the major breakdown product of nicotine—in their blood.[64]

The health risks to passive smokers are no less serious than if they were the ones lighting up a cigarette or puffing on a cigar. The U.S. Surgeon General has concluded that "the scientific evidence indicates that there is no risk-free level of exposure to secondhand smoke." In fact, secondhand smoke can kill.

Health Effects of Secondhand Smoke

Secondhand smoke, which can linger in the air for hours after cigarettes have been extinguished, can exacerbate—or cause—a number of health conditions, including cancer, respiratory infections, and asthma. On a basic level, it can irritate the eyes, nose, throat, and lungs. It can also cause chest pain, coughing, and production of excessive phlegm. In a report spanning more than 700 pages, the U.S. Surgeon General concluded that secondhand smoke can also:

- Cause premature death and disease in children and adults who do not smoke.

- Increase a nonsmoker's risk of heart disease by 25–30%.

- Cause lung cancer in people who have never smoked.

- Cause respiratory illnesses, including asthma, in children.

- Cause ear infections in children.

- Cause sudden infant death syndrome in some babies.[64]

"The health effects of secondhand smoke exposure are more pervasive than we previously thought," the report summarized. "The scientific evidence is now indisputable: secondhand smoke is not a mere annoyance. It is a serious health hazard that can lead to disease and premature death in children and nonsmoking adults."[64]

secondhand smoke (environmental tobacco smoke) The smoke nonsmokers are exposed to when someone has been smoking nearby; a combination of sidestream smoke and mainstream smoke.

sidestream smoke Smoke emanating from the burning end of a cigarette or pipe.

mainstream smoke Smoke exhaled from the lungs of smokers.

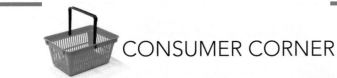
Are "Light" Cigarettes Safer to Use?

You have probably seen advertisements for cigarettes that are "low-tar," "mild," "light," or "lite." Some even purport to be "ultra-light." But are such cigarettes really any less dangerous than regular cigarettes?

Although it's true that some of these cigarettes deliver less tar or nicotine than regular cigarettes in machine-based tests, health experts say there is no convincing evidence

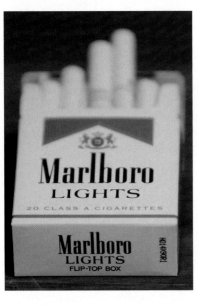

that they are less harmful to a person's health. On the contrary, studies have shown that when smokers switch to low-tar cigarettes, they often change the way they smoke, smoking more cigarettes, taking bigger puffs, and holding smoke in their lungs longer.[1]

- The U.S. Surgeon General has concluded that "light" cigarettes do not actually decrease the health risks of smoking, primarily because these changes did not reduce smokers' actual exposure to tobacco toxicants.[1]

- The National Cancer Institute has determined that people who switch to light cigarettes are likely to inhale the same amount of hazardous chemicals as those smoking regular or "full-flavored" cigarettes. They also remain at high risk for developing smoking-related cancers and other diseases.[2]

- There is no evidence that switching to light cigarettes actually helps smokers kick their habit.

The bottom line: "Light" cigarettes are still harmful to a person's health.

References: 1. How Tobacco Smoke Causes Disease: The Biology and Behavioral Basis for Smoking-Attributable Disease, a Report of the Surgeon General, by the U.S. Department of Health and Human Services, 2012. 2. Risks Associated with Smoking Cigarettes with Low Machine-Measured Yields of Tar and Nicotine [Monograph 13], October 2001, by the National Cancer Institute, retrieved from http://cancercontrol.cancer.gov/tcrb/monographs.

Health experts estimate that secondhand smoke causes 3,400 lung cancer deaths and between 22,700 and 69,600 heart disease deaths in adult nonsmokers in the United States each year.[65]

Because their bodies are growing and developing, infants and children are particularly vulnerable to the effects of secondhand smoke. Secondhand smoke causes more than 750,000 middle-ear infections in children and increases the number and severity of asthma attacks in more than 200,000 asthmatic children.[65] It also reduces lung function in children and promotes the development of persistent wheezing.

Other Forms of Tobacco

Cigars, clove cigarettes, bidis, pipes, and smokeless "spit" tobacco are other commonly used tobacco products. Like cigarettes, they are also associated with numerous health problems.

Cigars

Cigars contain many of the same addictive, toxic, cancer-causing substances that cigarettes do. The smoke from cigars also contains many of the toxins found in cigarette smoke, including ammonia, carbon monoxide, and benzene, but in much higher concentrations. A single cigar can contain as much tobacco as an entire pack of cigarettes.[66]

Because most cigar smokers do not inhale, their risk of developing lung cancer is lower than it is for cigarette smokers. However, cigar smokers still have higher rates of lung cancer, heart disease, and COPD than nonsmokers do.[67]

Clove Cigarettes

Clove cigarettes, which have a distinctly sweet, pungent odor, are shaped like traditional cigarettes and are imported from Indonesia or other Southeast Asian countries. Also called *kreteks*, they usually contain tobacco, cloves, and other additives. Although they may smell and taste different from conventional cigarettes, there is no evidence that they are any safer. Clove cigarette smokers have higher rates of asthma and up to 20 times the risk for abnormal lung function, compared with nonsmokers.[68]

New federal laws ban the sale of flavored cigarettes, including clove cigarettes. It is not illegal to smoke them, but it is illegal to sell them.

Bidis

Bidis (pronounced bee-dees) are thin, hand-rolled cigarettes that come in a variety of flavors, including cherry, chocolate, grape, and mango. Imported from India and other Southeast Asian countries, they are packed with tobacco and wrapped in leaf, sometimes tied at the ends by a colorful string.

>> **Check out this article on the history of baseball and chewing tobacco from** *Slate* **magazine:** www.slate.com/id/2234341.

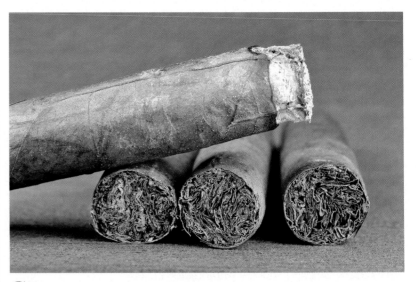

Cigars, clove cigarettes, bidis, and smokeless tobacco all increase the risk of cancer and heart disease.

Contrary to a popular misconception, bidis are *not* safer than cigarettes. Bidi smoke contains three to five times more nicotine than found in a regular cigarette.[68] Bidi smokers are at increased risk for several types of cancer, including oral, lung, stomach, and esophageal cancer, as well as coronary heart disease, emphysema, and chronic bronchitis.[68]

Smokeless ("Spit") Tobacco

For some young people, especially young men, the use of smokeless tobacco is almost a rite of passage, even though it carries dangerous health risks. Baseball fans are used to seeing their heroes use smokeless tobacco, also known as "spit" or "chew." Indeed, one in three major league baseball players uses smokeless tobacco.[69] In some communities, especially rural areas and small towns, younger men may pick up a tradition of using smokeless tobacco from fathers and older brothers.[70] No wonder, then, that many boys and young men have followed in the footsteps of their role models, using smokeless tobacco at alarming rates. One survey of teenagers found that in 2011, about 8% of high school seniors were using smokeless tobacco.[71]

Smokeless tobacco use is far higher among men than women, and highest in the states of Wyoming, West Virginia, and Mississippi.[72] One survey of college students in Texas found that white and Native American young men who played college sports and had friends and teammates who used "spit" were most likely to use it themselves.[73]

Smokeless tobacco comes in two forms. *Snuff* is a fine-grain tobacco that is often sold in teabag-like pouches that users "pinch" or "dip" between their lower lip and gum. *Chewing tobacco* comes in wads of shredded or "bricked" tobacco leaves that people put between their cheek and gum. No matter the type, smokeless tobacco is meant to stew in the mouth for minutes at a time. Users suck on the tobacco juices and then spit to get rid of the saliva that builds up, hence the nickname "spit."

Chewing tobacco is made from tobacco leaves that have had their stems removed. Snuff is made from both the leaf and stem. Both are typically loaded with sweeteners and flavorings to make them taste more pleasant. Although they don't emit harmful plumes of smoke like cigarettes and cigars do, smokeless tobacco contains plenty of addictive nicotine. It is absorbed into the bloodstream through the mucous membranes that line the mouth, and users can become physically hooked without ever swallowing the tobacco soup that builds up in their mouths. The average dose of smokeless tobacco, in fact, contains up to four times the amount of nicotine found in the average cigarette. One can of snuff is equivalent, nicotine-wise, to about four packs of cigarettes.

The health effects of using smokeless tobacco are varied. Regular use increases a person's risk for cancers of the lip, tongue, cheeks, gums, and mouth. The products stain and wear down the teeth, cause gums to recede, and can cause a condition called **leukoplakia**, characterized by whitish lesions in the mouth. These lesions may become cancerous and are frequently found in snuff and chew users in their 20s.

Electronic Cigarettes

A newer nicotine product often advertised as a smoking cessation aid is the so-called electronic cigarette (or e-cigarette), a battery-powered device that delivers a dose of nicotine in vapor form. Invented in China in 2003, it quickly became popular in the United States. In 2010, the Food and Drug Administration (FDA) classified the electronic

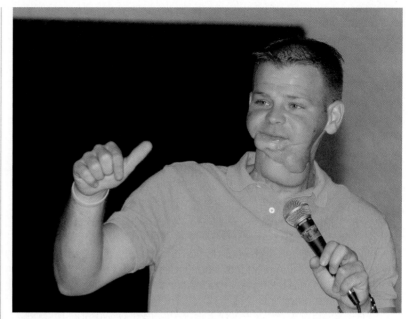

Gruen Von Behrens was hooked on chewing tobacco at age 14 and diagnosed with oral cancer at age 17. He has lost his jaw, lower teeth, and part of his tongue in his fight to beat the disease.

cigarette as both a drug and a "drug-delivery device" subject to FDA approval. It also announced that it had taken action against five manufacturers of electronic cigarettes because of health risks, poor manufacturing practices, and unsubstantiated claims of benefits.[74]

Getting Help to Quit Smoking

If you smoke, the odds are that you have thought about quitting. Perhaps you have already tried to quit. Usually they are unsuccessful. Indeed, more than half of all smokers make a determined effort to quit each year.[75] And for good reason. Researchers recently determined that if smokers quit before the age of 35, they can regain the entire 10 years of life expectancy that smoking takes away, and even after age 35, it is possible to gain back many years in life expectancy if you break the habit.[57]

Stopping smoking is not a simple matter. Nicotine activates the pleasure and reward centers of the brain and raises levels of the "feel good" neurotransmitter, dopamine. Consequently, nicotine can be as addictive as heroin or cocaine. Those attempting to quit often must deal with withdrawal symptoms such as restlessness, depression, hunger, insomnia, and headaches. A smoker's brain develops an abundance of nicotine-binding receptors to accommodate the large doses of nicotine. Recent research findings conclude that for up to 6 weeks after people stop smoking, these receptors still exist.[76] Unfortunately, these nicotine-receptor brain cells contribute to the cravings and other discomforts of smoking withdrawal and probably explain why the first months of smoking cessation are very difficult for many people. The good news is that after 6–12 weeks of abstinence, the former smoker's nicotine receptor levels match those of a nonsmoker and consequently relapse is less likely.

leukoplakia White spots on the mucous membranes in the mouth that may become cancerous.

The health benefits of quitting smoking begin almost immediately. Figure 8.6 illustrates the short- and long-term benefits of quitting.

>> View a video explaining the timeline for the beneficial health effects of quitting smoking: www.youtube.com/watch?v=fLbQfMmrlSE.

Treatment Options

Several products are available to aid smokers who wish to quit. Most of them, including nicotine gum, inhalers, lozenges, nasal sprays, and patches, are *nicotine replacement therapies* designed to help smokers gradually reduce their dependence on nicotine and reduce the severity of nicotine withdrawal symptoms. Others, such as bupropion (Zyban) and varenicline (Chantix), do not contain nicotine at all but reduce the smoker's craving for tobacco and ease withdrawal symptoms (note that serious safety concerns have recently arisen about both of these drugs). You should talk with your doctor or a pharmacist before taking any smoking cessation products, especially if you have any allergies, health problems, are taking any medications, or are pregnant or planning to become pregnant.

Note that nicotine replacement therapies are only available to those aged 18 and older. You should not continue smoking while taking a smoking cessation product. You should also avoid taking more than one smoking cessation product at the same time without consulting a doctor because improper use can result in nicotine overdose.

In addition to nicotine replacement therapies, smoking cessation programs are effective for approximately 20–40% of smokers.[64] There are several types of treatment options, including residential, individual or group therapy, and education and support groups.

> *If smokers quit before the age of 35, they can regain the entire 10 years of life expectancy that smoking takes away . . ."*

Dealing with Relapse

Smokers commonly experience withdrawal symptoms when they first quit smoking, including difficulty concentrating, a negative mood, and the urge to smoke. These symptoms usually peak within one or two weeks. Not surprisingly, smokers are most likely to relapse early in the quitting process, although sometimes relapse can occur months or even years after quitting. Any smoking—even taking one single puff—increases the likelihood of a full relapse.

Change Yourself, Change Your World

Smoking injures and kills. Whether you're a smoker and want to quit, or you just want to reduce the threat of secondhand smoke, there are powerful choices you can make to reach your goal.

QUIT SMOKING

First 48 hours:

20 minutes	8 hours	24 hours	48 hours
• Blood pressure drops to normal. • Pulse rate drops to normal. • Body temperature of hands and feet increases to normal.	• Carbon monoxide level in blood drops to normal. • Oxygen level in blood increases to normal.	• Chance of heart attack decreases.	• Nerve endings start regrowing. • Ability to smell and taste is enhanced.

First year:

2 weeks to 3 months	1 to 9 months	1 year
• Circulation improves. • Walking becomes easier. • Lung function increases up to 30%.	• Coughing, sinus congestion, fatigue, and shortness of breath decrease. • Cilia regrow in lungs, increasing ability to handle mucus, clean the lungs, and reduce infection. • Overall energy level increases.	• Excess risk of coronary heart disease is half that of a smoker.

Future years:

5 years	10 years	15 years
• Lung cancer death rate for average former smoker (one pack a day) decreases by almost half.	• Lung cancer death rate similar to that of nonsmokers. • Precancerous cells are replaced. • Risk of cancer of the mouth, throat, esophagus, bladder, kidney, and pancreas decreases.	• Risk of coronary heart disease is that of a nonsmoker.

FIGURE 8.6 Benefits of Quitting Smoking. The health benefits of quitting smoking begin the moment you stop.

Personal Choices

If your goal is to quit smoking and avoid relapse, you'll want to follow a plan that works. The plan here, adapted from the National Cancer Institute (NCI), is one you can trust.[77]

Quitting is more likely to succeed if you're prepared. Start by thinking about why you want to quit. Write down your reasons, and keep them with you. Make sure the reasons you list are meaningful to you. For instance:

• I'll have more stamina on the basketball court.

• I won't have to be embarrassed about bad breath and smelly clothes.

• I'll know that I'm the one in control of my life.

Next, take a good, hard look at how strong your addiction to nicotine really is. For instance, do you smoke only socially or by yourself as well? After you wake up in the morning do you crave your first cigarette? How many cigarettes do you typically smoke in a day? Your honest answers may help you to decide whether or not you need professional support to quit. Going "cold turkey" usually works for only a very small percentage of smokers who have a low level of nicotine dependency.[77] Others need support.

Then, identify your triggers—the activities, feelings, and other factors that make you want to smoke. Is it coffee? Being around other smokers? Feeling bored, unhappy, or depressed? List a strategy for avoiding each trigger entirely or for substituting a behavior other than smoking. For example, if you typically smoke when you drive, replace cigarettes in your car with a stash of chewing gum. If a craving still hits, take a long, deep breath and remind yourself that it will go away, usually in just a few minutes.

Finally, learn your options. Earlier in this chapter, we discussed campus and community-based support as well as medications and clinical smoking cessation programs. Stay open to the option of combining two or more of these methods. **Practical Strategies: Quitting Smoking** also summarizes a step-by-step strategy for taking the plunge to quit, prepared by the National Cancer Institute.

 Ready to quit smoking today? Visit the National Cancer Institute's www.smokefree.gov. **The American Cancer Society also offers helpful tips for quitting smoking at** www.cancer.org/Healthy/StayAwayfromTobacco/index.

Campus Advocacy

Many national public health organizations, from the U.S. Centers for Disease Control and Prevention to the American College Health Association, support not only indoor smoking bans on college and university campuses, but outdoor bans as well. This is in part because indoor smoking bans may encourage smokers to cluster just outside of buildings, saturating these areas with tobacco smoke, which can then drift back into the building.[78]

Quitting Cold Turkey

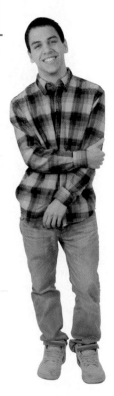

 "HI, I'M ADDISON. When I first started smoking I was 16 years old. I've tried to quit numerous times—always cold turkey. I'd last maybe a week if I was lucky. Recently I tried to quit again. This time I went cold turkey *and* I started working out too. I tried to replace a bad habit with a healthier habit. I go to the gym every day, I haven't smoked in two weeks, and I hope to keep it that way."

1. What stage of behavior change is Addison in? (Review Chapter 1 if you can't remember the stages of behavior change.)

2. What do you think of Addison's plan to "replace" smoking with working out?

3. How can Addison improve his chances of quitting smoking for good?

If you'd like to advocate for a smoke-free campus, the American College Health Association recommends you address the issue on multiple fronts. Specifically, it recommends a policy that includes the following provisions:[79]

• Prohibit smoking and all forms of tobacco on all campus grounds and in all campus-related facilities, including residence halls and fraternities and sororities, and at all indoor and outdoor campus events.

• Prohibit the sale, advertising, and the free distribution of tobacco products and tobacco-related merchandise on campus and at sporting events.

• Provide accessible tobacco treatment on campus, and promote it.

• Prohibit campus organizations, including athletic organizations, from accepting money or other forms of sponsorship from tobacco companies.

• Prohibit the university from holding stock in or accepting donations from the tobacco industry.

>> **Watch videos of real students discussing their experiences with alcohol and tobacco at** MasteringHealth™

Practical Strategies

Quitting Smoking

The National Institutes of Health promote the START method as an effective smoking cessation strategy.

S = Set a quit date.

Choose a date within the next 2 weeks as your official quit date. Smoking cessation experts suggest that you pick a special date as your quit date. Consider your birthday, a special anniversary, New Year's Day, 4th of July, "World No-Tobacco Day" (May 31st), or the "Great American Smokeout" (the third Thursday of November).

T = Tell family, friends, and coworkers that you plan to quit.

If you are going to be successful in your attempt to quit, you will need the help and support of others. So inform the important people in your life and let them know exactly how they can help you in your efforts.

A = Anticipate and plan for the challenges you'll face while quitting.

Studies show that most people who return to smoking do so within the first three months.

Make plans ahead of time for dealing with cravings and withdrawal symptoms when they hit.

R = Remove cigarettes and other tobacco products from your home, car, and work.

Get rid of everything you can that reminds you of smoking. Change your routine, so that certain events and places don't prompt a cigarette craving. Throw away all cigarettes and smoking paraphernalia such as lighters, matches, and ashtrays.

T = Talk to your doctor about getting help to quit.

Your health-care provider can prescribe medication that can help you quit. There are also effective over-the-counter products that are helpful in dealing with nicotine withdrawal. These products include:

- Nicotine gum
- Nicotine inhaler
- Nicotine lozenge
- Nicotine nasal spray
- Nicotine patch
- Bupropion SR pills (prescription only)
- Varenicline pills (prescription only)

For more help: Call 1-877-44U-QUIT (1-877-448-7848) to talk to a smoking cessation counselor from the National Cancer Institute. For help within your own state, call 1-800-QUITNOW (1-800-784-8669) or visit **www.smokefree.gov**.

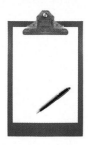

Choosing to Change Worksheet

To complete this worksheet online, visit MasteringHealth™

Alcohol and tobacco are highly addictive drugs that can be very difficult to curb or eliminate from your daily life. The following worksheet can help you work toward a healthier lifestyle. Or, if you are one of the many college students who do not use tobacco and do not drink alcohol or drink only moderately and infrequently, then use this worksheet to interview a friend who struggles with his or her alcohol or tobacco use.

Directions: Fill in your stage of change in Step 1 and complete Steps 2 or 3, depending on which one applies to your stage of change. Step 4 provides information for finding help with a drinking problem.

Step 1: *Your Stage of Behavior Change.* Check one of the following statements that best describes your feelings about your drinking or smoking habits.

_____I do not intend to quit or cut back on my drinking or tobacco use in the next six months. (Precontemplation)

_____I might quit or cut back on my drinking or tobacco use in the next six months. (Contemplation)

_____I am prepared to quit or cut back on my drinking or tobacco use in the next month. (Preparation)

_____I have cut back on my drinking or tobacco use less than six months ago. (Action)

_____I do not drink or use tobacco, or I have cut back on my drinking or tobacco use more than six months ago. (Maintenance)

Step 2: *Precontemplation and Contemplation Stages.* Reread the sections on the physical and behavioral effects of alcohol use or the effects of smoking on health on pages 180–184 or 191–194 and consider how you benefit from continuing your behavior or changing it.

Perceived Benefit of Continuing Excessive Drinking or Tobacco Use *What do I give up if I change?*	Perceived Benefit of Stopping or Modifying Excessive Drinking or Tobacco Use *How will this help me?*
1.	1.
2.	2.
3.	3.
4.	4.
5.	5.
6.	6.

Now, add up your totals: _____ reasons to change _____ reasons to stay the same

What one benefit do you think will motivate you the most? _____

What one barrier do you think will present the biggest obstacle for you? _____

Step 3: *Preparation, Action, and Maintenance Stages.* If you are ready to quit or cut back on your drinking, or have already started, complete the following.

1. What is your SMART goal? If you are in the Preparation stage, create a SMART goal for your change and write it down. If you are in the Action or Maintenance stages, write down the SMART goal you are working with.

_____

_____

2. Identify emotional or situational "triggers." What situations or emotions make you most want to drink or use tobacco? Common triggers include anxiety, boredom, meals, peer pressure, and socializing with friends.

_____

_____

3. Target one of the triggers and substitute an alternate healthier behavior instead of drinking or using tobacco. For example, if you know that you are more likely to drink at the end of a stressful day, instead decide to take a walk or go work out at the gym.

Target trigger: _____

Alternate healthy behavior response: _____

Step 4: Finding Help. If alcohol or tobacco is seriously disrupting your life, seek help. The following websites are two great places to start: **http://findtreatment.samhsa.gov** and **www.smokefree.gov**. Also, keep in mind that most college campuses have student health centers staffed with counselors who can help support you in breaking an alcohol or smoking habit.

Chapter Summary

- Alcohol and tobacco are the most commonly used drugs in the United States and on college campuses. People of traditional college age are among the heaviest users of both of these addictive substances.

- Alcohol is absorbed into the bloodstream from the stomach and small intestine. It is metabolized by the liver. If a person consumes alcohol at a faster rate than the liver can break it down, intoxication occurs.

- Blood alcohol concentration (BAC) is affected by numerous factors, including how much and how quickly alcohol is consumed, type of alcohol, sex, age, weight, physical condition, food intake, and medications.

- The short-term effects of alcohol use include lightheadedness, loss of inhibition, compromised motor coordination, slowed reaction times, slurred speech, dulled senses, dehydration, and hangover. Alcohol also impairs judgment and can lead to high-risk behavior, including impaired driving, unprotected sex, and assault.

- Long-term effects include increased risk of cancer, cardiovascular disease, liver disease, and neurological problems.

- Alcohol dependence is characterized by a tolerance to and craving for alcohol. Breaking the addiction can be challenging, but most people recover completely in time.

- Residential treatment programs, medications, Internet resources, and counseling can help problem drinkers quit drinking and avoid relapse.

- Students smoke for a variety of reasons. Both heredity and the environment are factors, including family and peer exposure, stress, and promotion of smoking in films and other media and advertising.

- The short-term effects of smoking include increased heart rate and blood pressure, shortness of breath, coughing, alertness, decreased skin temperature, increased blood sugar, dulled senses, bad breath, smelling like smoke, and decreased urine production.

- The long-term effects of smoking include increased risk of cancer, cardiovascular disease, respiratory disease, and erectile dysfunction as well as loss of bone density, gum disease, decreased fertility, and premature aging of skin.

- Secondhand smoke contains higher concentrations of some harmful chemicals than the smoke inhaled by smokers. People who inhale secondhand smoke can suffer from the same health problems as smokers. Infants and children are especially vulnerable.

- Nicotine replacement therapies (such as nicotine gums, inhalers, and patches) are designed to help smokers gradually reduce their dependence on nicotine and reduce the severity of withdrawal symptoms.

- Quitting smoking has numerous immediate and long-term health benefits. Many former smokers have found that getting assistance with quitting, often through a health-care provider, is most effective.

GET CONNECTED

 Visit the following websites for more information about the topics in this chapter:

- Rethinking Drinking: Alcohol and Your Health
  http://rethinkingdrinking.niaaa.nih.gov

- Alcoholics Anonymous
  www.aa.org

- Alanon-Alateen
  www.al-anon.alateen.org

- American Lung Association's Freedom from Smoking Online
  www.ffsonline.org

- Centers for Disease Control and Prevention
  www.cdc.gov/tobacco

- National Cancer Institute
  www.smokefree.gov

 MOBILE TIPS!
Scan this QR code with your mobile device to access additional tips about avoiding alcohol and tobacco abuse. Or, via your mobile device, go to **http://chmobile.pearson.com** and navigate to Chapter 8.

Website links are subject to change. To access updated web links, please visit MasteringHealth™

TEST YOUR KNOWLEDGE

1. Blood alcohol concentration can be affected by all of the following except
   a. how expensive the alcohol is.
   b. how much a person drinks.
   c. how fast a person drinks.
   d. how much a person has eaten prior to drinking.

2. A standard drink is
   a. equivalent to 1.5 ounces of 80-proof liquor.
   b. equivalent to 5 ounces of table wine.
   c. equivalent to 12 ounces of beer.
   d. all of these answers.

3. *Binge drinking* is defined as
   a. consuming five or more drinks within 2 hours for men, or four or more drinks within 2 hours for women.
   b. drinking once a day every day.
   c. consuming five or more drinks over the course of a week.
   d. drinking hard liquor.

4. Factors associated with an increased risk for alcohol dependence include
   a. female gender.
   b. poverty.
   c. Asian ethnicity.
   d. initiating drinking at age 21 or over.

5. The long-term effects of alcohol on the body include
   a. increased risk of cancer.
   b. increased risk of cardiovascular disease.
   c. increased risk of liver disease.
   d. all of the answers are correct.

6. What is the key psychoactive ingredient in cigarettes?
   a. ammonia
   b. carbon monoxide
   c. nicotine
   d. formaldehyde

7. The immediate physical effects of smoking include all of the following EXCEPT
   a. increased heart rate and blood pressure.
   b. increased skin temperature.
   c. increased level of blood sugar.
   d. shortness of breath.

8. Each year, how many deaths are due to smoking-related illness?
   a. 1 in 3
   b. 1 in 5
   c. 1 in 7
   d. 1 in 10

9. Quitting smoking
   a. is helped by the fact that nicotine lowers the "feel good" neurotransmitter dopamine.
   b. will provide health benefits as early as 6–12 weeks after smoking.
   c. is difficult in part because excess nicotine-binding receptors in the brain promote craving.
   d. can be aided by beginning a nicotine replacement therapy before you quit.

10. Smokeless tobacco is
    a. thought to be less addictive than cigarettes.
    b. used by about 18% of high school seniors.
    c. associated with an increased risk of cancer.
    d. all of these answers are correct.

Get Critical

What happened

You don't usually encounter a mouthful of yellowed teeth, a set of corroded lungs, or a dead body on product packaging, but in 2011, federal health officials presented these and other graphic images as a new set of warning labels on cigarette packages.[1] The U.S. Food and Drug Administration, in requiring the new labels, said they were needed to give renewed urgency to the dangers of smoking. Tobacco companies, however, sued, saying that mandatory use of the labels violated their right to free speech.[2] After several judges sided with the tobacco companies, the FDA said in 2013 that it would create a new, less dramatic set of warning labels.[3]

An example of the proposed tobacco labels, struck down by the courts.

What do you think?

- Do simple text-only warning labels on tobacco packaging with messages, such as "Smoking is hazardous to your health," go far enough in warning consumers?

- Would a graphic image of illness or death on a product stop you from buying it? Why or why not?

- How should the rights of tobacco companies be balanced against those of consumers, including those of smokers and those of people who inhale secondhand smoke generated by tobacco products?

References: 1. "FDA Unveils Final Cigarette Warning Labels," by the U.S. Food and Drug Administration, June 11, 2011, retrieved from http://www.fda.gov/NewsEvents/Newsroom/PressAnnouncements/ucm260181.htm. 2. "Tobacco Giants Suing FDA over Warning Labels Mandate," by M. Morgenstein, CNN.com, August 17, 2011, retrieved from http://www.cnn.com/2011/HEALTH/08/17/cigarette.labels.lawsuit/index.html. 3. "FDA Changes Course on Graphic Warning Labels for Cigarettes," by S. Almasy, CNN.com, March 20, 2013, retrieved from http://www.cnn.com/2013/03/19/health/fda-graphic-tobacco-warnings.

SOCIAL RELATIONSHIPS AND COMMUNICATION

More than **600 million** people use Facebook **every day**.[i]

Between 2006 and 2010, **48%** of unmarried women aged **15 to 44** lived with a partner for the first time. About **40%** of those couples living together transitioned to **marriage**[ii]

Just **over half** of all American adults are **married**, compared to more than **70% in 1960**.[iii]

Learning Objectives

IDENTIFY the characteristics of effective communication.

UNDERSTAND how self-perception, early relationships, and gender roles influence relationships.

IDENTIFY the benefit of healthy long-term friendships.

DISCUSS different forms of intimate relationships and Sternberg's Triangular Theory of Love.

DESCRIBE at least three different types of committed relationships.

EXPLAIN the factors that should be considered before starting a family.

DISCUSS strategies for building and maintaining healthy relationships.

We are social beings, craving connections with others and the support, love,

and sense of contentment they give us. Our families teach us and guide us through the highs and lows of life. Our friends listen to us, laugh with us, and share in our successes and failures. Our lovers provide us with intimacy, companionship, and comfort. Our relationships with others fulfill us, define us, nurture us, and make us feel safe. Good relationships can relieve stress and, indeed, help keep us healthy.

Relationships, however, take effort to maintain. Being able to speak up, listen well, and resolve conflicts are critical skills to develop for all personal relationships. In this chapter, we discuss the characteristics of effective communication, examine what constitutes a healthy relationship, identify signs of dysfunctional relationships, and explore various categories of committed relationships. Along the way, we will introduce methods of building relationship skills that strengthen healthy ties to friends, colleagues, family, and partners. We will emphasize that although there is no such thing as a perfect relationship or a perfect family, strong unions are based on mutual affection, respect, commitment, companionship, and honesty.

Communication in Relationships

The cornerstone of every successful relationship is effective communication. That idea seems straightforward enough, but in real life, true communication can be challenging. All of us, at times, will experience difficulty in making our thoughts, feelings, and needs known. In addition, understanding the intentions and concerns of others isn't always easy. Effective communication is a skill that can be developed and continually improved. Without it, many relationships fail.

Communicating Feelings

True communication entails much more than just making small talk. It involves sharing honest feelings and other personal information about ourselves—our hopes, our dreams, our secrets, our fears. This kind of sharing, called **self-disclosure,** was first described by psychologist Sidney M. Jourard in his 1971 work, *The Transparent Self*. "If we want to be loved, we must disclose ourselves. If we want to love someone, he must permit us to know him," he wrote. "This would seem to be obvious. Yet most of us spend a great part of our lives thinking up ways to avoid becoming known."[1]

It is not always comfortable to share one's feelings. To do so can leave a person feeling vulnerable and exposed. If you think back through your own life, odds are you have known someone who had difficulty saying "I love you" or telling you what he or she was feeling or thinking. In order to be truly close to another person, however, we need to

self-disclosure The sharing of honest feelings and personal information about yourself with another person.

> *In order to be truly close to another person, however, we need to occasionally let our guard down and speak freely and honestly about what is on our minds."*

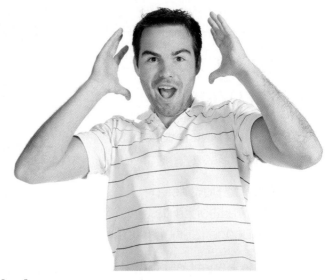

Body language can communicate a lot of information. Do you think this person is relaxed or surprised?

occasionally let our guard down and speak freely and honestly about what is on our minds.

Communication Skills

Especially when dealing with disagreements or other uncomfortable situations, certain communication strategies are helpful:

- **Stay focused.** Focus on the current issue, your feelings about it, and finding a solution.
- **Take responsibility.** Own what is yours and admit when you've made mistakes.
- **Use "I" messages.** Begin the discussion with an "I feel" statement. Making the discussion about the other person may make him or her feel attacked and trigger defensiveness.
- **Listen effectively.** A big part of being a good communicator is being a careful listener.
- **Be solution-focused.** Try to look for a win-win compromise. Effective communication requires that you find a resolution that both parties can be happy with.
- **Step away if necessary.** Sometimes the timing isn't right for resolving a relationship conflict. If tempers flare and the conversation is headed toward an unproductive verbal fight, take a break. But don't just forget about it. Problems don't disappear because you don't talk about them. So return to the issue when it can be approached with a more constructive attitude.
- **Avoid jumping to conclusions or making quick judgments.** Let the other person complete his or her thought before judging. If you have a question about what another person means, ask for a clarification.
- **Resist antagonizing the other person.** For example, resist correcting grammatical errors or nitpicking at other details that do not matter to the real issue at hand.
- **Seek help if you need it.** If you or your partner continues to have difficulty communicating about relationship issues in a constructive way, it may be time to seek help from a counselor or other professional who can help.

Nonverbal Communication

Sometimes you can get a message across without saying a single word. Imagine a teenager who has been out way past her curfew.

---

nonverbal communication
Communication that is conveyed by body language.

When she arrives home, she unlocks the front door and tiptoes inside, hoping to make it to her bedroom unnoticed. But in the living room, she sees her father, still awake in his easy chair, tapping his feet, arms crossed, face scowling. Message received.

Savvy communicators know that it isn't just what you say but *how* you say it that matters. Nonverbal cues such as posture, gestures, eye contact, and even touch help us broadcast our thoughts, whether we realize it or not. This is known as **nonverbal communication,** sometimes called *body language*. If a friend has a glazed-over look in her eyes or is yawning while you are talking, that body language can communicate that she is bored. A person with upright posture and good eye contact conveys confidence, whereas someone who is hunched over and whose eyes dart back and forth communicates nervousness and discomfort. Crossed arms can convey defensiveness—or simply that someone is cold. The ability to ensure that your body language is in tune with what you intend to say is a key characteristic of an effective communicator.

Being a Good Listener

Listening is an integral part of successful communication. Although it might seem like a simple skill, good listening actually requires concentration, focus, and attentiveness. Some strategies for effective listening include:

- **Be silent while another person is sharing his or her feelings or concerns.** Speak up only when you have a question or want to summarize what you have heard.
- **Empathize with what the other person is saying.** If you put yourself in the other person's shoes, you will gain a better perspective of his or her viewpoint.
- **Try to set aside any anger or resentment you may be feeling.** These emotions can interfere with your ability to truly listen.

- **Make other people feel comfortable speaking to you.** This can be done by maintaining eye contact, keeping a relaxed posture, and nodding and smiling so that others know you are listening.
- **Give the speaker your undivided attention.** Get rid of any distractions. Close the door and turn off your cell phone.

Resolving Conflicts

Put any relationship under a microscope and you will see conflicts arise. Conflict is a normal part of relationships because people have different needs, viewpoints, interests, and backgrounds. However, not everyone handles conflicts in the same way. Some people actively avoid discussing their concerns or annoyances, believing that it is better to keep the peace than start what could become an ongoing feud. This communication style is commonly referred to as **conflict avoidance**. Others prefer to be more direct and confrontational and have no problems making it clear when they are unhappy with a situation.

The most effective way to resolve conflict is for two people to voice their concerns maturely and engage in constructive criticism, rather than resort to name calling and finger pointing. Settling disagreements, of course, is not always easy. **Conflict resolution** is an acquired skill. To avoid **conflict escalation,** the opposing parties should agree to fight fair, be respectful, and stay away from personal attacks and put-downs. Strategies for effective conflict resolution include:[2]

- Strive to resolve conflict, rather than to "win."
- Voice your frustrations as soon as possible, rather than allowing them to build up.
- Approach the conflict as you would any other problem that needs to be solved: Define the problem, express the facts (and your feelings) regarding the problem, and listen to possible solutions. You should evaluate each possible solution, agree on one, and make specific plans on how and when to implement it. After a solution is adopted, evaluate it. Is everyone satisfied with the outcome, or would another solution work better?
- Communicate your concerns and opinions clearly, honestly, and directly, instead of expecting the other person to read your mind.
- Listen to the other person's feedback and summarize what you think he or she has said.
- Postpone a discussion to an agreed-upon time if one person is tired or not ready to work on the problem.
- Strive to "fight fair," rather than seeking a quick win by embarrassing the other person. For suggestions, see the **Choose This, Not That** feature on page 206.
- Forgive, forget, and start over.

Gender Roles and Communication

Although both men and women share a common need to communicate information, thoughts, and feelings, research reveals that there are often differences in how they go about it. One of the most fundamental differences is the motivation, or driving force, behind a man and a woman's communication. Men are more likely to communicate in order to perform tasks and seek social status, whereas women are more likely to communicate to build personal connections and seek social interactions.[3] Although individuals often vary, researchers have found that:

- Women seek to connect to others in conversation, whereas men want to be independent information givers.
- Women often want to build consensus before making a decision, whereas men prefer to make decisions expediently on their own.
- Women attempt to minimize differences, whereas men may prefer giving orders and pointing out areas of superiority.[4]

There are also gender differences in overall communication style. In general, these include the following:

- Men speak significantly fewer words each day than women, probably because men like to get to the bottom line and women like to build connections and share details.
- Women process their problems out loud. They will use conversation to think through a problem and work toward a solution. In contrast, men often think through a problem silently, and then verbalize their solution.
- Men are more likely to speak bluntly and state requests directly. Women are more likely to be tactful, use indirect speech, listen, and offer feedback or make requests.
- Women are more likely to use "circular" speech and may change the topic in the middle of a conversation, returning to it later to weave multiple topics together. Men are more likely to be linear communicators and thinkers; they want to finish one topic before going on to another.[5]
- Women are more frequent users of digital communication tools, and prefer directly interactive mediums that more immediately build connections and relationships, such as text messaging or online video calls, to technologies that are less immediately interactive, such as leaving a post in an online forum.[3]

Neither communication style is better or worse, just different. And understanding the differences can improve male-female communication and relationships.

Developing Relationships

Most of us are social creatures from the time we are born, craving closeness and connections to others. And whether we are at home, school, or work, we spend much of our time in the presence of other people. Several personal factors influence how we develop relationships with others, including our self-perception, our early relationships, and cultural gender roles.

conflict avoidance The active avoidance of discussing concerns, annoyances, and conflict with another person.

conflict resolution Resolving a conflict in a manner that both people can accept and that minimizes future occurrences of the conflict.

conflict escalation Increasing conflict to a more confrontational, painful, or otherwise less comfortable level.

Self-Perception

How we relate to others depends, in part, on how good we feel about ourselves, our self-concept. As discussed in Chapter 2, self-esteem is a sense of positive self-regard that results in elevated levels of self-respect, self-worth, self-confidence, and self-satisfaction. People with low self-esteem are more likely to feel lonely and socially isolated. They tend to be preoccupied with the thought of rejection and often behave agreeably toward others because they want to be liked.[6] One psychology professor found that college students with low self-esteem often blame themselves for a

When you want to resolve a **conflict**, you can find common ground productively, or make the problem worse. To settle conflicts in a healthy way:

CHOOSE THIS.

NOT THAT.

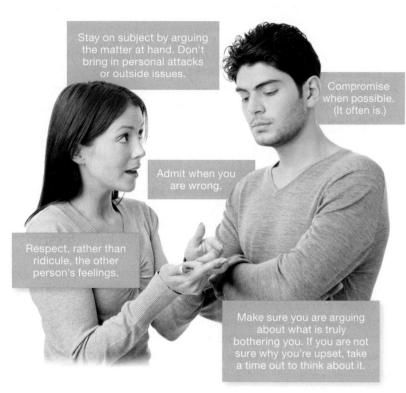

Stay on subject by arguing the matter at hand. Don't bring in personal attacks or outside issues.

Compromise when possible. (It often is.)

Admit when you are wrong.

Respect, rather than ridicule, the other person's feelings.

Make sure you are arguing about what is truly bothering you. If you are not sure why you're upset, take a time out to think about it.

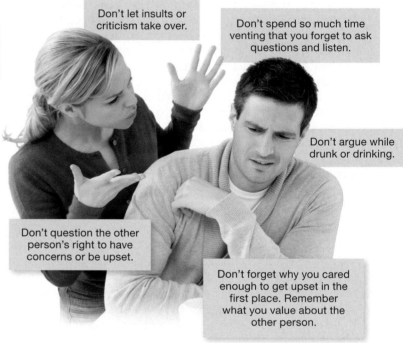

Don't let insults or criticism take over.

Don't spend so much time venting that you forget to ask questions and listen.

Don't argue while drunk or drinking.

Don't question the other person's right to have concerns or be upset.

Don't forget why you cared enough to get upset in the first place. Remember what you value about the other person.

A Fair Fight:

When you are feeling frustrated or angry with someone, it's easy to go on the offensive. But all you'll breed is more anger. Instead, try these tactics.

Full-On "Fight Club":

Do you argue to improve your relationships, or to prove you are right? Set some ground rules when you fight, and don't use fights as an excuse to be mean or hurtful.

boyfriend's or girlfriend's unhappiness, even when other factors are clearly responsible.[6] The finding is true not only of young lovers but of couples in long-term relationships. Researchers have found that even after a decade of marriage, people with low self-esteem misread subtle cues and believe their partners love them far less than they actually do.[7]

Early Relationships

The first relationship we ever experience is the family relationship. Early experiences with our families are important because they help form the template for all subsequent relationships we experience in our lives. Some experts theorize that our relationships with others are patterned after the attachment we had with parents and other caregivers when we were children, a concept known as **attachment theory**.[8] These early interactions may shape our expectations of adult relationships and be responsible for the individual differences in relationship behaviors and needs.[9]

Exactly what constitutes a "family" changes over time, but it is generally defined as a domestic group

attachment theory The theory that the patterns of attachment in our earliest relationships with others form the template for attachment in later relationships.

of people with some degree of kinship, be it through marriage, blood, or adoption. Families today take many different forms, including households headed by single parents, blended families with stepparents and stepsiblings, extended family households with relatives or family friends all living under the same roof, foster families, and gay and lesbian partnerships, to name just a few. There is no perfect or "right" kind of family, but in a healthful family environment, children are respected and nurtured and learn how to have strong relationships of their own.

Gender Roles

Gender roles are the behaviors and tasks considered appropriate by society based on whether we are a man or a woman. Just as many girls are trained at an early age to play with dolls and stuffed animals, boys are encouraged to appreciate cars and trains and to emulate seemingly all-powerful "super heroes." As we grow up, some experts think that beginning in adolescence, girls' tendencies to place greater value on interpersonal connections than boys do can even leave girls more vulnerable to depression and lower self-esteem.[10] In other words, while relationships are important, keeping them in perspective provides a more healthful balance.

Gender roles often extend into adulthood. However, we live in a time of changing gender roles. A generation ago, men were traditionally expected to work and support the family, whereas women were encouraged to stay home to raise the children. Today, many women opt to juggle both family and career, whereas some men make the decision to be stay-at-home fathers. Yet attitudes and stereotypes about gender roles remain. In addition, some research has shown that traditional gender roles become more pronounced in married couples after the birth of a child.[11]

Friendships

Do you have a "BFF" (Best Friend Forever)? If so, you benefit in more ways than one. Besides providing someone to hang out with and confide in, friendships can be important for good health.[12] For example, a study of college freshmen found that those who did not consider themselves lonely had a stronger immune response to a flu vaccine than students who had a small social circle and considered themselves more alone.[13] The quality of that social support matters: It must provide both a sense of belonging and intimacy and must help people to be more competent and feel more capable.

Friendships may be more complex and less immediate today than they have been in the past. One landmark study found that between 1985 and 2004, the number of Americans who felt they have someone to discuss important matters with dropped by almost a third. The study also found that the percentage of people who spoke about important matters only with family members jumped from 57% to 80%.[14] Other research, however, adds perspective to those findings, saying that friendships are shifting under the influences of technology, with weaker virtual friendships sometimes becoming more accessible than in-person contact.[15] The changing nature of friendship doesn't make it any less important, however; loneliness can harm your health. One study showed that college students with lower levels of social support were more likely to experience mental health problems, including a sixfold risk of depressive symptoms.[16] Loneliness is also associated with stress and poor life satisfaction.[16] See Chapter 2 for more on loneliness.

gender roles Behaviors and tasks considered appropriate by society based on whether someone is a man or a woman.

Good Friends

"HI, I'M BRITTANY and this is my friend Sandy. We're both freshmen and we've been friends for about a semester now, ever since we became neighbors in our dorm. We started eating dinner together occasionally and then began hanging out more and more often. We like the same music, we study together, go to the gym, and just hang out and have fun. Recently both of my parents were laid off, and Sandy has been really great in helping me deal with it; she listens to me talk and I feel like she's really there for me. In a few weeks, a group of us are going to Florida for spring break, and next year, we're even going to get an apartment together. I thought it was going to be difficult making friends in college but I'm so glad I've found such a good one already!"

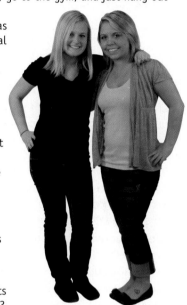

1. What are the benefits of Brittany and Sandy's friendship? What personal and environmental factors helped make them friends?

2. Why do you think Brittany confided in Sandy about her parents being laid off? How did Sandy help?

3. What can Brittany and Sandy do to make sure that they have a good living situation when they move in together next year?

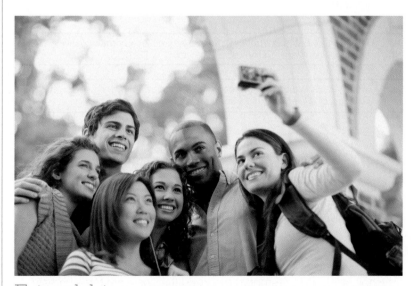

Friendships with others can boost emotional and physical health.

> ## "Friendships can be some of the longest, most-fulfilling relationships in your life, outlasting romantic relationships and even marriages."

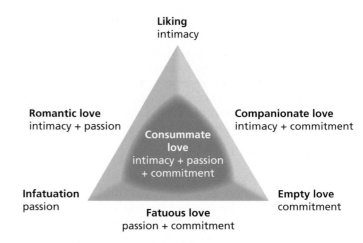

FIGURE 9.1 Sternberg's Triangular Theory of Love.

Source: Robert J. Sternberg, "A Triangular Theory of Love," *Psychological Review*, Volume 93(2), pp. 119–135, April 1986. American Psychological Association. Reprinted with permission.

Maintaining Old Friendships

Friendships can be some of the longest, most-fulfilling relationships in your life, outlasting romantic relationships and even marriages. But the demands of being a student can make it hard to keep up with older friendships. If you are struggling with maintaining your tried-and-true relationships now that you're in college, follow these tips:

- **Understand that you and your friends are changing.** Don't be afraid to show how you're changing, and don't expect your friends to stay exactly the same either.

- **Don't overwhelm old friends with information about your college life.** It's exciting to fill in your friends with what you are doing now, but be sure to listen to their stories as well.

- **Keep in touch.** Phone, email, voice over Internet services like Skype, instant messaging, and social networking applications like Facebook and Twitter are all great ways to update your friends about what you're doing and hear from them. However, if you really want to maintain a friendship with someone, take the time to send him or her a personal message or pick up the phone.

- **Don't be afraid to reconnect.** If you've lost touch with an old friend, research indicates that you can still rekindle the friendship even after years without contact.[17]

>> **Listen to this National Public Radio story on college friendships:** www.npr.org/templates/story/story.php?storyId=112330125.

>> **These videos explore the effects of social networking:** www.pbs.org/wgbh/pages/frontline/digitalnation/relationships/socializing.

Intimate Relationships

Intimacy is the emotionally open and caring way of relating to another person. An intimate relationship is usually one that is deep and has evolved over time, in which two people feel safe and comfortable sharing their innermost thoughts and secrets.

Sternberg's Triangular Theory of Love

Psychologist Robert Sternberg theorized that there are three primary components of healthy, loving relationships:

- **Intimacy.** The emotional component. Intimacy is the feeling of closeness and connectedness experienced in loving relationships.

- **Passion.** The motivational component. Passion is the intensity that fuels romance, physical attraction, and sex.

- **Commitment.** The cognitive component. Commitment is the short-term decision to love another person and the long-term decision to stay committed to maintaining that love.[18]

Sternberg used the shape of a triangle to illustrate his theory, which he called the Triangular Theory of Love **(Figure 9.1)**. Sternberg postulated that the type and intensity of love a couple experiences depends on the strength of each of the three components in their relationship. The factors can be combined to characterize seven different types of love:

- **Liking.** Liking is intimacy alone. A closeness to another person, without passionate feelings or a long-term commitment.

- **Infatuation.** Infatuation is passion alone. Also known as "love at first sight."

- **Empty love.** Empty love is commitment alone. The passion is not there and neither is the intimacy. This can be found in some stagnant relationships or just before a couple breaks up.

- **Romantic love.** Romantic love is passion and intimacy without commitment. Physical attraction with an emotional bond.

- **Companionate love.** Companionate love is commitment and intimacy without passion. It is essentially a committed friendship in which the passion has died down, as sometimes occurs in people who have been married a long time.

- **Fatuous love.** Fatuous love is commitment and passion without intimacy. A whirlwind romance that often does not last very long.

- **Consummate love.** Consummate love is the whole package: intimacy, passion, and commitment. The kind of love many of us strive for.[18]

Sternberg also identified an eighth category—nonlove—which is the absence of intimacy, passion, and commitment. This type of casual interaction makes up the majority of our relationships with other people.

---

intimacy A sense of closeness with another person formed by being emotionally open and caring.

Social Media, Communication, and CYBER-BULLIES

On February 4, 2004, Harvard computer science student Mark Zuckerberg launched "Thefacebook" and forever changed the world of social connections—and sometimes, unfortunately, social torment.[1]

Originally used only by Harvard students, Facebook has become a driving force in social media and an almost essential tool for socializing in our modern world. Despite lots of competition from Twitter, Google Plus, YouTube, and MySpace, Facebook (together with its subsidiary Instagram) is still the leading social networking site with more than one billion active members throughout the world.[2] More than half of its members actively use at least one of Facebook's platforms every day.[2] One study of college students found that Facebook made a meaningful difference in maintaining connections in a geographically mobile world, such as letting students stay close to friends from high school now going to school elsewhere.[3]

Despite the popularity of Facebook and other social media, they are not without critics. Privacy proponents worry that members' information is too easily accessed by those with both personal and business motives. Social critics say that real-world connections are being neglected for less meaningful ones online. On campuses, professors complain that students are wasting a tremendous amount of time on Facebook that could be spent studying and that students are distracted in class because they are using Facebook. Professors at some U.S. colleges have even banned laptops from classrooms because of social media such as Facebook.[4]

Using Social Media in a Healthy Way

Regardless of criticisms, social media such as Facebook is here to stay. You can communicate

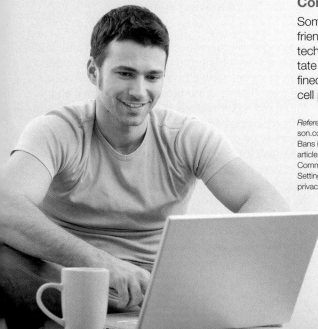

through social media in a healthy way by following a few tips:[5]

- **Limit your number of friends.** Limit your friends list to those you really care about, or use Facebook's tools to create a circle of truly close friends with whom you can maintain meaningful connections.

- **Don't tag friends in unflattering photos.** If you aren't sure, don't tag it.

- **Manage your profile settings.** You may not want your boss or professor seeing your photos from last weekend. So, if you have both personal and professional "friends," make sure you know how to use the custom settings to control what specific people can see.

- **Think before you post.** Don't post anything you wouldn't say in real life or don't want the entire Internet to read.

- **Don't list personal info.** Never post your address, phone number, class schedule, or any other personal information that you don't want thousands of people to know.

- **Activate privacy settings.** Most social media sites have several privacy settings that you can use to control the amount of information other people see. These often change, so stay on top of how your information can be used and shared.

- **Limit the amount of time you spend on social media.** Because information (even if it is trivial information) is updated constantly on social media, it can become addicting. Why not ignore your virtual friends for a while and spend some face-to-face time with your real live friends?

Confronting Cyber-Bullying

Sometimes, unfortunately, social media is far from friendly. Outlets such as Facebook, along with technologies like texting, have been used to facilitate *cyber-bullying*. This type of harassment, defined as repeated, deliberate harm inflicted through cell phones, computers, or other electronic

devices, is meant to inflict embarrassment and emotional pain, sometimes with tragic results. About 20% of 11- to 18-year-olds admit to harassing others in this manner.[6] One study of college students found that about 22% said they had been victims of cyber-bullying.[7] In high-profile cases around the country, teens and young adults have been victims of assaults related to cyber-bullying, and some victims have even committed suicide.[8, 9]

If cyber-bullying is affecting you or someone you know, a few quick actions can help confront the problem:[10]

- **Call out the bullying for what it is.** Don't assume the bullying is a one-time occurrence that will pass. Don't ignore the problem, which only encourages further harassment. Acknowledge the issue as something serious and harmful, and take it seriously.

- **Support the victim.** Let him or her know that the harassment is not his or her fault. Don't blame the target of the abuse.

- **Don't be a bystander.** Whether in person or online, bullies often seek an audience. Don't stand by and watch. Let the bully know that the harassment is not acceptable, and take steps to help the victim feel supported and safe.

- **Think before you post.** It's easy for comments to be taken out of context online and for situations to escalate with a simple click. Rather than going for an easy laugh at someone else's expense, think about what you are about to say. Would you want someone to say it about you, or post a similar photo of you?

- **Model how to treat others with respect.** In the online world, your actions and thoughts are visible to those in your circle. By avoiding bullying behavior, and calling out others who engage in it, you help create online spaces that are safer—and more fun—for everyone.

>> **Visit Facebook's anti-bullying page at** www.facebook.com/help/420576171311103.

References: **1.** "Hundreds Register for New Facebook Website," by Alan Tabak, February 9, 2004, *Harvard Crimson,* retrieved from http://www.thecrimson.com/article.aspx?ref=357292. **2.** *Key Facts,* Facebook Newsroom, retrieved April 6, 2013, from http://newsroom.fb.com/Key-Facts. **3.** "Laptop Bans in Classes Receive Mixed Reaction," by J. Luther, January 26, 2012, *The Chronicle,* Duke University, retrieved from http://www.dukechronicle.com/articles/2012/01/27/laptop-bans-classes-receive-mixed-reaction. **4.** Me and My 400 Friends: The Anatomy of College Students' Facebook Networks, Their Communication Patterns, and Well-Being," by A. Manago, T. Taylor, & P. M. Greefield, 2012, *Developmental Psychology, 48*(2), pp. 369–380. **5.** "10 Privacy Settings Every Facebook User Should Know," by N. O'Neill, February 2, 2009, *All Facebook,* retrieved from http://www.allfacebook.com/2009/02/facebook-privacy. **6.** "School-Based Efforts to Prevent Cyberbullying," by J. W. Patchin & S. Hinduja, 2012, *The Prevention Researcher, 19*(1), pp. 7–9. **7.** "Bullying Still Occurs in College, Professors Find," by Indiana State University, 2011, retrieved from http://www.indstate.edu/news/news.php?newsid=2904. **8.** "Ohio Teenagers Guilty in Rape That Social Media Brought to Light," by R. Oppel, March 17, 2013, *New York Times,* retrieved from http://www.nytimes.com/2013/03/18/us/teenagers-found-guilty-in-rape-in-steubenville-ohio.html?pagewanted=all&_r=0. **9.** "Rutgers Suicide: Man Who Filmed Gay Roommate Sentenced to 30 Days," by M. Hughes, May 21, 2012, *The Guardian,* retrieved from http://www.telegraph.co.uk/news/worldnews/northamerica/usa/9280850/Rutgers-suicide-man-who-filmed-gay-room-mate-sentenced-to-30-days.html. **10.** "Respond to Bullying," by the U.S. Department of Health & Human Services (publication date not provided), retrieved from http://www.stopbullying.gov/respond/index.html.

How to Be a Healthy Couple

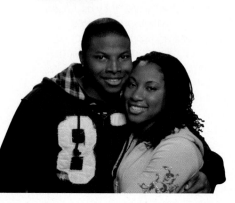

"HI, WE'RE JONATHAN AND YEANI, and we've been a couple for six months. There are a lot of obstacles that we face in our relationship, especially when it comes to juggling our schoolwork in addition to all the other aspects of our lives. At times, things seem hard. We each get stressed out by school and we can get on each others' nerves, but it's nice to have someone to lean on, and to know that you don't have to go through all your problems alone. For us, communication and trust have really helped make our relationship successful. Our best advice to new couples trying to make things work in college is to be open with one another, and don't be afraid to express your concerns, doubts, fears, or any other emotions with your partner."

1. Do you think juggling a relationship with school is a common source of stress for college couples? What can you do to help balance school and relationship time?

2. Why do you think Jonathan and Yeani chose to be in a relationship rather than just hooking up?

3. Do you agree with their advice for new couples in college? What else do you think college couples should do to keep their relationship healthy?

What Causes Attraction?

You have probably heard the saying "opposites attract," but scientists have found the opposite to be true. Studying the factors that bring two people together for a romantic relationship reveals that we tend to pick partners who are a lot like us—who are of similar economic class, educational level, religion, and racial or ethnic group and who share the same interests or values. This tendency to be attracted to people who share some of our characteristics is known as **assortative mating.** Some studies have also found that we look for people who share a similar level of physical attractiveness to us, with more attractive people being more particular about the physical attractiveness of their potential partners.[19]

Beauty, of course, is more than skin deep. Who we are and how we behave also influence whether others are attracted to us. One study found that men and women who were honest or helpful were perceived as better looking. Those who were rude or unfair or displayed other negative traits were generally considered to be less attractive.[20]

Although similarities in physique may bring us together, it is similarity in personality—and a generous attitude toward one's partner—that appears to be most indicative of whether the relationship will be a happy and lasting one.[21] Why? In one study, researchers found that when they asked members of couples to both describe their own personality traits and their partner's, it was those couples who described each other more generously than they described themselves who also had the highest levels of marital satisfaction.[21] In other words, not only sharing personality traits but seeing those positive traits magnified in one's partner appears to build enduring bonds.

Dating

Dating—that is, spending time with another person one-on-one to determine whether there is an attraction or a desire to see more of one another—has evolved over the years. In earlier generations, men would typically ask women out on a formal date, and steady dating would be considered a "courtship" intended to lead to marriage. But that linear path has been replaced by a less direct one, in which couples often meet through friends and get to know each other in groups or by spending time together more casually. If the relationship progresses, many young couples often live together before marriage.[22] A formal date is often now viewed as "the old way," or an event saved for special occasions.

Hooking Up

On campus, the concept of dating has largely been replaced with **hooking up**—casual, noncommittal, physical encounters that may range from kissing and "making out" to oral sex and intercourse. "Hooking up on college campuses has become more frequent than dating in heterosexual sexual interaction," noted one study.[23] However, although hooking up may be common, that does not mean it is popular with everyone. The same study found that men prefer this type of interaction, whereas women tend to prefer dating. Many students have had negative "hook-up" experiences. Because hooking up is often fueled by alcohol, your judgment during the encounter can be impaired. Some of the negative effects from hooking up include negative impact on psychological well-being and social status; regrets; decreased relationship skills; and sexual risk taking, including an increased likelihood of sexually transmitted infections (STIs) and unplanned pregnancy.[24, 25]

Some relationships experts are concerned that hooking up doesn't help today's singles learn the skills needed to build intimacy and test out whether someone would be a good marriage partner.

Online Dating

Online dating is now a dating mainstay, especially in the years after college, when life off-campus makes it harder to meet potential partners. Dating services are a booming business. Popular sites such as eHarmony.com, Match.com, and OKCupid report millions of users each month. These services assist members in finding suitable partners by providing a place where they can both advertise themselves online with a personal profile and view the profiles of others looking for partners. Members search profiles using criteria such as sex, age, location, and interests. Online dating easily and effectively increases the pool of potential partners. Also, because face-to-face meetings are not immediate, potential partners have the

assortative mating The tendency to be attracted to people who are similar to us.

hooking up Casual, noncommittal, physical encounters that may range from kissing and "making out" to oral sex and intercourse.

opportunity to build their relationships via phone calls, texting, email, and other technology before that first face-to-face encounter.

It's important to remember that online dates are basically strangers. So in order to stay safe while using an online dating service, keep these precautions in mind:

- Never give out your full name, address, or other personal information until you have met the person and are sure he or she is trustworthy.
- Make sure to meet your date in a public place, like a restaurant or café. Avoid going to isolated places with a new date, and don't arrange to meet at your home. Always tell a friend beforehand what you are doing and where you are going.
- If something doesn't feel right when you meet the person, don't be afraid to cut your date short.

Same-Sex Relationships

About nine million people in the United States identify as lesbian, gay, bisexual, transgender, queer or questioning, or intersex (LGBTQI).[26] Researchers estimate that about 3% of college students are gay or lesbian, although they caution that obtaining exact numbers is difficult because some students may not feel comfortable sharing information about their sexual orientation.[27] In many ways committed **homosexual** couples are similar to committed **heterosexual,** or straight, couples.[28] Studies conclude that long-term same-sex couples are just as committed and satisfied in their relationships as heterosexual married couples.[28, 29] In at least one study, same-sex couples reported more positive feelings toward their partners and less conflict than married straight couples.[29] Indeed, same-sex couples often have more egalitarian or equal relationships because they do not subscribe to traditional gender roles. If there is a major difference, it is seen in lesbian couples—whom scientists have found are "especially effective at working together harmoniously."[28]

>> **Online support for students struggling with their sexual identities can be found at** www.hrc.org/campaigns/coming-out-center#.UYMKkLVJOAh, www.glsen.org, **and** http://lgbtq.gmu.edu/coming-out/.

Yet one striking difference for LGBTQI couples is the disapproval and discrimination that same-sex couples often face from society or even from family. Many states do not allow homosexual couples to marry or adopt children, and some religions frown upon homosexuality. This can make homosexual couples feel stigmatized, isolated, and powerless. Societal attitudes and pressures against homosexuality, including **homonegativity**—unfavorable views of a person because he or she is, or is perceived to be, homosexual—or **homophobia**—a fear and hatred of homosexuality—can also discourage intimacy between same-sex friends if it makes them fear being labeled as gay or lesbian.[30]

Chapter 10 discusses issues related to homosexuality in more detail.

Healthy Relationships

Successful relationships are built on trust, respect, and communication. They enable each individual to retain his or her own identity and foster personal growth rather than smothering it.

Some people have an idealized view of healthy relationships, believing that they are free of conflict and require little effort to maintain. However, no deep, intimate relationship is without

homosexual A person sexually attracted to someone of the same sex.

heterosexual A person sexually attracted to someone of the opposite sex.

homonegative Having an unfavorable view of a person who is homosexual or who is perceived to be homosexual.

homophobia Fear and hatred of homosexuality.

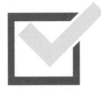

SELF-ASSESSMENT
Is My Relationship Healthy?

Check "Yes" or "No" in response to each of the following questions.

1. I am very satisfied with how we talk to each other. ____ Yes ____ No
2. We are creative in how we handle our differences. ____ Yes ____ No
3. We feel very close to each other. ____ Yes ____ No
4. My partner is seldom too controlling. ____ Yes ____ No
5. When discussing problems, my partner understands my opinions and ideas. ____ Yes ____ No
6. I am completely satisfied with the amount of affection from my partner. ____ Yes ____ No
7. We have a good balance of leisure time spent together and separately. ____ Yes ____ No
8. My partner's friends or family rarely interfere with our relationship. ____ Yes ____ No
9. We agree on how to spend money. ____ Yes ____ No
10. I am satisfied with how we express spiritual values and beliefs. ____ Yes ____ No

HOW TO INTERPRET YOUR SCORE
The more you replied "yes" to these statements, the more likely you are to be part of a happy couple.

To complete this Self-Assessment online, visit MasteringHealth™

Source: Adapted from *Empowering Couples: Building on Your Strengths* by D. H. Olson, & A. K. Olson. Copyright © 2000 by Prepare-Enrich / Life Innovations, Inc., Minneapolis, MN. Reprinted with permission.

challenges. Well-adjusted couples learn how to steer clear of avoidable problems and to be respectful, supportive, and sensitive to each others' feelings. With cooperation and compromise, as well as a commitment to work together, couples can help each other through some of the most trying times of life—the loss of a job, the death of a parent or child, or the onset of a chronic, debilitating disease. The **Practical Strategies** box on page 212 provides tips for maintaining a strong and healthy relationship.

How do you know if your intimate relationship is a healthy one? Are you at a point in your relationship where the negatives are outweighing the positives? Taking a step back and assessing the strength of your relationship with a boyfriend, girlfriend, or partner can be illuminating. The **Self-Assessment** above is one place to start.

Dysfunctional Relationships

Whereas some relationships are uplifting, others are toxic, becoming more of a burden than a joy. Dysfunctional relationships can come in many forms, with one or both partners being manipulative, controlling, mean, disrespectful, or even verbally or physically abusive.

This kind of negative behavior is often learned early in the home. Children observe how their parents relate to each other, and often think the hostile

Practical Strategies

Although there is no simple recipe for success, the following strategies can help you maintain a strong, healthy relationship with your boyfriend, girlfriend, spouse, or partner:

- **Be honest with the other person.** Strive to maintain a warm, comfortable relationship in which you can confide in each other about virtually anything.

- **Trust and respect each other.** Be able to disagree without using put-downs or threats. Try to understand the other person's feelings, even if you don't share his or her ideas.

- **Communicate effectively.** Ask how your loved one thinks and feels, rather than expecting him or her to be a mind reader. Offer empathy when needed.

- **Give your loved one freedom and encouragement.** Recognize that each person has the right to his or her own opinions, feelings, friends, and dreams.

- Encourage each other's enjoyment and success in life.

- **Encourage common interests and shared activities.** Engage in activities and hobbies you both like, including new ones. Discovering and learning new things together builds bonds and helps keep your relationship fresh.

- **Be kind to one another.** Help each other out and show care through consistent respect rather than abuse followed by apologies.

- **Be appreciative.** Remind yourself of all the good things that you admire about your loved one.

- **Be attentive, every day.** Each morning, try asking yourself, "What can I do for 5 minutes today to make my partner's life better?"

- **Share decision making.** Make decisions together, rather than tell each other what to do.[1, 2]

References: **1.** Adapted from *Characteristics of a Healthy and Enjoyable Friendship or Dating Relationship,* by Employee Assistance, retrieved from http://www.eap.partners.org/WorkLife/Relationships/Healthy_Relationships/Characteristics_of_a_Healthy_and_Enjoyable_Friendship_or_Dating_Relationship.asp. (Originally from Liz Claiborne, Inc.) **2.** "That Loving Feeling Takes a Lot of Work," by J. Brody, January 14, 2013, *New York Times,* retrieved from http://well.blogs.nytimes.com/2013/01/14/that-loving-feeling-takes-a-lot-of-work/?src=me&ref=general.

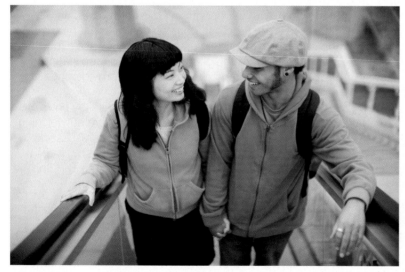

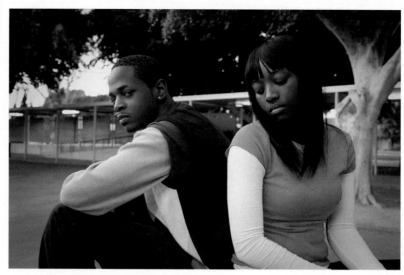

Addressing problems in relationships can help you fix them.

or unhealthy ways they interact are normal. Research has shown that adolescents who witnessed their parents' marital violence were more likely to be physically aggressive toward romantic partners themselves.[31] Similarly, adolescents exposed to marital discord tended to have conflict in their own marriages many years later.[31]

Often, the signs that a relationship is dysfunctional or somehow amiss are subtle:[32]

- You focus on the other person at the expense of yourself.
- You feel pressured to change to meet your partner's ideals.
- Your partner expects you to justify what you do and whom you see, or you expect your partner to.
- One of you makes all the decisions without listening to the other's input.
- You are afraid to disagree, and your ideas are criticized.
- You lie to each other.
- You feel stifled and trapped, unable to escape the pressures of the relationship.
- You or your partner is addicted to drugs or alcohol and it impacts your relationship.

If you have noticed any of these signs in your relationship, it may be time to think about whether it is indeed a good match for you.

Another problem that can damage relationships is **jealousy.** In relationships, jealousy is defined as the response to a threat to a relationship from an actual or imagined rival for a partner's attention.[33] Although it is natural to feel jealous once in a while, jealousy becomes serious when it is a precursor to domestic violence or interferes with the relationship in other ways. Jealousy is associated with low self-esteem, irrational thinking, depression, divorce, and physical violence. It is not a marker of true love, but rather insecurity, immaturity, and a need to be in control. An underlying cause of extreme jealousy is a fear of abandonment. Ironically, the behavior of extremely jealous partners often makes these fears come true.

jealousy The response to a threat to a relationship from an actual or imagined rival for a partner's attention.

Experts suggest that couples deal with jealousy directly and attempt to talk about the feelings underlying it. Often, talking about what sparks the jealousy may be enough to reduce it. If you are suffering from jealousy yourself, work on building your self-esteem because low self-esteem is one of the sources of jealousy. If your partner is jealous, be available and respond to his or her concerns, offer reassurance, and keep in mind that changes do not happen immediately and sometimes counseling may even be needed to help you and your partner move forward.[34]

There is one situation that demands that you immediately leave a relationship: physical abuse. If a partner is threatening you physically or is being physically abusive to you or your children, remove yourself and your children from the relationship as soon as possible. Chapter 14 discusses physical abuse and domestic violence in more detail.

When Relationships End

Despite our best efforts, many relationships eventually end. Those that lead to marriage are still vulnerable to the problems that can eventually result in a split: infidelity, jealousy, competitiveness, illness, money problems, and growing apart.

Breaking up, however, can be difficult, especially if you were not the initiator. Recovering from a failed relationship takes time and effort. Strategies that can facilitate the recovery process include:[35]

- **Talk about it.** Share your feelings with a good friend or family member.
- **Focus on what is good about you.** Resist the urge to blame yourself and exaggerate your faults while mending a broken heart.
- **Take care of yourself.** Exercise, eat well, and get plenty of sleep.
- **Let your emotions out.** Do not be afraid to cry.
- **Do things you normally enjoy.** Have some fun.
- **Keep yourself busy.** Get your mind off your pain for awhile.
- **Give yourself time to recover.** Recognize that your hurt will not go away overnight.

Committed Relationships

Most adults value having a committed relationship with another person. Nationwide surveys reveal that about two-thirds of unmarried adults say a long-term committed relationship is integral to having a fulfilling life.[36] Committed relationships come in various forms, including cohabitation, marriage, and domestic partnerships.

Cohabitation

One of the greatest transformations in family life in the United States during the last century has been the significant increase in **cohabitation**—unmarried couples living together under the same roof. Many couples today opt to live together before getting engaged or married. Some continue in long-term, committed relationships without ever tying the knot. Cohabitation is now so common and accepted in our society that researchers estimate more than 60% of couples in the United States now live together before getting married.[37] For some, cohabitation represents a chance to get to know each other better before taking marriage vows. Others choose to cohabit to benefit from the companionship, intimacy, and shared living costs cohabitation allows.

There is also a downside to cohabitation. Most cohabiting couples are denied the legal and financial benefits afforded to married couples. These

cohabitation The state of living together in the same household; usually refers to unmarried couples.

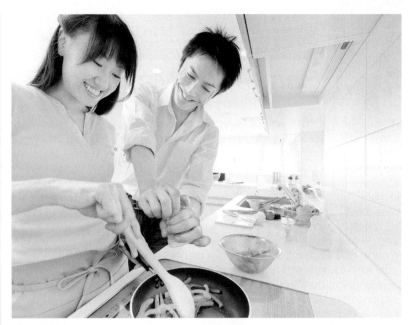

Cohabitation can have benefits, but it also has drawbacks.

include family leave, Social Security benefits after the death of a partner, and access to a lover's pension, health insurance coverage, and untaxed retirement savings.[38] In addition, cohabiting couples in the United States report the lowest levels of wealth among household types. Their relationships may also be less stable. One study found that nearly 40% of unmarried, cohabiting parents in their 20s who had a baby between 2000 and 2005 split up by the time their child was five, which is a separation rate three times higher than that for parents in their 20s who were married when they had a child.[39] One theory for these differences is that marriage fosters certain behavior changes by the couple and those around them that cohabitation just doesn't encourage.[40] The newest research is hopeful, however, indicating that these trends may be changing as cohabitation becomes more common and accepted in society. It also shows that cohabiting couples who are engaged before they move in together may be more successful than couples who live together but have no plans to marry.[41]

Marriage

Between 85% and 90% of Americans will marry during their lifetime.[42] Despite the increasingly casual nature of many of our romantic relationships, marriage remains so valued that it is the focus of a major social struggle: Same-sex couples have been waging an intense legal and political battle to have their unions recognized and legalized around the country. See the **Diversity & Health** box for more information.

Aside from its romantic associations, marriage has practical implications, benefits, and obligations. It is a legally binding contract, giving a sense of legitimacy to the relationship in the eyes of society and the law.[43] It signals to others that each spouse has entered into a long-term commitment that carries with it expectations of fidelity, mutual support, and lifetime partnership.

Benefits of Marriage

Study after study has shown that marriages in general—and good marriages in particular—provide a wealth of physical, psychological, and financial

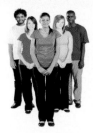

DIVERSITY & HEALTH

Same-Sex Marriage: The State of Our Current Debate

When, in early 2013, President Barack Obama, Vice-President Joe Biden, and former Secretary of State Hillary Clinton all voiced their support of gay marriage, they joined a growing group of politicians who have endorsed the rights of same-sex couples to marry. It also reenergized the discussion and debate about same-sex marriage in this country.

The issue of same-sex marriage can be polarizing. Perhaps that's because it exposes differences in our interpretation of certain doctrines we hold "sacred"—from the American ethic of fairness to religious and cultural teachings. For instance, some proponents of same-sex marriage argue that the guarantees of equal protection and due process in the United States Constitution require that same-sex couples be treated no differently from heterosexual couples. At the same time, opponents argue that marriage is an institution founded to promote

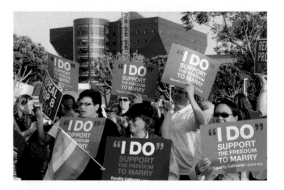

Same-sex marriage continues to be a controversial issue in the United States.

and protect the need to procreate and, therefore, can only occur between a male and a female.

What's at stake? Although the debate is certainly fueled by a clash of values, far more significant are the rights that marriage brings. In 2004, a federal report identified a total of 1,138 federal statutory provisions in which marital status is a factor in determining or receiving benefits, rights, and privileges.[1] A couple's status can affect whether they are entitled to certain tax advantages, health-care benefits, community property rights, and rights to surviving children. Moreover, homosexual couples have been denied the right to become foster parents and adoptive parents, to petition for their partners to immigrate, and to become residents in the same nursing home. Until recently, same-sex partners could even be denied the right to visit each other in the hospital: A ruling of the Department of Health and Human Services requiring hospitals to recognize gay and lesbian partners' visitation rights just took effect in 2011.

Recently, federal law has been changing with regard to same-sex marriages. The Defense of Marriage Act (DOMA), passed in 1996, allowed states to refuse to recognize same-sex marriages that were legal in other states.[2] Additionally, Section 3 of DOMA required that federal benefit programs define marriage as the union of one man and one woman, excluding same-sex partners from benefits they might otherwise have. However, in 2013, the U.S. Supreme Court overturned Section 3 of DOMA as unconstitutional.

Although same-sex marriages are now recognized by the federal government, individual states still have the right to decide whether they will recognize or grant gay and lesbian unions.

So, where in the United States is it possible for homosexual partners to marry? The answer to this question is continually changing due to shifts in the courts and at the ballot box. As of this writing, same-sex marriage is currently recognized in the District of Columbia and 14 states: California, Connecticut, Delaware, Illinois, Iowa, Maine, Maryland, Massachusetts, New Hampshire, New Jersey, New York, Rhode Island, Vermont, and Washington.

What is the future of same-sex marriage in the United States? Although no one can say for sure, dozens of polls conducted over the past decade show that the percentage of Americans who favor legal marriage between homosexual partners is inching upward. Despite generational, political, and regional differences, America's overall support for same-sex marriage is growing.

Critical-Thinking Questions

1. Do you think same-sex couples should have the legal right to marry? Why or why not?

2. Do you think same-sex marriages recognized in one state should be recognized in other states? What are the implications for couples if such marriages are not recognized state-to-state?

3. Why do you think younger Americans tend to be more supportive of same-sex marriage than older generations?

References: **1.** *Defense of Marriage Act: Update to Prior Report,* by the U.S. General Accounting Office, January 23, 2004, GAO-04-353R, Washington, DC. **2.** "Same-Sex Marriage: Legal Issues," by A. M. Smith, August 18, 2010, *Congressional Research Service,* 7-5700; RL31994, retrieved from http://assets.opencrs.com/rpts/RL31994_20100818.pdf.

benefits. The longer a person stays married, in fact, the more the benefits accrue.[43] The benefits include:

- **Better mental health.** Married people tend to be happier and more satisfied with their lives, on average, than unmarried people, according to an analysis of 22 studies.[44]

- **Better physical health and longer life expectancies.** Being married is linked to fewer sick days, less use of hospital facilities, and less likelihood of having chronic health conditions.[44] Married men can expect to live, on average, at least seven years longer than never-married men, whereas married women tend to live at least three years longer than their never-married counterparts.[44]

- **Better financial health.** Married couples tend to have higher household incomes than unmarried people.[45]

Are married people healthier because they are married? Or is it that healthier people are somehow more likely to get married? Although researchers suspect that both could be at play, there is evidence that marriage fosters healthful and helpful behaviors. For example, married couples generally drink less, exercise more, get more sleep, and visit the doctor more often than people who are not married.[46]

Separation and Divorce

"Till death do us part" is a phrase that is often included in marriage vows. For about half the couples getting married for the first time, however, the marriage will end not when one person passes away, but when one decides to file for divorce.[47] Divorce has become an increasingly common and accepted practice in the United States, as the moral and social stigmas surrounding it have greatly diminished. Divorce rates

> ❝ *Study after study has shown that marriages in general—and good marriages in particular—provide a wealth of physical, psychological, and financial benefits.* ❞

actually peaked in the early 1980s, and the rate of divorces and annulments has gone down slightly since then; over the past several years they have stabilized at just under 50%.[48]

Researchers attribute the divorce rate to a number of factors, including society's increasingly high expectations for marriage. During the 1950s and early 1960s, surveys of college students demonstrated that marriage was sought after because of the opportunities it afforded couples—namely, the chance to own a home, live a stable lifestyle, and have children. Nowadays, college students say they value marriage because they believe it will provide them with emotional fulfillment.[49]

Risk factors for divorce include a pattern of negative interactions between spouses, having parents who are divorced, marrying under the age of 21, and reacting strongly or defensively to problems and disappointments.[50] For those in really bad marriages, divorce can represent a relief, an end to seemingly never-ending marital woes.[51] For most people, though, divorce results in a crisis that causes severe emotional pain and distress to the entire family. Whereas adults often experience temporary stress and sadness, their children may develop long-term emotional problems that can get worse as they grow older.[52] Children of divorced parents are 50% more likely to get a divorce themselves one day.[53]

There are factors that decrease your risk of divorce. Divorce rates are lowest for people with at least some college, who have annual incomes over $50,000, who are religious, who have parents who are married, and who wait until the age of 25 to marry and have children.[42]

Domestic Partnerships

Although same-sex marriages are still not permitted in many states, **domestic partnerships** often are. In a domestic partnership, a couple lives together, stays in a long-term committed relationship, and legally registers as domestic partners. In return, they often have access to their partner's employer-sponsored benefits such as health insurance and bereavement leave. Domestic partnerships are also recognized by some states, counties, and cities, and give couples access to

> **domestic partnership** A legal arrangement in which a couple lives together in a long-term committed relationship and receives some, but not all, of the rights of married couples.

» This interactive map can help you learn about same-sex marriage and domestic partnership legislation for each state: www.npr.org/2009/12/15/112448663/state-by-state-the-legal-battle-over-gay-marriage.

other privileges, including the ability to visit a partner in the hospital. Yet the benefits vary widely by location and fall far short of those provided through marriage. In many states, domestic partnerships are open to committed couples—homosexual or heterosexual—who have lived together usually for more than one year.

Staying Single

In 1980, the median age at marriage was 22 years for women and 24.7 years for men. Fast-forward a quarter century and the age rose to 25.8 years for women and 28.3 years for men—the oldest in U.S. history.[54] In 2008, 22% of men aged 35 to 44 had never been married, and 17% of women that age had also never married.[55] The trend to stay single is occurring in all racial groups in the United States but is most pronounced in African Americans.[55]

Why are Americans waiting longer to marry or avoiding marriage entirely? Some opt to focus on their education and career. Rising cohabitation rates have also meant that many adults enjoy intimacy and companionship while remaining legally single. Women today are also much more financially independent and less pressured to marry in order to attain economic stability. Attitudes about marriage and childrearing have also changed, with far more couples having children out of wedlock. According to one study, 48% of first births now occur outside of marriage.[56]

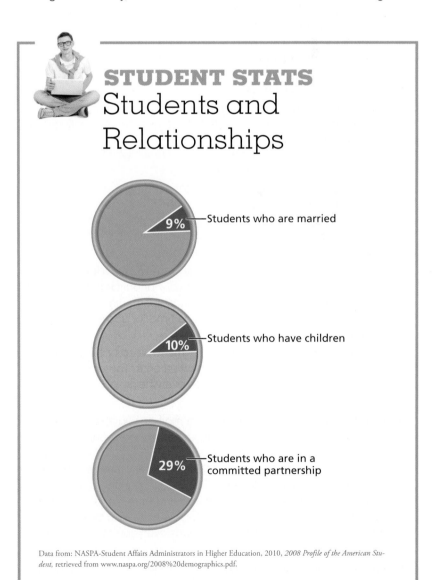

STUDENT STATS
Students and Relationships

- 9%—Students who are married
- 10%—Students who have children
- 29%—Students who are in a committed partnership

Data from: NASPA-Student Affairs Administrators in Higher Education, 2010, *2008 Profile of the American Student*, retrieved from www.naspa.org/2008%20demographics.pdf.

Singles can, and do, lead very fulfilled lives, enjoying successful careers, close personal friendships, and strong family ties. Some date frequently, others rarely. Some choose to live with a partner long-term. Singles are often stereotyped as being alone and lonely, but, in reality, they are likely to have networks of important people and friendships that have lasted years beyond many marriages.[57]

Starting a Family

Most people in the United States anticipate that they will be parents one day. For some, raising children is one of the life achievements they most look forward to. The American family, however, has undergone a dramatic transformation in recent decades. Women are waiting longer to have children, spacing births further apart, and ending their fertility at earlier ages than ever before. In addition, almost 9% of women now say they do not want to have any children.[58] Consequently, the U.S. birth rate is at an all-time low.

Nontraditional families are also on the rise, with single-parent households increasing more than sixfold since 1950, and unmarried-couple households more than quadrupling.[59] Only 67% of children in 2009 lived with two married, biological parents.[60] These changes in the traditional organization of the American family don't necessarily signal the decline of our social structure. They do, however, point to how flexible and complex American family arrangements have become and remind us that there is no such thing as a "typical" family.

Choosing Children

Having a baby can be one of the most rewarding experiences in life. It can also be one of the most difficult, trying a new parent's patience and testing a couple's relationship.

If you are considering parenthood, ask yourself whether you are ready for the following dramatic changes:

- **Relationship changes.** Caring nonstop for a newborn baby can leave little time for couples to focus on their own relationship. Especially during the child's first year, parents are likely to fight more and be intimate less. Married couples often experience a decrease in their overall satisfaction with their marriage.[61]
- **Changes in your relationships with family and friends.** Your parents may have ideas about what your priorities should be, and they may differ from yours. Your friendships could also change because new babies leave much less time for socializing with friends.
- **Less time for yourself.** Having little time to sleep or take good care of yourself is a complaint of many new parents. The amount of work it takes to care for a newborn can be overwhelming.[61]

In addition, assess the following:

- **Your health.** If you are a prospective mother, you should evaluate how healthy you are and what you should do to prepare your body for a pregnancy. If you smoke or drink, quit. Eat nutritious foods, get regular exercise, and begin taking prenatal vitamins right away. If you are a prospective father, you should also work at adopting a more healthful lifestyle including avoiding tobacco, alcohol, and recreational drugs because using these substances before conception could affect male fertility or perhaps even contribute to poor fetal health.[62]
- **Your finances.** Consider your monthly budget and the added expenses that come with a baby, including food, diapers, clothing,

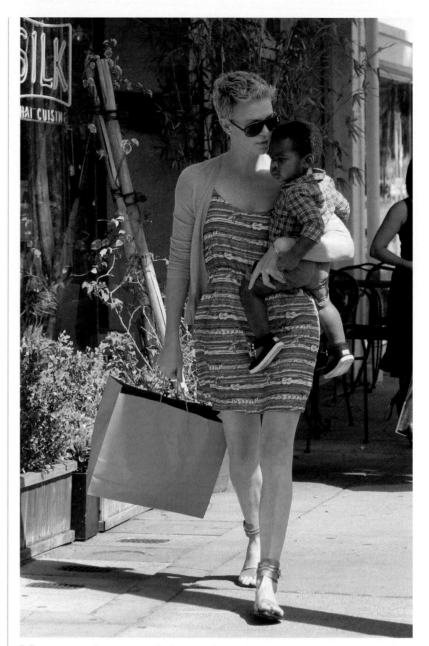

Nontraditional families are on the rise. For example, actress Charlize Theron adopted a son while unmarried.

furniture, and possibly a bigger place to live. Assess the decrease in income you will see if one of you takes time off work. Come up with a plan on how to cover the medical bills and the cost of child care, if you will need it.

- **Your childcare arrangements.** Agree on who will care for your child. You? Your partner? A family member? A daycare center? Are any of these options affordable?
- **Parenting styles.** What values do you want to emphasize? Do you have similar beliefs on discipline?

Stepfamilies

One out of every three Americans is now a stepchild, a stepsibling, a stepparent, or another member of a stepfamily.[63] These "blended families" have become commonplace in modern society, as more parents have opted to divorce and later remarry. Indeed, about three-fourths of divorced adults do go on to remarry, many of them within the first few years of their original marriage's end.[64] In about 65% of these remarriages, one or both partners have children from a previous relationship, according to the National Stepfamily Resource Center.[65]

When a stepfamily is first coming together, life can be unpredictable and chaotic. It can take several years for members of previously distinct families to integrate, and they do not always succeed.[66] Members of a stepfamily need to form new roles and norms within their new family, rather than trying to re-create the original family. Setting realistic expectations and encouraging open communication can be extremely useful in fostering strong stepfamily relationships.

Single Parenthood

Even if you were not raised by a single parent, odds are you know someone who was. Of the 74.2 million children living in the United States in 2009, 26% lived with only one parent.[67] This statistic reflects the high divorce rate, the small number of partners who are widowed, and the growing number of parents who have never been married. One-third of children today are born to unmarried mothers.[68]

One of the greatest hurdles single mothers face is economic hardship. An estimated 30% of women who have a child born out of wedlock live in poverty, compared with just 8% of women who were married at the time of their child's birth.[69] Single mothers, on average, also have lower levels of education than other women, which can hurt their job prospects and lower their earnings potential.

Just how children fare growing up in a single-parent household varies and has been the source of some controversy. Experts recognize that a family's structure is not as important as how it functions. Yet children from single-parent families have a risk of difficult life outcomes that is two to three times higher than children from married, two-parent families.[70] Children born out of wedlock are more likely to experience a wide range of behavioral and emotional problems, reaching adulthood with less education and earning less income. They are more likely to be "idle"—out of school and out of work—in their late teens and early 20s. They experience more symptoms of depression and have more troubled marriages and higher rates of divorce. They are also more likely to have a child out of wedlock themselves.[71]

But do these gloomy predictions hold for children born to women who deliberately choose single motherhood? A growing number of sociologists are saying no. Women who are financially independent and well-educated—whether lesbian or heterosexual—are increasingly choosing to have children without men. Sociologist Suzanne Bianchi of the University of Maryland explains that these women make sacrifices in their personal lives and careers to make single parenting work, putting their children first. Wellesley College sociologist Rosanna Hertz agrees: "The child really becomes the focal point of their lives."[72] A 2004 study involving 1,500 U.S. multiethnic 12- and 13-year-olds supports these observations: Cornell professor Henry Riciutti found that, when income and level of education are factored in, there's "little or no difference" between the intellectual development, academic achievement, and behavior of children in single-parent and two-parent families. The study also suggests that any risks of single parenting can be greatly reduced with increased access to economic, social, educational, and parenting support.[73]

Characteristics of Happy Families

Researchers have devoted a great deal of time to looking at strong families, measuring their affection and communication, trying to decipher their secrets for success. What they found is that a happy family is not one without trouble or weaknesses. Some have experienced financial difficulties, health problems, or other setbacks. But strong families learn how to adapt and endure, taking a constructive approach to dealing with crises, often because they have a shared agreement on what constitutes their own particular version of "success."[74]

Members of strong families share and value these traits:[75]

- **Commitment.** They are dedicated to the family and promoting each other's happiness. They are honest, faithful, and dependable.

- **Appreciation and affection.** They care for each other and are not afraid to express it. They give compliments and show their affection freely.

- **Positive communication.** They are good talkers and good listeners. They do argue but avoid blaming each other and are able to compromise.

- **Time together.** They spend quality time together as often as they can and arrange their schedules to ensure that this happens.

- **Spiritual well-being.** They have hope, faith, and compassion as well as shared ethical values.

- **The ability to manage stress and crises.** They see crises as both challenges and opportunities for growth. They pull together during tough times and give support to each other. They set their own definitions of success, and work together to take steps both large and small to reach their goals.

Change Yourself, Change Your World

Healthy relationships have many challenges, from misunderstandings and hurt feelings to episodes of significant emotional pain. Still, failing to build healthy relationships simply is not an option! In the words of civil rights leader Martin Luther King, Jr., "We must learn to live together as brothers, or perish together as fools."[76] The rewards of healthy relationships are abundant.

Personal Choices

If you want to build and maintain healthy relationships, a smart first step is to practice the skills—including effective communication and conflict-resolution skills—described earlier. In addition, it's important to adopt the following behaviors:

- **Stay true to who you are.** Everyone wants to experiment with different beliefs, values, and behaviors. But when you adopt attitudes and behavior patterns that don't feel authentic, just because you think doing so will help you fit in or keep a relationship going, you're doomed to dishonest, superficial relationships. Be yourself, right from the start.

- **Respect others for who they are.** Have you ever found yourself thinking about breaking off a relationship because you're just "too different"? If so, it might be time to think again. If you can learn to value your differences—in beliefs, standards, experiences, skills, behaviors, style—you might find that you're able to forge a highly energetic relationship in which you and your partner become more productive and creative. Sociologist Mark Granovetter refers to this phenomenon as "the strength of weak ties," and it's a key reason to value diversity in your relationships.[77]

- **Learn to give and receive.** This doesn't mean the two of you have to be rich! The most meaningful gifts in lasting relationships are gifts

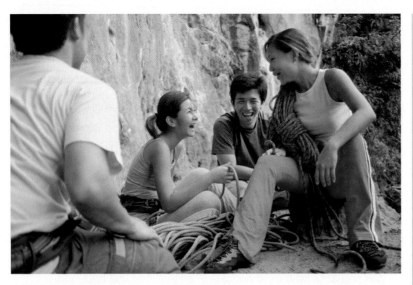

Taking the time to appreciate your friends and partners for who they are can strengthen your relationships.

of time, attention, listening, and emotional support. Give of these gifts unselfishly, and accept them from your partner with gratitude.

- **Lighten up.** Finally, make room in your relationship for fun! Take a break from studying and take a bike ride, or keep a Saturday free for a trip to the beach. Keep humor a part of your daily interactions.

Campus Advocacy

College students come together from regions all over the world not only to acquire knowledge, but to learn to respect and negotiate differences. These include differences in culture, religion, language, ability, sexual orientation, and much more. What can you do to build bridges to others on your campus? Here are some simple ideas.

Keep the Lines of Communication Open

One international student described her two years of study at an American university as "a challenging experience."[78] She noted that students on her campus tended to associate only with those like themselves and often avoided even speaking to students from other countries. She offered this advice for keeping the lines of communication open:[78]

- Initiate a conversation. If the person has difficulty speaking English, give him or her some time to think through a translation, or to take out the person's electronic dictionary and find the right words.
- Words are not the most important part of human communication. Observe the person's facial expression and gestures; take a look!
- During a conversation, empathize. Try to see the world through the other person's perspective.

Join a Campus Organization That Promotes Tolerance

Many different organizations provide training and tools to combat *bias*—unfair preferences—and promote an atmosphere of tolerance on campus. For example:

- The National Educational Association of Disabled Students (NEADS) has a network of 40 campus-based groups to support students with disabilities. Membership is open to all students, regardless of level of ability. For information about forming a group or becoming a member, go to **www.neads.ca/en/norc/ campusnet/leadership_starting.php.**
- Campus Pride is a national nonprofit group working to create a safer college environment for LGBT (lesbian, gay, bisexual, or transgender) students across the United States. Find out more about this organization at **www.campuspride.org.**

These are just a few examples, so find out what's happening on your campus and get involved.

Explore New Options

You don't have to join an organization to build diverse relationships on campus. Try attending a few services of a campus religious organization that you're not familiar with. Volunteer to help plan a social or cultural event sponsored by an international students' organization. Advocate for a culture of respect on campus, both among students and in the rules set by the administration, that discourages bullying (in person or online) and states that such behavior is not tolerated at your school.[79] You might argue that you're only one person, but in reality, you're part of a vast network of relationships. By reaching out in simple ways like these, you challenge the belief that differences can keep us from building strong, meaningful relationships.

>> **Watch videos of real students discussing communication and relationships at** MasteringHealth™

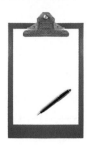

Choosing to Change Worksheet

To complete this worksheet online, visit MasteringHealth™

Successful healthy relationships are built on trust, respect, and communication. They enable each individual to retain his or her own identity and foster personal growth rather than smothering it. With this in mind, think about one relationship that is important to you and needs improvement. Write down this relationship in Step 1.

Directions: Fill in your stage of change in Step 1 and complete the remaining steps with your stage of change in mind.

Step 1. *Your Stage of Behavior Change.* My relationship with _____ is important to me and needs improvement. Please check one of the following statements that best describes your readiness to improve this relationship.

_____ I do not intend to participate in building a healthy relationship in the next six months. (Precontemplation)

_____ I might participate in building a healthy relationship in the next six months. (Contemplation)

_____ I am prepared to participate in building a healthy relationship in the next month. (Preparation)

_____ I have been building a healthy relationship for less than six months but need to do more. (Action)

_____ I have built a healthy relationship for more than six months and want to maintain it. (Maintenance)

Step 2. *Communication Skills.* It is important to know how to communicate effectively with others. Think about the communication skills listed on pages 203–204. List the skills that you feel you have mastered in your own life. Then, list one area in particular that you would like to improve.

Mastered: _____

_____

Needs improvement: _____

_____

Step 3. *Feedback on Your Communication Style.* Find someone close to you whom you trust and who you can have an open discussion with. Ask that person about your communication skills, that is, what your strengths are and what might need improvement. Try not to become offended if the person suggests areas for improvement; honest feedback is the hallmark of a true friend. What did that person say and how do you feel about it?

_____

_____

_____

Step 4. *Listening.* Listening is a major component of communication. Consider the good listening skills that were discussed on pages 204–205. Which techniques can you try to become a better listener? Provide examples of how you will apply these skills within your chosen relationship.

Techniques: _____

_____

Examples: _____

_____

Step 5. *Putting Yourself in Someone Else's Shoes.* Another way to improve a relationship is to try to see things through the other person's eyes. Take a moment to think about your chosen relationship and write down key factors in that person's life and situation. Answer the following questions: Who are the important people in his or her life and why? What other people is he or she having problems with and why? What are his or her current stressors? What is he or she looking forward to or worried about?

_____

_____

_____

Step 6. *Writing a Note.* Imagine that you are writing a note to the person with whom you want to improve relations. What would you say? Write it down.

_____

_____

_____

_____

Step 7. *Your Next Step.* Given your current stage of behavior change, what will be your next step in building the relationship you want to improve? If you are in the preparation stage of change, write down your SMART goal.

_____

_____

_____

Chapter Summary

MasteringHealth™

Build your knowledge—and health!—in the Study Area of **MasteringHealth**™ with a variety of study tools.

- Good communication includes being able to articulate your honest thoughts and feelings, being a good listener, and being aware of how body language can affect how others interpret what you are saying.

- Effective conflict resolution requires that both parties voice their concerns maturely and engage in constructive criticism, rather than resorting to personal attacks and put-downs.

- Self-perception, early relationships, and gender roles affect how we develop relationships throughout life.

- Strong friendships and social ties contribute to greater overall health. Although online friendships are common and fun, they often do not provide the same level of support and connection as in-person contact.

- Sternberg's Triangular Theory of Love identifies intimacy, passion, and commitment as the three primary components of healthy, loving relationships.

- Healthy relationships are based on trust, respect, and communication. Dysfunctional relationships are characterized by physical or verbal abuse, manipulation, disrespect, or cruelty.

- Cohabitation, marriage, and domestic partnerships are examples of different kinds of committed relationships. Same-sex couples are conducting an intense effort to gain the same right to marry that heterosexual couples enjoy.

- Raising children can be rewarding as well as stressful. Couples should ask themselves how having a baby would change their lives and whether they are truly ready for those changes.

- Strong families are characterized by commitment, appreciation, affection, positive communication, time together, spiritual well-being, and the ability to adapt to changes.

GET CONNECTED

>> Visit the following websites for further information about the topics in this chapter:

- Conflict Resolution Information Source
  www.crinfo.org
- American Psychological Association
  www.apa.org
- Human Rights Campaign
  www.hrc.org
- Loveisrespect.org
  www.loveisrespect.org
- The National Marriage Project
  http://nationalmarriageproject.org

MOBILE TIPS!

Scan this QR code with your mobile device to access additional tips about communication and relationships. Or, via your mobile device, go to **http://chmobile.pearsoncmg.com** and navigate to Chapter 9.

- American Association for Marriage and Family Therapy
  www.aamft.org
- Go Ask Alice
  www.goaskalice.columbia.edu

Website links are subject to change. To access updated web links, please visit MasteringHealth™

TEST YOUR KNOWLEDGE

1. Sharing your feelings and other personal information with another person is called
   a. self-assuredness.
   b. self-love.
   c. self-appreciation.
   d. self-disclosure.

2. All of the following are examples of nonverbal communication except
   a. eye contact.
   b. email.
   c. arm movements.
   d. facial expressions.

3. In Sternberg's Triangular Theory of Love, the primary components of healthy relationships include all of the following except
   a. passion.
   b. contentment.
   c. commitment.
   d. intimacy.

4. Assortative mating refers to the tendency of people to
   a. be attracted to people who have opposite interests to their own.
   b. fall in love at first sight.
   c. "hook up" instead of date.
   d. select romantic partners who are similar to themselves.

5. Attachment theory states that
   a. becoming close to a romantic partner weakens existing friendships.
   b. close friends will grow to be more and more like one another.
   c. the more attached you become to someone, the more healthy the relationship becomes.
   d. early childhood relationships shape our expectations of adult relationships.

6. Friendships are
   a. stronger today with modern technology.
   b. helpful in promoting health.
   c. difficult to rekindle if you have been out of touch.
   d. all of these answers are correct.

7. All of the following will help you maintain relationships EXCEPT
   a. stay true to who you are.
   b. respect others.
   c. avoid conflict.
   d. be generous.

8. In general, married people
   a. enjoy better mental and physical health than unmarried people.
   b. live longer than unmarried people.
   c. are financially better off than unmarried people.
   d. all of these answers are correct.

9. The divorce rate in the United States is
   a. just under 50%.
   b. just under 75%.
   c. around 33%.
   d. increasing.

10. What proportion of people in the United States are part of a stepfamily?
   a. one in two
   b. one in three
   c. one in four
   d. one in five

Get Critical

What happened

When should the medical community take a stand on a social issue? The nation's most influential group of pediatricians, the American Academy of Pediatrics (AAP), raised that question anew when the organization stated its public support for gay marriage.[1] The group based its 2013 declaration on a four-year review of scientific studies, saying that allowing gay and lesbian parents to marry promotes relationship stability and is in the best interests of their children.

"Lack of opportunity for same-gender couples to marry adds to families' stress, which affects the health and welfare of all household members," the AAP's report stated. "Because marriage strengthens families and, in so doing, benefits children's development, children should not be deprived of the opportunity for their parents to be married."

The group's report also emphasized that parental competence, rather than sexual orientation, should be the focus of discussions about the aptitude of prospective parents. Some other scientists, however, countered that although the body of scientific evidence behind the AAP's statement may be growing, it is not yet sufficient enough to warrant such a clear-cut policy statement.[2]

What do you think?

- Do you think health organizations should make statements about social issues?
- What do you think are the most important factors in providing a secure, healthy environment for raising children?

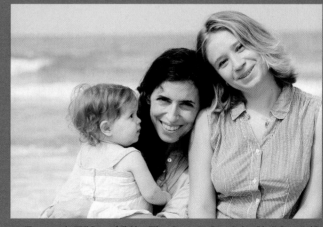

References: **1.** "Promoting the Well-Being of Children Whose Parents Are Gay or Lesbian," by E. Perrin and B. Siegel, 2013, *Pediatrics, 131*(4), e1374–e1383. **2.** "Pediatrics Group Backs Gay Marriage, Saying It Helps Children," by C. Saint Louis, *New York Times,* March 21, 2013, retrieved from http://www.nytimes.com/2013/03/21/health/american-academy-of-pediatrics-backs-gay-marriage.html.

SEXUALITY, CONTRACEPTION, AND REPRODUCTIVE CHOICES

About **34% of college students** report that they have never engaged in vaginal **intercourse**.[i]

In a recent study, **20% of teens** and 33% of young adults reported sending or **posting nude** or semi-nude **photos or videos** of themselves over their **cell phones**.[ii]

In the United States, **half** of all **pregnancies** are **unplanned**—about 3 million each year.[iii]

10

Learning Objectives

DESCRIBE the primary structures in male and female sexual anatomy.

DESCRIBE the key events in the female menstrual cycle.

IDENTIFY the phases of the sexual response cycle and discuss common sexual dysfunctions.

DEFINE *abstinence, non-intercourse sexual activity*, and *sexual intercourse*.

DISCUSS three basic sexual orientations.

COMPARE and contrast different methods of contraception.

DISCUSS surgical and medical abortion.

DESCRIBE the key stages of pregnancy and childbirth.

DISCUSS causes of infertility as well as ways to prevent it.

CONSIDER different ways of developing and promoting healthy sexuality, both for yourself and your community.

Sex is something people rarely think about intellectually.

Sure, you may fantasize about it, but pondering the physiological and wellness aspects of sex is usually not high on a college student's list of priorities. Yet sex is worth deeper thought than we often give it. Sex influences how we see ourselves and how we relate to others. It affects our health, our sense of pleasure, our romantic relationships, and our decisions about whether and when to have a family. Understanding your **sexuality,** knowing your reproductive options, and making choices that best fit your values and goals are important elements of your overall health and well-being.

Sexual Anatomy and Health

Whether we engage in sexual activity or not, our bodies are continually preparing for reproduction. A woman's ovaries release an egg each month, whereas a man's testes are constantly manufacturing new sperm. Given these biological realities, the sexual decisions we make in a split second can alter the course of our lives dramatically, sometimes by leading to an unplanned pregnancy or a sexually transmitted infection (see Chapter 11) that permanently affects fertility.

Female Sexual Anatomy

A woman's sexual anatomy includes both external and internal sex organs **(Figure 10.1)**. The term **vulva** refers to all of the female external organs collectively—also known as *genitals*. These include the following structures:

- **Mons pubis.** The fatty, rounded area of tissue in front of the pubic bone; covered in pubic hair after puberty.
- **Labia majora.** The fleshy, larger outer lips (*labia* means lips) surrounding the labia minora.
- **Labia minora.** The thin, inner folds of skin, which rest protectively over the *clitoris,* the *vaginal opening,* and the *urethral opening*, through which urine is released from the body.
- **Clitoris.** An organ composed of spongy tissue with an abundance of nerve endings that make it very sensitive to sexual stimulation. During sexual arousal, the clitoris fills with blood and plays a key role in producing the female orgasm. In fact, the clitoris is the only organ in either sex with the sole purpose of sexual arousal and pleasure.
  The internal organs include the following:
- **Vagina.** The tube that connects a woman's external sex organs with her *uterus*. It serves as the passageway through which menstrual flow leaves the body as well as the passageway through which sperm enters the body during heterosexual intercourse. During childbirth, it functions as the birth canal.
- **Uterus.** Also known as the *womb.* The uterus is a pear-shaped organ, normally about the size of a

sexuality The biological, physical, emotional, and psychosocial aspects of sexual attraction and expression.

vulva All of the female external organs collectively. Also called *genitals*.

mons pubis The fatty, rounded areas of tissue in front of the pubic bone.

labia Two pairs (majora and minora) of fleshy lips surrounding and protecting the clitoris and the vaginal and urethral openings.

clitoris An organ composed of spongy tissue and nerve endings that is very sensitive to sexual stimulation.

vagina The tube that connects a woman's external sex organs with her uterus.

uterus (womb) The pear-shaped organ where a growing fetus is nurtured.

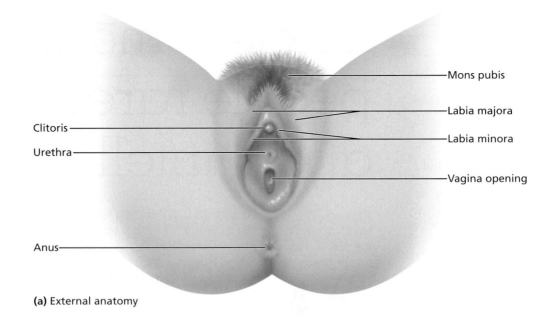

(a) External anatomy

Mons pubis
Labia majora
Clitoris
Labia minora
Urethra
Vagina opening
Anus

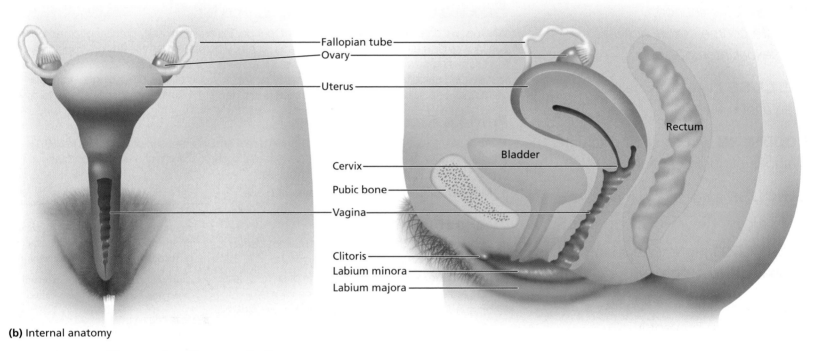

(b) Internal anatomy

Fallopian tube
Ovary
Uterus
Rectum
Bladder
Cervix
Pubic bone
Vagina
Clitoris
Labium minora
Labium majora

FIGURE 10.1 Female Sexual Anatomy.

fist. It is here that a growing fetus is nurtured. The innermost lining of the uterus is called the *endometrium*. It is shed monthly in nonpregnant women of **childbearing age,** a range often defined as being between 15 and 44 years old.[1] The narrowed end of the uterus that projects into the top of the vagina is called the *cervix*. Sperm deposited into the vagina swim through the opening of the cervix into the body of the uterus.

• **Ovaries.** The two chambers, one on either side of the pelvic cavity, where a woman's eggs, or *ova,* are stored. Every month, at approximately midway through her **menstrual cycle,** a woman *ovulates*; that is, one of her ovaries releases an egg. The ovaries produce the hormone *estrogen*.

• **Fallopian tubes.** The tubes— one on either side of the uterus—that connect the uterus to the ovaries. After ovulation, the egg is swept into the nearby fallopian tube. It then travels through the tube to the uterus. If it encounters sperm within the tube, the egg may become fertilized. Either fertilized or not, the egg will continue to be swept into the uterus.

childbearing age The age range at which a woman can become pregnant, often defined as between 15 and 44 years old.

ovaries The two female reproductive organs where ova (eggs) reside.

menstrual cycle A monthly physiological cycle marked by *menstruation*.

fallopian tubes A pair of tubes that connect the ovaries to the uterus.

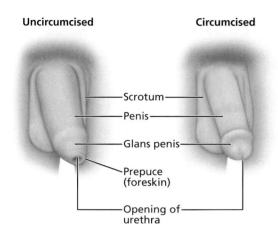

Uncircumcised **Circumcised**

Scrotum
Penis
Glans penis
Prepuce (foreskin)
Opening of urethra

(a) External anatomy

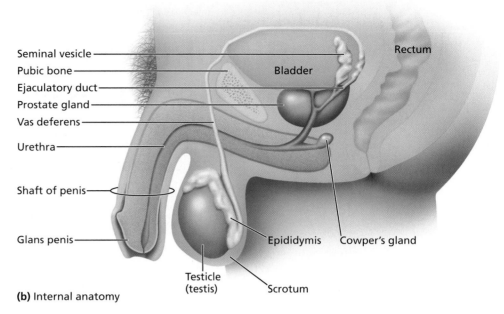

Seminal vesicle
Pubic bone
Ejaculatory duct
Prostate gland
Vas deferens
Urethra
Shaft of penis
Glans penis

Rectum
Bladder

Epididymis   Cowper's gland

Testicle (testis)   Scrotum

(b) Internal anatomy

FIGURE 10.2 Male Sexual Anatomy.

Common Sexual Health Problems in Females

Good sexual health includes good preventive care. According to the American Congress of Obstetricians and Gynecologists (ACOG), girls should have their first gynecologic visit between the ages of 13 and 15. Unless a girl is sexually active or is experiencing problems, these first visits will most likely not include a pelvic exam. New ACOG guidelines indicate that women should have their first pelvic exam and Pap test by age 21 and most women under 30 should receive cervical screening once every two years until the age of 30. Those aged 30 and older, who have had three consecutive negative Pap tests, can wait three years between Pap tests. Unfortunately, about half of all college-age women do not get screened regularly.[2] Not only does this reduce the odds that any medical problems will be detected early, it also deprives women of the opportunity to discuss important sexual health issues and reproductive concerns with a trusted expert.

Among the most common sexual health problems in women are menstrual irregularities, discussed on pages 228–229. Sexually transmitted infections (STIs) are another major health concern, not only for the harm they cause directly, but also because of their association with other serious disorders, including infertility and cervical cancer. (For detailed information on STIs, see Chapter 11.)

Another infection affecting females is *vulvovaginal candidiasis* (VVC), an inflammation of the vagina that can produce itching, pain, and discharge. Although it is not sexually transmitted, the condition is common and often referred to as a "yeast infection." It is typically caused by an overgrowth of *Candida albicans,* a species of yeast (a type of fungus) that is normally present in the vagina in controlled amounts. VVC most commonly occurs when a woman takes a broad-spectrum antibiotic that kills off the normal vaginal bacteria that usually compete with *Candida* for nutrients.

Male Sexual Anatomy

A man's reproductive anatomy also includes both internal and external organs **(Figure 10.2)**. The external organs are the following:

- **Penis.** The male sexual and reproductive organ, which consists of the shaft (body), and a slitted tip called the glans penis (head). Made up of soft, spongy tissue, the penis fills with blood during sexual arousal and becomes firm and enlarged, a state known as an **erection**. Boys are born with a hood of skin, known as the *foreskin,* covering the head of the penis. In more than half of boys born in the United States, parents opt to have the skin surgically removed through a procedure called **circumcision** (see **Myth or Fact?: Should Boys Be Circumcised for Health Reasons?**).

- **Scrotum.** The skin sac at the base of the penis that contains the *testes* (testicles). The scrotum is responsible for regulating the temperature of the testes, which need to be kept cool to facilitate production of *sperm*, the male reproductive cells.

The internal male organs are the following:

- **Testes (testicles).** The reproductive glands that manufacture sperm.

- **Epididymis.** The coiled tube—one above each testicle—where sperm are held until they mature.

- **Vas deferens.** The tube that ascends from the epididymis—one on each side of the scrotum—and transports sperm into the *ejaculatory duct*.

- **Accessory glands.** A set of glands that lubricate the reproductive system and nourish

penis The male sexual and reproductive organ.

erection The process of the penis filling up with blood as a result of sexual stimulation.

circumcision The surgical removal of the foreskin.

scrotum The skin sac at the base of the penis that contains the testes.

testes (testicles) The two reproductive glands that manufacture sperm.

epididymis A coiled tube on top of each testicle where sperm are held until they mature.

vas deferens A tube ascending from the epididymis that transports sperm.

accessory glands Glands (seminal vesicles, prostate gland, and Cowper's gland) that lubricate the reproductive system and nourish sperm.

Should Boys Be Circumcised for Health Reasons?

Infant boys are born with a hood of skin, known as the *foreskin*, covering the head of the penis. In more than half of boys born in the United States, parents opt to have the foreskin surgically removed through a procedure called *circumcision*.

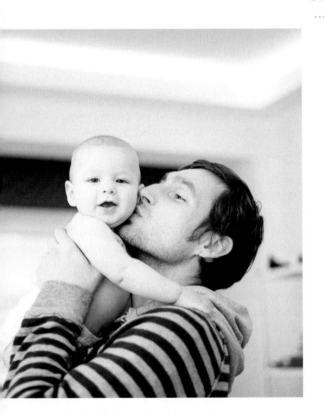

Circumcision rates vary greatly across the country and throughout the world, with the surgery performed on about 55% of newborn boys in the United States in 2007.[1] Circumcision is also widely performed in the Middle East and Canada, but in Europe, Latin America, China, and India it is uncommon.

In some families, the decision to circumcise is primarily a religious one. In both the Jewish and Muslim faiths, circumcision is a common rite of passage. In others, it is more of a cultural determination—boys are circumcised because their fathers were. What remains most controversial is circumcising for health-related reasons, although recent research is adding more weight to the procedure's potential health benefits.[1]

These benefits start with cleanliness. Circumcision boosts personal hygiene, making it somewhat easier to wash the penis. It also reduces the risk of urinary tract infections in infancy. Men who have been circumcised have lower rates of penile cancer, and several types of research studies have documented a reduced risk of

both acquiring and transmitting some sexually transmitted infections, including HIV.[1] Safer sex practices, however, are much more important at stopping the spread of those diseases than circumcision is. Still, one economic study determined, circumcision provides enough health benefits that if the U.S. circumcision rates were to fall to levels seen in Europe, the decline would add more than $4 billion to U.S. health care costs.[2]

Opponents of circumcision point out that the procedure can be painful. It also comes with risks, including the potential for infection and excessive bleeding. Rarely, the penis may not heal properly or a second surgery may be needed. Some opponents argue that circumcision reduces penile sensation and sexual function; however, well-designed studies of these issues are few and inconclusive.[3]

In 2013, the evidence pointing to the health benefits of circumcision led federal health officials to state, "Male circumcision is a proven effective prevention intervention with known medical benefits. Financial and

other barriers to access to male circumcision should be reduced or eliminated." The American Academy of Pediatrics revised its policy a few months prior, stating that the benefits outweigh the risks and "justify access to the procedure for families who choose it."[4] Although the prominent pediatricians' group stopped short of recommending circumcision for all newborns, the Academy stated that health insurance should cover the cost of the procedure.[5] When parents choose circumcision, the Academy advises that pain medication be given to the newborn.[5]

References: 1. *Male Circumcision,* by the Centers for Disease Control and Prevention, 2013, retrieved from http://www.cdc.gov/hiv/prevention/research/malecircumcision. 2. "Declining Rates of U.S. Infant Male Circumcision Could Add Billions to Health Care Costs, Experts Warn," by *Johns Hopkins Medicine,* August 20, 2012, retrieved from http://www.hopkinsmedicine.org/news/media/releases/declining_rates_of_us_infant_male_circumcision_could_add_billions_to_health_care_costs_experts_warn. 3. *Male Circumcision and Risk for HIV Transmission and Other Health Conditions: Implications for the United States* by the Centers for Disease Control, 2008, retrieved from http://www.cdc.gov/hiv/resources/factsheets/circumcision.htm. 4. "Circumcision Policy Statement," by the American Academy of Pediatrics, 2012, *Pediatrics, 130*(3), pp. 585–586. 5. "Technical Report: Male Circumcision," by the American Academy of Pediatrics, 2013, *Pediatrics, 130*(3), pp. e756–e785.

the sperm. They include the *seminal vesicles,* small sacs that store *seminal fluid,* which provides sugars and other nutrients that feed and activate sperm. The seminal vesicles secrete seminal fluid into the ejaculatory duct, which also receives sperm from the vas deferens.

semen The male ejaculate consisting of sperm and other fluids from the accessory glands.

This mixture of sperm and seminal fluid is called **semen.** Another accessory gland that contributes to semen is the *prostate gland,* a walnut-shaped structure below the bladder. It secretes into semen an alkaline fluid that helps protect sperm from the acidic environment of the vagina. Below the prostate are the *Cowper's glands,* pea-shaped glands on each side of the urethra that discharge a lubricating secretion into the urethra just before ejaculation.

- **Urethra.** Within the prostate, the ejaculatory duct joins the urethra, a much longer duct that travels from the bladder through the shaft of the penis, and carries fluids to the outside of the body. Both urine from the bladder and semen from the ejaculatory duct pass through the urethra, although not at the same time.

Common Sexual Health Problems in Males

Like women, men should take their sexual health seriously and get regular medical checkups. Sexually active men are also encouraged to perform self-exams of their genitals, looking in particular for any sores or warts. These may be signs of an STI (see Chapter 11). If you notice these—or any other changes to your genitals—be sure to discuss them promptly with a doctor. A hard lump in a testicle may be a sign of testicular cancer, which is most often diagnosed in young men in their 20s and 30s. For more information on testicular cancer, see Chapter 12.

Several common sexual health problems in men involve the prostate:

- **Prostatitis.** An infection or inflammation of the **prostate gland**. Symptoms range from the frequent need to urinate to pain in the pelvic region and lower back.

- **Prostate gland enlargement.** An excessive growth of prostate tissue that presses on the urethra, impairing or blocking the flow of urine. This usually develops in men over age 60.

- **Prostate cancer.** A typically slow growth of cancerous tissue from which cancer cells can spread to other parts of the body (see Chapter 12). Prostate cancer most commonly affects men over age 65.[3]

The Menstrual Cycle

A rite of passage for girls as they transition into womanhood is **menarche** (pronounced *me-NAR-kee*), the onset of **menstruation,** the discharge of blood and endometrial tissue from the vagina. Also called a *period* or *menstrual period,* menstruation usually lasts from 3 to 7 days. In the United States, the average age at menarche is 12, although it is considered normal to start as early as 8 or as late as 15.[4]

urethra A duct that travels from the bladder through the shaft of the penis, carrying fluids to the outside of the body.

prostate gland A walnut-sized gland that produces part of the semen.

menarche The first onset of menstruation.

menstruation The cyclical discharge of blood and tissue from the vagina.

menopause The time when a woman stops having menstrual cycles.

menstrual phase Phase of the menstrual cycle characterized by menstrual flow, the release of follicle-stimulating hormone from the pituitary gland to the brain, and the release of estrogen into the bloodstream.

proliferative phase Phase of the menstrual cycle characterized by a thickening of the lining of the uterus and discharge of cervical mucus. This phase ends when luteinizing hormone triggers the release of a mature egg.

secretory phase Phase of the menstrual cycle characterized by the degeneration of the follicle sac, rising levels of progesterone in the bloodstream, and further increase of the endometrial lining.

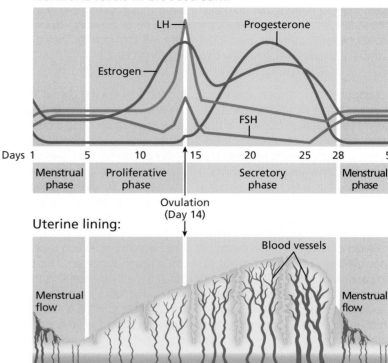

Hormone levels in bloodstream:

LH

Progesterone

Estrogen

FSH

Days 1 · · 5 · · · · 10 · · · · 15 · · · · 20 · · · · 25 · 28 · · · · 5

| Menstrual phase | Proliferative phase | Secretory phase | Menstrual phase |

Ovulation (Day 14)

Uterine lining:

Blood vessels

Menstrual flow

Menstrual flow

FIGURE 10.3 Phases of the Menstrual Cycle. The menstrual cycle consists of a menstrual phase, a proliferative phase, and a secretory phase.

Menopause, the time at which women stop menstruating, usually occurs in a woman's early 50s.

Menstruation is just one of several physiological events in a woman's *menstrual cycle* **(Figure 10.3).** Because it is controlled by hormones, the menstrual cycle can be interrupted by anything that affects hormone production. This includes illness, excessive dieting with or without excessive exercise, and breast-feeding. Of course the menstrual cycle also ceases during pregnancy. Otherwise, in women of childbearing age, it repeats approximately every month, spanning from 21 to 35 days (the average is 28 days) each time.[4]

 View an animation of the menstrual cycle at www.womenshealth .gov/publications/our-publications/fact-sheet/menstruation .html#flashmovie. **(Click Start in the lower right corner of the diagram.)**

Phases of the Menstrual Cycle

The menstrual cycle is characterized by a series of events involving both the uterus and the ovaries. As indicated in Figure 10.3, fluctuations in the levels of four female reproductive hormones control these events, which are typically grouped into three phases: the **menstrual phase**, the **proliferative phase**, and the **secretory phase**.

Menstrual Phase

The first day of a woman's menstrual flow is arbitrarily designated as day 1 of the menstrual cycle. Menstruation results from the breakdown of the endometrium after the body "recognizes" that a pregnancy has not occurred. During this phase, a hormone called *FSH— follicle-stimulating hormone*—is released from the pituitary gland in the brain. A woman's ovary contains thousands of egg sacs called *folli-cles*. FSH stimulates the maturation of the immature egg within a few of these follicles. As they develop, the follicles begin releasing an ovarian hormone, *estrogen,* into the bloodstream. As estrogen reaches the uterus, it causes menstruation to end (around day 6).

Proliferative Phase

Estrogen is also responsible for causing the lining of the uterus to thicken (proliferate) in preparation for the entry into the uterus of a fertilized egg. Also during this phase, a woman may notice a copious, slippery discharge of mucus from her vagina. This characteristic *cervical mucus* helps facilitate the mobility of sperm and protect them from the otherwise acidic environment of the vagina. Its presence also indicates that a woman is about to **ovulate,** that is, release an egg. In fact, the proliferative phase ends when, around day 14 of a 28-day cycle, the pituitary gland releases another hormone, *LH,* or *luteinizing hormone,* which triggers just one of the several maturing follicles to release a mature egg (an ovum). In some women, ovulation is accompanied by a sharp pain on one side of the lower abdomen. This pain is caused by irritation from the stretching of the ovary wall and the release of fluid into the lower abdominal cavity. Although it may last for several minutes to several hours, this "mid-cycle pain" is entirely normal and can help a woman pinpoint more precisely the time when she is fertile.

Secretory Phase

Once the ovum has been ejected, the remaining follicle sac degenerates into a *corpus luteum*, a tiny gland that begins releasing a fourth reproductive hormone, progesterone. Rising levels of progesterone enter the bloodstream and travel to the uterus, further thickening the endometrial lining in preparation for the arrival of a fertilized egg.

As noted earlier, the released ovum is swept into the nearby fallopian tube and begins to travel toward the uterus. If sperm are present in sufficient numbers in the fallopian tube, fertilization is likely to occur. The fertilized egg will then produce the hormone *human chorionic gonadotropin* (hCG), which is needed to sustain a pregnancy. In fact, over-the-counter pregnancy test kits work by detecting the presence or absence of hCG in a woman's urine. Within 3 to 4 days, the fertilized ovum reaches the uterus.

A woman's ovum is viable only for about 12 to 24 hours. If fertilization does not occur within this time period, it will quickly deteriorate, and the levels of all four reproductive hormones will begin to dramatically decrease. Thus, around day 25, the endometrium will start to degenerate. Within approximately 3 to 4 days, menstruation will begin and the cycle repeats itself again.

Disorders Associated with the Menstrual Cycle

Although normal menstruation is a sign of health and maturity, in some women it's accompanied by pain, excessive bleeding, or other problems that interfere with their ability to carry out their daily activities. We discuss the most common of these disorders here.

Premenstrual Syndrome

As many as 85% of women experience mildly disturbing emotional and physical symptoms just prior to menstruation.[5] These symptoms can include breast tenderness, fluid retention,

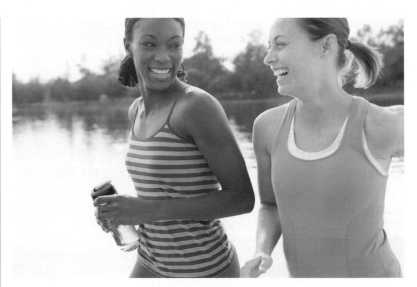

Exercise can help relieve the symptoms of premenstrual syndrome.

headaches, backaches, uterine cramping, irritability, mood swings, appetite changes, depression, and anxiety. Approximately 15% of women experience a constellation of the symptoms at a "sufficient severity to interfere with some aspect of life" and consequently are considered to have **premenstrual syndrome,** or **PMS.**[6] The symptoms of PMS typically appear in the week or two before the period begins and dissipate after menstrual bleeding starts.

Exactly what causes PMS isn't entirely clear. Some women may simply be more sensitive to the changes in female reproductive hormones that occur during the menstrual cycle. Chemical changes in the brain may also play a role. Stress and psychological problems do not cause the syndrome, although there is evidence that they can exacerbate it.[7]

Some lifestyle changes can reduce the symptoms of PMS. These include avoidance of smoking, alcohol, caffeine, salt, and sugary foods. A balanced diet rich in whole grains, fruits, and vegetables is important, along with regular exercise and adequate, restful sleep. In addition, some women find that a multivitamin and mineral supplement providing adequate levels of B vitamins, magnesium, and vitamin E is helpful, and women aged 19–50 should consume 1,000 milligrams of calcium daily. Over-the-counter remedies such as aspirin and ibuprofen can also relieve symptoms. In more severe cases of PMS in women who do not want to become pregnant, a woman's physician may prescribe birth control pills, which stop ovulation and reduce menstruation.[7]

Premenstrual Dysphoric Disorder (PMDD)

Some women experience the psychological symptoms of PMS in a more severe and debilitating way. This condition, known as **premenstrual dysphoric disorder (PMDD),** can interfere with daily functioning and social relationships. (*Dysphoria* refers to a generalized feeling of sadness, anxiety, or discontent.) Although any woman who has experienced a crying jag or a bout of irritability in the days before her period may assume her symptoms are severe, only 3–8% of

---

ovulate To release an egg from the ovary.

premenstrual syndrome (PMS) A collection of emotional and physical symptoms that occur just prior to menstruation.

premenstrual dysphoric disorder (PMDD) Severe and debilitating psychological symptoms experienced just prior to menstruation.

women actually suffer from true PMDD.[8] A diagnosis of PMDD means that a woman experiences at least five of its symptoms, which include:

- anxiety
- panic attacks
- mood swings
- feelings of despair
- persistent irritability or anger
- sleep disturbances
- food cravings
- low energy
- difficulty focusing
- a loss of interest in daily activities and relationships

As with PMS, engaging in regular exercise, getting adequate rest, and following a balanced diet may help. Treatment may also include vitamins and over-the-counter pain relievers. In addition, the woman's physician may prescribe a type of antidepressant called a *selective serotonin reuptake inhibitor*, or SSRI, to modulate the brain's level of the neurotransmitter serotonin.

Dysmenorrhea

More than half of all menstruating women experience some pain for 1 to 2 days each month.[9] In most of these women, the pain is mild; however, sometimes the pain is severe enough to interfere with normal activities. This is called **dysmenorrhea,** or painful menstruation, and can include severe abdominal cramps, back or thigh pain, diarrhea, or even headaches in the days immediately preceding and during menstruation.[10] Dysmenorrhea is the leading cause of absenteeism from school in adolescent girls.[10]

The cramping pain of dysmenorrhea is due to *prostaglandins,* chemicals that regulate many body functions, including contraction of smooth muscle—like the muscle in a woman's uterus. Prostaglandins cause uterine muscle cells to contract, expelling the uterine lining. This is why over-the-counter prostaglandin inhibitors like ibuprofen and naproxen are usually effective in treating dysmenorrhea. The discomfort also usually wanes spontaneously with age and often disappears after pregnancy.

Endometriosis

Endometriosis is a condition in which endometrial tissue grows in areas outside of the uterus such as the fallopian tubes, ovaries, and other structures in the pelvic region.[11] This tissue responds to the same hormonal signals that affect the uterus and so breaks down and bleeds monthly into the abdominopelvic cavity. The condition can cause severe pain in the pelvic region that may be associated with the menstrual cycle as well as scarring that can result in infertility. Endometriosis occurs most commonly in women in their 30s and 40s but can occur at any time during the reproductive years. Although a physician can evaluate a woman for endometriosis during a physical examination, it is confirmed by laparoscopic surgery, in which a thin, lighted tube is inserted into the abdominopelvic cavity. If endometrial tissue is found, it can often be removed during the same procedure.[11]

dysmenorrhea Pain during menstruation that is severe enough to limit normal activities or require medication.

endometriosis A condition in which endometrial tissue grows in areas outside of the uterus.

amenorrhea Cessation of menstrual periods.

human sexual response cycle Distinct phases extending from the first moment of sexual desire until the calm after orgasm.

excitement The first phase of the sexual response cycle, marked by erection in men, and lubrication and clitoral swelling in women.

plateau The second phase of the sexual response cycle, characterized by intense excitement, rapid heartbeat, genital sensitivity, the secretion of pre-ejaculatory fluid in men, and vaginal swelling in women.

Amenorrhea

As much as some young women would love to stop menstruating, lack of periods can be a sign that the body is in distress. Missed periods, also known as **amenorrhea,** can usually be traced to severe weight loss with or without excessive exercise, a hormonal imbalance, or significant stress. Some medications, including certain birth control pills, can also suppress menstruation.

Amenorrhea is clinically defined as having no periods for at least three consecutive months.[4] It occurs normally in women who are pregnant and usually throughout the first few months of breast-feeding. However, it can also signal a serious underlying disorder of the reproductive organs. Amenorrhea is also a common consequence of disordered eating. For example, it is somewhat common among athletes—especially gymnasts and long-distance runners—who train vigorously while restricting their calorie intake to maintain a competitive weight.

Amenorrhea is not without long-term consequences. Symptoms can include headaches and vaginal dryness, but doctors are most concerned about its effect on bone health. Recall that the female reproductive hormone estrogen is produced by the ovaries during the normal menstrual cycle. Estrogen plays a key role in building new bone tissue, so amenorrhea puts women at significant risk for low bone density. This means that women who experience long-term amenorrhea can suffer from osteoporosis and bone fractures at a relatively early age.

The Sexual Response Cycle

Famed sex researchers William H. Masters and Virginia E. Johnson were the first to scientifically study the body's physiological reaction to sexual stimulation and subsequent release through orgasm. They called this process the **human sexual response cycle.** According to Masters and Johnson's model, the cycle is made up of four distinct phases extending from the first moment of sexual desire until the calm after sexual fulfillment:

- **Excitement.** The first phase occurs as the result of any erotic mental or physical stimulation that leads to arousal. In both sexes it is characterized by increased heart and respiration rate and also increased blood pressure. Nipple erection, especially as the result of direct stimulation, occurs in almost all females and in approximately 60% of males. Both may also experience a "sex flush," which is the reddening of the skin due to vasocongestion (blood vessel engorgement). In males, the penis becomes mostly erect and the testicles draw upward. In females, the labia increase in size and the clitoris swells. Lubrication occurs as the result of vasocongestion of the vaginal walls.
- **Plateau.** This more intense excitement takes partners to the edge of orgasm, leaving hearts beating rapidly and genitals sensitive to touch. In males, the urethral sphincter, a valve at the base of the penis that prevents urination during ejaculation, closes. Muscles at the penis base also begin to contract rhythmically. Males also secrete a pre-ejaculatory fluid (that may contain small amounts of sperm) and the testicles rise closer to the body. In females, the outer third of the vagina

swells and the pelvic muscle tightens, creating what Masters and Johnson refer to as the *orgasmic platform.*

- **Orgasm.** This event concludes the plateau phase and is the peak or climax of sexual response. It is accompanied by rhythmic muscle contractions of the genitals and surrounding areas. Most describe it as an intensely pleasurable feeling of release of sexual tension. In men, orgasm is accompanied by ejaculation.

- **Resolution.** In this phase the body returns to normal functioning. It often includes a sense of both well-being and fatigue.[12]

Men usually experience a *refractory period,* a period of time when they are not immediately able to respond to stimulation with an erection and may actually find continued stimulation unwelcome, or even painful. Most women do not experience a refractory period and may be able to immediately return to the plateau stage, allowing for the possibility of multiple orgasms.

Sexual Dysfunctions

Sexual dysfunctions are problems that can occur during any stage of the sexual response cycle—curbing desire, interrupting arousal, reducing pleasure, or preventing orgasm. An estimated 43% of women and 31% of men report having had at least one symptom of sexual dysfunction at some point in their life.[13]

Female Sexual Dysfunctions

A variety of problems can keep a woman from enjoying sex. These include painful intercourse, low level of sexual desire, and inability to achieve orgasm:[14]

- **Painful intercourse.** Up to 20% of women experience episodes of pain just before, during, or after intercourse.[15] Often the pain occurs only under certain circumstances, such as when the penis first enters the vagina or during vigorous thrusting. In other cases, the woman experiences a general burning or aching sensation. The causes vary with the type of pain reported, but some of the most common are insufficient vaginal lubrication, prior injury, infection or inflammation, an allergic reaction to a birth control product such as a spermicide or a latex condom, or an underlying disorder. Emotional factors such as stress, low self-esteem, or a history of sexual abuse occasionally play a role. Often, simply a change in position or the use of a commercial lubrication product can correct the problem. Underlying infection or other disorders should also be treated. In some cases, hormonal medications or therapy can help.

- **Low level of sexual desire.** About 5–15% of women experience a persistently low sex drive.[16] Common physical causes include fatigue, medication side effect, alcohol abuse, pregnancy, breast-feeding, and menopause. In addition, psychological problems and unresolved issues within the relationship can be factors. Lifestyle changes such as regular exercise and stress management can help, as can couples counseling. Hormonal therapy is also available. Finally, some women find that *Kegel exercises*—tightening the pelvic floor muscles as if stopping the flow of urine, holding for a few seconds, and releasing—can help put them back in touch with their sexual anatomy and their sex drive.

- **Inability to achieve orgasm.** About 1 in 5 women worldwide have difficulty experiencing orgasm.[17] The problem can occur as a side effect of prescription medications, including certain antidepressants. Medical problems, relationship problems, embarrassment, or a history of sexual abuse or rape can also prevent some women from reaching orgasm. However, one common factor is simply insufficient stimulation of the clitoris. Switching sexual positions can produce more clitoral stimulation during intercourse. Masturbation or use of a vibrator during sex can also help.[17]

Male Sexual Dysfunctions

Being unable to perform sexually can be damaging to a man's self-esteem and place stress on the relationship. Problems related to male sexual function include the following:

- **Erectile dysfunction (ED)** is the inability of a man to get or maintain an erection firm enough for sexual intercourse.[18] The problem is most prevalent among older men. Erectile dysfunction most commonly results from injury or underlying disease, but it can stem from fatigue, stress, depression, use of certain medications, or excessive alcohol or tobacco use. As treatment, a physician may prescribe lifestyle modifications such as weight loss or quitting smoking. Oral medications such as Viagra, Cialis, or Levitra can help by boosting the flow of blood to the penis, enabling an erection to occur; however, they can have serious side effects and are not intended for men with certain underlying health conditions. Surgery may be recommended in cases of underlying injury, and counseling or sex therapy is also an option.

- **Premature ejaculation (PE)** is a condition in which a man ejaculates earlier than he would like to, or than his partner would like him to. Although in the past, sex researchers and therapists

orgasm The peak, or climax, of sexual response, characterized by rhythmic muscle contractions of the genitals and surrounding areas, and ejaculation in men.

resolution The stage of the response cycle in which the body returns to normal functioning.

sexual dysfunctions Problems occurring during any stage of the sexual response cycle.

erectile dysfunction (ED) The inability of a male to obtain or maintain an erection.

premature ejaculation (PE) A condition in which a male ejaculates earlier than he would like to.

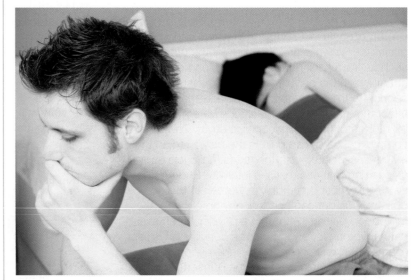

Sexual dysfunctions can occur in both men and women.

attempted to define PE based on a quantitative time frame (i.e., how long it took to ejaculate), today most agree that a male has a problem when poor ejaculatory control interferes with the sexual satisfaction of one or both partners. PE can result from physical factors, but in most cases it is due to psychological factors such as anxiety. In college-aged men it frequently occurs because of lack of experience, intense arousal, and alcohol use.[19] However, hormonal imbalance, infection, nervous system disorders, and other physical causes should be ruled out if PE is chronic. Treatment of any underlying physical problem is important. In many cases, sexual counseling and incorporating into sexual activity a delaying tactic called the "squeeze technique" can resolve the problem.[20]

>> For more information on the "squeeze technique," visit the Mayo Clinic website at www.mayoclinic.com/health/premature-ejaculation/DS00578/DSECTION=treatments-and-drugs.

Sexual Behavior

A wide range of human sexual behaviors and interests are considered "normal." Before biologist Alfred Kinsey's research in the late 1940s and early 1950s, Americans had no basis for determining what the norm was. Kinsey's research provided a basis for social comparison and helped answer a question many people wondered about: "Who's doing what with whom and how often are they doing it?" Since Kinsey, many researchers studying this question have concluded that the continuum of "normal" sexual behavior in our society is broad and varied.

Abstinence and Celibacy

Abstinence refers to the avoidance of sexual intercourse. Whether it is by active choice or as a matter of circumstance, many people find themselves abstaining from sexual activity for extended periods. This long-term abstinence is referred to as *celibacy*. Some choose celibacy for religious or moral reasons; others out of a desire to avoid becoming pregnant or developing an STI.[21] The **Spotlight** box on page 233 takes a closer look at abstinence and celibacy among young adults.

Non-Intercourse Sexual Activity

There are a number of ways people experience sexual pleasure without actually engaging in sexual intercourse. Among them are masturbation, sexual fantasies, kissing, "outercourse," and oral sex. Pornography, another form of non-intercourse sexual activity, is discussed in the **Media and Sexuality** box on page 234.

Fantasy and Masturbation

Sexual fantasies are sexual or romantic thoughts, daydreams, and imagined scenarios that can be very detailed and explicit, featuring fictional characters or actual people. They may reflect a person's unconscious desires, allowing the person to imagine sexual experiences that they may not feel comfortable acting out in real life.

> " *A wide range of human sexual behaviors and interests are considered 'normal.'* "

Masturbation is the manipulation of one's own genitals for sexual pleasure. Masturbation is a healthy and common expression of sexuality. Research indicates that 92% of male college students and nearly half (48%) of female college students have masturbated.[22]

"Outercourse" and Oral Sex

Although the definition can vary, **outercourse** generally refers to sexual intimacy without penetration of the vagina or anus. Outercourse includes everything from kissing and "making out" to manual stimulation of the genitals and mutual masturbation. Because no semen enters the vagina during outercourse, there is no risk of pregnancy. The risk of STIs is also minimized, although infections like herpes and HPV can still spread through simple skin-to-skin contact of the genitals.

Oral sex is the stimulation of the genitals by the tongue or mouth. **Fellatio** is oral stimulation of the penis, and **cunnilingus** is oral stimulation of the vulva or clitoris. Some couples use oral sex as *foreplay,* stimulation that is erotic and is intended to increase arousal prior to sexual intercourse. Others engage in oral sex in place of sexual intercourse. Still others avoid the practice. Although oral sex does not result in pregnancy, it is not necessarily "safer" sex. Unprotected oral sex can leave a partner vulnerable to the transmission of herpes, syphilis, hepatitis B, and gonorrhea. Using a condom or dental dam during oral sex can help prevent the spread of STIs. See Chapter 11 for more information on preventing STIs.

"Sexting"

Sexting is the use of cell phones or similar electronic devices to send sexually explicit text, photos, or videos. In a recent study, 20% of teens and 33% of young adults reported sending or posting nude or semi-nude photos or videos of themselves. In addition, 39% of teens and 59% of young adults reported they are sending or posting sexually suggestive messages. One-third of male teens and one-fourth of female teens report receiving nude or semi-nude images that were originally meant to be private.[23]

Sexting most frequently occurs in one of three circumstances:

- Exchanges of images only between two romantically involved partners.
- Exchanges between partners and shared outside the relationship.
- Exchanges involving people who are not in a relationship, but at least one of them hopes to be.[24]

Many states are enacting legislation to regulate sexting. Arizona passed a bill in March 2010, making it a class-two misdemeanor for minors to possess or send sexually explicit text messages to another minor.[25] This law sets an important precedent because it is specific to the offense. Before its passage, prosecutors could only use child pornography laws, which were written long before the development of wireless technologies and were thus difficult to apply. It is likely that the new bill will prompt more prosecutions and more research examining sexting among college students.

abstinence The avoidance of sexual intercourse.

masturbation Manipulation of one's own genitals for sexual pleasure.

outercourse Sexual intimacy without penetration of the vagina or anus.

oral sex Stimulation of the genitals by the tongue or mouth.

fellatio Oral stimulation of the penis.

cunnilingus Oral stimulation of the vulva or clitoris.

sexting The use of cell phones or similar electronic devices to send sexually explicit text, photos, or videos.

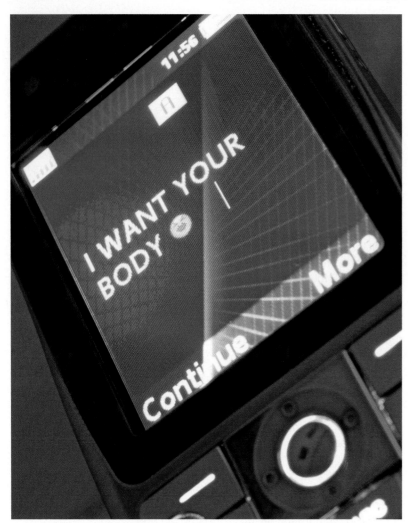

"Sexting" can leave you vulnerable to privacy breaches and embarrassment.

>> Do you have questions about sex that you are afraid to ask? *Go Ask Alice* is a website sponsored by Columbia University that answers many frequently asked questions: www.goaskalice.columbia.edu.

Sexual Intercourse

Sexual intercourse, or *coitus,* is sexual union involving genital penetration. For many heterosexuals, the term is synonymous with **vaginal intercourse,** the insertion of the penis into the vagina. Unless they are trying to conceive, couples engaging in vaginal intercourse are encouraged to practice "safer sex." The use of condoms is advised to avoid unintended pregnancy while reducing the couple's risk for STIs.

Long considered a taboo in U.S. society, **anal intercourse** has increasingly become accepted, especially among younger generations. According to surveys from the Centers for Disease Control and Prevention (CDC), about 40% of men and 35% of women aged 25–44 have had anal sex with a partner of the opposite sex.[26] The CDC also reports that 6% of men aged 15–44 have had anal sex with another man at some point in their lives. The practice involves penile penetration of the anus and rectum. Because these tissues are much more fragile than

those of the vagina, anal intercourse is one of the riskiest of sexual behaviors in terms of both injury and transmission of infectious disease. It represents one of the primary risk factors for acquiring HIV, the virus that causes AIDS, and is also associated with the spread of syphilis and gonorrhea. Condoms can be used, but they tend to break during anal sex. Sex educators advise couples engaging in anal sex to use a lubricant along with a condom.

Communicating About Sex

Each year, there are more than 15 million STIs among people in the United States and well over 1 million terminations of unplanned pregnancies.[27] Given these statistics, it seems obvious that practicing safer sex is crucial. But before you can practice it, you have to talk about it. It's also important to communicate what you're comfortable with in terms of sexual behaviors, frequency, and other potentially sensitive issues. So how do you get up the nerve to talk candidly about sex? See **Practical Strategies: Communicating Effectively About Sex and Birth Control** on page 244.

Sexual Orientation and Gender Identity

At a very early age, humans begin to develop their **sexual orientation,** their romantic and physical attraction toward others. Experts believe that our natural tendency to be attracted to men or women—or both—is shaped by a confluence of biological, environmental, and cognitive factors, with sexual orientation being neither a conscious choice nor something that can be readily changed.

Sex researcher Alfred Kinsey theorized that sexual orientation could be delineated on one basic continuum, broken down into seven parts. At one end of the Kinsey Scale are **heterosexuals,** "straight" people who are solely attracted to the opposite gender. On the other end are **homosexuals,** *gays* or *lesbians* who are attracted to people of the same gender. In the middle are **bisexuals,** individuals who are attracted to members of their own sex as well as the opposite sex. In between these points on the scale are varying levels of bisexuality.

Heterosexuality

Throughout the world, the majority of people describe themselves as heterosexual. In the United States, 95.9% of men and women aged 18–44 identify themselves as heterosexuals, and 4.1% of men and women identify themselves as homosexual or bisexual, according to a survey conducted by the CDC.[26]

Heterosexuality is the only sexual orientation that receives full social and legal legitimacy in most countries, including the United States. As a result of this and other cultural factors, homosexuals and bisexuals can be subjected to "heterosexism," a system of negative

vaginal intercourse Intercourse characterized by the insertion of the penis into the vagina.

anal intercourse Intercourse characterized by the insertion of the penis into a partner's anus and rectum.

sexual orientation Romantic and physical attraction toward others.

heterosexuals People who are sexually attracted to partners of the opposite sex.

homosexuals People who are sexually attracted to partners of the same sex.

bisexuals People who are attracted to partners of both the same and the opposite sex.

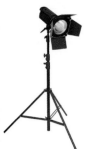

Celibacy: The New Sexual Revolution?

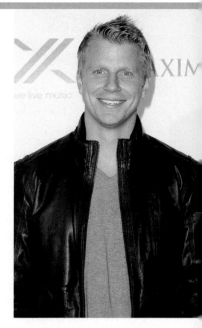

Bachelor Sean Lowe.

Recently, the hit series *The Bachelor* took a sudden break from being quite so steamy—and featured a potential groom who turned out to prefer celibacy. Bachelor Sean Lowe kept his dates on the show fairly chaste and, after the finale, stated that after some sexual experience in college, he decided to abstain from sex until marriage. When bloggers and tabloids responded with surprise, even dubbing him a "born-again virgin," Lowe gave the equivalent of a polite shrug. "That's my personal opinion," he said in one interview. "For me, it's a non-story."[1]

For once, reality TV seems to be mirroring the real world. Today more young adults are waiting before having sex. In a national survey released in 2013, about 34% of college students reported that they have never had vaginal intercourse, and about 31% said they had never had oral sex.[2] This modest increase in abstinence correlates with the statistics from surveys of high school students: in a 2010 survey, 53% identified themselves as virgins (someone who has never had intercourse), up 7% from 1991.[3]

At the same time, celibacy programs are increasingly visible on college campuses. A campus newspaper at the Lutheran Gustavus Adolphus College in Minnesota recently ran an article titled "Celibacy: The New Hipster Trend?"[4] It proposed that, "On a campus where condoms are handed out like candy . . . celibacy is becoming as hip as organic coffee." But Christian colleges are not alone in reporting the trend: Recently, "abstinence clubs" have emerged at Ivy League schools, including the Anscombe Societies at Princeton University and MIT, and True Love Revolution at Harvard. The clubs include among their members not only students from conservative religions, but also so-called new feminists and philosophy students who use ethical arguments to ground their choice of celibacy.[5]

Not everyone agrees that celibacy is compatible with feminism—or a superior ethical choice for single adults. The movement has drawn a fair amount of controversy, with opponents claiming that the clubs perpetuate gender stereotypes that value women who are virgins and denounce those who are not. Some have accused the clubs of manipulating statistics about unplanned pregnancies and sexually transmitted infections to frighten students into celibacy.

Still, even opponents admit that the clubs provide a valuable service to students who want to abstain from sexual behavior during their college years, giving them a safe space—via meetings and a club website—where they can debate social, scientific, philosophical, and religious positions on celibacy, and simply share information. Perhaps most importantly, they give members a circle of companions who know and respect their choices—and who might not have been as surprised as the blogosphere by Sean Lowe's personal decision on abstinence.

References: **1.** "Why Did 'The Bachelor' Hide Sean Lowe's Born-Again Virginity?" by Ramin Setoodeh, March 11, 2013, *The Daily Beast*, retrieved from http://www.thedailybeast.com/articles/2013/03/11/why-did-the-bachelor-hide-sean-lowe-s-born-again-virginity.html. **2.** *American College Health Association-National College Health Assessment (ACHA-NCHA II) Reference Group Executive Summary, Fall 2012*, by the American College Health Association, 2013, retrieved from http://www.acha-ncha .org. **3.** "QuickStats: Never-Married Females and Males Aged 15–19 Years Who Have Ever Had Sexual Intercourse—National Survey of Family Growth, United States, 1988–2008," by the Centers for Disease Control, 2010, *Morbidity and Mortality Weekly Report, 59*(26), p. 819, retrieved from http://www.cdc.gov/mmwr/preview/mmwrhtml/mm5926a8.htm?s_cid=mm5926a8_w. **4.** "Celibacy: The New Hipster Trend?" by Elizabeth Folsom, from The Campus Majority website, Thursday May 13, 2010. Reprinted by permission of the author. **5.** "Students of Virginity" by Randall Patterson, March 30, 2008, *The New York Times*, retrieved from http://www.nytimes.com/2008/03/30/magazine/30Chastity-t.html.

attitudes, bias, and discrimination in favor of heterosexual relationships. Those with a heterosexist view think that their orientation is the only "normal" one.

Homosexuality

Homosexuality is deep-rooted in many world cultures, having been an accepted practice in some parts of the ancient world. In other regions it has been and is still shunned. For example, psychiatrists in some countries, including China, India, and Brazil, still consider it a mental illness.

In the United States, the American Psychiatric Association removed homosexuality from its manual of psychiatric disorders in 1973, in response to a growing understanding of homosexuality as an entirely normal variant of sexual orientation. Correspondingly, there has been an increasing acceptance of homosexuality in U.S. culture. For example, in a 1973 survey, 70% of people in the United States reported believing that homosexual relations are always sinful; but in 2009, only

> " *In the United States, the American Psychiatric Association removed homosexuality from its manual of psychiatric disorders in 1973.*"

49% expressed this belief.[28] As of 2011, 52% of all employers offered domestic partner health benefits, a quick jump up from 31% in 2010.[29]

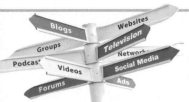

media and SEXUALITY

Is Porn a Problem?

Pornography, explicit sexual material that is used for sexual excitement and erotic stimulation, has never been easier to find. Porn appears in a host of media, including books, magazines, photos, animation, film, sculpture, painting, and video games; however, the two top revenue generators are video sales and rentals and Internet sites. Of all websites, approximately 12% (4.2 million) are pornographic, and 25% of all search engine requests (68 million) are related to pornography.[1] In the United States alone, pornography is estimated to be a $12 billion business.[1]

With porn so ubiquitous in our society, college campuses are far from exempt. A study conducted by East Carolina University found that 43% of college students reported looking at pornography at least once or twice a week. Almost 32% of college men reported viewing pornography three to five times per week, whereas less than 4% of women reported doing so. The findings from this study also suggest that the Internet is the primary source of pornography for college students.[2]

Along with commercial pornography websites, there has been an increase in noncommercial, free sites where visitors can post their own photos and videos. Some of these sites are devoted to college students and are referred to as "dorm porn." Some experts contend that such noncommercial pornographic websites reflect a larger trend toward digital self-exploitation.[3]

In the East Carolina University study, men expressed greater approval of pornography, and women reported feeling more threatened by it. Is there anything behind these concerns? Pamela Paul, a prominent researcher and author on the effects of pornography, cites several issues surrounding pornography that can be problematic.[4, 5] Looking at porn wastes time: Studies are delayed or cut short, work is interrupted, and relationships are put on hold. It also wastes money: Once users become "acclimated" to free sites, they move to expensive services. Porn has addictive elements, claiming increasing amounts of time and money; interfering with activities of daily living, goals, and relationships; and involving a sense of compulsion. Particularly on the Internet, users find themselves turning more and more often to increasingly violent and shocking images, including those involving abuse, torture, or children. Many users report feeling increasingly debased by their porn use; images that once would have disgusted them come to seem "routine," and ever harder-core porn becomes a requirement for sexual arousal.

Porn has specific effects on romantic relationships as well. Porn is essentially a form of voyeurism, involving looking at but not interacting with the model or actor. As such, it elevates the physical—body parts and acts—while ignoring all other qualities that make us human. Viewers learn to relate to others as objects rather than to form and maintain relationships with them. Not surprisingly, porn reduces the viewer's ability to be close to others—including their current partner. Many find that their sex lives deteriorate and their relationships collapse. In a 2004 poll, one in four divorced respondents said Internet pornography and chat had contributed to the breakup. Some psychologists view pornography use as a hallmark of disconnection and a risk factor for developing a true intimacy disorder.

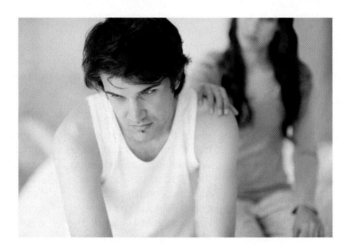

Excessive use of pornography can interfere with relationships in real life.

Critical-Thinking Questions

1. Do you agree that men and women often have different views about porn? If so, what do you think are some of the factors behind these differences?

2. What are some common stereotypes about men and women depicted in pornography?

3. How might these stereotypes be detrimental to a person's real-life relationships?

References: **1.** *National Pornography Statistics,* by Brigham Young University, 2010, retrieved from https://wsr.byu.edu/pornographystats. **2.** "College Student Attitudes Toward Pornography Use," by S. O'Reilly, D. Knox, & M. E. Zusman, 2007, *College Student Journal, 41,* pp. 402–404. **3.** "Editorial: Sexting: A New Form of Victimless Crime?" by K. Jaishankar, 2009, *International Journal of Cyber Criminology, 3*(1), pp. 21–25. **4.** "The Cost of Growing Up on Porn," by Pamela Paul, March 7, 2010, *The Washington Post,* retrieved from http://www.washingtonpost.com/wp-dyn/content/article/2010/03/05/AR2010030501552.html?sid=ST2010030502871. **5.** "Why the Government Should Care About Pornography," by the United States Senate, November 10, 2005, Senate Judiciary Committee: Testimony of Pamela Paul, retrieved from http://judiciary.senate.gov/hearings/testimony.cfm?id?1674&wit_id?4824.

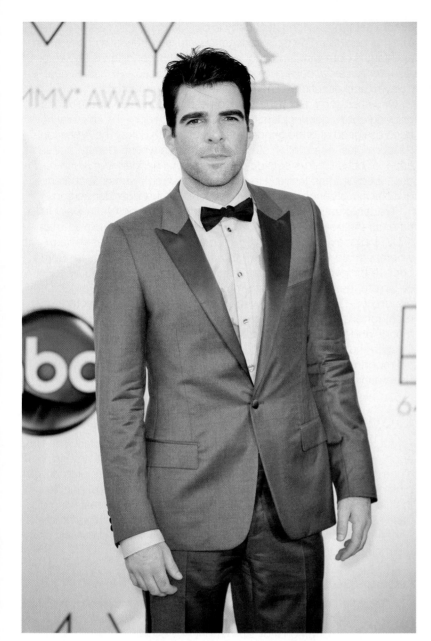

Actor Zachary Quinto came out in 2011.

Still, many homosexuals continue to face discrimination and harassment in the United States, a fact acknowledged by 64% of the population.[28] This discrimination can take many forms: **homonegativity,** having a negative attitude toward homosexuality, or **homophobia,** an irrational fear of, aversion to, or discrimination against homosexuals or homosexuality. The harassment often begins at an early age. In one study, researchers found that homosexual and bisexual students "are at greater risk of suicidal thoughts, suicide attempts, victimization by peers, and elevated levels of unexcused absences from school," with 84.6% of such students reporting verbal abuse and 40.1% reporting having been physically assaulted because of their sexual orientation.[30] They were also twice as likely to have skipped school in the previous month out of a concern for their own safety. Homonegativity and homophobia sometimes erupt into criminal violence: In 2012, the FBI reported more than 1,300 incidents of hate crimes against homosexuals.[31]

Bisexuality

One common, and often inaccurate, definition of bisexuality is having romantic or sexual relations with people of the same and opposite genders, often outside a monogamous relationship. Yet, as the Kinsey Scale indicates, sexual orientation may often be experienced as a continuum, rather than a set of rigid rules, and many bisexual people may find that their preference on this continuum can vary over

homonegativity Having a negative attitude toward homosexuality.

homophobia The irrational fear of, aversion to, or discrimination against homosexuals or homosexuality.

Deciding to Get on the Pill

"HI, I'M BETTY. When discussing contraceptives with my mom, she gave me so many options. She works in maternal health care, so she had this huge planner out and she was like 'this is a female condom and this is this and that'—and it was just like, I don't even want to know all the other stuff. I didn't want an IUD and I didn't want a female condom or anything like that . . . I was like, let me go to the simplest form. That way if I decide 'OK, if I don't want to take this anymore, then I can get rid of it.' I ended up deciding to get on the pill. The pros are that you always know when your period is going to arrive, it lessens PMS and cramping, and you won't get pregnant. The cons—you have to continuously stay on it. You have to keep it as a ritual: like, get in the shower, brush your teeth, and before you brush your teeth, take your pill. Sometimes it can make you nauseous. That's another con, but other than that, it's great."

1. Given what you've learned in this chapter, do you think birth control pills alone are enough to protect you (or your partner) against pregnancy? How about STIs? Explain your answer.

2. Betty was able to turn to her mom for advice on what contraceptive was right for her. Think about the resources available to you. Where will you go to learn more about contraceptive options and decide which one is right for you?

time.[32] Some bisexuals may choose not to act on their innate impulses, whereas others have not had the opportunity to do so. Some may pursue a monogamous relationship with a man at one point in their lives and a committed relationship with a woman later. A better gauge of bisexuality is having an attraction to both men and women. The intensity of the attraction can change over time, but bisexuality should not be seen as a "phase" that a person is going through. In one long-term study of bisexual women, the subjects reported being attracted to both sexes throughout the 10-year study period.[33] Bisexuality, the experts wrote, is a "stable identity" rather than a "transitional stage."

Transgenderism and Transsexuality

Whereas the term *sex* refers to an individual's biological status as male or female, *gender* includes the ways people act, interact, and feel about themselves. **Transgenderism** is the condition where someone's *gender identity* (sense of his- or herself as male or female) or gender expression is different from his or her *assigned sex*. Sex assignment

transgenderism The state in which someone's gender identity or gender expression is different from his or her assigned sex at birth.

transsexual A transgendered individual who lives as the gender opposite to his or her assigned sex.

conception The fertilization of a female egg with male sperm.

occurs at birth—as long as a baby is born with typical male or female external genitalia. The term *transgenderism* is not used in cases when an infant is born with ambiguous genitalia. This condition is known as a *disorder of sexual development*, and in such cases, sex assignment is delayed until genetic and hormonal testing is conducted.

Once assigned, sex usually becomes a profound component of a growing child's gender identity. But for some people, the sex they have been assigned and the gender they identify with differ. The American Psychological Association states that "Anyone whose identity, appearance, or behavior falls outside of conventional gender norms can be described as transgender. However, not everyone whose appearance or behavior is gender-atypical will identify as a transgender person."[34]

Transsexuals are transgendered individuals who live, usually full-time, as the gender opposite to their assigned sex. Female-to-male (FTM) transsexuals are biological females who now live as males, whereas male-to-female (MTF) transsexuals are the opposite. Some choose to have hormonal treatments and surgical procedures to complete the physical transformation from one sex to the other. Others do not. One study of FTM transsexuals who were attracted to men, for example, found that "most were 'out' as transgender among friends and family, but not on the job or within the gay community."[35] Despite the complexities of such considerations, many transsexuals report feeling comfortable with their gender identity and sexual orientation.[35]

Conception and Contraception

About half of pregnancies in the United States are unintended. The U.S. abortion rate, although off its all-time high, continues to be among the highest in the industrialized world. In addition, failure to use protective birth control options, such as condoms, exposes millions of people in the United States each year to STIs that can cause life-threatening disease as well as infertility. So whether you are planning to have children or not, it is important to understand your fertility, how to protect it, and the methods for family planning.

Conception

At birth, a female's ovaries are filled with more than 1 million ovarian follicles, each containing an immature egg. After puberty, a woman's body prepares itself for pregnancy each month by ovulating—releasing one egg. Meanwhile, a man's testes are constantly creating sperm, millions of which are released into the woman's vagina during ejaculation. The vast majority of these sperm will never find their way to their target—millions will leak from the woman's vagina or be destroyed in its acidic environment. The few thousand sperm that do reach the egg—typically while it is still within the fallopian tube—next face the difficult task of penetrating the egg's tough outer layer. Thousands more of these remaining sperm are "used up" secreting enzymes that dissolve a region of the egg's membrane. As soon as a minute portion of the egg is exposed, the next sperm that approaches will be able to make contact with the egg and will be pulled into the egg cell interior. The egg will then undergo a chemical change that will block any further sperm from penetrating its membrane. The "winning sperm" then travels to the egg's nucleus, and fertilization—or **conception,** the combination of the genetic material (DNA) of an egg and sperm cell—occurs.

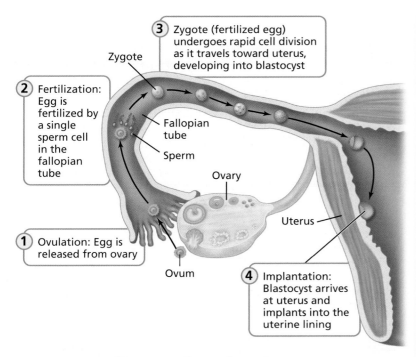

③ Zygote (fertilized egg) undergoes rapid cell division as it travels toward uterus, developing into blastocyst

Zygote

② Fertilization: Egg is fertilized by a single sperm cell in the fallopian tube

Fallopian tube

Sperm

Ovary

① Ovulation: Egg is released from ovary

Ovum

Uterus

④ Implantation: Blastocyst arrives at uterus and implants into the uterine lining

FIGURE 10.4 Events Involved in Conception. The process of conception includes ovulation, fertilization, and implantation.

Source: Thompson, Janice; Manore, Melinda; and Vaughan, Linda, *The Science of Nutrition,* 3rd Ed., © 2011, p. 621. Reprinted and electronically reproduced by permission of Pearson Education, Inc., Upper Saddle River, New Jersey.

Even then, pregnancy is not guaranteed. The fertilized egg, now called a **zygote,** must complete its journey through the fallopian tube and emerge into the uterus, where it can implant in the endometrium (**implantation**). Any scar tissue within the tube can "snag" the zygote so that it attaches to the wall of the tube, where it cannot grow. In some cases the zygote will make it into the uterus but fail to implant, and the entire process from menstruation to ovulation will begin all over again.

Figure 10.4 summarizes the processes of conception through implantation.

Contraceptive Options

Contraception is any method used to prevent pregnancy. Contraceptive options differ in technique, price, effectiveness, and side effects, but they all have the same goal: to keep eggs and sperm apart. They do this in a number of ways:

- *Natural methods* involve no pills or devices and are therefore always available and cost-free.
- *Barrier methods* work to prevent sperm from reaching an egg.
- *Hormonal methods* deliver hormones to a woman that prevent ovulation. If no egg is released it can't be fertilized.
- *Surgical methods* are available for women and for men and are the most permanent of options.

Table 10.1 on pages 238–239 summarizes different forms of contraception, organized into four

general categories: cost-free methods, methods available over the counter, methods requiring a prescription, and surgical methods. As we take a closer look at these methods, take note of differences in availability, cost, effectiveness, ease of use, and whether or not the method provides protection against STIs. Meanwhile, the **Student Stats** box on page 240 illustrates the most popular forms of contraception reported by college students.

Cost-Free Methods

Three methods of contraception are always available and are cost-free. They are intimacy without intercourse, fertility awareness, and withdrawal. Note that none of them are 100% reliable.

Intimacy without Intercourse. Some couples who desire a sexual relationship yet want to avoid the risks of pregnancy and STIs opt for non-intercourse sexual activities like kissing, "making out," manual stimulation of the genitals, and mutual masturbation. Because intercourse doesn't occur, the chance of pregnancy or STIs is theoretically zero. However, in reality, this method requires a high level of commitment, self-discipline, and mutual cooperation and trust.

Fertility Awareness (Rhythm or Calendar Method). With **fertility awareness (rhythm or calendar method),** a woman tracks on a calendar the day her period begins each month. Ideally, she also logs the days on which she had copious, slippery cervical mucus because its presence indicates that she is fertile (the mucus occurs as ovulation approaches). Finally, if possible, she makes a note of the day on which she experienced mid-cycle pain (indicating ovulation). **Figure 10.5** on page 240 provides an example of fertility tracking over the course of a month. Because most women's cycles vary somewhat from month to month, it's essential that a woman using the fertility awareness method track her cycles for several months (a full year is ideal) before relying on this method. Also, keep in mind that this method is not fail-safe, and that women with irregular menstrual cycles should rely on other methods of contraception.

Using the data from several months, the woman next calculates her average cycle length (for example, 28 days, 32 days, etc.). Because sperm can survive for 5 days in the vagina—possibly more, and an egg is viable for up to 2 days, a woman is theoretically able to conceive as many as 5 days before she ovulates and as many as 2 days afterward. However, to be on the safe side, women should avoid intercourse for 7 days prior to ovulation and for 4 days afterward.

Some women also track their body temperature, which typically rises slightly after ovulation. However, because the temperature increase is so slight—usually less than 1 degree—and must be recorded at the same time every morning before getting out of bed, many women do not have success with this method.

In addition to the careful planning required, the fertility awareness method requires couples to abstain from sexual intercourse for 11 days out of each cycle. If couples also abstain during the first few days the woman is having her period, this can eliminate half of all days each month. During that time, the couple can use other forms of contraception or engage in non-intercourse sexual activity. Also note that when the couple does engage in unprotected intercourse, both partners may be at risk for STIs.

zygote A fertilized egg.

implantation The lodging of a fertilized egg in the endometrium of the uterus.

contraception Any method used to prevent pregnancy.

fertility awareness (rhythm or calendar method) The tracking of a woman's monthly menstrual cycle; may be used as a method of preventing pregnancy if the woman tracks carefully and has regular periods, although it is not fail-safe.

TABLE 10.1 A Summary of Contraceptive Options

Method	Description	Advantages	Disadvantages	Failure Rate*	Average Cost
Cost-Free Methods					
Intimacy without intercourse	Engaging in sexual or sensual behavior without vaginal penetration	Prevents pregnancy and STIs	Requires mutual commitment, trust, and self-control	No statistics available	No cost
Fertility awareness (rhythm or calendar method)	Understanding the monthly menstrual cycle and avoiding intercourse on fertile days	No cost	No protection against STIs; not as effective if cycle is irregular; high possibility of failure	1–25	No cost
Withdrawal	Withdrawing the penis before ejaculation	No cost	No protection against STIs; high risk of pregnancy; requires physical and psychological control and awareness	19	No cost
Over-the-Counter Methods					
Male condom (such as Durex, Lifestyles, Trojan)	Very thin sheath that fits over an erect penis to prevent semen from entering vagina	No medical exam required; side effects are uncommon; latex condoms protect against many STIs	Only about 80–94% effective at preventing pregnancy; if not used correctly, unintended pregnancies can occur; requires planning	2–15	$0.50–$3.00 each use
Female condom (such as Reality, F.C.)	A thin sheath with a soft outer ring and a pliable inner ring; the condom covers the inside of the entire vagina	Protects against STIs	Some users may have difficulty inserting the condom correctly	5–21	$0.50–$3.00 each use
Contraceptive sponge (such as Today Sponge)	A round, soft foam sponge containing spermicide with a nylon loop for removal	Easy to obtain, no medical exam required; easy to carry; can be left in place for up to 30 hours	No protection against STIs and increases risk of STIs and other infections; may cause irritation in some women	9–16	$9–$15 for a packet of three sponges
Spermicides (such as Encare, VCF, Gynol)	Chemical compounds that immobilize sperm	Easy to obtain, no medical exam required; variety of forms for convenience	May leak; high failure rate if used alone; doesn't protect against STIs; increases risk of some STIs	18–29 if used alone, but spermicides increase protection when used with other barrier methods	$0.50–$3.00 each use
Emergency contraception (EC) (Also known as the "morning-after pill," such as Plan B One-Step and Next Choice)	A single pill or two pills containing a synthetic form of progesterone that can suppress ovulation and disrupt implantation	Effective when used within 72 hours after unprotected intercourse to prevent pregnancy, although it is most effective within the first 24 hours following intercourse	Not effective if woman has already ovulated prior to using; begins to lose effectiveness 24–72 hours after intercourse; does not protect against STIs	No statistics available	$35–$60
Methods Requiring Prescriptions					
Diaphragm	A soft dome-shaped cup with a flexible rim that is filled with spermicide and fits inside the vagina, covering the cervix	Does not require the ingestion of hormones; may be left in place for up to 24 hours	No protection against STIs; cannot be used during menstruation; some women find insertion difficult; may become dislodged; requires an exam and fitting by a health-care provider; may cause urinary tract infection or vaginal irritation in some users	6–16	$100–$200 for device, fitting, and spermicide
Cervical cap	A pliable cup filled with spermicide that fits inside the vagina, covering the cervix	Does not require the ingestion of hormones; may be left in place for up to 48 hours	No protection against STIs; cannot be used during menstruation; some women find insertion difficult; may become dislodged; requires an exam and fitting by a health-care provider; may cause urinary tract infection or vaginal irritation in some users	6–16	$100–$200 for device, fitting, and spermicide
Intrauterine Device (IUD)					
ParaGard	A small T-shaped plastic device that releases copper	No action necessary before, during, or after sex; can be left in place for 10–12 years	No protection against STIs; in rare cases, may cause infections or the device may slip out	Less than 1	$200–$300
Mirena	A small T-shaped plastic device that releases progestin	No action necessary before, during, or after sex; may lessen periods or they may cease; can be left in place for up to 5 years	No protection against STIs; in rare cases, may cause infections or the device may slip out	Less than 1	$200–$300
Birth control pills *A variety of combination pills are available.*	Pills containing the hormones estrogen and progestin, which prevent pregnancy; one pill should be taken at the same time each day	Convenient; helps protect against cancer of the ovaries and uterus; some women have lighter periods and milder cramps	No protection against STIs; requires taking a pill each day, which may be hard to remember; refills must be on hand; requires ingesting artificial hormones; adverse effects possible; consultation with health-care provider is essential	1–8	$20–$35 per month

TABLE 10.1 **A Summary of Contraceptive Options** (continued)

Method	Description	Advantages	Disadvantages	Failure Rate*	Average Cost
Emergency contraception (EC)/ella	A "morning-after pill" that can be taken up to 5 days after sexual intercourse to suppress ovulation and prevent pregnancy	Unlike OTC EC, can be taken up to 5 days after sexual intercourse and still be effective	Not effective if woman has already ovulated prior to using; does not protect against STIs; requires a prescription	No statistics available	No information available at press time
"Mini-pill"	Pills containing the hormone progestin, which prevents pregnancy	Convenient; helps protect against cancer of the ovaries and uterus; some women have lighter periods and milder cramps; better choice for women who are at risk for developing blood clots	No protection against STIs; requires taking a pill each day, which may be hard to remember; refills must be on hand; requires ingesting artificial hormones; several adverse effects possible; consultation with health-care provider is essential	1–8	$20–$35 per month
Transdermal patch	A thin plastic patch that is placed on the skin, which releases the hormones estrogen and progestin slowly into the body	Convenient—woman does not have to remember to take a pill every day; may reduce risk of endometrial cancer and other cancers, relieve PMS and menstrual cramping, and improve acne	No protection against STIs; may cause bleeding between periods, breast tenderness, or nausea and vomiting; may cause skin irritation at patch site; may alter a woman's sexual desire; may be less effective in women who weigh more than 198 pounds; several long-term adverse effects possible; consultation with health-care provider is essential	1–8	$25–$30 per month
Vaginal ring (NuvaRing)	A small flexible ring that releases the hormones estrogen and progestin slowly into the body	Convenient—woman does not have to remember to take a pill every day; may reduce risk of endometrial cancer and other cancers, relieve PMS and menstrual cramping, and improve acne	No protection against STIs; may cause bleeding between periods, breast tenderness, or nausea and vomiting; may increase vaginal discharge and lead to irritation or infection; may alter a woman's sexual desire; several long-term adverse effects possible; consultation with health-care provider is essential	1–8	Cost of initial health-care appointment plus $15–$50 per month
Monthly injections	An injection containing the hormones estrogen and progestin	Convenient, may help reduce risk of certain cancers and promote lighter, shorter periods	No protection against STIs; requires monthly visit to health-care provider; side effects may include bloating/weight gain, headaches, vaginal bleeding, and irregular periods; women over the age of 35 or who smoke or have certain health conditions are at risk for serious adverse effects	1–3	$30–$35 month
Quarterly injections	An injection containing the hormone progestin	Convenient; requires only one injection four times a year; helps protect against endometrial cancer; reduces monthly bleeding and anemia; in most cases, women stop having their periods	No protection against STIs; side effects may include amenorrhea, headaches, depression, loss of interest in sex, and bone loss; fertility may be delayed for many months after discontinuing; not advised for women who want less than a year of birth control	1–3	$60–$75 for 3 months
Implant	A thin plastic rod containing the hormone progestin	Convenient; lasts for 3 years; helps protect women from endometrial cancer	No protection against STIs; insertion and removal of implants requires a small cut in the skin, and scarring may occur; if implants fail, there is a greater chance of ectopic pregnancy; side effects may include acne, headaches, weight gain	1	$450–$750 for 5 years
Surgical Methods					
Tubal ligation	The fallopian tubes are surgically tied or otherwise sealed	Convenient; no hormonal effect; permanent solution to birth control	No protection against STIs; invasive; permanent	Less than 1	$1,500–$6,000
Hysterectomy	Surgical removal of a woman's uterus, sometimes along with her ovaries and fallopian tubes	May be necessary to treat health conditions such as excessive menstrual bleeding or tumors	Irreversible	No statistics available	No information available
Vasectomy	A minor surgical procedure performed at a hospital or clinic in which the vas deferens is tied off and cut on both sides of the scrotum	Convenient; procedure does not affect sexual desire or hormone levels; male may resume sex as soon as it is comfortable; permanent solution to birth control	No protection against STIs; after the procedure the male will still have viable sperm for a period of time; sterilization is considered permanent	Less than 1	$350–$1,000, including sperm count

*Number of women out of 100 likely to become pregnant during the first year of use. Number ranges indicate perfect versus typical use.

Source: Data from: *"Comparing Effectiveness of Birth Control Methods"* from Planned Parenthood website, accessed 2013.

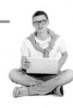

STUDENT STATS
Sex and the College Student

Number of sexual partners college students reported having over the past year

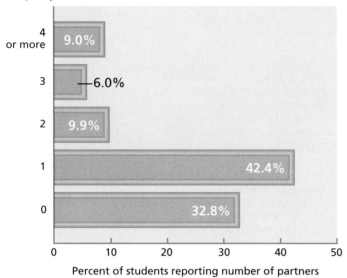

- 4 or more: 9.0%
- 3: 6.0%
- 2: 9.9%
- 1: 42.4%
- 0: 32.8%

Percent of students reporting number of partners

Top methods of contraception used by college students*

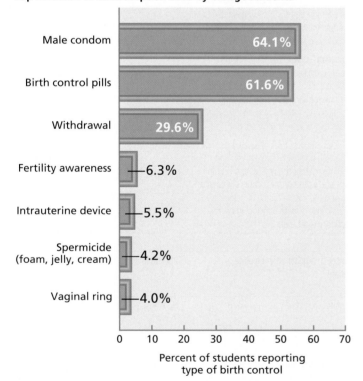

- Male condom: 64.1%
- Birth control pills: 61.6%
- Withdrawal: 29.6%
- Fertility awareness: 6.3%
- Intrauterine device: 5.5%
- Spermicide (foam, jelly, cream): 4.2%
- Vaginal ring: 4.0%

Percent of students reporting type of birth control

* Who engaged in vaginal intercourse and used contraception

Data from: *American College Health Association-National College Health Assessment (ACHA-NCHA II) Reference Group Executive Summary, Fall 2012,* by the American College Health Association, 2013, retrieved from www.acha-ncha.org.

Sunday	Monday	Tuesday	Wednesday	Thursday	Friday	Saturday
1	2	3	④ Start of period	5	6	7
8	9	10	11	12	13	14
15 Cervical mucous spotted	16	17 Sharp pain, ovulation?	18	19	20	21
22	23	24	25	26	27	28
29	30	① Start of period	2	3	4	5

Start of period: ○   Avoid sex: ✕

FIGURE 10.5 Fertility Awareness Tracking. Jotting down key events in the menstrual and ovulatory cycles can help couples identify which dates to avoid intercourse.

> ❝ *In addition to the careful planning required, the fertility awareness method requires couples to abstain from sexual intercourse for 11 days out of each cycle.*❞

Withdrawal. Also called *coitus interruptus*, the **withdrawal** method requires the man to withdraw his penis from his partner's vagina before he ejaculates. Often the man is unable to do this, and withdrawal is associated with a very high failure rate (see Table 10.1). Even if the man can exert the required self-control, pregnancy can still occur because the pre-ejaculate fluid may contain sperm. This method also provides no protection against STIs and can be unsatisfying for both partners.

Over-the-Counter Methods

Over-the-counter methods are available without a prescription or examination. They include condoms, which may be available from campus health clinics and other

withdrawal The withdrawal of the penis from the vagina before ejaculation.

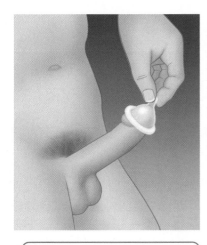

① Pinch the tip of the condom to expel any air.

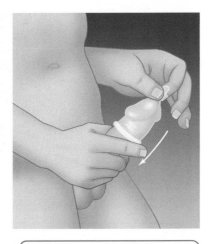

② Keep the tip pinched with one hand. Use the other hand to roll the condom onto the penis.

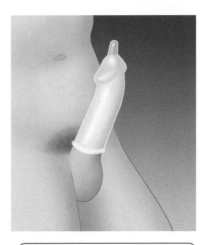

③ Make sure the condom smoothly covers the entire penis.

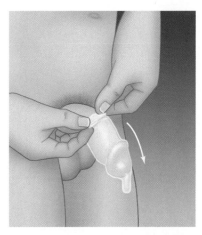

④ After ejaculation, hold on to the base of the condom as you withdraw. Remove the condom carefully so that semen does not spill.

FIGURE 10.6 Applying a Male Condom.

sources free of charge; the contraceptive sponge; spermicides; and emergency contraceptives.

Condoms. The **condom (male condom)** is a thin sheath, typically made of latex, polyurethane, or lambskin, which is unrolled over the erect penis prior to vaginal penetration (**Figure 10.6**). If used correctly and consistently, it offers excellent protection against pregnancy and STIs. Either can occur, however, if the condom breaks or comes off during sex. Most condoms are lubricated. However, note that lambskin condoms do not provide as much protection against infection as do latex and polyurethane.

Some men feel that wearing a condom decreases their level of stimulation and pleasure. Experimenting with different sizes, types, and brands, as well as using a water-based personal lubricant, may help.

When using condoms, it's important to check the expiration date on the packet. Discard a condom if the expiration date has passed. When the penis is erect, squeeze the air out of the tip of the condom and place it over the glans (head) of the penis. Roll the condom down over the shaft of the penis as far as possible. After ejaculation, but before the penis has become flaccid, grasp the condom at the base of the penis and withdraw. Throw the condom away.

The female condom is a lubricated latex or polyurethane sheath with flexible rings on either end (**Figure 10.7**). Using a special applicator, the woman inserts it into the vagina until the inner ring rests against the cervix. The outer ring remains outside the body, partly covering the labia. The female condom can be inserted several hours before sex and provides protection against both pregnancy and STIs. However, some women find it awkward to insert, and it can cause some discomfort during sex. It can also get pushed upward into the vagina. Finally, it is associated with a higher pregnancy rate than is the male condom.

Contraceptive Sponge. A flexible foam disk (**Figure 10.8** on page 242) containing spermicide, the **contraceptive sponge** is moistened with water and inserted into the vagina until it rests

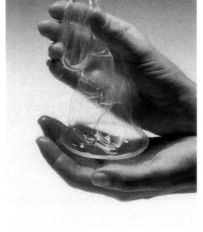

(a) Female condom

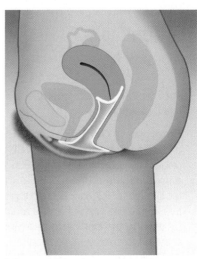

(b) Female condom in place

FIGURE 10.7 The Female Condom. **(a)** The FC2 is made of synthetic latex. **(b)** A female condom properly inserted.

condom (male condom) A thin sheath typically made of latex, polyurethane, or lambskin that is unrolled over the erect penis prior to vaginal penetration.

contraceptive sponge A flexible foam disk containing spermicide that is inserted in the vagina prior to sex.

spermicide A substance containing chemicals that kill or immobilize sperm.

against the cervix. The sponge can cause irritation and dryness. It does not protect against STIs; in fact, it slightly increases the risk of contracting one. It must be left in place for 6 hours after intercourse and is associated with an increased risk for a urinary tract infection, vaginal infection, and toxic shock syndrome.

Spermicides. A **spermicide** is a substance containing nonoxynol-9, a chemical that kills or immobilizes sperm. Spermicides are available as foams, gels, film, and suppositories. They are not very effective in preventing pregnancy and don't prevent STIs when used alone (see Table 10.1). In fact,

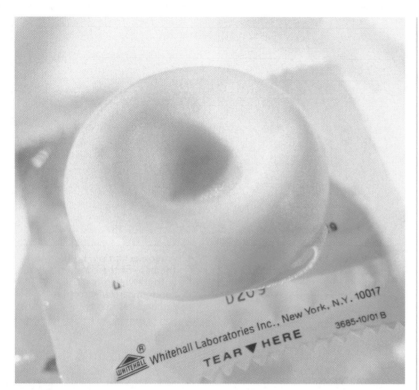

FIGURE 10.8 A Contraceptive Sponge.

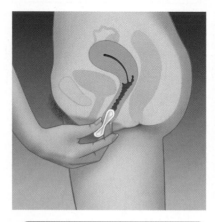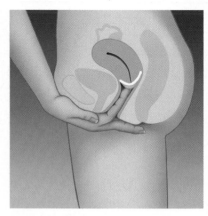

(1) After filling the diaphragm with spermicide, hold it dome-side down and squeeze the opposite sides of the rim together.

(2) Insert the diaphragm into the vagina, pushing it along the vaginal floor as far back as it will go. Make sure the diaphragm completely covers the cervix (the bump at the back of your vagina.) Tuck the front rim of the diaphragm up against your pelvic bone.

FIGURE 10.9 Inserting a Diaphragm.

spermicide use can increase a woman's chance of developing a urinary tract infection.

Emergency Contraception (EC). Also called the **"morning after" pill, emergency contraception (EC)** is currently available over the counter under the brand name Plan B. Plan B is a pill containing levonorgestrel, a synthetic hormone similar to those found in birth control pills. It is effective up to 72 hours after unprotected sex. However, it is most effective within the first 24 hours after intercourse.[36] It prevents pregnancy by tricking the body into believing that pregnancy has already occurred, preventing ovulation, fertilization, or implantation. It should not be confused with *RU-486,* the so-called abortion pill. If a woman is already pregnant, Plan B will do nothing to stop the pregnancy.

See page 243 for a discussion of ella, a recently approved, prescription-only form of EC that can be effective 120 hours after intercourse.

Methods Available by Prescription

Many more sophisticated methods of contraception are available by prescription. Prescription barrier methods include the diaphragm, cervical cap, and IUD. Prescription hormonal methods are available in various delivery methods. Notice that all of these options are for women. Research into such methods for males is ongoing.

Diaphragm and Cervical Cap. The **diaphragm** and cervical cap are small, flexible, silicone cups that the woman fills with spermicide and inserts into the vagina **(Figure 10.9)**. They must be fitted by the woman's health-care provider, and some devices must be replaced annually. These devices

emergency contraception (EC; "morning after" pill) A pill containing levonorgestrel, a synthetic hormone that is used to prevent pregnancy after unprotected sex.

diaphragm A flexible silicone cup filled with spermicide and inserted in the vagina prior to sex to prevent pregnancy.

intrauterine device (IUD) A plastic, T-shaped device that is inserted in the uterus for long-term pregnancy prevention.

birth control pills Pills containing combinations of hormones that prevent pregnancy when taken regularly as directed.

must be left in place for at least 6 hours following intercourse and may be left in place for up to 24 hours. However, they do not reliably protect against STIs and are associated with an increased risk of urinary tract infection and toxic shock syndrome.

IUD. An **intrauterine device (IUD)** is a plastic, T-shaped device that is inserted by a health-care provider into the uterus for long-term pregnancy prevention. There are two types, both of which are highly effective in preventing pregnancy:

- The ParaGard copper IUD continually releases copper, which works either by preventing sperm from reaching the fallopian tubes, or by preventing implantation of a fertilized egg, should conception occur. It can be effective for up to 10 years. Side effects include cramps, nausea, severe menstrual pain and bleeding, painful sex, and anemia.[37]

- The Mirena hormonal IUD releases progestin, which works either by thickening the cervical mucus—blocking sperm transit—or by suppressing ovulation. It can be effective for up to five years. Side effects include weight gain, acne, headaches, ovarian cysts, and abdominal pain.[38] Neither of these devices guards against STIs, and both can be expelled from the uterus.

Pharmaceutical Hormones. Synthetic hormones, including estrogen and progestin, are combined in **birth control pills,** typically referred to simply as "the pill" **(Figure 10.10)**. A progestin-only "mini-pill" is also available. However, synthetic hormones don't only come in pill form; they're also available as a skin patch that is replaced weekly, a vaginal ring replaced monthly,

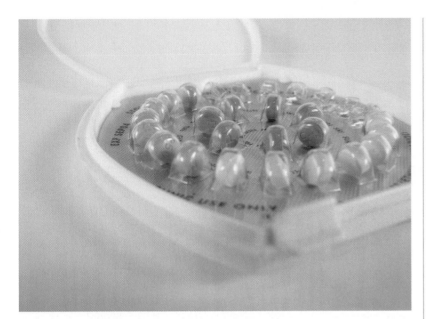

FIGURE 10.10 A Typical Pack of Birth Control Pills.

injections given monthly or quarterly, and an under-the-skin implant that can last for up to three years. To compare these hormonal methods, see Table 10.1.

Bear in mind that, although all of the hormonal methods are convenient and highly effective at preventing pregnancy, they do not protect against STIs; thus, condom use is still important. Also, because they release reproductive hormones into the body, these methods can provoke symptoms that mimic those of early pregnancy, including nausea, weight gain, breast tenderness, and moodiness.

In addition, women who have taken the pill for several months can experience long-term adverse effects. These include post-pill amenorrhea that can last for three to six months as well as increased blood pressure and an increased risk of cardiovascular disease, especially in smokers. Long-term use can also increase a woman's risk for cervical and liver cancer. On the upside, pill use can decrease a woman's risk for ovarian and endometrial cancer. The relationship between pill use and breast cancer is not clear.[39]

Other forms of hormonal contraceptives can have similarly serious adverse effects. For example, the skin patch can increase the risk for blood clots, heart attack, and stroke, whereas the injection form can lead to loss in bone mineral density. Thus, anyone considering the hormonal methods should carefully weigh the risks and benefits with her health-care provider.

In 2010, the Food and Drug Administration (FDA) approved a new EC pill called ella. Unlike Plan B, which begins to lose effectiveness within 24 hours after sexual intercourse, ella is effective for up to 120 hours (5 days) after unprotected sex, and its effectiveness does not diminish with time.

Surgical Methods

The surgical methods discussed here are classified as *sterilization*; that is, they permanently prevent conception by involving surgical manipulation of the reproductive organs.

Tubal ligation is a surgical procedure in which a woman's fallopian tubes are tied off or sealed to prevent the egg from traveling toward the uterus.

failure rate The percentage of women who typically get pregnant after using a given contraceptive method for one year.

continuation rate The percentage of couples who continue to practice a given form of birth control.

Sperm also cannot reach the egg; thus, fertilization cannot occur. Tubal ligation can sometimes be reversed but should not be undertaken if a woman thinks she may change her mind.

A *hysterectomy* is a procedure in which a woman's uterus is surgically removed, sometimes along with her ovaries and fallopian tubes. It is considered a method of permanent, absolute, irreversible sterilization and is not an option for women who merely desire contraception. However, if a woman has other factors, such as excessive menstrual bleeding, or benign or malignant tumors in the uterus, and she desires to permanently cease childbearing, then the procedure may be considered.

A *vasectomy* is a surgical procedure in which a man's vas deferens is tied off and cut on both sides of the scrotum. This makes it impossible for sperm—which are manufactured in the testes—to make their way upward and into the semen. The man typically notices no difference in the quantity of semen he ejaculates, and although there is some swelling, bruising, and discomfort immediately after the surgery, long-term complications are rare. The procedure is nearly 100% effective at preventing pregnancy; however, it is difficult to reverse. Thus, men who choose vasectomy should consider the procedure permanent.[40]

Which Method Is the Best?

The answer to this question depends on each individual and each couple. When deciding which type of birth control to use, individuals and couples should consider how comfortable they are with the method, how many side effects it has, how well it works, and how likely they are to use it correctly.

It is important to note that although every method has a published **failure rate** (indicating the percentage of women who typically get pregnant after using that method for one year), the figures are a bit misleading. That's because failure rates indicate pregnancy rates if the method is used exactly as directed, a concept known as "perfect use." In reality, couples do not always use birth control perfectly. Women forget to take their pills. Men put condoms on improperly. The end result is what is known as "typical use," which has substantially higher pregnancy rates. Another critical factor is the **continuation rate,** or the percentage of couples who continue to practice that form of birth control. Often, couples will stop using one method and, before choosing a new method, will have unprotected sex.

When making a decision about the right birth control, either proactively on your own or as part of a couple, here are some factors to consider:

- Are you with one-long term sexual partner? Or are you currently not in a committed relationship, or do you have more than one partner? Be sure your birth control considerations account for protection you may need against STIs as well as pregnancy.

  - How good are you at sticking to routine? If you are a woman, will you remember to take a pill every day? If you are a man, will you always carry condoms—and use them—when sexual encounters might be possible?

  - Do you need or want a birth control method you can use without getting a doctor's prescription? Some people, for reasons of cost or privacy, may prefer not to visit a doctor to seek birth control. However, as a student, you may have access to low-cost appointments and contraceptives through your student health center.

Practical Strategies

Communicating Effectively About Sex and Birth Control

If you are thinking about beginning a sexual relationship with someone, it's important to be able to communicate effectively about topics like sexual history, sexual health, contraceptive preferences, and how comfortable you each are with different types of sexual activity.

- **Know your preferences.** What do you hope for out of a sexual relationship? Are there certain sexual experiences that you aren't comfortable with? Do you know which type of contraception is right for you? Answer these types of questions for yourself first, before you discuss them with a potential partner. Keep in mind that if you aren't ready for parenthood, contraception is a critical part of your decision-making.

- **Prepare to talk.** Once your preferences are clear to you, jot down thoughts, concerns, and questions in advance. For instance, it's important to know your partner's sexual history. It's also important to share your own. What can you do to feel more comfortable asking about your partner's history, including experiences with contraceptives? Rehearsing the words in advance doesn't commit you to following a script, but it can help you frame your message in the moment with greater ease, clarity, and sensitivity.

- **Set a time to talk.** Once you're secure about the content of the conversation you want to have, reserve a time when you're both relaxed and not distracted and a place that's comfortable and private. You might

want to tell your partner that there are some things you'd like to talk about, and suggest that the two of you get together in a private place. Have the conversation before you are in a situation where you might have sex. Once you are "in the moment," it's especially hard to stop and have a detailed conversation about sexual history, STIs, and contraception.

- **Express your questions, concerns, and desires from a personal perspective.** Use "I" statements consistently, as in, "I'd like to know about your sexual history, and I will be honest in sharing mine." Pay attention to your partner's responses. Take in not only the words used, but your partner's body language as well.

- **Be honest and clear.** Especially when it comes to deciding on a birth control method and agreeing on the sexual experiences you're comfortable with, it's important that you stand up for your values and desires, even if they don't match with your partner's. Make sure your partner understands your preferences.

- **Near the end of the conversation, recap any decisions you've mutually made.** Include steps that

you'll take, such as, "Okay, so tomorrow we'll both schedule appointments at the campus health center to get screened for STIs." If you've made shared decisions about birth control, talk to each other to make sure that necessary steps get followed up. If you decide you'll use condoms, for example, it's helpful to buy a few to keep in each of the places where you are likely to have sex. Make sure that your words are followed up with actions that reflect the experiences and preferences the two of you have shared.

Source: Adapted from *Talking with Your Partner About Birth Control by PT+3 Partnership*, by the Alabama Medicaid Agency (no date provided), retrieved from www.medicaid.state.al.us/. . .5. . ./3C-8-4-Talk.About.BC-partner.pdf?; and *Tips to Talk to Your Partner About Sex*, by the Society of Obstetricians and Gynaecologists of Canada, 2006, retrieved from http://www.sexualityandu.ca/adults/tips-1.aspx#.

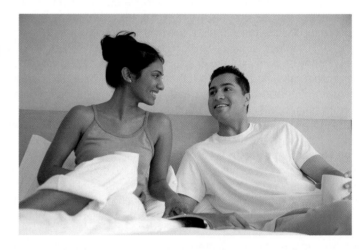

- Do you have any health risks, such as smoking? This is an especially important factor for women considering hormonal contraceptive methods such as birth control pills.

- Do you want to have children in the future? Your answer to this question can help you make decisions on relatively effective but invasive contraception methods, such as tubal ligation or a vasectomy.

If you are not yet in a sexual relationship, but are considering one, talking to potential sexual partners is another important step in choosing contraception. For suggestions on how to make these conversations more effective and less awkward, see **Practical Strategies: Communicating Effectively About Sex and Birth Control.**

>> **Which contraceptive method is right for you? To find out, log onto** www.plannedparenthood.org/all-access/my-method-26542.htm **and take the MyMethod quiz. It's written for women, but men can take it as well, by answering the questions from the perspective of their partner.**

Abortion

Birth control failure—and the failure to use birth control—combine to create a large number of unintended pregnancies, as we noted at the beginning of this chapter, about 3 million in the United States every year.[41] Many women experiencing an unplanned pregnancy decide to keep their baby. Some—typically fewer than 2%—maintain the pregnancy but relinquish the baby for adoption. About 14% miscarry, and about 42% choose abortion each year.[42]

Abortion is a medical or surgical procedure used to terminate a pregnancy and involves removing the embryo or fetus from the uterus. The number of abortions performed has been declining in recent years, and the abortion rate is at its lowest level since 1974. Nevertheless, an estimated 1.2 million abortions were performed in the United States in 2008, indicating that more needs to be done to help couples avoid unintended pregnancy.[43]

Methods of Abortion

There are two types of procedures for terminating a pregnancy: medical and surgical abortion. *Medical abortion*, which involves the administration of medications (via pill or injection) to end a pregnancy, has been gaining in popularity since its approval by the U.S. Food and Drug Administration in 2000. About 13% of women who underwent an abortion in 2005 used the medical method, up from 1% just a few years before. Moreover, 22% of abortions performed in the first nine weeks of pregnancy used the medical method.[43] *Surgical abortion* has a much longer history in the United States and remains the prevailing option, with 87% of women who sought an abortion in 2005 ultimately selecting it.[43]

Which method is advised? The World Health Organization has stated, "There is little, if any, difference between medical and surgical abortion in terms of safety and efficacy. Thus, both methods are similar from a medical point of view and there are only very few situations where a recommendation for one or the other method for medical reasons can be given."[44]

Medical Abortion

Medical abortions are intended for women in the earliest stages of pregnancy, within nine weeks of the start of their last menstrual period (seven weeks of pregnancy). There is no surgery and no anesthesia. The medical route is recommended if the woman has health risks that make surgery unadvisable, such as obesity or uterine malformations.

The process starts with the administration—either by pill or injection—of the medication *mifepristone*, also known as *RU-486*. The medication blocks progesterone, which is needed to support a pregnancy. Two days later, the woman takes a pill containing the drug *misoprostol*, which causes the uterus to contract and expel the fertilized egg along with the endometrial lining. The pregnancy usually terminates within hours after the second drug is ingested but sometimes can take up to 2 days. Two weeks after the process is initiated, women are instructed to return to their physician's office for a follow-up exam. The procedure successfully terminates pregnancy in more than 96% of cases.[43] If the pregnancy was not successfully terminated, a surgical abortion is then recommended.

The expulsion of the pregnancy from the uterus can cause severe cramping pain, nausea, heavy bleeding, fever, and diarrhea. Nevertheless, many women choose medical abortion because it allows them to end an unwanted pregnancy in privacy at home and without the trauma of an invasive surgical procedure.

Surgical Abortion

Suction curettage, or vacuum aspiration, is the surgical abortion method most commonly chosen. Typically used in the first 6 to 12 weeks of pregnancy, it involves an injection to numb the cervix,

abortion A medical or surgical procedure used to terminate a pregnancy.

suction curettage A method of surgical abortion characterized by vacuum aspiration; typically used in the first 6 to 12 weeks of pregnancy.

dilation and evacuation (D&E) A multistep method of surgical abortion that may be used in pregnancies that have progressed beyond 12 weeks.

Talking Honestly About Sex

"HI, I'M ABBEY. I absolutely think that people have a responsibility to tell someone if they have a sexually transmitted disease before they have sex. That is definitely something that their partner should know ahead of time, and it's deceitful to hide that from them. If someone asked me if I had an STI right before sex, I would answer honestly. I wouldn't be put off. I would understand why they would want to know that, and respect that they want to be safe and responsible with their body. How would I ask someone if they had an STI? I would just straightforwardly ask them."

1. Why is it so important to discuss sexual histories and exposure to sexually transmitted infections with a new partner prior to sex?

2. Why is it risky for sexually active individuals to skip regular medical checkups?

followed by the insertion of a series of rods of increasing thickness to dilate (widen) the opening of the cervix. Once the cervix is adequately dilated, the physician inserts a hollow tube through the cervix into the uterus. The tube is attached to a pump, which generates suction to remove tissue from the uterine walls. Usually performed in a doctor's office or outpatient clinic, suction curettage is a relatively quick procedure, often taking just minutes to complete.

Manual vacuum aspiration is similar to suction curettage but can be performed much earlier in the pregnancy. Doctors use thin flexible tubing attached to a handheld syringe and insert it through the cervix into the uterus. The syringe—rather than a machine—creates enough suction needed to strip the uterine lining and terminate the pregnancy.

For pregnancies that have progressed beyond 12 weeks, **dilation and evacuation (D&E)** may be performed. This procedure requires multiple trips to the health-care provider. During the first visit, the health-care provider performs an ultrasound scan to determine the status of the pregnancy and eligibility for the procedure. Then, 24 hours before the surgery, the cervix is numbed and a medication administered that will dilate it slowly. At the final appointment, either at a clinic or a hospital the woman is given a local anesthetic or, in some cases, spinal or general anesthesia, and the physician uses instruments and suction to remove the pregnancy. The procedure can produce pain and heavy bleeding and is associated with a variety of possible complications. Follow-up care is important.

Physical and Psychological Complications of Abortion

The earlier an abortion is performed, the lower the risk of complications; however, at every gestational stage, abortion is safer than carrying the pregnancy to term.[45] Serious complications of abortion are extremely rare but may include hemorrhage, fever, adverse effects from anesthesia, perforation of the uterus, injury to the bladder or the intestines, infection, and a disorder characterized by coagulation within the blood vessels. In some abortions, the embryo or fetus is not completely removed from the uterus and the procedure must be done again.

Deaths caused by abortion are rare. For example, of the more than 784,000 legally induced abortions in the United States in 2009, there were 12 known fatalities.[46]

For the vast majority of women who get an abortion, physical complications are not an issue. But what about psychological ones? Some research studies have found that some women may experience an increased risk of mental health problems after an abortion.[47] Abortion critics have argued that women who undergo an abortion are at risk for a constellation of mental health problems they call *postabortion traumatic stress syndrome*. Yet this is not recognized as a legitimate mental health condition by either the American Psychological Association or the American Psychiatric Association.

Still, recognizing that abortion can be stressful for some women, causing feelings of sadness or guilt, the American Psychological Association convened a task force on abortion and mental health and concluded that there is no credible evidence that terminating a single unwanted pregnancy creates mental health problems for adult women.[48] The risk, they found, was no greater than if the women had opted to give birth.

Just as the decision to have children is deeply personal, so is the choice to end a pregnancy. Reactions may vary widely from one individual to another. Some women, unprepared for an unplanned pregnancy, may feel a sense of relief after an abortion. Others may experience a sense of loss or guilt. If a woman chooses to terminate a pregnancy, it is important to recognize that a range of emotional reactions is possible, and to seek support as needed.

Legal Status of Abortion

Abortion has long been a contentious issue in the United States. Despite largely being legal during the nation's founding years, both abortion and contraception gradually fell out of favor. The Federal Comstock Act of 1873 criminalized the distribution or possession of devices, medication, or even information used for abortion or contraception. For an entire century, many women who wanted to terminate an unwanted pregnancy resorted to "back-alley" abortions, performed in unsterile locations, often by untrained personnel using rudimentary instruments. These procedures were dangerous, and many women died attempting to end an unwanted pregnancy.

In 1973, the U.S. Supreme Court made a landmark decision in the case of *Roe v. Wade* that all women had a constitutional right to an abortion in the first six months of their pregnancy. The legislation trumped all state laws limiting women's access to an abortion, and

TABLE 10.2 Arguments in Opposition and Support of Abortion Rights

Arguments in Opposition to Abortion Rights	Arguments in Support of Abortion Rights
Life begins at conception, and abortion is therefore murder.	Legal abortion is performed when the embryo or fetus is not capable of sustaining life independently and is therefore not murder.
Performing an abortion violates medical ethics, which require health-care providers to promote and preserve life.	If safe clinical abortions were no longer legal, women would again resort to "back-alley" abortions, resulting in cases of permanent infertility, serious disease, and death.
Abortion exposes girls and women to significant risk of physical and psychological harm.	Carrying an unwanted pregnancy to term exposes girls and women to significant risk of physical and psychological harm.
Women with an unwanted pregnancy should relinquish their baby for adoption, because many people are on waiting lists to adopt a child.	Carrying an unwanted pregnancy to term and then relinquishing the newborn for adoption can promote physical and emotional harm.
Highly reliable forms of contraception are readily available. Abortion should not be available as a form of birth control.	Among sexually active couples, no method of contraception is 100% reliable. Although the rate of unintended pregnancies can be reduced, some are inevitable, and women should not be forced to carry them to term.

stipulated that individual states could only ban abortions during the final three months of pregnancy, when a fetus would have a chance at surviving outside the womb. From the fourth through the sixth month of pregnancy, however, states could regulate the abortion procedure in the interest of maternal health.

Abortion continues to be legal in the United States, but a number of rulings have chipped away at *Roe v. Wade,* placing new restrictions on who can get an abortion, and when. More than 30 states now require that minors notify their parents before getting an abortion, often needing parental permission to continue with the procedure. Others impose a mandatory waiting period on women, requiring them to read information on alternatives to abortion before being allowed to terminate their pregnancy. The U.S. Congress has also blocked the use of federal Medicaid funds to pay for elective abortions except when a pregnancy would endanger a woman's life, or in cases of rape or incest.

Some of the main arguments commonly advanced for and against abortion rights are listed in **Table 10.2.**

Pregnancy and Childbirth

Among the milestones in life that people cherish the most is the journey to becoming a parent and the birth of their child. The following sections provide an overview of the stages of pregnancy and childbirth as well as an examination of the choices available to couples struggling with infertility.

Pregnancy

For young, healthy couples having unprotected sex, there is about a 20% chance the woman will get pregnant during any given menstrual cycle.[49] Pregnancies are divided into three trimesters, each lasting about three months. Women may experience vastly different symptoms during each phase of their pregnancy, with the second trimester often being referred to as the "golden age" because women tend to have more energy and less nausea at this point.

A woman who suspects she might be pregnant can find out for certain with the use of a simple pregnancy test. There are two types on the market: a urine test available over the counter and a blood test offered only in physicians' offices. Both look for the presence of hCG, a hormone that is only made in the body during pregnancy.

The blood test can detect hCG about a week after ovulation. But many women opt for a home urine test, which is painless, inexpensive, and private. It's able to detect hCG levels about two weeks after ovulation—approximately the day a woman's period is due. For the most accurate results, however, health experts recommend waiting until a few days later before taking a home pregnancy test. In one study of six popular home pregnancy kits, researchers found that only one, the First Response Early Result Pregnancy Test, was consistently able to provide correct results the day a woman's period was due.[50]

Because home pregnancy tests are not 100% accurate, women who get a negative result are encouraged to test again one week later if they still have not started menstruating.

Preconception Care

Many women recognize that **prenatal care**, including nutritional counseling and regular medical screenings throughout pregnancy, is important for the growth and development of the unborn baby. So, too, is preconception care, initiated before a woman has even gotten pregnant. Obstetricians encourage their patients who are attempting to start a family to first take care of any health problems that could affect the pregnancy, including type 2 diabetes and high blood pressure. Prenatal vitamins containing a sufficient amount of folic acid are also recommended because they significantly reduce the risk of birth defects.

During a preconception visit, a doctor may also suggest changes in a woman's nutrition or exercise patterns and will instruct women not to use tobacco, alcohol, or illegal drugs, or take certain medications while they attempt to conceive. Because women do not learn they are pregnant until several weeks after conception, it is critical to make positive lifestyle changes long before that faint positive sign first appears on a home pregnancy test.

Early Signs of Pregnancy

Pregnancy symptoms can begin to surface before a woman even misses her period, although the first signs could also be indicative of an illness or even impending menstruation. Still, women who begin to experience many of these symptoms should consider taking a home pregnancy test or visiting their gynecologist:

- A skipped period
- An extremely light "period" known as implantation bleeding that occurs when a fertilized egg implants itself in the uterus
- Frequent urination
- Nausea
- Swollen breasts
- Fatigue
- Food aversions or cravings
- Mood swings
- Abdominal bloating or pressure
- Dizziness

Some women will experience none of these symptoms in the early weeks of their pregnancy. Others may notice a few signs but not right away.

prenatal care Nutritional counseling and regular medical screenings throughout pregnancy to aid the growth and development of the fetus.

Changes in a Pregnant Woman's Body

A woman's body undergoes a series of physical changes throughout the course of pregnancy **(Figure 10.11)**. Some go unnoticed by the mother-to-be. For example, the heart begins to work harder, and a physician may notice fluctuations in the woman's blood pressure. Breathing patterns change slightly, with breaths becoming deeper and faster. The kidneys kick into high gear, filtering an increasing volume of blood. Ligaments and muscles stretch. The cervix becomes thinner and softer.

Myriad other changes, however, are difficult for women to miss. Hormone changes, especially in the first trimester, can cause bouts of

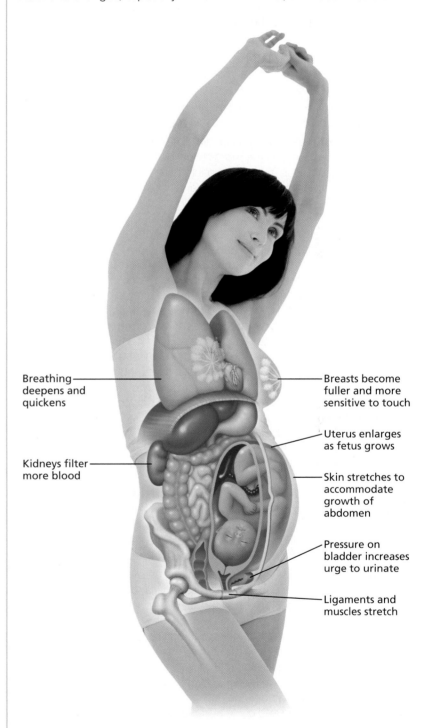

Breathing deepens and quickens

Breasts become fuller and more sensitive to touch

Uterus enlarges as fetus grows

Kidneys filter more blood

Skin stretches to accommodate growth of abdomen

Pressure on bladder increases urge to urinate

Ligaments and muscles stretch

FIGURE 10.11 Changes in a Pregnant Woman's Body.

nausea and vomiting called "morning sickness," a misnomer because women afflicted with it often find that it persists throughout most of the day. Breasts become fuller and tender to the touch as they get ready for milk production. The uterus enlarges as the fetus grows, ultimately extending up to the woman's rib cage. The growing uterus presses on the bladder, creating the constant urge to urinate. It also shifts the woman's center of gravity, exaggerating the curve in her lower back and giving her a characteristic "waddling" walk. The skin stretches to accommodate the growing breasts and abdomen and sometimes darkens at points on the face and in a thin line near the navel. As the pregnancy draws near a close, women may also develop heartburn or hemorrhoids. By the time the baby is born, the average woman will have gained between 25 and 30 pounds—or more if she is carrying twins or triplets. Not surprisingly, as a result of all these physical changes, many women report experiencing significant fatigue during their pregnancy.

Development of the Fetus

The fetus also undergoes significant physical changes as it transforms from a microscopic fertilized egg into an average 7.5-pound newborn.

First Trimester. The first trimester, which accounts for the first 13 weeks of pregnancy, is the most critical period in the baby's development. At this stage, it is most susceptible to any substances a woman ingests, including drugs, alcohol, and certain medications, and any environmental toxins, from pesticides to the chemicals in cigarette smoke.

Recall that when an egg and sperm combine, they form a single-celled organism known as a zygote. As the zygote makes its way from a woman's fallopian tube to her uterus, it rapidly divides and becomes a cluster of dozens of cells called a *blastocyst*. The blastocyst, which is no larger than a pinhead, implants itself in the uterine wall, where it begins to receive nourishment. About two weeks after fertilization—around the time a woman first misses her period—the growing collection of cells is known as an **embryo** and is already beginning to differentiate into three tissue layers. One layer becomes the fetal nerves, brain, and spinal cord. The second layer becomes bone, muscle, and skin. The third develops into the fetal respiratory, digestive, and urinary organs.

The growing embryo has a powerful support system. It receives its nutrients and oxygen—and gets rid of its waste products—from the **placenta,** the tissue that connects mother and baby. The **umbilical cord** also plays a key role, linking the bloodstream of the placenta to that of the embryo and enabling the exchange of gases, nutrients, and wastes. The embryo is surrounded and protected by **amniotic fluid,** which keeps the baby's temperature regulated and allows it to move freely.

At eight weeks after fertilization, the embryo is called the **fetus,** a name it will keep until childbirth. By the time the first trimester comes to a close, the fetus is much larger than the pinhead it once was, measuring 3 to 4 inches in length. Still, it weighs only the equivalent of two dozen paper clips. The bulk of the fetus's growth will occur in the trimesters to come.

Second Trimester. The second trimester is an exciting time for many women. Fatigue and nausea tend to dissipate, and the fetus provides them with a few welcome signs of the life developing within. During this trimester, the woman begins to feel the fetus moving and kicking, and the fetal heartbeat can be heard through an obstetrician's stethoscope. All major organs and physiological systems become fully formed. The fetus continues its rapid growth, measuring 13 to 16 inches by the end of the second trimester and weighing around 2 or 3 pounds. A fetus might survive if born at the end of this trimester but would require a lengthy hospitalization and could suffer long-term health effects.

Third Trimester. During the last three months of pregnancy, the fetus gains most of its weight, including a layer of fat needed for insulation during the first weeks of life outside the womb. Its organs continue to mature, and it moves into position—head down—as it gets ready for birth. Throughout the last trimester, the mother may experience *Braxton Hicks contractions,* irregular movements of the uterus that may be confused with the signs of premature labor. Braxton Hicks contractions, however, are simple tightenings of the uterus, nothing more than false labor.

Although a standard pregnancy lasts about 40 weeks, babies are considered full term if they are born between 37 and 42 weeks. Babies born before 37 weeks' gestation are considered preterm and are at risk for developmental delays and other complications. Babies born after 42 weeks' gestation are post-term and may stop growing in the uterus. In some instances, post-term pregnancies result in stillbirth.

Figure 10.12 illustrates the various stages of fetal development.

Prenatal Care

The health of the baby depends in part on the health of the mother and the measures she takes during pregnancy to protect them both. Prenatal care, which includes regular checkups during pregnancy and counseling about nutrition, exercise, sleep, and other topics, should be an integral part of every pregnancy. Babies born to mothers who receive no prenatal care are five times more likely to die than those whose mothers do get regular care.[51] As soon as a woman learns she is pregnant, she is encouraged to:

- **Get regular checkups.** Select an obstetrician or certified nurse midwife and schedule an initial appointment. This is followed by regularly scheduled appointments at which the woman is monitored for many factors, including blood pressure, blood sugar, weight gain, and fetal well-being.

- **Follow good nutrition advice.** It is commonly said that a pregnant woman is "eating for two," but that is only partially accurate. During pregnancy, the body only needs an extra 300 calories per day—not exactly a doubling of food. Yet what is true is that what a woman consumes, her growing fetus consumes, be it fruits, vegetables, lean meats, and whole grains—or cake, cookies, drugs, and alcohol.

- **Exercise regularly.** Fitness is important to the health of the mother and her growing baby. Exercise can help relieve some of the symptoms of pregnancy and may prevent gestational diabetes. It can also help prepare a woman for labor and childbirth. Kegel exercises are recommended for strengthening the muscles of the pelvic floor, which support the uterus and bladder. By repeatedly contracting the muscles used to stop the flow of urine, women can reduce their risk of incontinence, a common complaint during and after pregnancy.

- **Avoid drugs, including alcohol and tobacco.** These substances, including some prescription and over-the-counter medications, can be harmful to the growth and development of the unborn fetus. A pregnant woman should always check with her physician before taking any medications. The same holds true for dietary supplements, including herbs.

embryo The growing collection of cells that ultimately become a baby.

placenta The tissue that connects mother and baby.

umbilical cord A vessel linking the bloodstream of the placenta to that of the baby and enabling the exchange of gases, nutrients, and wastes.

amniotic fluid Fluid that surrounds the developing fetus that aids in temperature regulation and allows the baby to move freely.

fetus The name given to the developing embryo eight weeks after fertilization.

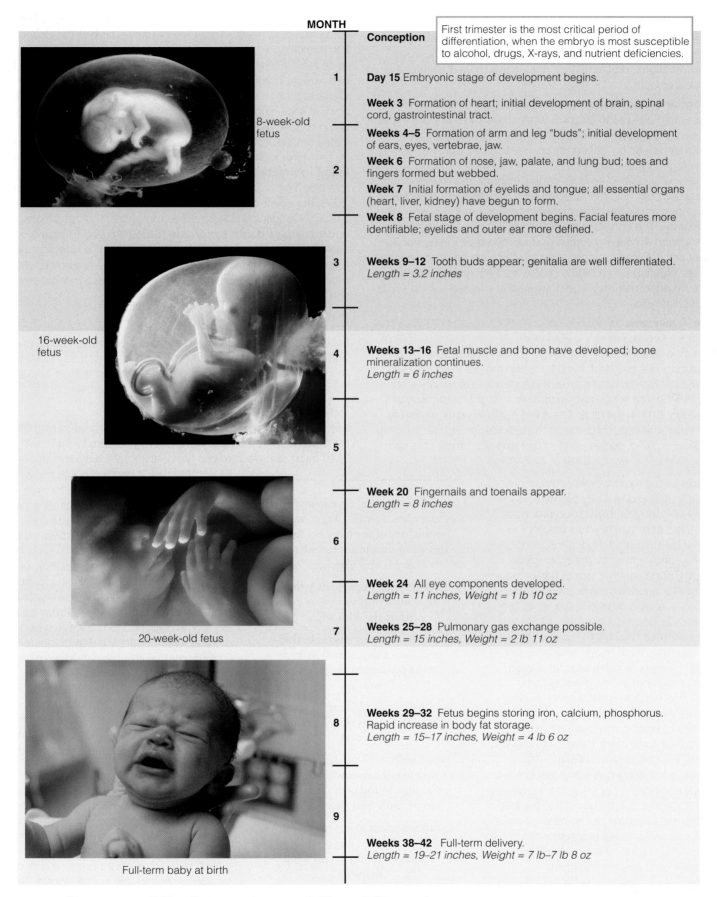

MONTH

Conception

First trimester is the most critical period of differentiation, when the embryo is most susceptible to alcohol, drugs, X-rays, and nutrient deficiencies.

1

Day 15 Embryonic stage of development begins.

Week 3 Formation of heart; initial development of brain, spinal cord, gastrointestinal tract.

8-week-old fetus

Weeks 4–5 Formation of arm and leg "buds"; initial development of ears, eyes, vertebrae, jaw.

2

Week 6 Formation of nose, jaw, palate, and lung bud; toes and fingers formed but webbed.

Week 7 Initial formation of eyelids and tongue; all essential organs (heart, liver, kidney) have begun to form.

Week 8 Fetal stage of development begins. Facial features more identifiable; eyelids and outer ear more defined.

3

Weeks 9–12 Tooth buds appear; genitalia are well differentiated.
Length = 3.2 inches

16-week-old fetus

4

Weeks 13–16 Fetal muscle and bone have developed; bone mineralization continues.
Length = 6 inches

5

Week 20 Fingernails and toenails appear.
Length = 8 inches

6

20-week-old fetus

Week 24 All eye components developed.
Length = 11 inches, Weight = 1 lb 10 oz

7

Weeks 25–28 Pulmonary gas exchange possible.
Length = 15 inches, Weight = 2 lb 11 oz

8

Weeks 29–32 Fetus begins storing iron, calcium, phosphorus. Rapid increase in body fat storage.
Length = 15–17 inches, Weight = 4 lb 6 oz

9

Weeks 38–42 Full-term delivery.
Length = 19–21 inches, Weight = 7 lb–7 lb 8 oz

Full-term baby at birth

FIGURE 10.12 Stages of Embryonic and Fetal Development.

Complications

Most pregnancies progress without a hitch, with the fetus developing properly and the birth being trouble-free. For some women, however, there are complications, problems that pose a risk to the health of the mother or baby, or both.

Ectopic Pregnancy. An **ectopic pregnancy** occurs when a fertilized egg implants within one of the fallopian tubes. It can also implant in the cervix or an ovary, although much less frequently. Between 2% and 3% of all pregnancies in the United States are ectopic, with that rate increasing slightly in recent years.[52]

As the improperly located embryo begins to grow, the woman may experience severe pain, and the fallopian tube may rupture. An ectopic pregnancy can never develop normally and survive and is a threat to the mother's life. The condition accounts for 3–14% of all maternal deaths, with African American women and women over the age of 35 at the highest risk.[53] Ectopic pregnancies can also cause scarring in the fallopian tubes, creating future fertility problems. Risk factors include smoking, having endometriosis, and having been infected with the STIs gonorrhea or chlamydia.

Miscarriage. A **miscarriage,** or *spontaneous abortion*, is a pregnancy that suddenly ends on its own before the 20th week. An estimated 10–15% of known pregnancies end this way, but because many losses occur before a woman realizes she is pregnant, experts believe the true number could be closer to 40%.[54] Exactly what causes a pregnancy to terminate is not always clear, but the majority of miscarriages are thought to be caused by chromosomal problems in the fetus. The risk is higher in women who are over age 35, have a history of diabetes or thyroid disease, or have a history of miscarriages. Smoking, drinking alcohol, or using illicit drugs while pregnant may also increase a woman's risk of miscarriage.

Hypertension. A pregnant woman's blood pressure is normally checked at every prenatal visit to screen for hypertension (high blood pressure), which is the most common medical disorder in pregnancy.[55] If left untreated, hypertension during pregnancy can progress to **preeclampsia,** a serious health condition that can threaten the life of both mother and fetus. Characterized by high blood pressure and protein in the urine, preeclampsia typically develops after the 20th week of pregnancy. Women may begin experiencing headaches, swelling of the hands and face, excessive weight gain, abdominal pain, and even vision changes. Without skilled medical care, preeclampsia can result in seizures and multiple organ failure as well as fetal death.

About 5–8% of pregnant women develop preeclampsia.[56] Unfortunately, there is no way to prevent it, and the only cure is childbirth. Physicians will often admit a woman with preeclampsia to the hospital so she and her fetus can be closely monitored. Although it can be harmful to the baby to be born prematurely, often it can be even more dangerous for a preeclamptic pregnancy to go full term. Doctors may decide to induce labor early in an effort to save both mother and child.

Low Birth Weight and Infant Mortality. We noted earlier that the average birth weight in the United States is about 7.5 pounds. Newborns weighing less than 5 pounds, 8 ounces at birth are called **low birth weight** babies and are at risk for serious health problems, including death. About 8% of babies born in the United States fall into this category, and the number has been on the rise for the past few decades.[57] Preterm labor is the leading cause, with two out of three low birth weight babies arriving before the 37th week of pregnancy.[57] Low birth weight babies are vulnerable to a host of health problems and disabilities, including learning disabilities, cerebral palsy, hearing loss, and vision problems. Women are more likely to have a low birth weight baby if they smoke, drink alcohol, or use illicit drugs during pregnancy.

Low birth weight and prematurity are two factors influencing the **infant mortality rate,** a calculation of the ratio of babies who die before their first birthday to those who survive until their first birthday. In 2008, the infant mortality rate in the United States was 6.7 per 1,000 births.[58] Congenital abnormalities, pregnancy complications, and **sudden infant death syndrome (SIDS)** are also to blame. SIDS is the sudden death of a seemingly healthy infant while sleeping. Although researchers still do not entirely understand the phenomenon, they recognize that putting a baby to sleep on its stomach or side increases its risk for the condition.

Childbirth

For expectant parents longing to meet their unborn baby, pregnancy and its 40 weeks of waiting can seem like an eternity. Childbirth is a moment they await with anticipation—and sometimes apprehension—knowing that their lives are about to change forever.

Childbirth Options

Pregnant women have many choices about where to give birth, ranging from hospitals to alternative birthing centers to their own home. They must also decide who will be their care provider—for example, an obstetrician, a certified nurse midwife, or a lay midwife. Some parents-to-be even draft birth plans, documents that spell out their preferences on everything from the use of pain relievers during labor to the number of people they would like in the birthing room.

Even with so many choices, 99% of women still opt to have their baby in a hospital, attended by a physician or certified nurse midwife.[59] Fortunately, many U.S. hospitals today have birthing rooms designed to resemble a bedroom in a home, with comforting wall colors, pictures, a rocking chair, soft lighting, and even music.

Women whose pregnancies are considered high risk because of their age, health problems, or concerns about the health of the baby may be encouraged to give birth in a medical center that has a neonatal intensive care unit. This is also true of women carrying twins, triplets, or quadruplets.

Labor and Birth

Anywhere from several hours to several days before labor begins, many women experience a discharge of copious, red-tinged mucus commonly called the "bloody show." This mucous plug has been blocking the cervix throughout the pregnancy, protecting it from bacteria and other harmful agents, and its discharge signals that the cervix is beginning to dilate in preparation for labor.

Onset of Labor. The precise events signaling the onset of **labor** differ for every woman and every

---

ectopic pregnancy A pregnancy that occurs when a fertilized egg implants within one of the fallopian tubes instead of the uterus; considered a medical emergency.

miscarriage A pregnancy that suddenly terminates on its own before the 20th week.

preeclampsia A serious health condition characterized by high blood pressure in the pregnant woman.

low birth weight The term given to birth weights less than 5 pounds, 8 ounces.

infant mortality rate A calculation of the ratio of babies who die before their first birthday to those who survive until their first birthday.

sudden infant death syndrome (SIDS) The sudden death of a seemingly healthy infant while sleeping.

labor The physical processes involved in giving birth.

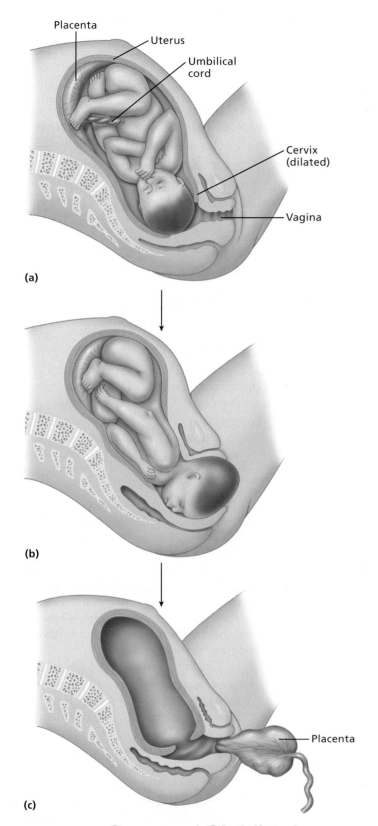

Placenta
Uterus
Umbilical cord
Cervix (dilated)
Vagina

(a)

(b)

Placenta

(c)

FIGURE 10.13 Stages of Childbirth. **(a)** The first stage is characterized by cervical dilation and contractions of the uterus that begin to move the baby toward the birth canal. **(b)** In the second stage, the woman pushes until the baby is born. **(c)** In the third stage, the placenta is expelled.

Source: From Stanfield, Cindy, *Principles of Human Physiology,* 4e, Figure 22.24, p. 662. © 2011. Pearson Education.

pregnancy. Some women begin to experience regular, mild contractions—caused by the release of a hormone called oxytocin—that become more frequent and intense over several hours. Other women don't experience contractions until their "water breaks"; that is, until the sac holding the amniotic fluid ruptures and amniotic fluid flows out from the vagina. Some women may experience vague abdominal cramps and lower back pain that do not go away. Such symptoms are a sign that a woman is experiencing the first of three stages of the birth process **(Figure 10.13)**.

First Stage of Labor. First-time mothers spend an average of 12 to 14 hours in labor, although some progress much more quickly and others more slowly.[60] The first stage of labor is the longest: 9 or more hours. Those who have already had one vaginal birth tend to experience a faster first stage during subsequent pregnancies.

During early labor, contractions of the uterus begin to move the fetus toward the birth canal. Contractions also cause the cervix to begin to open—or dilate—and thin out, a process known as *effacement*. Between each contraction, the pain typically abates completely and the woman can rest. If the sac holding the amniotic fluid has not already broken, it may do so now. During active labor, the cervix dilates further and contractions strengthen, lengthen, and become more frequent. Many women request pain medication during this time. The final phase of this first stage of labor is known as **transition.** Amidst strong and prolonged contractions, the cervix dilates to about 10 centimeters, usually large enough for the baby's head to fit through. A woman may begin to feel shaky, sweaty, and weak. Physical and emotional support from care providers and the woman's partner are important during this phase.

Second Stage of Labor. Once the cervix has dilated to 10 centimeters, the woman will be encouraged to help move the fetus further into the birth canal by actively pushing; that is, bearing down with each contraction. Many women find this stage of labor, which can last an average of 30 minutes to 3 hours, more rewarding than the first stage because they can feel that their efforts help the birth to progress.[60] Others, however, view this as the hardest stage of labor. When the baby's head "crowns," or appears at the vaginal opening, labor is almost over. The woman stops pushing, and after one or two further contractions, the baby is born, slick and sticky from the amniotic fluid. The birth attendant removes mucus and fluid from the newborn's mouth and nose, and dries him or her off with a towel. The umbilical cord, which still attaches the newborn to the placenta, is clamped and cut.

Third Stage of Labor. Although the baby has been born, the body still has one important task to do: expel the placenta. This is typically accomplished by a few more contractions. The woman continues to bleed, but massaging the abdomen or breast-feeding the newborn can control the bleeding within about 5 to 15 minutes. The final stage of labor is over.[60]

For the baby, the work has just begun. Just 1 minute after birth, the baby is given his or her first test, a measurement of how well the baby tolerated the stresses of birth.[61] This test is known as the APGAR and the resulting score, from 1 to 10, is an **Apgar score.** Babies are assessed on five characteristics: their muscle tone, their heart rate, their reflexes, their skin coloration, and their breathing. Five minutes after

transition The final phase of the first stage of labor, characterized by the dilation of the cervix and strong, prolonged contractions.

Apgar score A measurement of how well a newborn tolerated the stresses of birth as well as how well he or she is adapting to the new environment.

birth, the test is repeated to see if the baby's score has improved. A final score between 7 and 10 is considered normal. Babies who receive a lower rating may need additional medical assistance.

Doctors will also take a sample of blood from the infant's heel to test for hidden disorders that are not always apparent at birth. Rare metabolic disorders such as phenylketonuria, or PKU, can be successfully controlled if detected early but can cause mental retardation or even death if left undiagnosed.

Cesarean Birth. In consultation with their health-care provider, some women decide during pregnancy to give birth via a scheduled **cesarean section (C-section)**.

This surgery involves making an incision through the woman's abdominal and uterine walls in order to deliver the baby. A C-section may be necessary if the mother is experiencing hypertension or another disorder, if the placenta is covering the cervix, or if the fetus is very large or in the wrong position in the birth canal. Also, women who have had a prior C-section may be encouraged to have one during subsequent pregnancies to avoid the small but serious risk of uterine rupture. An emergency C-section may be warranted if labor is not progressing, if the fetus appears to be in distress during labor, or if there is a problem with the umbilical cord or placenta, putting the baby's life in jeopardy.

The rate of C-sections doubled between 1996 and 2006, according to national statistics.[62] Nearly one in three babies, 31.1%, are now delivered via C-section, a statistic that has troubled critics, some of whom argue that the increase is caused by financial incentives and fear of malpractice suits rather than concern for the patients. Although the surgery is relatively safe, it has a higher rate of complications and involves a longer recovery time for mothers than a vaginal birth.

Infertility

Many couples attempt to get pregnant only to find that it is not always easy to do. An estimated 12% of women and 14% of couples in the United States experience **infertility,** or the inability to conceive after trying for one year.[63] The problem becomes more prevalent with age, and so doctors recommend that a woman in her 30s get checked for underlying health issues if she has been trying unsuccessfully to get pregnant for more than six months. Doctors will also examine her partner because infertility can be caused by a low sperm count or other factors involving the male. Fortunately, there are many treatment options available, and about two-thirds of couples who have difficulty conceiving ultimately go on to have their own biological children.[64]

Causes of Infertility

Roughly one-third of infertility cases are due to health problems in the woman, another third are due to problems in the man, and the final third are either caused by problems in both partners or simply cannot be explained.[64]

For women, the most common causes of infertility are:

- A failure of ovulation prompted by hormonal problems, advanced age, premature menopause, or scarred ovaries.
- Blocked fallopian tubes, stemming from a prior ectopic pregnancy, surgery, or, most commonly, an untreated STI such as chlamydia or gonorrhea that caused scarring in the fallopian tubes and/or progressed into pelvic inflammatory disease (PID). Endometriosis, discussed earlier, also can block the tubes.

- A deformed uterus, which can not only cause infertility but may lead to miscarriage.
- Uterine fibroids and other noncancerous growths, which can obstruct both the uterus and the fallopian tubes.

The most common causes of infertility in men include:

- A low sperm count, defined as less than 10 million sperm per milliliter of semen. This can be caused by smoking cigarettes or marijuana.
- Incorrectly formed sperm, which are not able to penetrate the egg.
- Poor sperm motility, or the inability of sperm to move quickly and effectively.
- Prior infection. Contracting mumps during adulthood is a common culprit. STIs such as gonorrhea can also cause scarring that hinders sperm movement.
- Environmental exposure to pesticides, lead, and other substances that disrupt hormones in the body.

Options for Infertile Couples

The type of medical treatment ultimately used by couples to get pregnant depends to a large degree on the root cause of their troubles. Options for infertile couples include:

- Surgery to repair blocked fallopian tubes, remove scarring or uterine growths, and treat endometriosis in women. Occasionally, surgery may be indicated if there is a problem with a man's sperm.
- Fertility drugs, which promote ovulation in women. Side effects can include headaches, nausea, hot flashes, and breast tenderness. Because the medications can spur the body to release more than one egg at a time, couples using fertility drugs have a higher chance of having twins, triplets, or quadruplets.
- Intrauterine insemination, to boost the odds that an egg will be fertilized. Sperm are collected from a woman's partner or a donor and processed in a laboratory, enabling a higher concentration of sperm to be injected into the vagina or uterus through a syringe.
- *In vitro fertilization (IVF),* a procedure that dramatically transformed the field of fertility treatment when the first "test-tube baby" was born in 1978. Egg and sperm are retrieved from a woman and a man and combined in a laboratory dish (*in vitro* means "in glass"), where fertilization may occur. If eggs do become fertilized, they are implanted in the uterus. When multiple eggs are transferred, multiple births may occur.
- *Gamete intrafallopian transfer (GIFT),* a process similar to IVF. The egg is not fertilized in a laboratory, however. Instead, sperm and several eggs are placed in a woman's fallopian tube. There is no guarantee, though, that the sperm will penetrate at least one of the eggs.
- *Zygote intrafallopian transfer (ZIFT),* fertilization of an egg or eggs in a laboratory setting. Unlike IVF, however, the fertilized eggs are transferred to a fallopian tube rather than the uterus.
- *Intracytoplasmic sperm injection (ICSI),* the direct injection of a single sperm into an egg. The fertilized egg is then implanted in the uterus through normal IVF technology. ICSI may be considered when men have low sperm counts or when fertilization failed to occur in previous IVF attempts.
- Surrogate motherhood, which requires an agreement with a third party—a fertile woman—to carry a pregnancy to term. In some cases the surrogate's egg is fertilized through intrauterine

cesarean section (C-section)
A surgical procedure involving the incision of a woman's abdominal and uterine walls in order to deliver the baby.

infertility The inability to conceive after trying for at least a year.

insemination with the prospective father's sperm. In other cases, she is impregnated through IVF with the couple's embryo. The woman is paid for her service to the couple, and immediately following the baby's birth, she relinquishes the infant to them.

Not all couples choose medical treatment. Many opt for adoption, either domestically or internationally. In 2008, there were 55,000 adoptions in the United States involving public child-welfare agencies.[65] Statistics on adoptions involving private agencies do not have to be reported by states and are therefore not available. The adoption experience can be as satisfying to parents as pregnancy and childbirth. It can also cost less—or much more. Adoptions from foster-care agencies typically cost very little or are free of charge. Domestic adoptions using private agencies can cost several thousand dollars, and costs for international adoptions can reach $30,000 or more and take several years to be approved. Not all couples who want to adopt a baby are successful.

Prevention remains one of the best options for infertility. Although many couples in their late teens and early 20s are more interested in *avoiding* pregnancy, steps should be taken to preserve fertility for the years to come. Practicing safer sex can reduce the spread of STIs, which are often the cause of fertility problems. Getting timely treatment for an STI is also important. Because fertility drops and the risk of birth defects and miscarriages rises when a woman is in her 30s, couples who want to have a child are encouraged to start their family planning before the woman turns 35.

Change Yourself, Change Your World

We've presented a lot of facts about sexual health—but how do you integrate cold facts with the complex desires you feel? And how can the decisions you make about whether, when, and with whom to have sex stay aligned with your goals and your dreams? Healthy sexuality requires not only protecting the health of your body, but also accepting and supporting your sexual orientation, contraception preferences, possible plans for children one day, and personal values—and those of your partners and peers.

Personal Choices

First, know yourself before you become intimate with others. Clarify what you want—and that requires you to distinguish your own values from those of the people around you. Second, talk with your partner before things get physical. You can make an awkward situation easier by being the one to start the dialogue and share your own experiences. Treat potential partners with the same respect you show yourself, and be honest about who you are and what you want. Discuss your expectations for the relationship, what you do and don't want physically, and the practical matters of your sexual history, STI prevention, and contraception. Third, if you become sexually active, consistently practice safer sex and have a backup plan if your primary method fails. Finally, if an intended or unintended pregnancy happens, visit a health-care provider right away and talk with your partner about your options, if you're not ready to be parents, or your plans, if you are.

Campus Advocacy

How can we avoid the trap of labeling ourselves or others based on our sexual histories, behaviors, or orientation? How can we develop tolerance in ourselves and promote healthier sexuality in our community? Different methods have arisen on different college campuses across the United States. Here are just a few ideas:

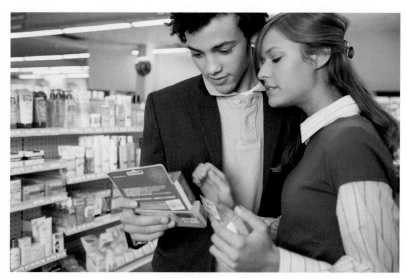

Choose a contraceptive with your partner and make sure you both understand how to use it.

- Over 200 U.S. colleges and universities have programs fostering alliances among heterosexual and lesbian, gay, bisexual, transgender (LGBT) students. These programs typically have names such as Safe Zone, Safe Space, Safe Harbor, and Safe On Campus. The hallmark of these "Safe" programs is the public identification of "allies" by placing a "Safe" symbol—usually a pink triangle or a rainbow—on doors or walls of offices or living spaces.

- CollegeTown is a diversity immersion program modeled after the National Conference for Community and Justice's (NCCJ) AnyTown high school program. In this 4-day/3-night retreat, students explore issues of discrimination, including racism, sexism, and homophobia, as well as ways to build community. CollegeTown graduates return to their campuses empowered to act as leaders, promoting respect for all. To see how it works, check out the CollegeTown group at Arizona State University, Tempe, on Facebook.

- Visit your campus health services center and confirm that it offers a variety of low-cost contraceptives. In 2009, Congress reinstated a program enabling college health centers to purchase and sell prescription medications, including hormonal contraceptives, at a discounted rate.[66] Make sure your campus health center is taking advantage of this program.

- You can also consider supporting free condom distribution on your campus. The Great American Condom Campaign (GACC) is a youth-led grassroots movement. Each year, GACC members give out 1,000,000 male condoms on college campuses across the United States, educate their peers about sexual health, and organize to improve the policies that affect young people's health and lives. Find out more about GACC at **www.amplifyyourvoice.org/gacc.**

If activism isn't your thing, you can still make individual choices to promote tolerance and respect for different orientations and reproductive choices. If someone is on the opposite side of the abortion issue from you, or holds different views on gay marriage, take a moment to dialogue about what values you hold in common—responsible sexual decision-making, for instance, or a secure and loving home for every child.

>> **Watch videos of real students discussing sexuality, contraception, and reproductive choices at** MasteringHealth™

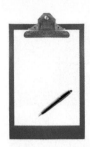

Choosing to Change Worksheet

To complete this worksheet online, visit MasteringHealth™

Each safer sex method has its pros and cons. Keep in mind that even the most effective methods can fail. But your chances of getting an STI or becoming pregnant are lowest if the method you choose always is used correctly and consistently every time you have sex.

Directions: Fill in your stage of change in Step 1 and complete Steps 2, 3, or 4 depending on which ones apply to your stage of change.

Step 1: *Your Stage of Behavior Change.* Please check one of the following statements that best describes your readiness to follow your selected safer sex method correctly and every time you have sex. Keep in mind that abstinence and intimacy without intercourse are forms of safer sex.

_____ I do not plan to practice safer sex consistently and correctly in the next six months. (Precontemplation)

_____ I might practice safer sex consistently and correctly in the next six months. (Contemplation)

_____ I am prepared to begin practicing safer sex consistently and correctly in the next month. (Preparation)

_____ I have been practicing safer sex consistently and correctly for less than six months. (Action)

_____ I have been practicing safer sex consistently and correctly for six months or longer. (Maintenance)

Step 2: *Precontemplation and Contemplation Stages.* What is holding you back from practicing safer sex correctly and consistently every time?

_____

_____

If a pregnancy or STI were to occur due to inconsistent or incorrect use of a safer sex method, what would be the effects on you and your partner? Think of emotional, financial, school, and family effects.

_____

_____

Even if you don't think you're ready, what could you do to move toward practicing safer sex correctly and consistently?

_____

_____

Step 3: *Preparation, Action, and Maintenance Stages.* *Correct use:* Read the packaging of the contraceptive or safer sex method you are using. Or, for cost-free methods, re-read the section on these methods. Are you using the method correctly? If not, what have you been doing incorrectly or what are you confused about? How can you begin to use the method correctly?

_____

_____

Consistent use: If you are in the preparation stage, write down a SMART goal for using this method consistently every time. If you are in the action or maintenance stages, how are you making sure you use the method consistently every time?

_____

_____

Step 4: *Maintenance Stage.* What motivates you to continue practicing correct and consistent safer sex?

_____

_____

Are there obstacles you face in practicing safer sex correctly and consistently? If so, how are you dealing with them?

_____

_____

_____

Chapter Summary

- Good sexual health requires knowledge, effort, and appropriate medical care.

- Male and female sexual anatomy includes both external and internal organs. Among the female organs are the paired ovaries, one of which releases an egg cell monthly, and the uterus, where a fertilized egg implants and grows. Among the male organs are the paired testes, which constantly manufacture sperm—the male reproductive cells—which travel through a series of ducts to contribute to the man's semen.

- The menstrual cycle is an approximately monthly series of events in a nonpregnant woman of childbearing age. These events, which include the buildup and shedding of the uterine lining, are controlled by hormones, which simultaneously coordinate the maturation and release of an egg cell from a woman's ovary.

- The sexual response cycle consists of a series of phases from arousal to orgasm to resolution.

- Sexual dysfunction is fairly prevalent in the United States, with a sizable portion of men and women having difficulty enjoying sex at some point in their lives.

- Abstinence is the avoidance of sexual intercourse and has gained greater social acceptance in recent years.

- Sexual behavior includes much more than just sexual intercourse, with hugging, kissing, masturbation, and other forms of non-intercourse sexual activity all being a healthy part of a sexually active lifestyle.

- Humans develop their sexual orientation at a very early age, and it is theorized that sexual orientation is a result of the interaction of biological, environmental, and cognitive factors. Heterosexuality, homosexuality, and bisexuality are variations of a broad spectrum of sexuality.

- About half of all pregnancies in the United States are unplanned, despite the wide variety of contraceptive options available.

- Among the choices in contraceptive methods, only male and female condoms provide protection against sexually transmitted infections. Different methods offer varying rates of efficacy in preventing pregnancy.

- Abortion is the purposeful termination of a pregnancy. There are two types of abortion: medical and surgical. Serious physical complications from abortion are extremely rare, but it can cause feelings of sadness or guilt in some women.

- Pregnancy involves three trimesters, each with unique stages of development for a fetus and physical effects for the mother.

- Women planning a pregnancy need preconception health care.

- Regular prenatal care can lead to a healthier pregnancy and a healthier baby.

- The first stage of labor is characterized by uterine contractions and cervical dilation. The fetus descends into the birth canal. During the second stage, the woman bears down with each contraction until the baby is born. The third stage of labor is expulsion of the placenta.

- Fertility declines with increasing age. Males and females have about an equal rate of infertility.

- You can protect and promote your sexual health—and that of your partners and peers—by being honest about what you want out of sexual relationships, planning ahead for pregnancy and STI protections, and promoting open, tolerant conversations about sexual issues on campus.

GET CONNECTED

>> Visit the following websites for further information about the topics in this chapter:

- Planned Parenthood
  www.plannedparenthood.org

- FDA Birth Control Guide
  www.fda.gov/ForConsumers/ByAudience/ForWomen/
  WomensHealthTopics/ucm117971.htm

- Abstinence
  www.stayteen.org/waiting

- Go Ask Alice (advice about sexuality and sexual health)
  www.goaskalice.columbia.edu

MOBILE TIPS!

Scan this QR code with your mobile device to access additional tips about sexuality, contraception, and reproductive choices. Or, via your mobile device, go to **http://chmobile.pearsoncmg.com** and navigate to Chapter 10.

Website links are subject to change. To access updated web links, please visit MasteringHealth™

TEST YOUR KNOWLEDGE

1. What is a woman's first period called?
   a. menstruation
   b. ovulation
   c. menarche
   d. menopause

2. Which of the following is/are NOT part of the internal male genitals?
   a. glans penis
   b. epididymis
   c. vas deferens
   d. testes

3. What is the name for the last phase of the sexual response cycle?
   a. finality
   b. resolution
   c. conclusion
   d. climax

4. What is a transgendered individual?
   a. a person whose assigned sex differs from the gender he or she identifies with
   b. a person born with both male and female genitalia
   c. a person who is about equally attracted to both males and females
   d. a person who is only attracted to people of the opposite sex

5. Which of the following is NOT considered non-intercourse sexual activity?
   a. oral sex
   b. anal sex
   c. mutual masturbation
   d. fantasy

6. Of the following methods of birth control, which provide(s) protection against sexually transmitted infection?
   a. diaphragm
   b. female condom
   c. cervical sponge
   d. spermicides

7. What is the average annual percentage of unplanned pregnancies in the United States?
   a. 20%
   b. 30%
   c. 40%
   d. 50%

8. What is the approximate chance of getting pregnant in any given month for young, healthy couples who are having unprotected sex?
   a. 5%
   b. 10%
   c. 20%
   d. 30%

9. What is the developing baby called after the first eight weeks of a pregnancy?
   a. embryo
   b. blastocyst
   c. fetus
   d. zygote

10. Which of the following is not an infertility treatment?
    a. ZIFT
    b. ICSI
    c. GIFT
    d. PIXY

Get Critical

What happened

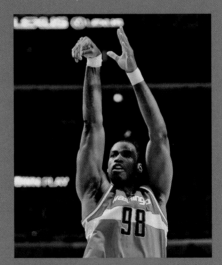

In the spring of 2013, everyone was talking about the big news in basketball, but it wasn't on the court. Twelve-year NBA veteran Jason Collins came out of the closet, the first male professional major league athlete to do so. "I didn't set out to be the first openly gay athlete in a major American team sport," Collins wrote in the *Sports Illustrated* essay that carried his announcement. "But since I am, I'm happy to start the conversation."[1] Some critics questioned Collins's decision, wondering if it would harm his career. Many prominent supporters, however, applauded his bravery, including basketball superstar Kobe Bryant, who Tweeted his support, telling Collins not to suffocate who he is because of the ignorance of others.[2]

What do you think?

- Why do you think professional athletes have been reluctant to come out as gay?

- Given the many dimensions of professional sports, including media appearances and product sponsorships, do you think sexual orientation should be an important factor in a player's career?

- What types of changes would help make the professional sports world more comfortable for athletes of any sexual orientation?

References: 1. "12 Year NBA Veteran Jason Collins Comes Out," by J. Collins & F. Lidz, April 29, 2013, *Sports Illustrated*, retrieved from www.si.com/2854464/an-nba-player-comesout. 2. <Twitter post, no title>, By K. Bryant, April 29, 2013, retrieved from twitter.com/kobebryant.

PREVENTING INFECTIOUS DISEASES & SEXUALLY TRANSMITTED INFECTIONS

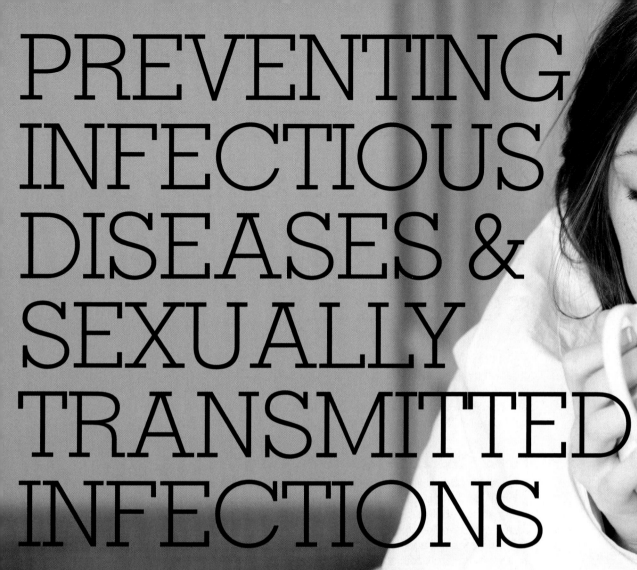

Each year in the United States, **5% to 20%** of the population gets the **seasonal flu**, resulting in 200,000 hospitalizations and as many as 49,000 deaths.[i]

About 20 million people in the United States are infected each year with a **sexually transmitted infection** and **half** of these cases occur in young people aged 15 to 24.[ii]

Approximately **25%** of the people in the United States infected with **HIV do not** realize it.[iii]

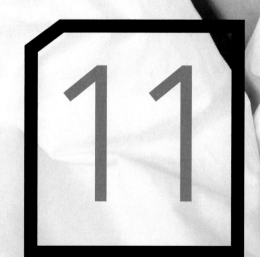

11

Learning Objectives

IDENTIFY the causes of infectious diseases and recognize how they are transmitted.

DESCRIBE how the body's immune response works against infections.

UNDERSTAND how immunization prevents infectious disease, both in individuals and in communities.

DISCUSS the most common infectious diseases, how they affect the body, and how they can be treated.

LIST common sexually transmitted infections (STIs), their causes, risk factors, symptoms, and treatment.

UNDERSTAND how to prevent infectious diseases and sexually transmitted infections.

The air we breathe, the food we eat, and even everyday items we handle constantly,

like door handles and cell phones, carry tiny microorganisms. They may be small, but microorganisms have a large impact on human health. Some of these microbes are harmless or even helpful, but others are capable of causing disease. Millions of people die each year from infectious diseases such as influenza, malaria, tuberculosis, and acquired immunodeficiency syndrome (AIDS). Knowing how to protect yourself from infection is critical to your health.

How Are Infections Spread?

Despite our best intentions to stay free of illness, it is impossible to make it to adulthood without ever having battled an infection. An **infection** is an invasion of body tissues by microorganisms that use the body's environment to multiply. In the process, these organisms damage and weaken the body and make us sick.

Pathogens are agents that cause disease. Common pathogens are harmful bacteria, viruses, fungi, protozoa, and parasitic worms. The natural environment for any particular pathogen, where it accumulates in large numbers, is called a **reservoir.** Pathogens move from a reservoir to a **host**—a person, a plant, or an animal in which or on which they can live and reproduce. The mode of transmission, or the way a pathogen moves from reservoir to host or from host to host, depends on the pathogen.

For infections to spread in a population, six conditions have to be met. These are collectively referred to as the **chain of infection (Figure 11.1).** Some of the ways infections are transmitted include:

Direct Transmission

- **Contact with infected people.** Close person-to-person contact with someone who has an infection is a common mode of disease transmission. Even if a person does not have any symptoms, he or she can still be infectious and considered a **carrier.** Many infections are spread sexually or even through simple touch. Contact with blood, saliva, or other bodily fluids can directly transmit infection from one person to another as well. Follow safer sex practices, avoid kissing sick people or direct contact with blood, and thoroughly wash your hands often to reduce your risk of infection. See the **Spotlight** box on page 260 for tips on hand washing and hand sanitizer use.

infection The invasion of body tissues by microorganisms that use the body's environment to multiply and cause disease.

pathogen An agent that causes disease.

reservoir The natural environment for any particular pathogen, where it accumulates in large numbers.

host A person, plant, or animal in which or on which pathogens live and reproduce.

chain of infection Group of factors necessary for the spread of infection.

carrier A person infected with a pathogen who does not show symptoms but who is infectious.

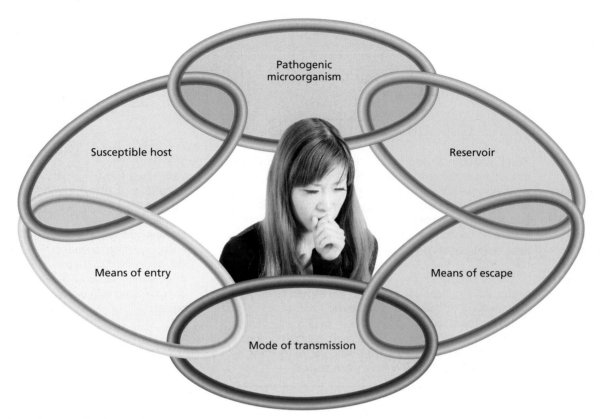

FIGURE 11.1 Chain of Infection. To cause infection, a pathogen such as a cold virus has to have a reservoir, such as a college student's body, in which to multiply and a means of escape, such as a cough. This enables the virus to be transmitted—for instance, by air to another student's eyes (the means of entry). If the student is susceptible—that is, if he or she has no immunity to the particular virus—he or she will experience infection.

- **Contact with infected animals.** The recent outbreaks of avian influenza showed us that people living and working closely with certain animals can risk catching infections from them. The Centers for Disease Control and Prevention (CDC) estimates that approximately 60% of human pathogens originated in animals and that 75% of emerging diseases involve transference from animals to humans.[1] It doesn't take an exotic animal to spread disease either. Pets can carry rabies, meningitis, salmonella, or other infections that can be passed on to humans. Vaccinating your pets, washing your hands after handling animals, and avoiding contact with animal feces greatly reduce the risks of transmission.

Indirect Transmission

- **Touching contaminated objects.** If you have an infection and then cough or sneeze on an object—or touch it with your dirty hands— you leave pathogens behind for the next unwitting person to pick up. Bacteria adhere to both natural and manufactured surfaces, often as a survival mechanism, and once adhered can be harder to destroy than free-floating bacteria.[2] Touching a contaminated object, and then touching your mouth, nose, or eyes, can move pathogens into your body.

- **Breathing airborne pathogens.** When you cough and sneeze, tiny droplets of mucus tainted with pathogens waft in the air, which can be inhaled by another person. Viruses and bacteria that cause colds, influenza, and tuberculosis are commonly spread in this manner.

- **Bites from infected insects.** Pathogens can hitch a ride to a host onboard a **vector,** an animal or insect that transports pathogens from one point to another. Classic examples of vectors are

vector An animal or insect that transports pathogens from one point to another.

" *If you have an infection and then cough or sneeze on an object—or touch it with your dirty hands—you leave pathogens behind for the next unwitting person to pick up.*"

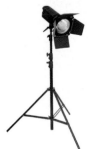

Hand Washing and Hand Sanitizers

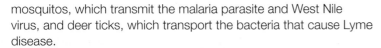

Keeping your hands clean is one of the best ways to prevent infections. The most effective method is to wash your hands with soap and water. Be sure to wash them thoroughly and frequently, especially during cold and flu season. Wet your hands with running water, lather up to your wrists with soap, and scrub for at least 20 seconds. Dry your hands on a clean towel or disposable paper towel. You do not need to use antibacterial soap when washing your hands; regular soap is just as effective, and antibacterial soaps can lead to antibiotic resistance (discussed later in the chapter).[1]

Unlike antibacterial soaps, alcohol-based hand sanitizers will not cause antibiotic resistance. If you don't have access to a sink, using hand sanitizer that contains at least 60% alcohol is a good backup. When using a hand sanitizer, apply enough to wet your hands completely and rub them together until dry. If your hands are ever visibly dirty, however, you should opt for hand washing instead.

You should clean your hands:

- before and after handling food, eating, treating wounds, or touching a sick person.
- after using the toilet, changing a diaper, touching an animal or animal waste, blowing your nose, coughing, sneezing, or handling garbage or anything that could be contaminated with dirt or germs.

Reference: **1.** *Hand Washing: Do's and Don'ts,* by the Mayo Clinic staff, 2011, retrieved from http://www.mayoclinic.com/health/hand-washing/HQ00407.

---

mosquitos, which transmit the malaria parasite and West Nile virus, and deer ticks, which transport the bacteria that cause Lyme disease.

- **Drinking or eating contaminated water or food.** Viruses, protozoa, and bacteria from animal or human feces can get into lakes, rivers, oceans, swimming pools, hot tubs, water slides, and public fountains. Chlorine can help kill pathogens but not entirely. Food can also become contaminated with pathogens when handled or processed in unsanitary ways.

Protecting Against Infections

Your body is not defenseless against infectious microorganisms. Even if you are exposed to pathogens, your body's defenses may protect you.

The Body's First Line of Defense

One of the most powerful barriers between you and pathogens is your skin. Your skin keeps the millions of bacteria that live on it from entering your body. Breaches can occur, however, if you get a cut, bad scrape, or puncture wound—one of the reasons why doctors encourage you to thoroughly cleanse and cover a wound immediately after sustaining it.

Skin doesn't shield your entire body, of course. Openings such as your mouth and nose need other forms of protection. Mucous membranes line the mouth, airways, vagina, and digestive tract, trapping many unwanted microorganisms. *Cilia*, tiny hairlike projections, line the airways and help sweep away tiny pathogens. Bodily fluids such as saliva, tears, earwax, vaginal fluid, and digestive acid trap and kill or expel many potential invaders. Coughing, sneezing, vomiting, and diarrhea are other ways the body expels foreign intruders.

immune system Your body's cellular and chemical defenses against pathogens.

inflammatory response A response to damaged body tissues designed to kill any pathogens in the damaged tissue, promote healing, and prevent the spread of infection to other parts of the body.

If any of the systems that provide these first defenses becomes damaged, for instance if your skin is severely burned or your cilia are damaged from smoking, you become more susceptible to infection. Even with healthy first defenses, however, pathogens can occasionally enter your body and infect you, at which point your immune response kicks in.

The Body's Immune Response

The **immune system** is the set of your body's cellular and chemical defenses against pathogens. Key players in the immune system are white blood cells, which patrol the circulatory system and body tissues looking for microscopic enemies **(Figure 11.2)**.

Nonspecific Response

Some white blood cells respond to a broad range of foreign invaders and attack and destroy them in what is called a *nonspecific response*. These cells are neutrophils, natural killer (NK) cells, and macrophages. Neutrophils, the most common type of white blood cells, conquer bacteria and other foreign invaders traveling in the blood by ingesting and destroying them. NK cells eliminate body cells that are infected by viruses. Macrophages survey our tissues and gobble up bacteria and wounded and dead cells.

Another essential component of nonspecific response is the **inflammatory response.** If body tissue is damaged, the inflammatory response kicks in. Neutrophils and macrophages migrate to the area of damage. They release chemical signals, called cytokines, which attract additional white blood cells to the location, increase blood flow to the area (promoting the delivery of immune cells), and induce fever. This response is designed to kill any pathogens that reside in the damaged tissue, promote healing, and prevent the spread of infection to other parts of the body.

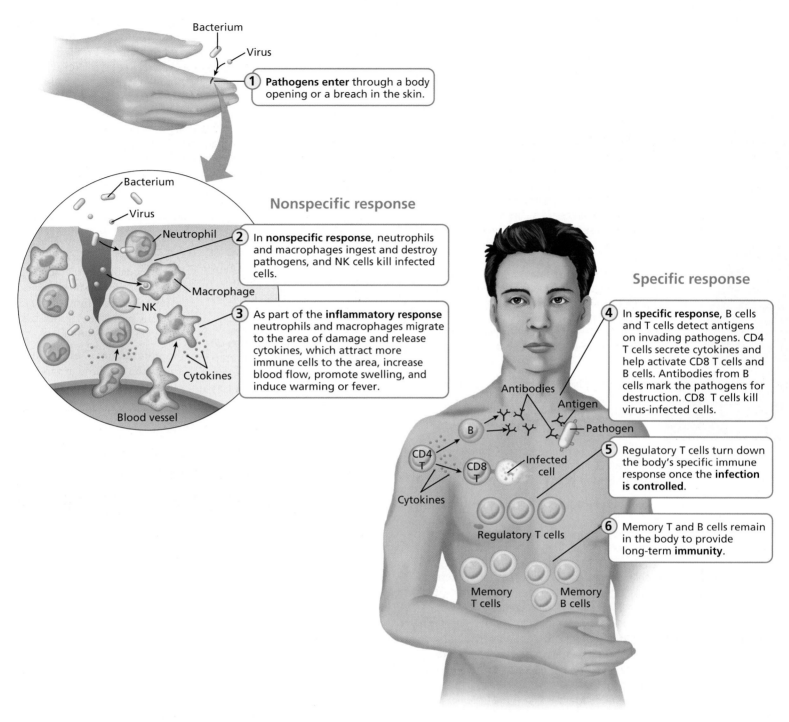

FIGURE 11.2 Your Body's Immune Response.

Specific Response

Other white blood cell types, the lymphocytes, mount a *specific response* in which they recognize and attack specific pathogens. The lymphocytes consist of B cells and T cells and are mostly found in the body's lymph fluid, lymph nodes, and other lymph organs such as the spleen. Both B cells and T cells bear surface receptors that detect **antigens,** tiny regions on the surface of a pathogen.

In response to an antigen, B cells release **antibodies,** proteins that bind tightly to invaders and

antigen Tiny regions on the surface of an infectious agent that can be detected by B cells and T cells.

antibodies Proteins released by B cells that bind tightly to infectious agents and mark them for destruction.

mark them for destruction. In fact, the term *antigen* is a contraction of *anti*body-*gen*erator. Antibodies are highly specialized, with each type targeting only one specific antigen, just as a key will only fit one lock.

How T cells respond to an antigen depends on the T cell type. There are three types of T cells. Cytotoxic T cells (CD8 T cells) kill virus-infected cells. Helper T cells (CD4 T cells) secrete cytokines that help activate B cells,

How I Avoid Infections

"HI, I'M JESSICA. As a germaphobe, I'm constantly sanitizing my hands after touching doorknobs, ATMs, or anything in a store. I absolutely have to keep clean everywhere I go. I always have little hand sanitizer bottles in my bag, and I have a gigantic one in my room. I use it when I don't have access to a sink to wash my hands. It's really easy just to dab some on your hand and just go and it's quick. I also get the seasonal flu vaccine every year.

Living on campus, you're always around people and touching everything everyone else touches. Your chance of getting sick is always way higher than if you were to live on your own somewhere. So I'm just really careful to keep my hands clean—it's the best solution to prevent getting a cold every other week."

1. Will using hand sanitizer and getting a flu vaccine prevent Jessica from getting all infections? What other ways might Jessica get an infection?

2. Do you think Jessica is right that living on campus increases your chances of getting sick? Why?

---

cytotoxic T cells, and NK cells. Regulatory T cells help turn down the specific immune response once the infection is under control.

The antigen-activated B cells and T cells also create long-lived *memory B cells* and *memory T cells*. These cells stay in the body and quickly identify and attack that specific pathogen should it enter the body again in the future. This is why successfully defeating an infection leaves us with **acquired immunity,** which in some cases leads to lifelong protection against the same infection. For example, if you have ever had chickenpox, you are unlikely to get it again.

Immunization

Acquired immunity can protect you against infections that your immune system recognizes, but what about diseases that your body has never seen before? In the past, the primary way people developed immunity was by contracting a disease and surviving it, a process known as *naturally acquired immunity*. Many diseases such as polio, whooping cough, measles, mumps, and rubella commonly killed or crippled victims before their bodies could fight them off. Widespread adoption of immunizations turned that tide. The advent of immunizations has been recognized as one of the most monumental developments in modern medical history, effectively eradicating some diseases such as smallpox and limiting others significantly.

Immunization often involves exposing a person to a pathogen through a vaccine, which allows the body to develop immunity

to the pathogen without actually falling ill. This is called *artificially acquired immunity*. Vaccines are composed of pathogens—or parts of pathogens—that have been killed or weakened. When they are introduced into the body, these dead or weakened microbes pose little threat, yet the body believes it is under attack and sounds the alarm to battle them. The immune system then produces memory B cells and memory T cells that can stave off that particular type of infectious disease for years to come, perhaps for a lifetime. This is known as *active immunity* because it induces an immune response.

In other instances, injections can provide temporary *passive immunity*, when ready-made antibodies specific to a particular pathogen are introduced into the body to fight off an infection. Passive immunity is used, for example, in the case of exposure to the hepatitis A virus. The injected antibodies immediately target the virus for destruction. Passive immunity lasts only as long as the injected antibodies survive, a few months at most.

The Centers for Disease Control and Prevention has developed recommended immunization schedules for children, teens, and adults **(Table 11.1)**, and all states require certain

acquired immunity The body's ability to quickly identify and attack a pathogen that it recognizes from previous exposure. In some cases acquired immunity leads to lifelong protection against the same infection.

immunization Creating immunity to a pathogen through vaccination or through the injection of antibodies.

TABLE 11.1 Vaccines Recommended for College Students[α]

Vaccine	Number of Doses
Tetanus, diphtheria, pertussis (Tdap, Td)[a]	Single dose of Tdap then boost with Td every 10 years
Measles, mumps, rubella (MMR)[a]	2 doses recommended for college students
Polio (IPV)[a]	4 doses if given in childhood; 3 doses if given in adulthood
Varicella (Var) (chicken pox)[a]	2 doses
Human papillomavirus (HPV)[a, b]	3 doses
Hepatitis B (Hep B)[a]	3 doses
Meningococcal disease[c]	1 dose
Pneumococcal polysaccharide (PPV)[d]	1 dose with revaccination after 5 years for those with elevated risk factors
Hepatitis A (Hep A)[d]	2 doses
Annual influenza (and H1N1)[d]	1 dose annually

[a]Recommended for those who lack documentation of past vaccination with all recommended doses and have no evidence of prior infection.
[b]Recommended for those aged 26 and under.
[c]Recommended for previously unvaccinated college freshmen living in dormitories.
[d]Recommended if some other risk factor is present.

Source: Adapted from *Recommended Immunizations for Adults* by the U.S. Department of Health and Human Services, Centers for Disease Control and Prevention, 2013. Retrieved from http://www.cdc.gov/vaccines/schedules/downloads/adult/adult-schedule-easy-read.pdf.

Do Vaccines Cause Autism?

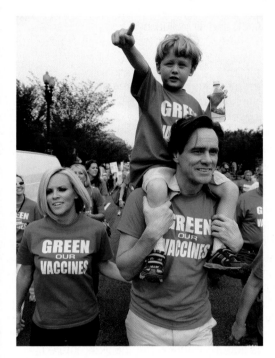

In 1998, an article appeared in the British medical journal *The Lancet* that claimed that autism—a developmental brain disorder that causes problems in communication, social interaction, and behavior—was caused by the childhood vaccine for measles, mumps, and rubella (MMR).[1] In response, some parents' groups began a movement against vaccinations, and more and more parents stopped vaccinating their children.

Anti-vaccine groups claim that autism is linked to the recommended number and schedule of childhood vaccinations and the use of thimerosal, a preservative that contains mercury, in some vaccines. As evidence of the damage of vaccinations, parents of autistic children publicized "before" and "after" home videos of their children displaying autistic characteristics only after the date of vaccination. Celebrities such as Jenny McCarthy advocated for vaccination reform.

However, after much research, there is no evidence of a link between autism and vaccines.[2] Thimerosal, which was never present in the MMR vaccines most blamed for autism, was removed from most common childhood vaccines by 2001 and autism rates have not declined.[3, 4] And in February 2010 *The Lancet* retracted the original paper linking autism to the MMR vaccine, citing a recent British medical panel ruling that the lead author had been deceptive and violated basic research ethics in his study.

The causes of autism remain unknown. However, one thing is clear: It is dangerous to become infected with a disease that could be prevented by a vaccine.

References: **1.** "Ileal-Lymphoid-Nodular Hyperplasia, Non-Specific Colitis, and Pervasive Developmental Disorder in Children," by A. J. Wakefield, S. H. Murch, A. Anthony, J. Linnell, D. M. Casson, M. Malik, . . . J. A. Walker-Smith, 1998, *The Lancet, 351*(9103), pp. 637–641. **2.** *Vaccine Studies: Examine the Evidence,* by the American Academy of Pediatrics, retrieved from http://www.aap.org. **3.** "Thimerosal Content of Vaccines Routinely Recommended for Children 6 Years of Age and Younger," Table 1 in "Thimerosal in Vaccines," in *Vaccines, Blood & Biologics* by the U.S. Food and Drug Administration, 2010, retrieved from http://www.fda.gov/BiologicsBloodVaccines/SafetyAvailability/VaccineSafety/ucm096228.htm#t1. **4.** "Prevalence of Autism Spectrum Disorders—Autism and Developmental Disabilities Monitoring Network, 14 Sites, United States, 2008," by the Centers for Disease Control and Prevention, 2012, *Morbidity and Mortality Weekly Report Surveillance Summaries, 61*(3), pp. 1–24, retrieved from http://www.cdc.gov/mmwr/pdf/ss/ss6103.pdf.

>> *Frontline: The Vaccine War* **explores both sides of the vaccine debate:** www.pbs.org/wgbh/pages/frontline/vaccines/view.

---

immunizations before children can enter school. Exemptions to immunization laws can be given if a child has certain medical conditions, for religious reasons, and sometimes for other beliefs. In addition, some people are not immunized because they don't know or understand the recommendations, don't have access to health care, or cannot afford the shots. When groups of people are not immunized it can compromise **herd immunity.** Herd immunity occurs when greater than 90% of people in a community or group are fully vaccinated against a disease, leaving that disease with little ability to spread through the population. Herd immunity is important because it offers some protection against the disease for individuals who cannot be vaccinated (due to medical conditions) or who haven't been vaccinated yet (such as newborns).

Immune Disorders

Not all immune systems are strong. Newborns do not yet have fully developed immune systems, and seniors tend to have weak ones, which grow less and less effective as they age. This leaves these groups more vulnerable to infection and disease. Chronic stress can also impair the immune system, a topic discussed in more detail on page 54 of Chapter 3. In addition, the immune system can sometimes develop disorders. Two common problems are allergies and asthma.

Allergies

More than 50 million people in the United States have **allergies,** abnormal immune system reactions to substances that are otherwise harmless. Allergies are widespread on college campuses, with 21.5% of students in one survey stating that they had been treated for allergies in the last year.[3]

Allergies are caused by a hypersensitive immune system, which mistakenly perceives substances such as pollen, peanuts, pet dander, and pest droppings to be serious threats.[4] If you have allergies, you may suffer from itching, sneezing, coughing, watery eyes, difficulty breathing, and congestion. When allergic people come into contact with substances they are sensitive to, their

herd immunity The condition where greater than 90% of a community is vaccinated against a disease, giving it little ability to spread through the community, providing some protection against the disease to members of the community who are not vaccinated.

allergies Abnormal immune system reactions to substances that are otherwise harmless.

immune systems begin to produce antibodies called immunoglobulin E, or IgE. IgE molecules bind simultaneously to the allergen and to a **mast cell,** a type of cell in the skin and mucous membranes. As a result of these interactions, the mast cell releases powerful chemicals such as histamine into the bloodstream. It is these chemicals—and not the allergens themselves—that make allergy sufferers miserable.

In some instances, allergens cause a rare, serious allergic reaction known as *anaphylaxis*. In this case, the wave of histamine and chemicals released by mast cells occurs throughout the body and can cause **anaphylactic shock.** Blood pressure drops and airways swell. If not treated immediately with an injection of epinephrine, a person can lapse into unconsciousness and even death.

Fortunately, there are strategies for coping with allergies. Allergists recommend you steer clear of the things you are allergic to whenever possible. Your doctor may recommend prescription or over-the-counter medications that can help alleviate symptoms. Immunotherapy, in which patients are given repeated shots containing increasing amounts of the allergen to desensitize them, is also an option.

 The American Lung Association provides more information on how to manage asthma and minimize triggers of an asthma attack: www.lung.org/lung-disease/asthma.

The incidence of allergies has increased steadily in recent years. Ironically, this increase may be the unintended result of our antiseptic, health-conscious lifestyle. A possible explanation, the *hygiene hypothesis*, contends that early childhood exposure to microbes can prevent the development of allergies, and, conversely, reduced exposure to microbes can increase the chances of developing allergies. Many factors in developed countries today reduce exposure to microbes: smaller family size (fewer siblings means fewer family members bringing microbes into the home); less exposure to animals, specifically farm animals; use of vaccines and antibiotics; and less exposure to general dirt and microorganisms.

The hygiene hypothesis may also contribute to the increasing rates of asthma, a condition that we'll look at next.

 This video explores the hygiene hypothesis of developing allergies: www.pbs.org/wgbh/evolution/library/10/4/l_104_07.html.

Asthma

Asthma occurs when the airways of the lungs become constricted and inflamed, making breathing difficult. The symptoms and severity of asthma range from shortness of breath and wheezing (a whistling-type noise produced during exhalation) to the life-threatening inability to effectively move air in and out of the lungs. There are two general types of asthma. *Allergic asthma* is caused by exposure to allergens such as those in the air (e.g., pollen), in the blood (e.g., bee venom), or in food (e.g., peanuts). *Intrinsic asthma*, on the other hand, can be induced by exercise or cold temperatures and is not associated with an allergy. It isn't clear why some people have asthma and others do not, but it is likely a combination of genetics and the environment in which you live.

An asthma attack is the result of three main physiological changes: the constriction of the airway muscles, known as *bronchoconstriction;* the overproduction of mucus in the airway; and inflammation of the airway lining. All of these changes can lead to a terrifying result—the inability to breathe. Prevention of asthma includes avoiding known triggers and, in some cases, taking regular doses of medicines that prevent bronchoconstriction and inflammation. Once an attack has begun, fast-acting bronchodilators, administered through inhalers, and oral anti-inflammatory medicines help open the airways and ease breathing.

Nearly 1 in 10 school-aged children in the United States suffers from asthma, reflecting a doubling of asthma rates over the last 30 years.[5] Also notable is the racial disparity in asthma rates. About 17% of African American children have asthma, compared to about 11% of children of other racial and ethnic backgrounds. This is thought to reflect socioeconomic conditions, with poorer children more likely to be exposed to mold, diesel soot, and air pollution.

Infectious Diseases

Even with advances in modern medicine, infections remain the world's leading killer of children and young adults. The burden on society from even minor infections is immense. Infectious disease costs the United States more than $120 billion per year.[6]

Infections can be categorized by the types of pathogens that cause them: viruses, bacteria, fungi, protozoa, and parasitic worms **(Table 11.2)**.

Viral Infections

Viruses are microscopic organisms that cannot multiply without invading body cells. They hijack the cellular machinery and force it to crank out duplicate viruses at the expense of the cells' normal functions—and at the expense of your health. Viruses cannot survive for long periods outside of a host, but once inside a host cell they can multiply very quickly. For example, a cell infected with the common flu virus begins to release new flu viruses only 6 hours after the virus enters the cell, and it produces enough new viruses to infect another 20 to 30 cells. In the process, the infected cell dies about 11 hours after the virus entered.[7]

Colds

More than 200 different viruses cause cold symptoms. Common culprits are groups of viruses called rhinoviruses and coronaviruses. They are typically spread by touching contaminated objects, through personal contact, or by breathing airborne pathogens. Symptoms appear about 2 or 3 days after infection and can include a runny nose or congestion, sneezing, cough, sore throat, headache, and mild fever. There is no known cure, but over-the-counter pain relievers, antihistamines, and decongestants may provide some relief from symptoms.

Colds generally end in about a week and cannot be treated with antibiotics because antibiotics are designed to fight bacteria, not viruses. However, sometimes viral infections leave the body susceptible to secondary bacterial infections of the sinuses, ears, or respiratory tract, in which case antibiotics would be prescribed. Wash your hands frequently, keep your hands away from your face, and stay away from people who have colds to help keep from getting one.

Influenza

The flu is a contagious respiratory condition caused by a

mast cell A type of cell in the skin and mucous membranes that releases histamine and other chemicals into the bloodstream during an allergic reaction.

anaphylactic shock A result of anaphylaxis where the release of histamine and other chemicals into the body leads to a drop in blood pressure, tightening of airways, and possible unconsciousness and even death.

asthma Chronic constriction and inflammation of the airways, making breathing difficult and causing shortness of breath, wheezing, coughing, and chest tightness.

virus A microscopic organism that cannot multiply without invading body cells.

TABLE 11.2 Pathogens and the Diseases They Cause

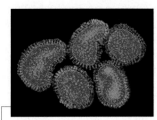

Influenza viruses
(32,000 ×).

Pathogen: Viruses

Description: Microscopic infectious agents that are composed not of cells but of small amounts of genetic material covered by a protein coat. They cannot multiply unless they invade living cells and hijack those cells' metabolic machinery.

Examples: Rhinoviruses; coronaviruses; Influenza viruses; Epstein-Barr virus; Hepatitis A–E; HIV; Herpes simplex virus types 1 and 2 (HSV-1 and HSV-2); Human papillomavirus

Diseases Caused: Common cold, flu, mononucleosis, hepatitis, AIDS, herpes (oral or genital), cervical cancer, warts, genital warts

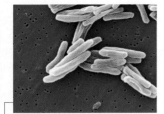

Mycobacterium tuberculosis bacteria (15,549 ×).

Pathogen: Bacteria

Description: Single-celled microorganisms that have genetic material but lack a distinct cell nucleus. They invade and reproduce inside a host, sometimes releasing toxic enzymes and chemicals.

Examples: *Neisseria meningitidis, Staphylococcus aureus, Group A Streptococcus, Streptococcus pneumoniae, Borrelia burgdorferi, Mycobacterium tuberculosis, Chlamydia trachomatis, Treponema pallidum*

Diseases Caused: Meningitis, staph infection, food poisoning, toxic shock syndrome, strep throat, pneumonia, Lyme disease, tuberculosis, sexually transmitted infections

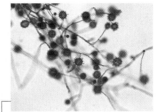

Histoplasma capsulatum (400 ×).

Pathogen: Fungi

Description: Organisms with sophisticated cellular structures, including a true nucleus and a strong, flexible cell wall. Fungi include yeasts and molds. They feed on organic matter, including human tissue.

Examples: *Candida albicans, Histoplasma capsulatum, Trichophyton*

Diseases Caused: Candidiasis (yeast infections), thrush, diaper rash, infections of nail beds, histoplasmosis, *tinea pedis* (athlete's foot), jock itch, ring worm, nail infections

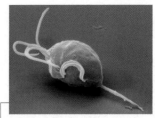

Trichomonas vaginalis (9,000 ×).

Pathogen: Protozoa

Description: Single-celled parasites that rely on other living things for food and shelter.

Examples: *Plasmodium, Toxoplasma gondii, Trichomonas vaginalis*

Diseases Caused: Malaria, toxoplasmosis, trichomoniasis

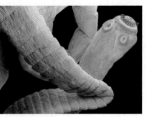

Taenia tapeworm (15 ×).

Pathogen: Parasitic worms (helminths)

Description: Multicellular parasitic creatures that are ingested as eggs or burrow through the skin and compete with a host body for nutrients.

Examples: *Taenia solium, Taenia saginata, Hymenolepis nana, Enterobius vermicularis, Ancylostoma duodenale*

Diseases Caused: Tapeworm, pinworm, hookworm infection

---

number of **influenza** viruses. Between 5% and 20% of the U.S. population get the flu every year, suffering from high fever, body aches, fatigue, and a dry cough. Although it often is a moderate illness, lasting a little longer and making people a little more miserable than the common cold, the flu can cause a medical emergency in some infants, seniors, or people with weakened immune systems. The flu can also lead to bacterial pneumonia, dehydration, sinus infections, and ear infections and tends to exacerbate underlying medical conditions such as asthma and diabetes. Every year, more than 200,000 people in the United States are hospitalized with flu complications, and as many as 49,000 die from an influenza infection.[8]

As with colds, influenza viruses are spread through personal contact, airborne pathogens, or touching inanimate objects covered with a virus. There is no known cure—although antiviral medications may be prescribed to reduce symptoms—and so prevention remains the best medicine. In addition to proper hand washing and coughing and sneezing into the bend of your arm rather than your hand, federal health officials recommend that children, pregnant women, health workers, people over age 65, and people of all ages with chronic medical conditions such as asthma and diabetes get an influenza vaccine annually. "Flu shots" are available at many campus health centers, doctors' offices, pharmacies, and even grocery stores every fall.

When a flu is able to pass quickly from person to person unchecked and eventually spreads worldwide, it is called a **pandemic.** Pandemics can occur when a new influenza virus emerges that humans have not been exposed to before. This lack of exposure leaves people with no acquired immunity to help defend against the virus, and it can become very contagious. Often, animals are the reservoir for flu viruses that mutate into new strains that cause pandemics. The most recent pandemic, the 2009 H1N1 flu pandemic, was caused by a virus that started in pigs. When a pandemic virus is also deadly the casualties can be staggering. In 1918 an influenza pandemic killed approximately 40 million people.

>> **This CDC video explains how to "Take 3" to avoid catching or spreading influenza:** www.cdc.gov/CDCTV/IR_Take3/index.html.

Mononucleosis

Infectious **mononucleosis,** or *"mono,"* is often called "the kissing disease" and is caused by the Epstein-Barr virus. It is transmitted through contact with an infected person's saliva, mucus, or tears. Sharing drinking glasses or straws, eating utensils, or toothbrushes can expose you to the Epstein-Barr virus. Common among teens and young adults, mono causes fatigue, weakness, sore throat, fever, headaches, swollen lymph nodes and tonsils, and loss of appetite. The condition usually is not serious, although some people may experience complications such as hepatitis or enlargement of the spleen. Most symptoms dissipate within two or three weeks, but the fatigue, weakness, and swollen lymph nodes can persevere for months. Blood tests may be used to

influenza A group of viruses that cause the flu, a contagious respiratory condition.

pandemic A worldwide epidemic of a disease.

mononucleosis A viral disease that causes fatigue, weakness, sore throat, fever, headaches, swollen lymph nodes and tonsils, and loss of appetite.

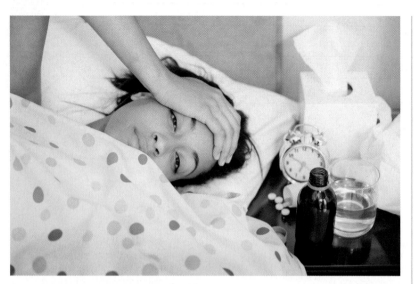

Many infections cause *fatigue*.

diagnose mononucleosis, and the primary treatments are as basic as getting lots of rest and drinking plenty of fluids.

Hepatitis

Hepatitis is an inflammation of the liver. It causes **jaundice,** fatigue, fever, nausea, abdominal pain, and muscle and joint pain. In some cases it can be deadly. Viral infections are the primary cause of hepatitis, although alcohol, drugs, and some underlying medical conditions can be blamed. There are several types of hepatitis. Hepatitis A, hepatitis B, and hepatitis C are the most common forms in the United States, but there are also rarer hepatitis viruses, known as D and E. Hepatitis B is transmitted mostly through sexual contact and is discussed on page 273.

Hepatitis A is the most widespread form of hepatitis. It is contracted through consuming microscopic amounts of feces that can lurk on contaminated fruits, vegetables, and ice cubes. The virus can also be spread during oral-anal sexual contact, or by changing dirty diapers and failing to thoroughly wash your hands afterward. Symptoms can last for weeks or months, although some people never feel ill. Although the virus can cause liver failure and death in a small portion of the population, most people make a full recovery, sustaining no permanent liver damage. Rates of hepatitis A have decreased in recent years. A vaccine for hepatitis A was introduced in 1995, and doctors recommend that children, travelers to certain countries, and other at-risk individuals get the vaccine, which has led to a reduction in infections.

Hepatitis C is the primary reason for liver transplants in the United States. More than three-fourths of those who are infected with this highly destructive virus go on to develop chronic infections that can last a lifetime, scarring the liver or triggering liver cancer. Unfortunately, early symptoms of this form of hepatitis are mild or nonexistent, and many people do not realize they have it until liver damage has occurred. Hepatitis C kills between 8,000 and 10,000 people in the United States every year

hepatitis Inflammation of the liver that affects liver function.

jaundice A yellowing of the skin, mucous membranes, and sometimes the whites of the eyes often caused by liver malfunction.

bacteria (singular *bacterium*) Single-celled microorganisms that invade a host and reproduce inside. Harmful bacteria release toxic enzymes and chemicals.

antibiotic resistance When a bacterium is able to overcome the effects of an antibiotic through a random mutation, or change in the bacterium's genetic code.

and typically is spread through sharing syringes and other drug-related paraphernalia.[9] It can also be passed on by unsterilized tattoo needles and piercing equipment or sexual contact. Before screening tests were developed and made available in the United States, it was also spread through blood transfusions and organ transplants. It is still possible to pick up the infection from needles or other medical instruments in other parts of the world where sterilization practices may not be as rigorous.

Treatment for hepatitis is usually nothing more than rest, fluids, and proper nutrition for acute cases of hepatitis, but chronic cases sometimes benefit from medications. If you have chronic hepatitis, your doctor should regularly screen you for liver disease.

Bacterial Infections

Bacteria are single-celled microorganisms that are found throughout nature. They can exist independently or as parasites, drawing their nourishment from other forms of life. Harmful bacteria release toxins or damaging enzymes that disrupt the body. However, less than 1% of the many types of bacteria are actually harmful.[10] Some bacteria are even beneficial, helping us digest food, synthesize vitamins, and fight off disease. Manufacturers even add the *Lactobacillus acidophilus* bacteria to many yogurt and cheese products because of their healthful properties.

Unlike viruses, bacteria are able to replicate on their own without the help of a host cell by dividing in two. Antibiotics help defeat bacteria by blocking key steps in this process. However, bacteria can also develop **antibiotic resistance** to these important drugs. This occurs when a random mutation, or change in a bacterium's genetic code, enables the bacterium to overcome the effects of the antibiotic. Perhaps only 1 bacterium in 10 million gains this advantage, but that cell rapidly grows and divides, even in the presence of the antibiotic, and the resistant bacteria take over. This is why it is very important to take antibiotics only when they have been prescribed by a physician, to take them for the full course, and only for bacterial infections!

Meningitis

Meningitis is an infection of the meninges, the thin membranes that surround both the spinal cord and brain. The infection can be caused by a number of viral and bacterial strains and is characterized by high fever, stiff neck, headaches, and even confusion or seizures. When caused by a virus, meningitis tends to be much less severe and dissipates on its own. Bacterial meningitis, however, can be life-threatening and may cause hearing loss, brain damage, and other disabilities. The bacteria that most commonly cause meningitis are *Streptococcus pneumoniae* and *Neisseria meningitidis*; most often, meningitis occurs when these bacteria have infected another part of the body and then enter the bloodstream and migrate to the meninges. Even when treated promptly with the proper antibiotics, bacterial meningitis kills between 5% and 10% of patients worldwide, usually within a day or two of the onset of symptoms.[11]

Adolescents and young adults account for nearly one-third of all cases of bacterial meningitis in the United States, and college students—especially those living in dormitories—are at moderately increased risk. To reduce their risk, the CDC recommends that all youths between the ages of 11 and 18 receive the meningococcal vaccine, an inoculation that protects against some but not all of the bacterial strains that cause meningitis. Several states now require that students receive a meningococcal vaccine before entering college or university.

Staphylococcal Infections

There are more than two dozen types of *Staphylococcus* bacteria, but one—*Staphylococcus aureus*—is responsible for the bulk of all "staph" infections. It causes boils and other minor skin ailments, especially in people with eczema (a chronic, itchy skin rash) or burned skin. Sometimes staph can cause more serious infections of the blood, lungs, heart, or urinary tract, most often in those whose immune system is compromised because of illness or other conditions.

Staphylococcus aureus also releases toxins that can trigger food poisoning and **toxic shock syndrome.** Toxic shock syndrome is a rare yet serious disease that resembles a bad cold or flu in the first few hours but can quickly progress to a medical emergency. Fever, chills, nausea, and diarrhea give way to seizures, low blood pressure, and organ failure and, in about 5% of cases, death.[12] In 1980, more than 800 menstruating women developed the condition, and 38 died from it. Federal investigators linked the cases to use of a highly absorbent tampon that was subsequently taken off the market. Menstruating women can avoid toxic shock syndrome by changing their tampons every 4 to 8 hours, using the lowest absorbency tampon possible, and alternating between tampons and pads.

Some staph bacteria are resistant to the antibiotics typically used to treat them. Known as **methicillin-resistant *Staphylococcus aureus,* or MRSA,** these bacteria cause skin infections and are responsible for many cases of pneumonia. See the **Spotlight** on MRSA on page 268.

Streptococcus Infections

Chances are you or someone you know has been infected with the bacteria *Streptococcus*, perhaps more than once. Group A *Streptococcus* is behind all bouts of strep throat, a relatively mild illness that causes throat pain, swollen tonsils, fever, headache, and stomachache. Particularly common in children and teens, strep throat is highly contagious through airborne droplets or touching contaminated objects. Strep throat usually requires a course of antibiotics to treat. If left untreated, it can lead to scarlet fever or rheumatic fever. Strains of *Streptococcus* bacteria can also cause other types of infections, including skin infections and pneumonia.

Lyme Disease

If you have ever been hiking in the northwestern, midwestern, or northeastern states, you may have seen warning signs about Lyme disease. The infection is caused by the bacterium *Borrelia burgdorferi* and is transmitted to people through the bite of infected deer ticks and blacklegged ticks. Early symptoms are headache, fatigue, fever, and muscle or joint pain. Within 4 weeks of infection, 70–80% of victims also experience a bull's-eye-shaped skin rash that starts small and grows larger **(Figure 11.3)**. If the infection goes untreated, it can cause swelling and pain in the joints, rapid heartbeat or other heart problems, partial facial paralysis, and neurological problems such as memory loss, which can last for years. Antibiotics are usually successful at treating Lyme disease if used in the early stages, but some people will have recurring symptoms of the disease for years. Prevention remains the best medicine. Hikers should avoid wooded areas and overgrown grass

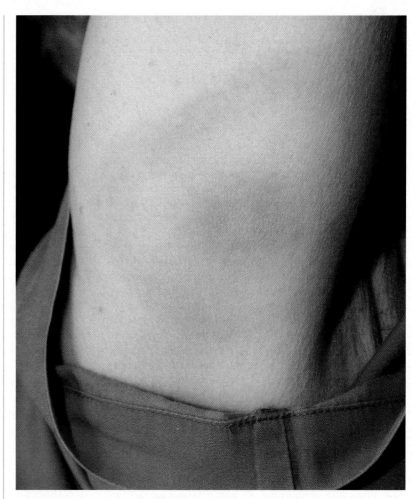

FIGURE 11.3 Lyme Disease "Bull's-Eye" Rash.

and brush, and wear long pants, long sleeves, and long socks to help keep ticks off their skin. Checking your body for ticks after being outdoors is also advised, and should you ever find one, pull it straight out with a pair of tweezers. Ticks normally will not transmit the bacterium until after they have fed, which can take anywhere from 36 to 48 hours.

Pneumonia

Pneumonia ranks as the ninth leading cause of death in the United States, and the number-one cause of death for children worldwide.[13,14] It is an inflammation of the lungs that can be caused by bacteria, viruses, fungi, or parasites. Pneumonia can vary from mild to deadly. Bacterial pneumonias are the most common in adults, and usually the most severe, causing high fever, chest pain, shortness of breath, chills, and a cough with green, yellow, or bloody mucus. Pneumonia tends to occur in conjunction with a cold or flu and is often mistaken by patients for these lesser infections. You should see a doctor immediately if you suddenly experience pneumonia symptoms.

The most common bacterial cause of pneumonia is the *Streptococcus pneumoniae* bacterium. Antibiotics are used to treat bacterial pneumonia

toxic shock syndrome A rare, serious illness caused by staph bacteria that begins with severe flu symptoms but can quickly progress to a medical emergency.

methicillin-resistant *Staphylococcus aureus* (MRSA) A strain of staph that is resistant to the broad-spectrum antibiotics commonly used to treat staph infections.

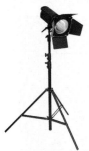

SPOTLIGHT

MRSA

MRSA, or methicillin-resistant *Staphylococcus aureus*, is a strain of staph that is resistant to the broad-spectrum antibiotics commonly used to treat staph infections. MRSA is responsible for serious skin infections, which first appear as painful, red, pus-filled lesions, and can also cause other infections, including pneumonia. Because it is not treatable with many antibiotics, it poses a threat to anyone who is infected. The Centers for Disease Control and Prevention estimates that nearly 100,000 people in the United States develop a serious MRSA infection in any given year and that about one-fifth of them die from it.

These statistics reflect a drastic rise in MRSA: In 1974, 2% of all staph infections were MRSA; in 1995, 22%; and in 2004 MRSA accounted for 64% of all staph infections.[1] It

is thought that the development of bacteria like MRSA, which are resistant to multiple antibiotics, is in part due to the misuse of antibiotics.

The infection can be spread by direct skin-to-skin contact or by touching something that has been touched by an infected person. Most people with MRSA become infected when in the hospital or in other health-care settings. Recent data indicates that the number of cases of MRSA acquired in health-care settings is declining. One study found that between 2005 and 2008, MRSA infections that began in hospitals declined 28%.[2] However, MRSA is becoming more common in schools and on college campuses. School athletes are especially susceptible due to frequent skin-to-skin contact with others, the higher possibility of cuts or abrasions on the skin,

and the use of facilities like locker rooms that may harbor MRSA. Unlike MRSA acquired in health-care settings, health officials are not seeing declines in rates of such "community-acquired" MRSA infections.[3]

Frequent hand washing, especially when in a clinical setting, is critical to limiting the spread of this infection. The following steps will also help you avoid catching or spreading MRSA:

- In addition to hand washing, keep open wounds covered with dry, sterile bandages.

- Shower immediately after exercise or participating in a close contact sport.

- Do not share personal items such as towels or razors with others.

- If you have a skin infection that does not appear to be getting better after a day or so, see a doctor and request that you be tested for MRSA.

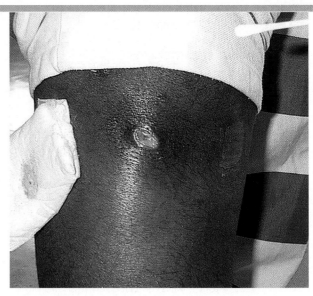

A sore due to MRSA.

Early detection is important, especially because some MRSA strains, at least for now, respond to the antibiotic vancomycin, and small skin infections can be treated by draining and cleaning the lesion.

References: 1. "Overview of Healthcare-Associated MRSA," in *Healthcare-Associated Methicillin Resistant Staphylococcus aureus (HA-MRSA)*, by the Centers for Disease Control and Prevention, 2010, retrieved from http://www.cdc.gov/ncidod/dhqp/ar_mrsa.html. 2. "Health Care–Associated Invasive MRSA Infections, 2005–2008," by A. Kallen, Y. Mu, S. Bulens, A. Reingold, S. Petit, K. Gershman, . . . S. Fridkin, 2010, *Journal of the American Medical Association, 304*(6), pp. 641–647. 3. "MRSA Statistics," in *MRSA Infections*, by the Centers for Disease Control and Prevention, 2011, retrieved from http://www.cdc.gov/mrsa/statistics/index.html.

---

infections, but as antibiotic-resistant strains have become more common, these drugs are less effective. Prevention remains the best measure. Health-care experts recommend that people get an annual flu shot to reduce their risk. Seniors and infants are at higher risk for pneumonia, as are younger people with asthma and other chronic respiratory problems, impaired immune systems, or who have been exposed to certain chemicals and environmental pollutants. High-risk individuals are encouraged to get the pneumococcal pneumonia vaccine.

Tuberculosis

Tuberculosis, or TB, is a serious disease caused by the bacterium *Mycobacterium tuberculosis* that is spread through the air. The bacteria typically attack the lungs, where they create holes in the airways and hinder breathing. They can also settle into the brain, spine, or kidneys, and without proper treatment can prove fatal.

Symptoms of TB include weight loss, fatigue, fever, night sweats, and a persistent cough that does not go away after three weeks. But not everyone with a TB infection will become ill from it. Many have what is called a *latent* TB infection that does not cause any symptoms, is not infectious, and may never progress to active TB disease. In fact, only about 5–10% of people with TB develop the active form of the disease.[15] Medication, taken for many months, can help keep latent TB infections from evolving into active TB disease, although drug-resistant strains of TB are emerging.

Once the leading cause of death in the United States, TB cases have been declining in recent years and reached an all-time low in 2008. Infection rates continue to be highest among immigrants and racial and ethnic minorities, the poor, the homeless, and those infected with HIV. Although there were only 10,528 new cases reported in 2011, millions of people in the United States are estimated to be living with a TB infection. Worldwide, about 2 billion people are infected.[16,17]

EMERGING
infectious
diseases

Although some diseases have plagued humankind for as long as records have been kept, others have only become a human health threat in recent years or have reemerged as worldwide travel has spread them. Some of the more troubling emerging infections are described here.

H1N1 ("Swine flu"). H1N1 is a new influenza virus first detected in the United States in April 2009. The virus contains genes not only from pigs, but also from birds and humans. H1N1 spreads from person to person similarly to the seasonal flu, and in June 2009, the World Health Organization declared it a worldwide pandemic. That pandemic warning was lifted in 2010, but health officials say the virus is still circulating, and protection against it is now included in seasonal flu vaccines in the United States. The virus causes cough, sore throat, congestion, body aches, headaches, chills, and fatigue. Most people recover on their own without treatment, but in some cases the illness can cause severe respiratory problems and even death.

H5N1 and H7N9 (Avian influenza or "bird flu"). H5N1 has been diagnosed in hundreds of people in more than a dozen countries since November 2003.[1] Most of them contracted the serious infection after coming into direct contact with infected poultry. It causes conjunctivitis (pink eye), pneumonia, and for more than half its victims, death. The virus has, in a few rare instances, spread from person to person, and it would only take a slight mutation for it to spread very easily. If that were to occur, H5N1 would have the potential of becoming the next influenza pandemic. In 2013, a similar avian influenza virus, H7N9, sickened more than 130 people in China, killing about 30% of victims. As with H5N1, this newer viral strain did not appear to spread from person to person but was being watched closely by international health authorities.

West Nile Virus. This infectious disease is spread through the bite of an infected mosquito. Although it appeared in other parts of the world earlier, it was not discovered in the United States until 1999. Since then it has spread rapidly, infecting tens of thousands of people across the country and killing more than 1,000.[2] Rates of West Nile virus are growing in the United States, and 2012 experienced the highest U.S. infections on record. Although 80% of infected people feel no effects, about 1 in every 150 people infected experience severe symptoms ranging from muscle weakness and disorientation to vision loss, paralysis, coma, and death. The only way to avoid getting the virus is to avoid mosquito bites.

Close contact with poultry or other animals can pass new diseases to humans.

References: **1.** *Number of Confirmed Human Cases of Avian Influenza A (H7N9) Reported to WHO,* Report 8 Data in WHO/HQ as of May 30, 2013, by the World Health Organization, retrieved from http://www.who.int/influenza/human_animal_interface/influenza_h7n9/08_ReportWebH7N9Number.pdf. **2.** "Statistics, Surveillance, and Control Archive" in *West Nile Virus,* by the Centers for Disease Control and Prevention, June 5, 2012, retrieved from http://www.cdc.gov/ncidod/dvbid/westnile/surv&control.htm#maps.

Practical Strategies

Protecting Yourself Against Infectious Diseases

To avoid contracting an infection:

- Wash your hands often, or use hand sanitizer with at least 60% alcohol.
- Keep your hands away from your eyes, nose, and mouth. Touching your face is a common way to transmit pathogens from your hands into your body.
- Avoid close contact with people who are sick.
- Routinely clean and disinfect surfaces, including keyboards, phones, and kitchen counters.
- Keep up to date on your vaccinations and get an annual flu shot.
- Avoid contact with wild animals. Rodents, bats, raccoons, skunks, and foxes can all spread harmful bacteria or viruses. Make sure your pets are up to date on their vaccinations as well.
- Avoid mosquito bites. In mosquito-dense areas, wear insect repellent when you are outdoors, particularly at dusk and dawn;

eliminate standing water in flower pots, bird baths, or other containers left outdoors; make sure you have intact window screens; and wear long-sleeved shirts and pants to avoid bites.
- Avoid walking barefoot in locker rooms or on dirt.
- Don't smoke, and avoid second-hand smoke.
- Don't drink alcohol or drink only in moderation.
- Get enough sleep. Lack of sleep can impair the immune system.
- Eat well. Proper nutrition supports your immune system.
- If you are feeling under the weather, take steps to prevent infecting others. Stay home when you are sick, cover your mouth or nose with a tissue when you cough or sneeze, or cough or sneeze into the bend of your elbow, and wash your hands after coughing or sneezing.

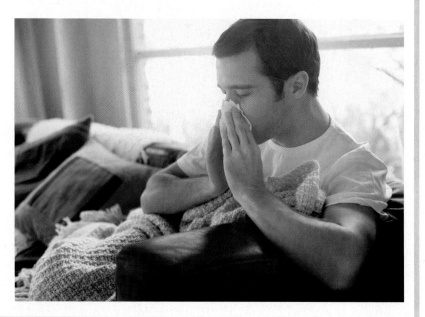

Fungal Infections

Fungi are organisms that obtain their food from organic matter, in some cases human tissue. Common examples of fungi are multicellular mold, mildew, and mushrooms, and single-celled yeast.

Some of the thousands of fungi that exist are quite beneficial. Penicillin, the powerful antibiotic used to treat a number of bacterial infections, is made from fungi. Yeast is used in making bread and cheese. Other types are not so helpful. Fungi are behind many minor infections of the skin, scalp, and nail beds but can also cause life-threatening systemic infections, especially for people with weakened immune systems.

Yeast infections are some of the most common types of fungal infections. Small amounts of a yeast called *Candida albicans* are always present in a person's body, but if imbalances occur—after taking antibiotics, for example, or, for women, during the normal hormonal changes that come with menstrual periods—this fungus is able to multiply out of control. It can cause infections in various parts of the body, such as the intestinal tract or vagina. Yeast infections, although uncomfortable and unpleasant, are usually not serious. In women, they are marked by itching in the vagina and around the genitals and are often accompanied by an abnormal vaginal discharge that can resemble cottage cheese. Sexual intercourse can also be painful. Treatment involves inserting a cream or suppository into the vagina or taking an oral medication. Other *Candida* infections include thrush (an overgrowth in the mouth), diaper rash, and infections of the nail beds.

Protozoan Infections

Protozoa are single-celled organisms that, like fungi, obtain nutrients from feeding on organic matter. Although some are free-living, and even helpful—consuming harmful bacteria or serving as food for fish and other animals—protozoan parasites rely on other living things, such as humans, for food and shelter. These protozoa are capable of causing serious diseases in humans, especially in people living in developing countries. In the United States, where sanitation and food-handling standards have reduced our exposure to them, protozoan infections are less common.

One of the protozoan diseases of most concern is **malaria,** which kills nearly 1 million people every year, primarily infants, children, and pregnant women.[18] The infection is caused by the protozoa *Plasmodium* and is typically transmitted to humans through the bites of infected mosquitoes. Malaria is a serious threat throughout much of sub-Saharan Africa and parts of Latin America, Asia, and the Middle East, and fully 50% of the world's population is at risk of contracting it.[18] Although it was controlled in the United States more than five decades ago, occasional outbreaks still occur here.

Initial symptoms include fever, chills, vomiting, and headache. If not treated with antimalarial drugs promptly, the infection can be fatal. Some strains of malaria have become resistant to drugs, making treatment much more difficult. Malaria can be prevented by preventing mosquito bites. Antimalarial drugs can also be taken during trips to malaria-rich areas to reduce the risk of contracting the disease.

fungi Multicellular or single-celled organisms that obtain their food from organic matter, in some cases human tissue.

protozoa Single-celled parasites that rely on other living things for food and shelter.

malaria A serious disease that causes fever and chills that appear in cycles. In some cases malaria can be life-threatening.

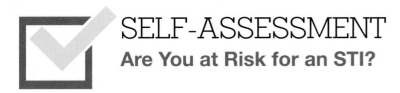

SELF-ASSESSMENT
Are You at Risk for an STI?

If you engage in sexual activity, then you are at risk for contracting an STI. However, your level of risk depends on certain behaviors.

"Sex" includes oral, vaginal, or anal sex, and a sexual partner is somebody with whom you have had oral, vaginal, or anal sex.

1. In the past 12 months, have you been diagnosed with any STI?*
   ☐ Yes ☐ No

2. In the past 12 months, have you had more than one sexual partner?
   ☐ Yes ☐ No

3. In the past 12 months, do you think your sexual partner(s) had any other partners?
   ☐ Yes ☐ Not sure ☐ No

4. In the past 12 months, have you had sex with a new partner?
   ☐ Yes ☐ No

5. Are you currently planning on having sex with a new partner?
   ☐ Yes ☐ Not sure ☐ No

6. In the past 12 months, how often have you used condoms during vaginal or anal intercourse or latex barriers during oral sex?
   ☐ Always ☐ Some of the time ☐ Most of the time ☐ Never

7. Do you discuss sexual history and testing with your partner(s)?
   ☐ Always ☐ Sometimes ☐ Never

HOW TO INTERPRET YOUR SCORE

If you answered "Yes" or "Not sure" to questions 1–5, you may be at higher risk for STIs. If you answered anything other than "Always" to questions 6 and 7, you may be at higher risk for STIs.

Consider making an appointment at your campus health center for STI screening and/or to discuss prevention strategies.

To complete this Self-Assessment online, visit MasteringHealth™

*Having had an STI recently may put you at higher risk for other STIs.

Source: Adapted from *UC Berkeley Sexually Transmitted Infection (STI) Risk Assessment*, from UC Berkeley University Health Services Tang Center website. Reprinted with permission.

Parasitic Worm Infections

Parasitic worms (helminths) are creatures that compete with a host body for nutrients. Some tiny worms burrow through the skin, whereas others are contracted from eating microscopic eggs in undercooked foods. Once inside the body, some can grow up to 10 to 15 feet in length. Others can live for up to 15 years. They are most frequently found in tropical regions and are a problem in areas with poor sanitation. Infections are most common in travelers, refugees, migrant workers, children, and the homeless. Two of the more common parasitic worms in the United States are tapeworms and pinworms, both of which can be treated with oral medications.

Sexually Transmitted Infections

Sexually transmitted infections (STIs) are commonplace. There are more than 30 different sexually transmissible bacteria, viruses, and parasites.[19] It is estimated that worldwide nearly a million people acquire an STI every day, and there are approximately 20 million new cases of STIs every year in the United States, costing the U.S. health-care system nearly $16 billion.[19,20,21]

The CDC estimates that although 15- to 24-year-olds represent only 25% of the sexually active population, they account for half of all new STI cases.[21] Among sexually active U.S. teens, the STI prevalence is 40% and those with three or more partners have a prevalence of more than 50%. Even among girls aged 14 to 19 reporting only one lifetime partner, approximately 20% have at least one STI.[22] Because many cases of STIs may go unrecognized or untreated, and some STIs can be treated but not cured, the CDC estimates that there are more than 110 million STI cases overall among men and women nationwide, including both new and existing infections.[21]

> These videos discuss STIs: www.cdc.gov/std/Be-Smart-Be-Well/default.htm.

Risk Factors for STIs

The college years can be a time of elevated risk for contracting an STI. Your likelihood of contracting an STI depends a lot on your behaviors. Some activities that increase risk are:

- Having unprotected vaginal, anal, or oral sex.
- Having sex with multiple partners, especially strangers, and not discussing STIs before sex.
- Exchanging sex for drugs or money.
- Participating in sex while drunk or high on drugs.
- Coming into direct skin-to-skin contact with someone who has infections such as human papillomavirus (HPV), herpes, pubic lice, or scabies.
- Injecting drugs or steroids with dirty needles or syringes—or having unprotected sex with someone who has.
- Sharing needles for tattoos and body piercings.
- Failing to be vaccinated against HPV or hepatitis B.

Are you at risk for a sexually transmitted infection? Take the **Self-Assessment** to find out.

parasitic worms (helminths) Multicellular creatures that compete with a host body for nutrients.

sexually transmitted infections (STIs) Infections transmitted mainly through sexual activity, such as vaginal, anal, or oral sex.

Sexual Conduct and Risk

Only abstinence provides 100% protection from STIs. If you choose to have sex, the safest sex is between two completely monogamous partners who have been tested and are uninfected with any STIs. Although condoms are not 100% effective against STIs, when used correctly and consistently they significantly reduce risk and make sex safer.

If you or your partner is not monogamous or has not been tested, it is considered high risk to have vaginal, anal, or oral sex with that person without a condom. Unprotected anal sex carries the highest risk, especially for the receiving partner. Unprotected vaginal sex is next highest risk. Unprotected oral sex is also considered high risk, although it is less risky than unprotected anal or vaginal sex. If you or your partner has any type of STI, doctors recommend avoiding sex until treatment has been completed and symptoms are no longer present.

Talking About Safer Sex

It may feel awkward to talk about sexual history or STIs with a new partner, but it's important. Before you have sex with a new person, ask:

- Does he or she have any STIs?
- Has he or she participated in risky activities in the past?
- Has he or she been tested for STIs in the past? If so, has he or she participated in any risky activities since then?
- Is he or she prepared to use a condom? Are there any other safer sex measures he or she wants to take?

Be prepared to answer these questions yourself as well. In many cases, you will find that your partner is concerned about these issues too. If your partner is unwilling to discuss safer sex or does not want to participate in the same level of safer sex that you do, reconsider sex with that person.

HIV and AIDS

Accounting for more than 1.7 million deaths worldwide every year, the human immunodeficiency virus (HIV) is the most serious of all sexually transmitted pathogens.[23] Worldwide, there are more than 34 million people with the infection, with infection rates in sub-Saharan Africa, India, southeast Asia, and Russia especially high (**Figure 11.4**). In 2011, 71% of new HIV infections in adults and children were in sub-Saharan Africa.[23] Although intensive public health efforts in this region have helped reduce new HIV infections in this region by 25% between 2001 and 2011, it remains the part of the world hardest hit by this devastating disease.[23] First identified in the United States in 1981, today more than 1.4 million people in North America live with HIV infection and the condition it causes, acquired immunodeficiency syndrome or AIDS (also called advanced HIV disease). African Americans are disproportionately infected, as are sex workers, intravenous drug users, and men who have sex with other men. Each year, 1,200,000 people in sub-Saharan Africa die from AIDS-related illnesses. In North America, that number is about 21,000 people yearly.[23]

HIV infection severely damages the body's immune system. In particular, the virus infects and destroys helper T cells (CD4 T cells), important players in the body's specific immune response. HIV enters CD4 T cells and multiplies within them, generating millions of new HIV viruses and destroying the CD4 T cells in the process. The new viruses go on to infect more CD4 T cells and begin the replication process all over again. The immune system mounts a vigorous response, with B cells multiplying and secreting antibodies, and CD4 T cells multiplying and secreting cytokines. After years or decades, however, CD4 T cell levels begin to decline, the immune system is progressively weakened, and the body loses its ability to fight off illness.

The first few weeks after contracting HIV are called the primary infection stage. During that period, some—but not all—people experience initial symptoms that resemble those of a cold or flu. Fatigue, fever, headache, sore throat, swollen lymph glands, and muscle aches are reported, as are diarrhea, yeast infections, rashes, and mouth sores. The

opportunistic diseases Infections and other disorders that take advantage of a weakened immune system.

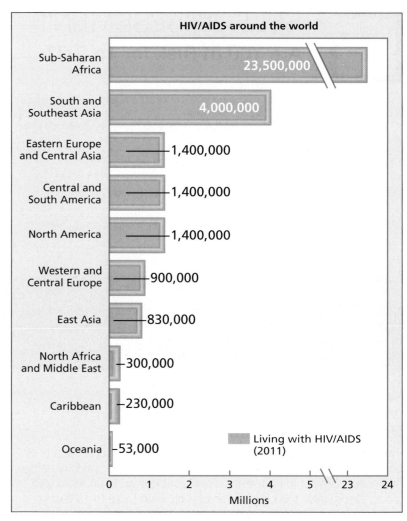

FIGURE 11.4 HIV/AIDS Around the World.

Source: Data from *Global Report: UNAIDS Report on the Global AIDS Epidemic,* by the Joint United Nations Programme on HIV/AIDS (UNAIDS) and World Health Organization (WHO), 2012.

primary infection is followed by an asymptomatic stage and new symptoms may not occur for another 8 to 10 years. However, during this period the virus is still reproducing rapidly and the immune system is fighting it. Eventually, with the loss of CD4 T cells, the person will become more vulnerable to **opportunistic diseases**—infections and other disorders that take advantage of a weakened immune system—like pneumonia, tuberculosis, eye infections, yeast infections, and cancer, including Kaposi's sarcoma. An HIV-positive person is diagnosed with AIDS when at least one opportunistic disease has developed or when that person's CD4 T cell count drops below 200 cells per microliter of blood (a healthy CD4 count is between 450 and 1,200 cells per microliter). Once AIDS develops, additional complications can arise, including severe weight loss, dementia, brain tumors, and a protozoan infection called toxoplasmosis.

Transmission of HIV

Once infected with HIV, people can transmit it to others regardless of the stage of the disease or whether or not they have experienced symptoms. HIV can be found in blood, seminal fluid, vaginal secretions, and breast milk. It can be transmitted during unprotected vaginal, oral, or anal sex or when sharing needles for intravenous drug use, tattoos, or piercing (**Figure 11.5**). You cannot catch the virus through sneezing, handshakes, insect bites, sharing food, or any other type of casual contact. Among

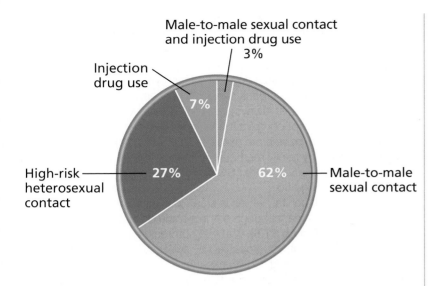

Male-to-male sexual contact and injection drug use **3%**

Injection drug use **7%**

High-risk heterosexual contact **27%**

Male-to-male sexual contact **62%**

FIGURE 11.5 Transmission Categories for New HIV/AIDS Cases in Adolescents and Adults in the United States.

Source: Data from *Diagnoses of HIV Infection in the United States and Dependent Areas, 2011 HIV Surveillance Report, Volume 23,* by the U.S. Department of Health and Human Services, Centers for Disease Control and Prevention, 2013.

the sexual transmission paths for HIV, unprotected anal sex is one of the most high-risk behaviors for spreading the virus. (See the "Sexual Conduct and Risk" section on page 271 for more about the relative risks of various sexual activities.) If you already have another STI, such as herpes or syphilis, your risk of becoming infected with HIV increases significantly. In the past, HIV was occasionally transmitted to recipients of blood transfusions; however, due to reforms, all donated blood in the United States is now screened for the virus and is considered safe.

Infected mothers are at risk of giving the virus to their infants, which is called *mother-to-child-transmission* (MTCT). This can occur during pregnancy, childbirth, and breast-feeding. The World Health Organization estimates that worldwide 430,000 children are newly infected each year, 90% through MTCT.[24] Untreated, approximately 50% of these infected children will die before age 2. The risk of MTCT of HIV ranges from 20% to 45%; however, with targeted prevention interventions, this risk can be reduced to less than 5%.[25]

HIV Testing and Treatment

The CDC estimates that about one-fourth of the people in the United States infected with HIV do not realize it. Because early HIV infections can have no or few symptoms, HIV screening is very important. Early diagnosis of HIV and prompt treatment is critical to slowing the virus's progression to AIDS. Knowing you have the virus can also help you take measures to avoid giving it to others.

The HIV test looks for the presence of antibodies to the virus rather than the virus itself—the presence of antibodies to HIV indicates that HIV is present in the body. The most common test is the EIA, or enzyme immunoassay, which is used to examine blood, saliva, or urine for antibodies to HIV. If an EIA test is positive, it is followed by an additional test such as the Western blot before a positive diagnosis of HIV infection is made. HIV antibody tests only work after a person's immune system has begun to develop antibodies to HIV. Because this can take up to six months in some people, testing too quickly after potential exposure to the virus is considered ineffective.

The CDC recommends that all people between the ages of 13 and 64 be tested for HIV at least once. People at high-risk for HIV

(intravenous-drug users, people engaging in unprotected sex or with multiple sex partners) should be tested annually, and pregnant women should be tested as part of their routine prenatal testing. Despite these recommendations, only 25.7% of college students report having ever been tested for HIV.[3]

HIV and AIDS are not curable, but they are treatable. Treatments called antiretroviral therapies can dramatically slow the deterioration of a person's immune system and are responsible for a dramatic decrease in AIDS deaths in recent years. There are three main types of antiretroviral drugs: reverse transcriptase inhibitors, protease inhibitors, and fusion inhibitors. The medications are frequently prescribed in combinations of three or four in a regimen often referred to as a *highly active antiretroviral therapy*, or HAART. For many living with HIV, HAART has changed the condition from a life sentence to a chronic manageable disease. The average life expectancy of a person newly diagnosed with HIV is approaching that of most uninfected people. Recent projection models suggest that a 39-year-old entering HIV care can expect to live until 63.[26] Unfortunately, HIV drugs are very expensive, have toxic side effects, and may not work for everyone.

Preventing HIV Infection

To avoid getting HIV and AIDS, you need to keep the blood, seminal fluid, vaginal fluids, or breast milk of an infected person from entering your vagina, penis, anus, mouth, or breaches in your skin. The surest way to protect yourself from HIV or any other STI is to avoid any sexual behavior that could transmit the disease. See **Practical Strategies: Reducing Your Risk of STIs** on page 274 for information on how to avoid STIs.

Intravenous drug users are at very high risk of contracting HIV if they share needles or syringes with other users. Efforts to sterilize equipment, including washing with bleach, are not always successful at killing HIV. Having intercourse while high on drugs is also risky because you are less likely to think clearly and practice safer sex.

 These podcasts discuss HIV testing and prevention: www.cdc.gov/hiv/library/podcasts/index.html.

Hepatitis B

Hepatitis B—which is more than 50 times as infectious as the virus that causes HIV—is most commonly spread through unprotected sex.[27] It can also be caught through sharing needles, razors, or syringes with an infected person. Symptoms generally occur two to three months after infection and involve abdominal and joint pain, nausea, dark urine, weakness and fatigue, and jaundice. Although the virus can cause immediate symptoms that go away on their own, for some people it can also remain in the body forever, resulting in long-term health problems ranging from liver damage to liver cancer and death. If you know you have been exposed to hepatitis B, contact your doctor right away. An injection of hepatitis B immune globulin (antibodies specific for hepatitis B; a passive immunization) within 24 hours of exposure may reduce your risk of developing hepatitis B. Because health-care providers began to routinely immunize children against hepatitis B in 1991, infection rates have dropped by an estimated 80%.[27] However, for as many as 1.4 million people in the United States currently living with a chronic hepatitis B infection, the vaccine became available too late.[27]

Genital Herpes

Genital herpes affects 16.2% of adults in the United States.[28] More than 80% of infected people do not realize they have the condition because they don't have symptoms or their symptoms are mild or mistaken for something else, such as jock itch, a yeast infection, or even insect bites. There are two types of herpes simplex virus: herpes simplex

Practical Strategies

Reducing Your Risk of STIs

A few simple steps can dramatically reduce your risk of contracting an STI.

- **Consider abstinence.** Abstinence from sexual intercourse is the most effective method for avoiding STIs.

- **Be faithful.** If you have sex, do it with one uninfected partner who is not having sex with others.

- **Be picky.** Limit the number of sex partners you have in your lifetime.

- **Use a condom or latex barrier.** Use latex or polyurethane condoms correctly and consistently for all vaginal or anal sexual encounters. Condoms, dental dams, or latex squares should be used for oral sex.

- **Talk with your partner.** Discuss STIs and prevention before you ever have sex. If you or your partner does not feel comfortable having that conversation, consider it a sign that you may not want to have sex with that person.

- **Get tested.** If you are sexually active, the only way to know for sure whether you have an infection is to be tested by a health practitioner. Many STIs have no noticeable symptoms and can go undetected for years, when treatment may be too late. It is a good idea for both partners to be tested before beginning a new sexual relationship.

- **Get annual checkups.** Annual checkups are a good time to discuss your sexual practices with your doctor.

- **Get vaccinated.** Ask your doctor about vaccines for HPV and hepatitis B. Men who have sex with other men should be vaccinated for hepatitis A as well.

- **Be alert to symptoms.** Should you develop any signs of an STI, get checked out by a physician right away. Prompt treatment can make all the difference between an effective treatment and long-term problems.

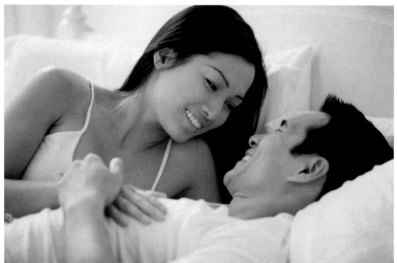

virus type 2 (HSV-2) and herpes simplex virus type 1 (HSV-1). Genital herpes is usually caused by HSV-2, whereas HSV-1 is the virus most often responsible for cold sores around the mouth. Herpes is extremely contagious. Genital herpes most often results from direct skin-to-skin contact, usually through vaginal, oral, or anal sex. Oral sex can pass both types of herpes virus back and forth between the mouth and the genitals. HSV-2 is almost always transmitted through sexual contact so most people do not contract it until they have become sexually active, whereas many people are exposed to HSV-1 in childhood, through nonsexual kisses by family members or friends. HSV-1 is very common; 50–80% of people in the United States have it, and as many as 90% of people have it by age 50.[29]

The hallmark of genital herpes is small, painful blisters or sores in the genital or anal area, although some people do not experience any symptoms at all **(Figure 11.6)**. The first outbreak usually occurs within 2 weeks of infection, is accompanied by flulike symptoms, and takes about three weeks to heal. Outbreaks can recur but tend to become less severe and less frequent over time. Stress, illness, poor diet, inadequate rest, and friction in the genital area can trigger outbreaks. The virus usually stays in the body forever, lying dormant in nerve cells, until the next recurrence. Herpes is most infectious when blisters or sores are present on an infected person. However, the herpes virus can be shed and passed on to others even when a person shows no symptoms. If you have ever had an outbreak of genital herpes, you should consider yourself contagious even if you have not had an outbreak for years. It is important to tell any potential partners that you have genital herpes and for both partners to remember that transmission, whether genital to genital or oral to genital, is possible even when the infection is in remission. Genital herpes can leave the body vulnerable to other STIs. The risk to a herpes patient of becoming infected with HIV if exposed to it is two to three times that of people who do not have herpes.[29] It can also make people with an HIV infection more infectious. Genital herpes can be fatal to a newborn baby if passed along during childbirth.

To diagnose herpes, a doctor takes a swab from a blister within the first 48 hours after it appears. If there is a sufficient amount of virus in the blister it is possible to distinguish it as either HSV-1 or HSV-2. Tests are also available that look for antibodies to the herpes virus in the blood.

Treatments for genital herpes are targeted toward alleviating symptoms. Antiviral medications such as acyclovir can reduce pain, hasten the healing of sores, and reduce the number of recurrences. Sex should be avoided when one partner has visible herpes sores, but the partner can still be contagious even when the sores have healed. Condoms or dental dams should always be used if a partner has genital herpes. They can reduce the risk of passing on the virus but are not foolproof because contagious sores can appear on areas not covered by the barrier. When taken daily to suppress herpes outbreaks and viral shedding, antiviral medications can also reduce the risk of transmitting herpes to a sexual partner, although condoms or dental dams should still be used.

Human Papillomavirus

Human papillomavirus (HPV) causes all types of warts, wherever they may be on your body. There are over 100 types of HPV. More than 40 types can infect the genitalia, although only 4 are responsible for most genital HPV infections. HPV is the most reported STI on college campuses. Most sexually active Americans will become infected with HPV at some point in their lives.[30] An estimated 79 million people in the United States are currently infected with HPV, and an additional 14 million develop the infection every year.[31] The infection is spread through skin-to-skin contact, usually during vaginal, oral, or anal sex.

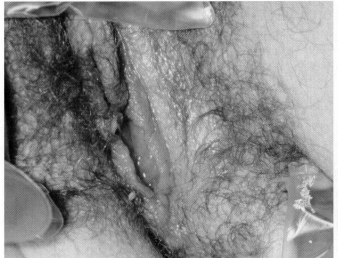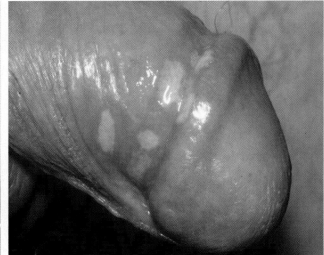

FIGURE 11.6 Genital Herpes Sores.

> ❝ *Most sexually active Americans will become infected with HPV at some point in their lives.*"

Most people do not realize they are infected with HPV. With the exception of the few HPV types that cause genital warts, HPV does not have any symptoms. For those who do experience warts, they can arise weeks or even months after infection. Warts can be raised or flat, pink or flesh-toned, and there may be only a single wart or multiple ones **(Figure 11.7)**. These warts can be treated with topical medications that are applied directly to the skin. They can also be frozen off through cryotherapy, burned off through electrocauterization, or removed by laser surgery. Warts can return even after treatment because these treatments do not cure HPV infection; they just help symptoms.

In about 90% of cases, the body's immune system overcomes an HPV infection naturally. However, some infections linger and cause cells to become abnormal or even cancerous. The types of HPV that cause cancer of the cervix, vagina, throat, penis, and anus are called "high-risk" strains of HPV. These strains do not cause warts and must be tested for. Cervical cancer is the biggest concern. Highly treatable when detected early, it can be fatal when left undetected. That is why the Pap test, which is used to screen for abnormal and potentially cancerous cervical cells, now typically includes a test for HPV. More than 11,000 women are diagnosed with cervical cancer every year.[32]

In 2006, the Food and Drug Administration (FDA) approved the first vaccine for HPV, Gardasil, for females aged 9 to 26. A second brand, Cervarix, has recently been added to the market as well. The vaccines protect against the two most common types of HPV associated with high-risk cervical cancer (types 16 and 18) and the two most common types of HPV associated with genital warts (types 6 and 11).

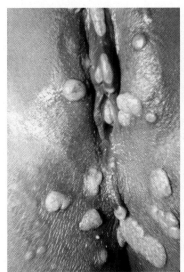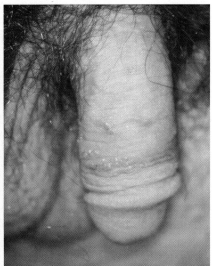

FIGURE 11.7 Genital Warts.

The vaccine is highly effective in women who were previously uninfected with those types of HPV. In October 2009, the FDA also approved the use of Gardasil for the prevention of genital warts caused by HPV types 6 and 11 in males aged 9 to 26.[33]

Chlamydia

Chlamydia, which is caused by the bacterium *Chlamydia trachomatis*, is extremely common in the United States. Young women are especially at risk, with an estimated 1 in 10 adolescent girls testing positive for the infection.[34] The infection can be spread during vaginal, anal, or oral intercourse, and it can be passed from mother to newborn baby during childbirth. Chlamydia can infect the vagina, penis, anus, cervix, urethra, and even the eyes or throat. Chlamydia is called the "silent disease" because the majority of those infected with it do not notice any unusual signs. Men, however, are more likely to show symptoms, often a burning sensation while urinating, as well as a discharge from their penis. Women who develop symptoms often notice an abnormal vaginal discharge and pain during urination. Symptoms usually develop within one to three weeks of infection.

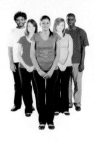

DIVERSITY & HEALTH

Rates of STIs for Different Sexes, Ages, Races, and Sexual Orientations

STIs may affect people of various sexes, ages, races, and sexual orientations differently. Certain groups are at higher risk for particular STIs or STIs in general.

Sex

- Women are biologically more susceptible to becoming infected with STIs than men are. Young women, especially, are at high risk because the cells lining the cervix are more immature and vulnerable to infection.

- Women are less likely than men to experience symptoms of STIs, which can postpone detection and treatment.

- Women are more likely than men to experience long-term, severe side effects of STIs, such as infertility and cervical cancer.

- Women account for 77% of all reported chlamydia cases.[1]

- Men accounted for 74% of new HIV/AIDS cases in 2007; women accounted for 26%.[2]

- Men account for 75% of all reported cases of syphilis.[1]

Age

- People aged 15–24 make up 74% of all reported chlamydia cases.[1]

- People aged 15–24 make up 61% of all reported cases of gonorrhea.[1]

- People aged 20–29 made up 25% of new HIV/AIDS cases in 2007.[2]

Race

- African Americans continue to experience an epidemic of HIV/AIDS, comprising 44% of all new infections of HIV in the United States in 2010.[2]

- African Americans—especially young African American women—are at disproportionately high risk for other STIs as well.

- Hispanics are disproportionately affected by HIV/AIDS, gonorrhea, chlamydia, and syphilis.[1] Although Hispanics made up 16% of the U.S. population in 2009, they comprised 20% of new HIV/AIDS cases in the United States.[3]

- Native Americans/Alaska Natives are at a disproportionately high risk for gonorrhea and chlamydia.[1]

- Asian and Pacific Islander groups are disproportionately affected by hepatitis B in the United States, accounting for more than 50% of Americans living with chronic hepatitis B in the United States.[4]

Sexual Orientation

- Young men who have sex with men, especially those of minority races or ethnicities, are at high risk for HIV infection, syphilis, and other STIs.

- The risk of female-to-female HIV transmission is low but possible, especially if one or both partners have sores on their genitals, if partners share sex toys, or if they participate in rough sex. Women can pass other STIs to one another as well.

Critical-Thinking Questions

1. Does young women's higher risk for contracting STIs make them especially motivated to follow safer sex practices and ask their partners to do the same? Why or why not?

2. Why do you think the rates of some STI infections are especially high among teens and younger adults?

3. What changes or new attitudes might encourage wider adoption of safer sex practices among young people?

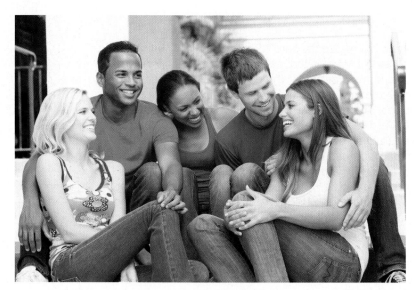

Young people are one of the groups at elevated risk for STIs.

References: **1.** Data from *Sexually Transmitted Disease Morbidity for Selected STDs by Age, Race/Ethnicity, and Gender 1996–2009*, by the Centers for Disease Control and Prevention, National Center for HIV, STD, and TB Prevention (NCHSTP), Division of STD/HIV Prevention 2011, CDC WONDER On-line Database, retrieved from http://wonder.cdc.gov/std-std-race-age.html. **2.** "HIV Among African Americans," in *HIV/AIDS*, by the Centers for Disease Control and Prevention, 2013, retrieved from http://www.cdc.gov/hiv/risk/racialethnic/aa/facts/index.html. **3.** "HIV Among Latinos," in *HIV/AIDS*, by the Centers for Disease Control and Prevention, 2013, retrieved from http://www.cdc.gov/hiv/risk/racialethnic/hispaniclatinos/facts/index.html. **4.** "Asian Americans and Hepatitis B," in *CDC Features*, 2013, retrieved from http://www.cdc.gov/features/AAPIHepatitisB.

If left untreated, chlamydia can have serious health consequences and lead to infertility. In 10–15% of the women whose chlamydia is not treated promptly, pelvic inflammatory disease occurs.[35] This condition damages the fallopian tubes and uterus, resulting in pelvic pain, infertility, and **ectopic pregnancies** that can be deadly to mother and fetus. Chlamydia can also leave men infertile, inflaming the prostate gland and epididymis and scarring the urethra.

The U.S. Preventive Services Task Force recommends that all sexually active women aged 24 or younger undergo regular screening for chlamydia.[36] As a result, many pediatricians offer routine testing to their adolescent patients. Women who are 25 and older and at increased risk because of unsafe sex practices or intercourse with multiple partners are also encouraged to get screened regularly. A simple urine test or swab taken from the penis or cervix can detect a chlamydia infection. Chlamydia can be cured with antibiotics. All sexual partners should be treated at the same time to avoid reinfection.

Gonorrhea

Gonorrhea, sometimes referred to as "the clap," is a common and highly contagious sexually transmitted infection. It is caused by the bacteria *Neisseria gonorrhoeae* and most often afflicts teenaged girls and men aged 20 to 24.[37] The bacteria are spread through intimate contact with an infected penis, vagina, anus, or mouth and can be passed on to a newborn baby during childbirth. Most women infected with gonorrhea experience no symptoms at all. Those who do may mistake the painful urination or increased vaginal discharge for a bladder or yeast infection. Men are more likely to have noticeable signs of the condition, including sore testicles, colored penile discharge, or a burning sensation while urinating. Symptoms usually occur within the first week after infection.

Without proper treatment, the bacteria can spread to the blood or joints, which can be life threatening. Pelvic inflammatory disease can also occur, causing pain and infertility. Women are at risk of having an ectopic pregnancy. Men can be left sterile. People with gonorrhea are also at greater risk of getting HIV.

Several laboratory tests can be used to diagnose gonorrhea, including a urine test or swab samples taken of the cervix, urethra, rectum, or throat. If you have the condition, your sexual partners should also be tested and treated. Antibiotics can often cure gonorrhea, but drug-resistant strains have been on the rise, making treatment more complicated. Because many people who have gonorrhea are infected with chlamydia at the same time, treatment often includes antibiotics for both. Avoid sexual contact until treatment is finished.

Pelvic Inflammatory Disease

Pelvic inflammatory disease, or PID, is an infection of a woman's uterus, fallopian tubes, and other reproductive organs that occurs when bacteria travel up from the vagina and spread. It affects an estimated 750,000 women in the United States every year, causing infertility in about 10%.[38] PID is caused by bacteria, most often from the bacteria associated with two of the most common sexually transmitted infections, chlamydia and gonorrhea.

With PID, bacteria infect the fallopian tubes, turning normal tissue into scar tissue. This can cause chronic abdominal pain. It also may block eggs from moving into the uterus, causing ectopic pregnancies or leaving a woman infertile.

Women may have no idea that they have PID, even as their reproductive system is being damaged. When symptoms do occur, they may be subtle or vague, including fever, irregular menstrual bleeding, painful intercourse, or lower abdominal pain. The condition often goes unrecognized by patients and physicians alike.

No single test detects the presence of PID. Doctors typically perform a pelvic examination and test for chlamydia and gonorrhea. However, an abdominal ultrasound and even laparoscopy (minimally invasive surgery) may be needed to confirm the diagnosis. Antibiotics can cure the infection but cannot undo any of the damage already done to a woman's reproductive organs. For that reason, prompt treatment is always critical. A woman's sex partners also should be treated—even if they have no symptoms—to keep from spreading the bacteria that cause PID back and forth. In some cases, a woman may need surgery to reduce the scarring. However, she may still remain infertile.

Avoiding STIs—or getting immediate medical care should one occur—will help protect women from developing PID. Because chlamydia and gonorrhea often have no noticeable symptoms, young sexually active women should undergo regular pelvic examinations and annual chlamydia testing. Sexually active women under the age of 25 have a higher risk of PID. In addition, women increase their risk of PID by douching, having recently had an IUD for birth control inserted, and having multiple sex partners.

Syphilis

Although syphilis is less widespread than other STIs, almost 14,000 cases of syphilis were reported in the United States in 2009.[39] Syphilis is especially prevalent in parts of the South and in urban areas, with men who have sex with men disproportionately affected. The infection can be transmitted from mother to child during pregnancy or childbirth. Syphilis is caused by the bacterium *Treponema pallidum*, which enters the body through irritated skin or mucous membranes, including the vagina, anus, penis, lips, and mouth.

If left untreated, syphilis can progress through three different stages. In the first stage, 10 days to three months after infection, primary syphilis appears. A painless sore called a *chancre* appears where the bacteria entered the body, around the genitals, inside the vagina or rectum, or on the lips or mouth **(Figure 11.8)**. The chancre will go away without treatment, but the infection itself

ectopic pregnancy A pregnancy where the embryo implants outside of the uterus, often in the fallopian tubes.

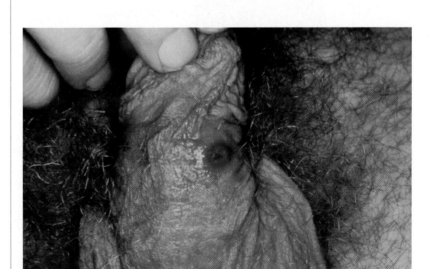

FIGURE 11.8 A Syphilis Chancre.

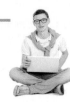

STUDENT STATS
STIs in People Aged 15–24

Of the total new syphilis, gonorrhea, and chlamydia cases between 1996 and 2009, these graphs show what percentages were in 15- to 19-year-olds and 20- to 24-year-olds.

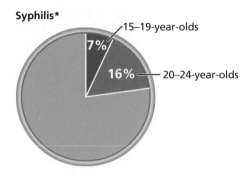

Syphilis*

- 7% — 15–19-year-olds
- 16% — 20–24-year-olds

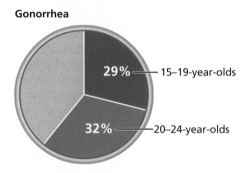

Gonorrhea

- 29% — 15–19-year-olds
- 32% — 20–24-year-olds

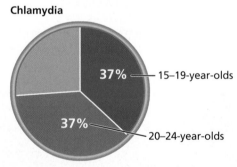

Chlamydia

- 37% — 15–19-year-olds
- 37% — 20–24-year-olds

*Primary and secondary syphilis.

Source: Data from *Sexually Transmitted Disease Morbidity for Selected STDs by Age, Race/Ethnicity, and Gender 1996–2009*, by the Centers for Disease Control and Prevention, National Center for HIV, STD, and TB Prevention (NCHSTP), Division of STD/HIV Prevention, 2011, CDC WONDER On-line Database.

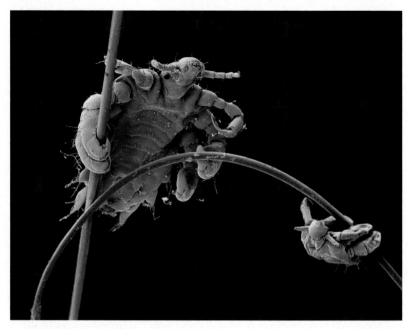

FIGURE 11.9 Pubic Lice.

to the nervous system occurs. Tertiary syphilis can also cause severe problems with the heart, brain, and eyes, causing blindness, paralysis, brain damage, dementia, and even death. Syphilis also increases the chances of contracting HIV.

Examination of a fluid sample taken from a chancre or swollen lymph nodes can confirm infection during primary or secondary syphilis. Two types of blood tests are also available to detect the bacteria during any of its stages. Antibiotics are the first line of defense against syphilis. If treatment is not initiated until the final stage, the bacteria can be killed but the internal damage that has already occurred cannot be reversed.

Pubic Lice and Scabies

Pubic lice, or *Pthirus pubis*, are tiny six-legged creatures that infest pubic hair **(Figure 11.9)**. Commonly known as "crabs," they can also attach themselves to eyebrows, eyelashes, beards, mustaches, or chest hair. Scabies is caused by tiny, eight-legged mites that burrow into the top layer of a person's skin and lay eggs. Scabies generally occurs in and around folds of skin but can affect other parts of the body as well. Pubic lice and scabies are usually transmitted through sexual contact but occasionally are spread through contact with clothing, towels, sheets, or toilet seats that have been used by an infected person.

The most common symptom of pubic lice and scabies is itching, especially during the night. In some instances, the infested area also becomes inflamed, and scabies can sometimes cause allergic reactions. The pests themselves do not spread disease, but excessive scratching of the skin can cause a bacterial infection.

A pubic lice or scabies infestation can be easily diagnosed with a doctor's visit. Prescribed creams or lotions can usually clear up these conditions, although an oral medication may be used for cases that are harder to treat.

Trichomoniasis

Trichomoniasis, or "trich," is caused by a protozoan called *Trichomonas vaginalis*. It is the most common curable STI in young women, although a recent study shows that the incidence is even higher in women over the age of 40.[40] Men can be infected as well. More than 7.4 million infections occur annually in the United States.[41]

will not. During the next stage, secondary syphilis, symptoms may include a rash on the hands or feet, neck, head, or torso, wart-like growths around the genitals, and grayish sores in the mouth. Hair loss may occur. The infection will then enter a latent stage, which lacks symptoms, and can last for years. If syphilis isn't treated, about 15% of people will develop the late or tertiary stage, where small tumor-like growths called *gummas* appear on internal organs and damage

The most common route of transmission is vaginal-penile inter-course. However, an infected woman can transmit *T. vaginalis* to a female sex partner during vulva-to-vulva contact. Fortunately, women often experience symptoms, typically within 5 to 28 days, so they seek medical treatment. Symptoms include painful urination, pain during intercourse, vaginal itching and irritation, and a greenish-yellow, strong-smelling vaginal discharge. Men often do not experience symptoms, but if they do they include irritation inside the penis and slight discharge. Infected women are at increased risk for HIV infection and are more likely to pass HIV to a partner. Studies also suggest that infected men and women are at increased risk for infertility.

Trich in women is diagnosed with laboratory analysis of a vaginal swab. In women, a pelvic exam will reveal small red sores on the vaginal wall or cervix. Infection can be cured with oral antimicrobial drugs, usually metronidazole. Both partners must be treated and must avoid sex until treatment is finished and all symptoms have cleared.

Change Yourself, Change Your World

Pathogens are all around us. This may leave you feeling that it's you against the world. But that's not true. When it comes to breaking the chain of infection, we work best when we work together.

Personal Choices

Help protect yourself from infections by keeping your immune system strong. Don't smoke. If you do, you're setting out the welcome mat to pathogenic microbes. Stay up to date on your vaccinations. Limit your alcohol. Eat right, don't short-change your sleep (short sleep reduces the number of functioning T cells), and exercise regularly.

When it comes to STIs, take these additional precautions:

- **Get vaccinated.** The CDC recommends that men who have sex with men receive the hepatitis A vaccine. All people need immunization against hepatitis B (HBV). The CDC also recommends vaccination against HPV for both males and females aged 9 to 26.

- **Use condoms.** One of the most important ways to protect yourself from STIs is to use latex condoms correctly and consistently—with every sex act. Always use a new condom. Never use an unapproved lubricant such as massage oil or petroleum jelly.

- **Get tested.** If you're sexually active, discuss STI testing with your health-care provider at each routine visit. If you don't have a regular health-care provider, visit your campus health center, which may offer free or low-cost testing. If you're concerned about high-risk exposure to HIV, see your physician immediately! A course of treatment with HAART can significantly reduce your risk for developing an active infection.

  If you find out that you've tested positive for any STI, tell your current partner and anyone you've had sex with during the past year. Encourage them to seek testing, too. If you're uncomfortable revealing your test results, talk with your health-care provider. Most states require that certain STIs be reported to public health authorities, who can then notify partners, anonymously and confidentially, about exposure to STDs. Some public health departments now use email notification.[42]

>> **To find a local clinic where you can be tested for STIs, just type in your zip code at** http://hivtest.cdc.gov/STDTesting.aspx.

Unprotected Sex

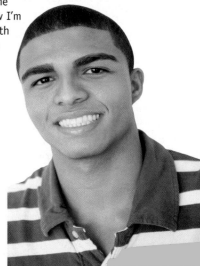

"HI, I'M GABE. Last weekend I did something really stupid. I went to a party with my friends and was flirting with this girl. We both got pretty drunk and ended up going back to my room and having sex. I was so drunk I didn't use a condom. She said it was OK, she's on the pill, but now I'm freaking out about STIs. She's friends with one of my friends, and he says he thinks she doesn't have anything, but I'm still worried. Do you think it makes it any better that it was only once?"

1. What STIs is Gabe now at risk for?

2. What could Gabe have done differently to reduce his risk for STIs?

3. Do you think Gabe can rely on his friend for information about whether his partner is healthy or not?

4. Do you think Gabe is at less risk because he only had unprotected sex once?

- **Get treated.** Bacterial STIs are usually curable with antibiotics. Trichomoniasis can also be cured with drug therapy. Taking the entire course of prescribed medication is essential, as is partner treatment. You must both avoid sex until the treatment is finished and you no longer have any symptoms.

  In general, viral STIs are not curable, but antiviral medication can suppress herpes outbreaks, and HAART can keep HIV infection in check for many years. Both herpes and HIV can be transmitted while the person is taking medication, so condom use is still essential.

Campus Advocacy

Because infections are spread among networks of people, the actions you take to reduce your own risk will benefit others in your campus community.

But there's more you can do:

- Stay home if you're feverish, have conjunctivitis, or can't control your coughing, sneezing, or runny nose. If you think you might have an STI, don't have sex until you've been checked by your health-care provider.

- Encourage your friends to check their immunization status and to get the annual flu vaccine.

- Work with your student health center to organize an STI awareness event. Need some inspiration? Check out Get Yourself Tested (GYT), a collaborative effort from MTV, the Kaiser Foundation, the CDC, and other national partners. Visit **www.itsyoursexlife.com/toolkit**.

>> **Watch videos of real students discussing STIs and other infections at** MasteringHealth™

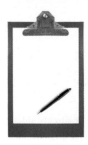

Choosing to Change Worksheet

To complete this worksheet online, visit MasteringHealth™

Your likelihood of contracting an STI depends primarily on your behaviors. To reduce your risk of contracting an STI, follow the steps below.

Directions: Fill in your stage of change in Step 1 and complete Steps 2, 3, or 4, depending on which one applies to your stage of change.

Step 1: *Your Stage of Behavior Change.* Please check one of the following statements that best describes your readiness to reduce your STI risk.

_____I do not intend to reduce my STI risk in the next six months. (Precontemplation)

_____I might reduce my STI risk in the next six months. (Contemplation)

_____I am prepared to reduce my STI risk in the next month. (Preparation)

_____I have been reducing my STI risk for less than six months. (Action)

_____I have been reducing my STI risk for more than six months. (Maintenance)

Step 2: *Precontemplation and Contemplation Stages.* Increasing your knowledge of the risk factors for contracting an STI can help motivate you to change. If you answer "Yes" or "Don't Know" to any of the 10 items below you may be at a higher risk for STIs.

1. I have had oral, vaginal, or anal sex without using a latex condom.	Yes	No	
2. I have had sex with multiple partners and not discussed STIs before having sex.	Yes	No	
3. I have had sex after consuming alcohol.	Yes	No	
4. I have had sex while under the influence of illegal drugs.	Yes	No	
5. I have exchanged sex for drugs or money.	Yes	No	
6. I have come into direct contact with someone who has infections such as HPV, herpes, pubic lice, or scabies.	Yes	No	Don't Know
7. I have injected substances with dirty needles or syringes—or have had unprotected sex with someone who has.	Yes	No	Don't Know
8. I have shared needles for tattoos or body piercings—or have had unprotected sex with someone who has.	Yes	No	Don't Know
9. I have not been vaccinated against hepatitis A, hepatitis B, or human papillomavirus.	Yes	No	
10. I have had sex while infected with an STI.	Yes	No	Don't Know

What might be some barriers holding you back from taking action on reducing your STI risk factor(s) and how could you overcome them?

Barrier	Strategy for Overcoming Barrier
Example: My partner doesn't want to wear a condom.	*I will explain to him why it is important to wear one and how I feel about his lack of wanting to use one.*
_____	_____
_____	_____
_____	_____
_____	_____
_____	_____
_____	_____
_____	_____

Step 3: *Preparation and Action Stages.* For each of the risk reduction guidelines listed below, indicate one action you can take (or have already taken) to meet that guideline in your own life. Be specific.

Reducing Your Personal STI Risk

STI Risk Reduction Guideline	Specific Action to Meet Guideline
Become more educated about the risks, symptoms, treatment, and prevention of STIs.	*Example: Talk to my nurse practitioner about safer sex practices and/or any STI symptoms I should watch out for.*
For STIs with an available vaccine (HPV and hepatitis B), get vaccinated.	
Be alert for signs or symptoms of STIs.	
Get tested.	
Communicate with sexual partners about your sexual histories, including histories of STIs.	
Don't impair your judgment before participating in sexual activity by using drugs or alcohol.	
Always use a latex condom from start to finish.	
Practice safe oral sex by using condoms, dental dams, or latex squares.	
Limit your number of sexual partners.	

Write down your **SMART goal** for reducing your STI risk, including a timeline, below.

_____

_____

Step 4: *Maintenance Stage.* Your goal is to stay focused and maintain your commitment to preventing STIs. What benefits of practicing STI prevention are most important to you and why?

_____

_____

How easy has it been to practice STI prevention? Is it truly a habit or do you need to expend some effort to do it? How can you keep yourself on track?

_____

_____

Chapter Summary

- Pathogens are the agents that cause infections. Pathogens include viruses, bacteria, fungi, protozoa, and parasitic worms.
- Infectious diseases can be spread by personal contact with an infected person, touching inanimate objects that are contaminated with pathogens, inhaling airborne pathogens, or contact with infected animals, insects, water, or food.

- Your body's first line of defense against infection is your skin, mucous membranes, cilia, and bodily fluids, which prevent pathogens from entering the body or trap and expel them if they do.
- Your immune system, a powerful network of cellular and chemical defenses, fights pathogens that enter the body. Neutrophils, natural killer cells, and macrophages are key nonspecific defenders. B cells and T cells work

with precision and focus to produce antibodies and kill specific pathogens. Memory B cells and T cells sometimes provide long-term immunity to an infection, which makes getting the same infection again unlikely.

- Sometimes the immune system mistakes common substances, such as nuts, pet dander, or pollen, as harmful agents, triggering allergies. Allergies are sometimes relatively mild but can also cause asthma or other dangerous reactions.

- HIV/AIDS is the most serious of the sexually transmitted infections. It targets and destroys the immune system and, left untreated, leads to death. Early detection is important because proper treatment can significantly prolong life.

- Other common sexually transmitted infections are hepatitis B, genital herpes, human papillomavirus (HPV), chlamydia, gonorrhea, syphilis, pubic lice, scabies, and trichomoniasis.

- It is up to you to help protect yourself from STIs and other infections by keeping up to date on your immunizations, properly washing your hands, and engaging in safer sexual practices.

- Prevention is the best medicine for sexually transmitted infections. Many may not show symptoms until irreparable damage has been done. Among other things, certain sexually transmitted infections can cause infertility or death. If you are sexually active, discuss STI testing with your health-care provider at every annual checkup.

GET CONNECTED

>> Visit the following websites for further information about the topics in this chapter:

- Mayo Clinic
  www.mayoclinic.com
- Medline Plus
  www.nlm.nih.gov/medlineplus
- The Centers for Disease Control and Prevention
  www.cdc.gov
- American Social Health Association
  www.ashastd.org
- Planned Parenthood
  www.plannedparenthood.org/health-topics/stds-hiv-safer-sex-101.htm
- Center for Young Women's Health, College Health: Sexual Health
  www.youngwomenshealth.org/collegehealth10.html
- The Body: The Complete HIV/AIDS Resource
  www.thebody.com

MOBILE TIPS!

Scan this QR code with your mobile device to access additional tips about infectious diseases and STIs. Or, via your mobile device, go to **http://chmobile.pearsoncmg.com** and navigate to Chapter 11.

- Smartersex.org
  www.smartersex.org
- Go Ask Alice
  www.goaskalice.columbia.edu

Website links are subject to change. To access updated web links, please visit MasteringHealth™

TEST YOUR KNOWLEDGE

1. Pathogens
   a. cannot be stopped by your body's first line of defense.
   b. are agents that cause disease.
   c. infect animals but not humans.
   d. die once they enter your body.

2. A person who spreads infectious disease to others is called a
   a. reservoir.
   b. carrier.
   c. contaminator.
   d. pathogen.

3. Your first line of defense against infection is
   a. your immune system.
   b. antibiotics.
   c. immunization.
   d. your skin.

4. Acquired immunity
   a. develops when your body creates memory B cells and memory T cells.
   b. develops when your body creates regulatory T cells.
   c. only lasts a few months, at most.
   d. develops only when your body contracts a disease and survives it.

5. Lyme disease is spread by
   a. fleas.
   b. ticks.
   c. mosquitoes.
   d. mice.

6. Antibiotics are appropriate treatments against
   a. bacteria.
   b. viruses.
   c. fungi.
   d. none of these pathogens.

7. The most commonly reported sexually transmitted infection among college students is
   a. genital warts/HPV.
   b. genital herpes.
   c. chlamydia.
   d. HIV/AIDS.

8. What percentage of new STI infections in the United States each year occur in people between the ages of 15 and 24?
   a. 15%
   b. 25%
   c. 30%
   d. 50%

9. Which of the following practices will NOT reduce risk of contracting HIV?
   a. correct use of condoms
   b. abstinence
   c. avoiding multiple partners and getting tested with new partners
   d. avoiding partners who look sick

10. Cervical cancer is caused by
    a. pelvic inflammatory disease.
    b. vaccines.
    c. human papillomavirus (HPV).
    d. gonorrhea.

Get Critical

What happened

In January 2011, while on a trip to Sudan to support a peaceful voting process on the question of independence for South Sudan, actor and activist George Clooney contracted malaria. After an acute 10-day illness, he spoke out to advocate for malaria prevention and treatment. While expressing gratitude that his own recovery from the illness had been quick, Clooney pointed out that the average Sudanese lacks access to effective medications. "I had drugs to take before, during, and after . . . Life-saving drugs for diseases that kill millions needlessly belong to mankind, not to companies to profit from."[1]

What do you think?

- Do you agree with Clooney that pharmaceutical companies should donate the medications they make to impoverished populations when lives are at stake? Why or why not?

- Malaria is a preventable disease, and prevention efforts, including the use of insecticide-treated bed nets, have helped reduce malaria rates as much as 90% in some regions. Yet the organization Malaria No More reports that malaria still kills one child every minute worldwide. What actions could college students in the United States take to provide bed nets for poor families in malaria-ridden areas? Go to **www.malarianomore.org** and find out.

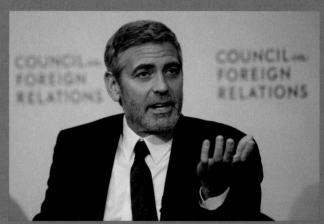

Actor George Clooney.

Reference: **1.** "George Clooney Answers Your Questions About Malaria," by N. Kristof, February 8, 2011, *The New York Times.*

DIABETES, CARDIOVASCULAR DISEASE, AND CANCER

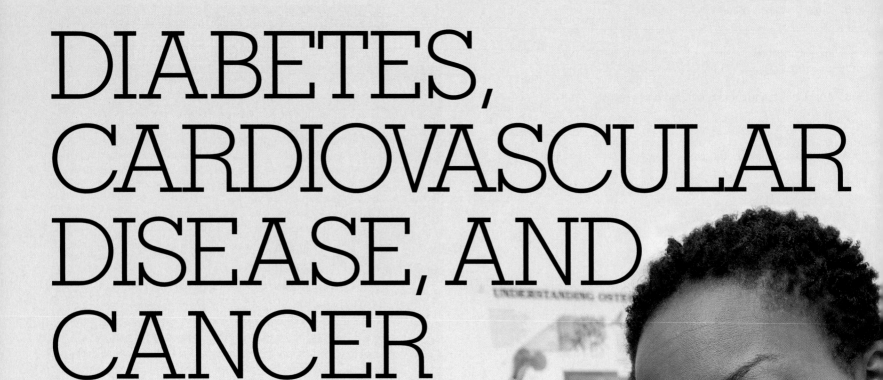

More than 25 million Americans have **diabetes**.[i]

Cardiovascular disease is the number 1 **cause of death** in both **men and women** in the United States.[ii]

The **five-year survival rate** for Americans with cancer has now **increased to 68%**.[iii]

12

Learning Objectives

DISCUSS the burden of chronic disease in terms of personal health and costs to society.

DISTINGUISH between type 1 and type 2 diabetes.

IDENTIFY several consequences of uncontrolled diabetes.

COMPARE and contrast the four major types of cardiovascular disease.

LIST the nine factors associated with cardiometabolic risk.

DESCRIBE the initiation and progression of cancer.

DISCUSS the most common cancers, including their major risk factors.

IDENTIFY the personal choices you can make to reduce your risk for chronic disease.

EXPLAIN how best to support a friend with a chronic disease.

College is all about preparing for your future.

Where will your major take you? Will you go to graduate school? What will your career be like? How will the friendships and relationships you make on campus shape your life in your post-college years?

To that list of questions, we'd like to add one more: Will the behaviors you practice today help maintain your health or lead you to chronic disease?

It's an important question because, when it comes to your risk of developing a chronic disease—like diabetes, cardiovascular disease, or cancer—the odds are against you. If 100 students were enrolled in your health course, and you all were to follow current U.S. health trends, here is where national statistics suggest you would wind up:

- About 14 people in your class would develop diabetes before reaching age 65.[1]
- About 30 class members would eventually die of diseases of the heart or blood vessels, such as a heart attack or stroke.[2,3]
- Roughly 40 class members would develop cancer, and 24 would die of it.[4]

These numbers are sobering. But they do not necessarily predict your fate. Just as you can use your time in college to shape your career, you can also use these years to start beating the odds of developing a chronic disease.

Overview of Chronic Diseases

A **chronic disease** is one that comes on gradually and lasts for a long time, causing either continual symptoms or recurring bouts of illness. The first two chronic diseases discussed in this chapter—diabetes and cardiovascular disease—usually resist complete cure. Instead, they're usually managed by a combination of lifestyle changes and medications focused on reducing the patient's *cardiometabolic risk*; that is, factors such as obesity, elevated blood pressure, and others that are associated with these two chronic diseases. We'll define cardiometabolic risk more precisely later in this chapter. Cancer, the third disease we'll focus on, can often be cured. The five-year survival rate for all cancers is now 68%.[4]

Scope of the Problem

Chronic diseases cause 7 out of every 10 deaths in the United States each year.[5] The chronic diseases discussed in this chapter—diabetes, cardiovascular disease, and cancer—are responsible for more than 54% of all deaths in the United States every year.[6]

Many of the deaths due to chronic disease occur prematurely; that is, at an earlier than expected age. But chronic diseases not only deprive us of years of life, they reduce our *health-related quality of life* because of the discomfort, pain, psychological distress, and activity limitations that accompany them. If you've ever seen someone with advanced diabetes walking with crutches because of an amputated foot, or heard someone struggling to speak because of the effects of a stroke, then you've witnessed some of the effects of reduced health-related quality of life.

Finally, the financial burden of chronic disease is tremendous: about 75% of the $2.2 trillion in health-care expenditures in the United States are for treatment of chronic disease.[7] Moreover, the economy of the United States loses hundreds of billions of dollars annually because of lost productivity due to chronic disease.[7]

> **chronic disease** A disease that comes on gradually and lasts a long time; many chronic diseases can be managed but resist a complete cure.

>> The Centers for Disease Control and Prevention have a comprehensive website covering chronic diseases, including strategies for prevention, statistics, fact sheets, and more: www.cdc.gov/chronicdisease/index.htm.

Influence of Four Key Behaviors

Diabetes, cardiovascular disease, and cancer might seem unrelated, but in fact they share some underlying physiological mechanisms and risk factors. That's because the functions of the chemicals, cells, and tissues of our bodies are interrelated, and certain factors that initiate disease in one body organ or system can initiate disease in another. For example, smoking can harm nearly every organ in your body.[8] It causes inflammation, reduced circulation, damage to blood vessels, genetic changes, and other problems that in turn are factors in diabetes, cardiovascular disease, and cancer—as well as chronic respiratory diseases.[8]

In fact, smoking is one of the four high-risk behaviors most strongly associated with the onset of chronic disease. These four behaviors, which we have discussed throughout this text, are:

- Poor nutrition. This includes a diet high in saturated and *trans* fats and low in fruits and vegetables as well as consumption of excessive calories. Obesity increases the risk for the most common form of diabetes as well as cardiovascular disease and certain cancers.[9]
- Lack of physical activity.
- Tobacco use, which is the single most avoidable cause of disease, disability, and death in the United States.
- Excessive alcohol consumption.[5]

In addition to lifestyle choices, socioeconomic and racial disparities are thought to play a role in the incidence of chronic disease. For more information on these disparities, see the **Diversity & Health** box.

Diabetes

Do you know someone with diabetes? Do you have it yourself? Your answer is far more likely to be "Yes" than was your parents' reply at your age.

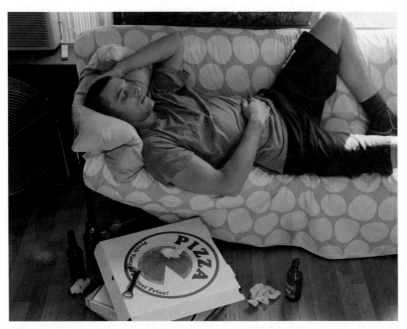

Risk factors for chronic disease include lack of physical activity and being overweight.

> " Once a condition seen mostly in adults over age 64, diabetes is now one of the most common serious illnesses in the United States, and the number of cases continues to grow rapidly."

Once a condition seen mostly in adults over age 64, diabetes is now one of the most common serious illnesses in the United States, and the number of cases continues to grow rapidly. More than 11% of Americans aged 20 or older has diabetes, and another 35% is on its way to developing it.[1] Between 1980 and 2011, the number of diagnosed cases more than tripled.[10]

Types of Diabetes

Diabetes, known formally as **diabetes mellitus,** is a broad term that covers a group of diseases characterized by high levels of sugar, or *glucose,* in the blood. In fact, the word *mellitus* is derived from the Latin word for honey. These high levels of blood glucose arise from problems with **insulin,** a hormone produced by the **pancreas** that is necessary for transportation of glucose into the body's cells.

Normally, when our blood glucose levels rise after we eat a meal or snack containing carbohydrate, the pancreas releases insulin into the bloodstream (**Figure 12.1**, first panel). Circulating insulin binds to the outer membrane of brain cells, muscle cells, and other body cells. There, it triggers proteins inside the cells to move to the membrane and take up glucose. Some people with diabetes simply don't make enough insulin to clear enough glucose from the bloodstream. Others make enough insulin, but their body cells don't respond to it effectively. In either case, glucose builds up in the bloodstream, while the body's cells—unable to take in glucose—suffer from lack of nourishment.

Type 1 Diabetes

Type 1 diabetes arises when the body's own immune system destroys the cells in the pancreas that make insulin (Figure 12.1, middle panel). Type 1 diabetes usually appears in childhood or adolescence, and researchers are investigating the role of specific genes in its development as well as the possible role of external factors such as viruses. People with type 1 diabetes must monitor their blood glucose level throughout each day and take supplemental insulin.

diabetes mellitus A group of diseases in which the body does not make or use insulin properly, resulting in elevated blood glucose.

insulin A hormone necessary for glucose transport into cells.

pancreas An abdominal organ that produces insulin as well as certain compounds helpful in digestion.

type 1 diabetes A form of diabetes that usually begins early in life and arises when the pancreas produces insufficient insulin.

Healthy person

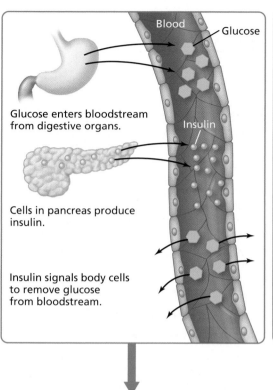

Glucose enters bloodstream from digestive organs.

Cells in pancreas produce insulin.

Insulin signals body cells to remove glucose from bloodstream.

- Blood glucose level is regulated.
- Body cells take in and utilize energy from glucose.

Person with diabetes

Type 1 diabetes

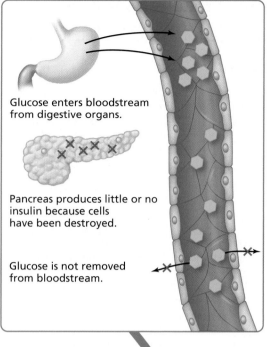

Glucose enters bloodstream from digestive organs.

Pancreas produces little or no insulin because cells have been destroyed.

Glucose is not removed from bloodstream.

Type 2 diabetes

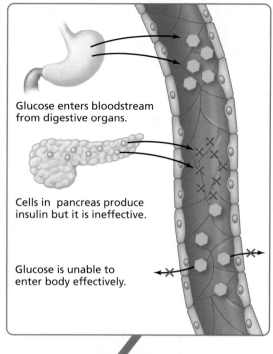

Glucose enters bloodstream from digestive organs.

Cells in pancreas produce insulin but it is ineffective.

Glucose is unable to enter body effectively.

- Glucose accumulates in blood and causes high blood sugar levels.
- Body cells lack energy.
- Nerves and blood vessels are damaged.

FIGURE 12.1 Two Types of Diabetes. In type 1 diabetes, the beta cells of the pancreas stop producing insulin entirely, or produce an amount insufficient for normal body functioning. In type 2 diabetes, the body is unable to use insulin properly. In advanced cases, the pancreas becomes exhausted and, as with type 1 diabetes, stops producing insulin. In either case, the body's cells are unable to take in glucose from the bloodstream.

For this reason, type 1 diabetes is often known as *insulin-dependent diabetes*.

Type 1 diabetes accounts for the majority of diabetes in children and up to 10% of diabetes cases in adults.[1] There is no cure for type 1 diabetes, but the condition is the focus of intense research, including studies into the use of stem cell therapy to replace the pancreas's insulin-making beta cells.

Type 2 Diabetes

Type 2 diabetes accounts for about 90–95% of all adult diabetes cases.[11] Once known as *adult-onset diabetes,* type 2 diabetes used to be extremely rare among children and teens. Now, about 3,600 Americans younger than age 20 are diagnosed with type 2 diabetes annually.[11] The incidence is also rising among young and middle-aged adults.

Whereas in type 1 diabetes the cells of the pancreas stop making insulin, most cases of type 2 diabetes begin as *insulin resistance.* The pancreas makes normal amounts of insulin, but the body's cells don't respond to it properly—they resist its effects (Figure 12.1, third panel). One factor in this resistance is interference due to an overabundance of fatty acids concentrated in fat cells. This explains why type 2 diabetes is linked not only to age but also to obesity. If the body's cells can't respond to insulin, they can't take up glucose, and it remains in the bloodstream. The resulting **hyperglycemia** (persistent high blood glucose) signals the pancreas to produce more insulin to get more glucose into the cells. As the demand for insulin continues to rise, the cells of the pancreas begin to fatigue. With continued high demand over time, they can lose their ability to produce insulin, just as in type 1 diabetes.

Other Forms of Diabetes

Less common varieties of diabetes resemble type 2 but also have differences that set them apart:

- *Gestational diabetes* develops in a woman during pregnancy and affects up to 2–10% of pregnant women. The condition usually disappears after childbirth, but researchers have learned that women who develop gestational diabetes have a

type 2 diabetes A form of diabetes that usually begins later in life and arises when cells resist the effects of insulin.

hyperglycemia A persistent state of elevated levels of blood glucose.

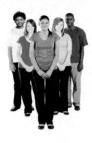

DIVERSITY & HEALTH

Socioeconomic, Racial, and Ethnic Disparities in Chronic Disease

Even as broad public health efforts focus on reducing the risks of chronic diseases, significant disparities remain. Consider the following:

- Poverty is an obstacle to receiving quality health care. Poor Americans are more likely to lack health insurance, to lack access to health screenings and other preventive measures, and to engage in behaviors that increase chronic disease risk, such as smoking, physical inactivity, and poor diet. According to the U.S. Census Bureau, in 2010, 9.9%

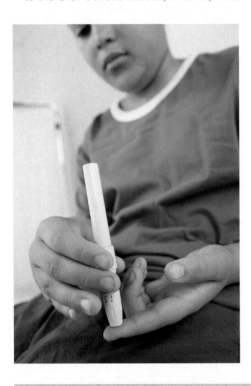

of Caucasian Americans lived in poverty. In contrast, 12.1% of Asian Americans, 26.6% of Hispanic Americans, and 27.4% of African Americans lived in poverty.[1]

- Among American adults, Caucasian Americans have the lowest rate of diabetes: 7.1%. The rate within certain Hispanic subgroups, including Cuban Americans and Central and South Americans, is only slightly higher, 7.6%, but it climbs to more than 13% among Mexican Americans and Puerto Ricans. The rate for Asian Americans is 8.4%. African Americans also have a high rate of diabetes— 12.6% for non-Hispanic blacks—and are more likely to die of diabetes than members of other groups. Native Americans have the highest rate in the world: More than 16% of Native American adults have diagnosed diabetes.[2]

- African Americans have the highest rate of deaths due to cardiovascular disease (both heart disease and stroke) of all racial and ethnic groups. Caucasian Americans have the second highest death rates from CVD. Hispanic Americans, Native Americans, and Asian Americans have lower rates of death due to CVD; in fact, among both Hispanics and Asian Americans, cancer has overtaken heart disease as the leading cause of death.[3]

- African Americans have the highest rates of cancer overall and are the most likely to die of cancer. Caucasian Americans have the second highest incidence and death rate, followed by Hispanic Americans and Asian Americans. Cancer statistics among Native Americans are thought to be unreliable.[4]

Regardless of racial or ethnic group, Americans living in poverty have much higher cancer death rates than more affluent Americans.[4]

If your socioeconomic bracket, race, or ethnicity puts you at higher risk for chronic disease, talk to your health-care provider. Maintaining a healthy weight, exercising, eating a nutritious diet, not smoking, and limiting your alcohol intake can go a long way toward reducing your risk.

Critical-Thinking Questions

1. Asian Americans have the lowest rates of obesity, binge drinking, and tobacco use of any ethnic group. How might these factors contribute to their risks for chronic disease as identified here?

2. In this chapter, we noted that chronic stress is a risk factor for both diabetes and CVD. How might stress be related to some of the statistics discussed above?

3. Type 2 diabetes, CVD, and cancer are all complex, multifactorial diseases. How might social determinants, policy-making, and access to health services influence differences in disease and death rates among these racial and ethnic groups? (See Chapter 1.)

References: **1.** *Income, Poverty and Health Insurance Coverage in the United States: 2010*, by the U.S. Census Bureau, September 13, 2011. http://www.census.gov/newsroom/releases/archives/income_wealth/cb11-157.html. **2.** *National Diabetes Fact Sheet, 2011*, by the Centers for Disease Control and Prevention, 2011. http://www.cdc.gov/diabetes/pubs/pdf/ndfs_2011.pdf. **3.** "CDC Health Disparities and Inequalities Report—United States, 2011," by the Centers for Disease Control and Prevention, January 14, 2011, *Morbidity and Mortality Weekly Report, 60*(Suppl.). http://www.cdc.gov/mmwr/pdf/other/su6001.pdf. **4.** "Cancer Disparities," from *Cancer Facts & Figures 2013* by the American Cancer Society, 2013, p. 40. http://www.cancer.org/acs/groups/content/@epidemiologysurveillance/documents/document/acspc-036845.pdf.

35–60% chance of developing type 2 diabetes within the next 10–20 years.[11]

- *Type 1.5* is a general term for several varieties of diabetes that blend aspects of type 1 and type 2. For instance, a physician may suspect type 1.5 in a newly diagnosed adult diabetic who is not overweight. Also called *latent autoimmune diabetes of adults* (LADA), type 1.5 is often revealed when blood tests show some

immune-system destruction of pancreatic beta cells—but healthy, insulin-producing beta cells as well. Researchers estimate that perhaps 10% of all diagnoses of type 2 diabetes are actually due to type 1.5, and the number of cases may be growing.[12]

>> **Watch a video showing how diabetes affects blood sugar at** www.mayoclinic.com/health/blood-sugar/MM00641.

Detecting Diabetes

The physical signs and symptoms of diabetes include:

- Frequent urination
- Excessive thirst
- Hunger
- Tendency to tire easily
- Numbness or tingling in the hands and feet
- In women, a tendency to develop vaginal yeast infections

These symptoms, although common across all types of diabetes, can develop differently from person to person. Also, early stages of diabetes may not be accompanied by any symptoms at all.

Two simple laboratory tests can reveal whether or not you have—or are developing—diabetes. One of the most common is the *fasting blood glucose test* (FBG), which requires you to fast (consuming nothing other than plain water) overnight. A technician then draws a blood sample, and the level of glucose in your blood is measured. Here is what the measurement values mean:

- A blood glucose level below 100 mg/dL is normal.
- A blood glucose level between 100 and 125 mg/dL means that you have **prediabetes.** That is, your FBG is higher than normal but not high enough to warrant a diagnosis of diabetes. Prediabetes indicates that your body is struggling to regulate your blood glucose, and you are at significant risk for developing diabetes.
- A blood glucose level of 126 mg/dL or higher indicates true diabetes.

A second test, known as the *glycated hemoglobin test*, or *A1C test*, measures how much glucose is attached to the hemoglobin—the oxygen-carrying compound—in your red blood cells. An A1C level of 6.5% or higher on two separate occasions indicates that you have diabetes, whereas 5.7% to 6.4% indicates prediabetes.[13]

If type 1 diabetes is suspected, the physician will order a further test to see whether or not there is evidence of an immune-system response against the beta cells of the pancreas. The urine may also be tested to look for waste chemicals suggesting that the body cells—given their inability to use glucose for energy—are breaking down fats or proteins for energy.

Long-Term Effects of Diabetes

Persistent hyperglycemia causes damage throughout the body, especially to blood vessels **(Figure 12.2)**. This damage in turn can lead to a variety of complications:[1]

- Damage to the blood vessels that supply the heart and brain at least doubles the risk of heart attack and stroke. And following a heart attack, patients with diabetes are twice as likely to die than patients without diabetes.[14]
- The kidneys have microscopic blood vessels that filter excessive glucose from the blood into urine. Hyperglycemia stresses this delicate filtration system, leading to kidney disease, a common and serious complication of diabetes. Kidney failure is a common cause of death among people with diabetes.
- Hyperglycemia also damages blood vessels that serve nerves, causing pain, loss of sensation, tissue breakdown, and poor wound healing, especially in the feet, ankles, and lower legs. This

prediabetes A persistent state of blood glucose levels higher than normal, but not yet high enough to qualify as diabetes.

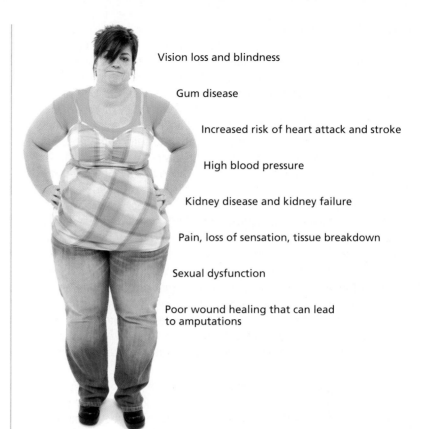

Vision loss and blindness

Gum disease

Increased risk of heart attack and stroke

High blood pressure

Kidney disease and kidney failure

Pain, loss of sensation, tissue breakdown

Sexual dysfunction

Poor wound healing that can lead to amputations

FIGURE 12.2 Long-term Complications Associated with Diabetes.

explains why more than 60% of toe, foot, and lower leg surgical amputations occur among people with diabetes.

- When hyperglycemia damages the tiny blood vessels serving the retina of the eye, vision deteriorates. In fact, diabetes is the leading cause of new cases of blindness among U.S. adults.
- Severe gum disease is also more common among people with diabetes.

Diabetes also increases the risk of death from infection, several cancers, and a variety of other disorders. Overall, diabetes is now the seventh most common cause of death in the United States, and a recent review study found that it shaves at least six years off a person's life.[6,15]

Risk Factors for Type 2 Diabetes

After age 50, body cells become increasingly less responsive to the effects of insulin. This explains in part the gradual increase in blood glucose levels that occurs as we age. But other risk factors are much more important than aging. These include the following:

- **Overweight.** About 85% of people with type 2 diabetes are overweight or obese, and two-thirds of obese people eventually develop diabetes.[16]
- **Disproportionately large waist.** People who carry more of their excess weight around their abdominal area are at greater risk for diabetes. Greater amounts of abdominal fat have been linked to insulin resistance.

- **Diet.** We've said that overweight increases your risk, but a few types of foods also play a role—independently of the number of calories. For instance, foods high in fiber slow the release of glucose into the bloodstream, so a high-fiber diet is thought to reduce your risk for diabetes. Foods high in saturated fats are also likely to be high in cholesterol, which further increases the vulnerability of your blood vessels to disease. These foods are also higher in calories so they contribute to being overweight. Beyond that, eating a nutritious diet with plenty of whole grains, vegetables, and lean protein foods is recommended. What about sweets? Eating a diet high in simple sugars does not directly cause type 2 diabetes because genetics, body weight, and many other factors play a role. However, epidemiological studies have revealed a relationship between the amount of sugar consumed within a population and that population's rate of diabetes.[17] Again, choosing fiber-rich carbohydrates over simple sugars is a healthful choice.

- **Lack of exercise.** When you have free time, do you opt for an activity like swimming or a bike ride? Exercise helps control weight, burns glucose, and makes your body cells more receptive to insulin. Physical activity also builds up muscle mass, and muscle cells absorb most of the glucose in your blood. In contrast, a sedentary lifestyle increases your risk for type 2 diabetes.

- **Chronic stress.** A recent study examined the influence of stress on diabetes risk in older adults. The researchers found that the participants who had the highest long-term levels of the stress hormone cortisol, as measured in scalp hair, also had the highest risk for diabetes. The influence of stress on diabetes risk was similar to that of traditional risk factors such as abdominal obesity.[18]

- **Genetic factors.** Do members of your family have type 2 diabetes? If so, you are at higher risk. Several common genetic variants that increase a person's risk of type 2 diabetes are found both within families and within ethnic groups. In addition, African Americans, Mexican Americans, Puerto Ricans, and Native Americans develop diabetes at higher rates than Caucasians, Asian Americans, and Hispanics from Cuba or Central or South America.[1]

You can also determine your risk for diabetes by taking the nearby **Self-Assessment**.

Clinical Management of Diabetes

If you are diagnosed with diabetes or prediabetes, your doctor will work with you toward one central goal—stabilizing your body's use of glucose. The approach prescribed will depend on the type and severity of diabetes you have.

Glucose Monitoring

To stay healthy, people with diabetes must maintain a continual awareness of their blood glucose levels. That means measuring and recording blood glucose levels as often as three times a day. In the past, blood glucose monitoring required pricking the finger. Now, devices are available that can read glucose levels through the skin or from a small needle implanted in the body.

Weight Loss

For people with prediabetes or type 2 diabetes who are overweight, weight loss is important. The good news is that losing just 5% to 7% of your body weight can significantly improve your cells' ability to respond to insulin.[16] In obese patients with diabetes, especially those with a body mass index (BMI) of 35 or higher who are at high risk for severe complications, bariatric (weight-loss) surgery may be an option.

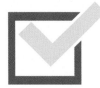

SELF-ASSESSMENT
Are You at Risk for Type 2 Diabetes?

Fill in the points that correspond to your answer on each line.

1. Are you age 45 or older? _____
   Yes (1 point)   No (0 points)

2. What is your weight status? (See the BMI chart in Figure 6.1 on p. 129.)
   _____
   BMI is less than 25 (0 points)
   BMI is 25–29.9 (1 point)
   BMI is 30–39.9 (2 points)
   BMI is 40 or above (3 points)

3. Do you have a parent, brother, or sister with diabetes? _____
   Yes (1 point)   No (0 points)

4. Is your family background African American, Alaska Native, American Indian, Asian American, Hispanic/Latino, or Pacific Islander American? _____
   Yes (1 point)   No (0 points)

5. Have you had gestational diabetes? _____
   Yes (1 point)   No (0 points)

6. Have you given birth to at least one baby weighing more than 9 pounds? _____
   Yes (1 point)   No (0 points)

7. Is your blood pressure 140/90 or higher, or have you been told that you have high blood pressure? _____
   Yes (1 point)   No (0 points)   Don't know (1 point)

8. Are your cholesterol levels higher than normal? Is your HDL, or good, cholesterol, below 35, or is your triglyceride level above 250? _____
   Yes (1 point)   No (0 points)   Don't know (1 point)

9. Are you fairly inactive? _____
   Yes (1 point)   No (0 points)

10. Do you have a history of cardiovascular disease? _____
    Yes (1 point)   No (0 points)

Add up your score: _____

HOW TO INTERPRET YOUR SCORE

The higher your score, the higher your risk for type 2 diabetes. If you scored 3 or higher, it is recommended that you take immediate action to reduce your risk for type 2 diabetes. If you answered "Don't know" to any questions, visit your health-care provider to get checked.

To complete this Self-Assessment online, visit MasteringHealth™

Based on *Am I at Risk for Type 2 Diabetes?* by the National Diabetes Information Clearinghouse, from NDIC website, June 2012; and *Diabetes Risk Test*, by the American Diabetes Association, from ADA website, accessed June 25, 2013.

Bariatric surgery reduces the size of the stomach and may also bypass the first section of the small intestine, so weight loss can be dramatic. However, patients will gradually begin to gain weight again if they do not follow a healthful diet and engage in regular exercise.

Exercise

During exercise, glucose is transported into body cells, especially muscle cells, for use as energy. Moreover, building muscle improves blood glucose control.[16] Exercise increases the sensitivity of body cells to insulin, so less insulin is needed to clear glucose from the bloodstream. For these reasons, a personalized program of aerobic exercise is typically prescribed.

Oral Medications

If someone with type 2 diabetes is not successful in losing weight, or weight loss doesn't reduce blood glucose significantly enough, the physician may prescribe an oral medication. Diabetes medications work in a variety of ways. Some, for instance, prompt the pancreas to manufacture and release more insulin, whereas others help increase the cells' response to insulin. If A1C tests continue to show, however, that medication isn't reducing blood glucose levels effectively, then the physician is likely to recommend a type 1 approach to treatment involving insulin therapy.

Insulin Therapy

All people with type 1 diabetes, and many with type 2, need insulin daily to survive. Insulin can't be taken by mouth because it is a protein and would be digested in the gastrointestinal tract. Many diabetics inject their insulin using a fine needle and syringe, or an insulin pen—a device that looks like an ink pen, except the cartridge is filled with insulin. Others use an insulin pump worn on the outside of the body. A tube connects the reservoir of insulin to a catheter inserted under the skin of the abdomen. The person programs the pump to dispense specific amounts of insulin **(Figure 12.3)**. Most of the new devices are about the size and weight of an MP3 player, and some are even free of tubing, delivering insulin via skin absorption from a "pod" attached to the skin with a gentle adhesive.

As you've seen, controlling diabetes requires consistent attention to diet, exercise, body weight, blood glucose levels, and all prescription therapies. But the rewards, including a longer life and a reduced risk of serious complications, are worth it.

Cardiovascular Disease

When an elderly acquaintance or loved one dies of a heart attack or stroke, you may not see any direct connection to your own health. After all, the person was a lot older than you. But even though heart attacks

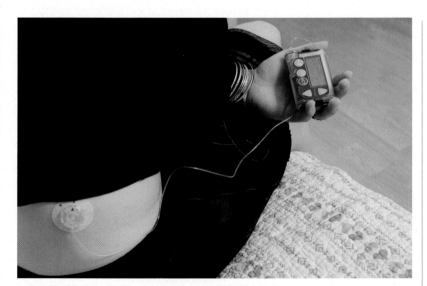

FIGURE 12.3 Controlling Diabetes. Insulin pumps allow many people to control their blood glucose levels throughout the day without painful injections.

A Family History of Diabetes

 "HI, I'M MICHAEL. Chronic disease runs in my family, particularly diabetes on both my mom's and dad's sides. Just recently, my mom, my sister, and my dad were all diagnosed with type 2. It has affected me because I have to watch them take all their pills and recover from injuries and sicknesses and see the pain that they're going through, particularly with the circulation in their legs.

I am doing things to stop the risk of getting diabetes. I'm eating better. I'm exercising. I'm studying diabetes and other chronic diseases just to make sure that I protect myself to the fullest. I'm also teaching my mom and my dad as well about it.

I would tell other students to eat right, eat your fruits and vegetables, and exercise a minimum of 30 minutes a day every day, to help you fight against chronic diseases such as diabetes."

1. Why is it that Michael's family members are having problems with pain and circulation in their legs? What are other short- and long-term effects of diabetes?

2. Michael is paying attention to his diet and staying physically active. What else could he do to lower his risk for developing diabetes?

and strokes do typically occur later in life, the conditions that trigger them begin to develop decades earlier.

Cardiovascular disease, or **CVD,** is a group of disorders that includes hypertension (high blood pressure), coronary heart disease (including heart attacks), congestive heart failure, and stroke. Diagnosed hypertension is present in 3.4% of college students, and heart disease in 3.2%.[19, 20] However, the prevalence of CVD among young adults in general is over 10%, and as we age, it skyrockets: More than a third of Americans in their 40s and 50s have CVD, and by age 80, the rate is almost 80%.[21] Not surprisingly, CVD is the leading cause of adult mortality in the United States, responsible for more than 3 in 10 deaths.[6]

Research shows that many college students don't realize their risks of joining this epidemic. Several surveys of undergraduates have found that most rate their risk of developing cancer as much higher than their risk of developing CVD. Female students in particular tend to overestimate their risk of breast cancer but underestimate their risk of CVD.[20]

A meaningful understanding of CVD requires that you become familiar with the structures and activities of your cardiovascular system.

cardiovascular disease (CVD)
Diseases of the heart or blood vessels.

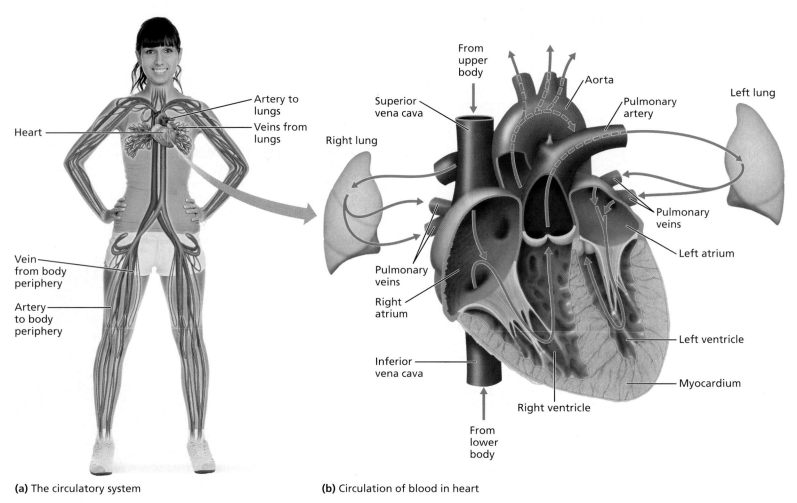

(a) The circulatory system

(b) Circulation of blood in heart

FIGURE 12.4 The Cardiovascular System.

The Healthy Cardiovascular System

The cardiovascular system is made up of blood vessels and the heart, which together form the blood-delivery network that keeps the body functioning. Blood, circulating through blood vessels, ferries oxygen, nutrients, and wastes to and from cells through **arteries,** which carry blood away from the heart, and **veins,** which carry blood back to the heart **(Figure 12.4a)**.

At the center of this system is the heart, which is only about the size of a fist, but is surprisingly strong. That's because it's almost entirely made up of a thick layer of muscle called the **myocardium.** The contractions of the myocardium keep blood moving, ensuring that it transports oxygen and nutrients to, and eliminates wastes from, every region of the body.

The interior of the heart consists of four hollow, muscular chambers **(Figure 12.4b)**. The two upper chambers are the **atria.** Each atrium is connected by a valve to one of the corresponding lower **ventricles.** A thick wall of tissue divides the right atrium and ventricle from the pair on the left, creating two side-by-side pumps. This division lets each side of the heart focus on

arteries Vessels that transport blood away from the heart, delivering oxygen-rich blood to the body periphery and oxygen-poor blood to the lungs.

veins Vessels that transport blood toward the heart, delivering oxygen-poor blood from the body periphery or oxygen-rich blood from the lungs.

myocardium The heart's muscle tissue.

atria The two upper chambers of the heart that receive blood from the body periphery and lungs.

ventricles The two lower chambers of the heart that pump blood to the body and lungs.

capillaries The smallest blood vessels, delivering blood and nutrients to individual cells and picking up wastes.

a different task—either sending oxygen-poor blood to the lungs for replenishment or pumping that reoxygenated blood back out to the rest of the body.

Here's how the blood circulates. The right atrium receives oxygen-depleted blood from the superior and inferior vena cava, the largest veins in the body, and then releases it into the right ventricle, which sends it into the pulmonary arteries, which take it to the lungs. There, blood cells collect freshly inhaled oxygen and unload carbon dioxide (a metabolic waste), which we exhale. Now the pulmonary veins bring the oxygen-rich blood to the left atrium and ventricle. They receive this blood and pump it out into the body via the aorta, a large artery that branches off into smaller arteries. These include the coronary arteries, which sustain the heart muscle itself.

The body's blood vessels divide into a network of smaller branches, eventually fanning out into **capillaries,** tiny blood vessels that deliver oxygen and nutrients to individual cells and collect their wastes. Once blood in the capillaries has exchanged oxygen and nutrients for wastes, it is returned to the heart via the veins. As with any system of pipes or tubes, the arteries, capillaries, and veins work best when they are free of blockage or damage, allowing blood to flow smoothly.

This complex process is remarkably quick. The average person has about five to six quarts of blood, all of which is pumped by the heart throughout the body in a single minute. In adults at rest, the heart typically beats 60–120 times per minute, pumping a few ounces of blood with each beat until all the blood has been circulated. To keep up this rapid rhythm, the heart relies on electricity. A bundle of specialized cells in the heart's sinus node, located in the right atrium, generate electrical impulses and transmit them throughout the myocardium at a steady, even rate, setting the heart to beat about 100,000 times a day.

If your cardiovascular system is healthy, circulation generally runs smoothly. But if damage occurs to even one part of the system, it will begin to struggle to perform its functions. Next, we'll look at the physiological mechanism that most commonly damages the cardiovascular system: atherosclerosis.

 Watch a video showing how the heart and blood vessels work at www.mayoclinic.com/health/circulatory-system/MM00636.

Atherosclerosis

Atherosclerosis is an arterial condition characterized by inflammation, scarring, and the buildup of mealy deposits along artery walls. In fact, the word's root, *athere,* is Greek for porridge! Together, these factors cause a narrowing of arteries, which restricts blood flow to cells and tissues "downstream" of the narrowed area. Cells starved of oxygen and nutrients cannot function; thus, when atherosclerosis affects the coronary arteries, the person can suffer a heart attack. When it affects arteries in the brain (cerebral arteries), the person can suffer a stroke.

Atherosclerosis begins when the delicate inner lining of an artery becomes damaged. Although the cause of this damage is not always known, in some cases it is thought to result when **blood pressure**— the force of blood pulsating against the artery walls—is excessive. In others, it reflects the lining's encounter with irritants, and as you now know, a high level of blood glucose is a major irritant of blood vessels. Excessive lipids in the bloodstream,

including triglycerides and cholesterol, can also irritate the vessel lining. In addition, the toxins in tobacco smoke and even certain types of infection can promote this initial damage.

The body responds to injury with inflammation, and at injured arterial sites, the resulting inflammation spreads into the artery wall. This leaves it weakened, scarred, and stiff (sclerotic). As a result, triglycerides and cholesterol circulating in the bloodstream can seep between the damaged lining cells and become trapped within the artery wall. Soon they are joined by white blood cells, calcium, and other substances. Eventually, this buildup, called *plaque,* narrows arteries significantly enough to impair blood flow **(Figure 12.5)**. When this occurs in a coronary artery, the person may experience chest pain (called *angina*), weakness, shortness of breath, and other symptoms.

Plaque may build up to the point where it significantly blocks or even stops the flow of blood through an artery. This causes death of the tissues that are normally served by that vessel. Sometimes plaque can become hardened and rupture, causing microscopic tears in the artery wall that allow blood to leak into the tissue on the other side. When this happens, blood platelets rush to the site to clot the blood. This clot can obstruct the artery. Alternatively, softer plaque can break off and travel through the bloodstream until it blocks a more distant, smaller artery. If either of these types of blockages occurs in a coronary or cerebral artery, the person will experience a heart attack or stroke.

As noted earlier, cholesterol, a lipid made by the body and found in the food you eat, is a major component of plaque. We all need cholesterol for our bodies to function, but excessive amounts can be a key contributor to atherosclerosis. In a national survey, over 3% of college students reported that they had been diagnosed with excessive blood cholesterol levels.[19] We'll look more closely at types of cholesterol, and what levels are considered healthful, later in this chapter.

Atherosclerosis is difficult to detect without specific medical tests, and most people who are developing the condition are unaware it is occurring. If your physician suspects that you're at risk, you'll likely be advised to improve the quality of your diet and increase your level of exercise. If your cholesterol levels are high and don't respond to lifestyle changes, cholesterol-lowering medications, most commonly *statins*, may help. Millions of people in the United States use statins to control cholesterol levels, but their use must be monitored for rare but serious side effects.

---

atherosclerosis Condition characterized by narrowing of the arteries because of inflammation, scarring, and the buildup of fatty deposits.

blood pressure The force of the blood moving against the arterial walls.

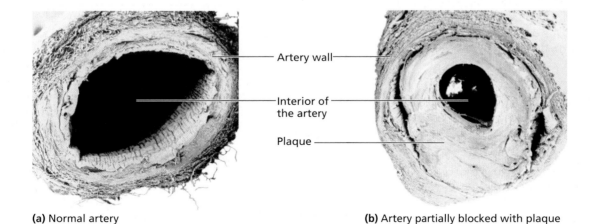

(a) Normal artery

(b) Artery partially blocked with plaque

FIGURE 12.5 Atherosclerosis. These light micrographs show a cross section of (a) a normal artery allowing adequate blood flow and (b) an artery that is partially blocked with plaque, which can lead to a heart attack or stroke.

Atherosclerosis is dangerous because it directly contributes to each of the forms of CVD discussed next: hypertension (high blood pressure), coronary heart disease, congestive heart failure, and stroke. As you read about these disorders, bear in mind that they rarely develop in isolation; rather, one condition typically contributes to or occurs simultaneously with another. In addition, as noted earlier, the damage to the body's blood vessels caused by diabetes also contributes to CVD.

Hypertension (High Blood Pressure)

Hypertension, more commonly known as *high blood pressure*, is a chronic condition characterized by consistent blood pressure readings above normal. (We'll define normal and hypertensive readings shortly.) Hypertension in and of itself is considered a form of CVD. In addition, it's also a risk factor for other forms of CVD, including coronary heart disease, congestive heart failure, and stroke.

Factors Influencing Blood Pressure

The level of your blood pressure is determined, in part, by the pumping actions of your heart. When your heart contracts, an action called *systole,* the pressure of the blood in your arteries momentarily increases. When it relaxes, an action called *diastole,* your blood pressure drops.

Blood pressure is also affected by the *compliance*—the ability to stretch and recoil—of your arteries. We noted earlier that atherosclerosis can lead to both narrowing and stiffening of the arteries. When it does, blood pressure rises. To appreciate why, imagine the difference between trying to pump a pulsing stream of water into a network of wide, soft tubes versus narrow, stiff pipes. The tubing would stretch and bounce back with each pulsation, absorbing some of the pressure and allowing the turbulence to quickly settle down and the water to flow. In contrast, the pipes would not accommodate the pulsating flow. This means the pump would have to work harder to propel the water against their resistance. When atherosclerosis has stiffened arteries and narrowed them with plaque, they impede blood flow and drive blood pressure up.

Blood pressure is also influenced by the volume of blood flowing through the vessels. Excessive glucose, sodium, or other solutes in the blood can increase its volume and stress the heart and blood vessels. In contrast, factors such as blood loss and dehydration can dangerously decrease the blood volume.

Signs and Symptoms of Hypertension

Most people with hypertension experience no symptoms. This fact, together with its contribution to heart attacks and strokes, explains the reputation of hypertension as a "silent killer." A very few people with dangerously advanced hypertension may experience headaches and dizziness.

Long-Term Effects of Hypertension

Left untreated, hypertension can lead to the other forms of CVD discussed in this section. It can also cause vision loss and kidney disease and can reduce your ability to think clearly, remember, and learn.[22]

Risk Factors for Hypertension

Almost 30% of the U.S. adult population, or about 73 million people, have hypertension.[21] Although atherosclerosis contributes to hypertension in many people, usually the causes aren't entirely clear. But your age, weight, ethnic background, and diet all play a role, with a high-sodium diet putting you at especially significant risk.

TABLE 12.1 Blood Pressure Classification

Classification	Systolic Reading (mm Hg)		Diastolic Reading (mm Hg)
Normal	< 120	and	< 80
Prehypertension	120–139	or	80–89
Hypertension			
Stage 1	140–159	or	90–99
Stage 2	≥ 160	or	≥ 100

Source: Data from *The Seventh Report of the Joint National Committee on Prevention, Detection, Evaluation, and Treatment of High Blood Pressure (NIH Publication No. 03-5233),* by the National Heart, Lung, and Blood Institute, 2005, Bethesda, MD: National Institutes of Health.

Clinical Management of Hypertension

Blood pressure is measured using a stethoscope and a device called a *sphygmomanometer.* Readings are recorded in millimeters of mercury (mm Hg). The systolic pressure—the pressure in your arteries as your heart contracts—is given first, and the diastolic pressure—the pressure when the heart is momentarily relaxed—is given second. So "125 over 70" means your systolic pressure is 125 and your diastolic is 70. Incidentally, this reading would qualify as prehypertension, even though, as you can see in **Table 12.1,** a diastolic reading of 70 is normal. In other words, if either number is elevated, the reading is considered abnormal.

Most physicians recommend that patients with hypertension follow a balanced, low-sodium diet. Sodium is an essential mineral, but if consumed in excess, it draws water out of cells and into the bloodstream. This increases the total volume of your blood and, therefore, the pressure that your blood exerts against the walls of your arteries. Sodium is bound to chloride in table salt but is also a prominent ingredient in most processed foods, from tomato soup to macaroni-and-cheese dinners. The 2010 *Dietary Guidelines for Americans* suggests that people with hypertension, as well as African Americans and all Americans over age 50, consume no more than 1,500 mg of sodium per day. To reduce your sodium intake, follow the DASH diet from the National Institutes of Health, which has been shown in numerous studies to reduce blood pressure.

>> **Download a colorful guide to the DASH eating plan at** www.nhlbi.nih.gov/health/public/heart/hbp/dash/new_dash.pdf.

In addition to a diet low in sodium, people with hypertension should follow a diet with an appropriate number of calories to help them achieve and maintain a healthy weight. Regular moderate exercise can also help reduce blood pressure and body weight. Smoking damages blood vessels, and anyone with hypertension who smokes should seek professional help to quit. Alcohol consumption should not exceed one drink per day for women and two drinks for men. Drinking in excess of this level raises blood pressure.[23]

Many patients with hypertension take prescription medications. Some of the most common are diuretics (commonly called "water pills"), which help the body to eliminate sodium and water, reducing blood volume. Other medications work by helping to relax and dilate blood vessels, and still others slow the heartbeat. Many doctors recommend a

hypertension (high blood pressure) A persistent state of elevated blood pressure.

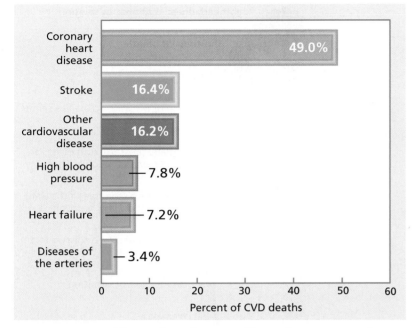

FIGURE 12.6 Deaths from Cardiovascular Disease in the United States. The majority of deaths resulted from coronary heart disease.

Source: Data from *Heart Disease and Stroke Statistics: 2013 Update,* by the American Heart Association, from *Circulation,* 2013, Volume 127. Used with permission.

remedy straight off the drugstore shelf: low-dose aspirin. Although better known as a pain reliever, aspirin also works as a mild blood thinner.

Coronary Heart Disease

Of all types of CVD, **coronary heart disease (CHD)** causes the most deaths **(Figure 12.6)**. In fact, CHD is the single leading cause of death in the United States. More than 15 million Americans have CHD, and the American Heart Association estimates that it causes about 1 out of every 6 deaths and kills almost 400,000 people each year.[24]

Also called *coronary artery disease,* CHD arises when plaque in the coronary arteries builds up to the point that it impairs the heart's ability to function. Partial coronary artery blockages can cause *angina,* or chest pain, that occurs when the heart muscle doesn't get enough blood. Larger or even total blockages can trigger a *myocardial infarction* (heart attack) or a disruption in heart rhythm known as *sudden cardiac arrest.* We'll look at these conditions next.

Angina

Narrowed coronary arteries can still deliver some blood to the heart—but not necessarily as much as this powerful muscle needs. Chest pain, or **angina pectoris,** occurs when the heart's need for nutrients and oxygen exceeds what the coronary arteries provide. Angina can feel like pressure or like a squeezing pain in the chest. These sensations can also radiate out to your shoulders, arms, neck, jaw, or back, or even resemble indigestion.

coronary heart disease (CHD) (coronary artery disease) Disease characterized by atherosclerosis of the arteries that feed the heart; angina; and reduced blood supply to the myocardium.

angina pectoris Chest pain due to coronary heart disease.

myocardial infarction (MI) (heart attack) A cardiac crisis in which a region of heart muscle is damaged or destroyed by reduced blood flow.

arrhythmia Any irregularity in the heart's rhythm.

bradycardia A slow arrhythmia.

tachycardia A fast arrhythmia.

sudden cardiac arrest A life-threatening cardiac crisis marked by loss of heartbeat and unconsciousness.

electrocardiogram (ECG) A test that measures the heart's electrical activity.

Angina itself may not be life-threatening, but it signals that a person is at significant risk of a life-threatening cardiac event. If angina isn't correctly recognized or treated, the arterial narrowing behind it may progress to a full blockage, leading to the next condition we'll discuss—heart attack.

Myocardial Infarction (Heart Attack)

When blockage of a coronary artery deprives a region of the myocardium of its blood supply, that region can stop working effectively. Its cells can even die if they go too long without blood and the oxygen and nutrients it carries. During a heart attack, or **myocardial infarction (MI),** the more time that passes without treatment to restore blood flow, the greater the damage. Warning signs of a heart attack include angina, discomfort in the chest or other parts of the upper body, shortness of breath, and sweating, nausea, or dizziness. Chest pain, which is a hallmark symptom in men, doesn't occur as often in women, who are somewhat more likely to experience less specific forms of pain and discomfort **(Figure 12.7)**.

According to the American Heart Association, more than a million people in the United States have a heart attack each year, and about one-third die as a result.[24] Those who survive often continue to face significant health risks and functional impairment.

Arrhythmia and Sudden Cardiac Arrest

If the heart is starved of blood, the nerve cells of the sinus node can also be affected, resulting in an irregularity of the heartbeat called an **arrhythmia,** in which the heart can beat too slowly, too quickly, or unevenly. Arrhythmias affect different aspects of the heart's function, and some are more serious than others. More than 2 million people in the United States live with some form of arrhythmia.[25]

A slow heart rate of less than 60 beats per minute is called **bradycardia.** A fast heart rate—more than 100 beats per minute—is called **tachycardia.** An especially dangerous type of tachycardia is *fibrillation*. In fibrillation, an improper electrical signal causes either the atria or the ventricles to contract so quickly and unevenly that they quiver rather than pump, unable to move blood effectively. Many people live with atrial fibrillation and have no symptoms at all, or symptoms that are troubling but not life-threatening, such as palpitations or fainting spells. In contrast, ventricular fibrillation completely stops heart functioning and is a medical emergency. It is the most common type of arrhythmia seen in cases of **sudden cardiac arrest.** The person's heart must be restarted within 6 minutes via electrical shock to prevent death. Even if the heart is restarted within 6 minutes, the patient may sustain irreversible brain damage from lack of oxygen to the brain.

Many factors increase the risk for arrhythmias. These include stress, smoking, genetic factors, heavy alcohol use, strenuous exercise, certain medications, and even air pollution. Coronary heart disease—because it deprives the heart of blood—is the most important risk factor.[25]

Clinical Management of CHD

The diagnosis and treatment of CHD depends on the precise form it takes, so let's look at each separately.

Management of Angina. An **electrocardiogram,** also called an *ECG* (or *EKG*), measures the heart's

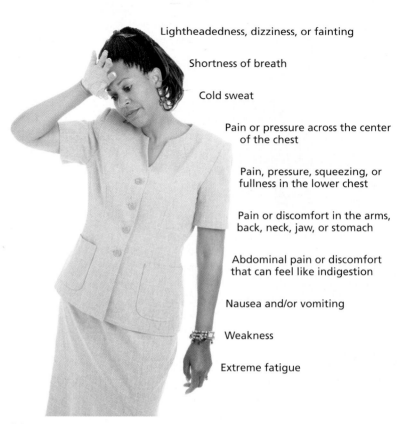

Lightheadedness

Pain across the center of the chest

Pressure, squeezing, or fullness in the chest

Pain or discomfort in the arms, back, neck, jaw, or stomach

Shortness of breath

Cold sweat

Nausea

Lightheadedness, dizziness, or fainting

Shortness of breath

Cold sweat

Pain or pressure across the center of the chest

Pain, pressure, squeezing, or fullness in the lower chest

Pain or discomfort in the arms, back, neck, jaw, or stomach

Abdominal pain or discomfort that can feel like indigestion

Nausea and/or vomiting

Weakness

Extreme fatigue

(a) Warning signs in men

(b) Warning signs in women

FIGURE 12.7 Warning Signs of a Heart Attack Differ Somewhat in Men and Women. These warning signs can occur individually, or several can occur simultaneously.

electrical activity and is commonly used to detect arrhythmias as well as the restricted blood flow that causes angina. An ECG conducted with the patient resting provides a baseline measurement, or the test can be done while the patient is exercising. This form, called a *stress test*, shows how the heart performs under increased physical demands. An *echocardiogram* may be done during the stress test to produce images of the heart using sound waves.

Whether angina is mild or severe, lifestyle changes can help. These include weight loss, eating a healthy diet, engaging in prescribed exercise, avoiding smoking, and managing blood glucose levels. The first medication a physician might try is aspirin, which helps prevent blood clots and improves blood flow. You may also have heard of people with angina placing nitroglycerin tablets under their tongue or using a nitroglycerin spray: These work by dilating blood vessels. Medications may be prescribed to reduce blood cholesterol, slow the heartbeat, or relax the muscles of the blood vessel walls.

Management of an MI. When a person arrives in a hospital emergency department (ED) complaining of chest pains, the ED team typically hooks the person up to a heart monitor, administers oxygen so that the heart doesn't have to work as hard, and provides medication—typically intravenous (IV)—to relieve the pain. A variety of tests may then be performed. A special blood test can determine if there is damage to the heart muscle indicative of an MI, and a test of the blood vessels, called *coronary angiography* (*angio-* refers to a vessel), may be done

balloon angioplasty An arterial treatment that uses a small balloon to flatten plaque deposits against the arterial wall.

coronary artery bypass grafting (CABG) A procedure to build new pathways for blood to flow around areas of arterial blockage.

to see how and where the blood is being blocked from flowing through the heart.[26]

In patients whose arteries are dangerously obstructed, procedures are available to open them. A **balloon angioplasty** involves threading a catheter through the artery and inflating a small balloon at the obstructed spot, flattening plaque against the arterial walls and opening the vessel. **Coronary artery bypass grafting (CABG)** circumvents the blocked vessel rather than opening it. Using a healthy blood vessel from another part of the body, the surgeon creates an alternative route for blood to flow around the arterial obstruction. If more than one artery is blocked, multiple bypasses can be performed.

Once the immediate crisis has been resolved, a special program of *cardiac rehabilitation* may be advised. In "cardiac rehab," patients learn to make lifestyle changes to improve their cardiovascular health. Counseling and support are also offered, and low-dose daily aspirin or other medications may be prescribed.

Management of Sudden Cardiac Arrest. In cases of sudden cardiac arrest, there is rarely time for transport to a hospital. The person's heart must be restarted within minutes with a device called an *automated external defibrillator* (*AED*), or the person will die. This device sends an electric shock to the heart and can restore a normal heartbeat, allowing time for transport to a medical center. Public places, including college campuses, usually have AEDs, but for obvious reasons, their location must be generally known and immediately accessible. Police,

Helping Someone in a CVD Emergency

We all know that someone showing signs of a heart attack, cardiac arrest, or stroke needs to head for the nearest hospital. But before the person is under medical care, you can take steps to help.

If you see someone showing the signs of a heart attack, cardiac arrest, or stroke, the first thing you should do is call 911. If possible, make this call from a land line, not a cell phone. Land line calls to 911 are usually routed straight to local emergency dispatch centers, whereas calls from cell phones are often routed to local highway safety agencies, who must then reroute the call to the correct dispatch center, sometimes costing valuable time.

Once you call 911, wait with the person until emergency medical services arrive rather than driving to the hospital yourself. Paramedic and ambulance units have life-saving equipment and skills that they can deploy immediately and sustain during the trip to the hospital. If you drive the person to the hospital, he or she can't benefit from this faster access to medical help.

In addition, here are ways you can help in specific types of emergencies:

Heart Attack

- Although the symptoms of a heart attack aren't always clear cut, don't hesitate to call 911 if you suspect one is occurring. Trying a "wait and see" approach could cost the person's life.

- Have the person chew an aspirin, unless he or she is allergic to aspirin or is under medical orders to avoid it. Aspirin has blood-thinning properties that can help in a heart attack. The drug used must be aspirin, not another type of pain reliever.

- Have the person take nitroglycerin if already prescribed. This drug is often used in people with CVD.

- If the person falls unconscious, begin "hands-only" CPR. If you don't know how, ask the dispatcher to instruct you on the proper technique until help arrives.

Sudden Cardiac Arrest

- If you suspect cardiac arrest, call 911 immediately. People in cardiac arrest need their heart restarted within 6 minutes or they will die.

- Check the unconscious person for a pulse *after* you call 911. The side of the neck is a more reliable place to feel for a pulse than the wrist.

- If you don't find a pulse, begin "hands-only" CPR. If you need help, the 911 dispatcher will instruct you on the proper technique until help arrives.

- If you are in a public place such as a campus or office building, an airport, or a shopping mall, ask someone nearby to look for a device called an *automated external defibrillator*, or AED. AEDs are electrical heart-starting machines, and they are designed for anyone to use. Just open the box and follow the instructions. Don't worry about shocking someone unnecessarily—AEDs are designed to scan for a heartbeat and not deliver a shock if a heartbeat is detected.

Stroke

- The classic signs of a stroke are face drooping, arm weakness, and slurred speech. If you suspect a stroke, call 911 immediately. The faster medical help arrives, the more likely it is that permanent brain damage can be avoided.

- Make note of the time you first noticed the symptoms. This information is vital for paramedics and doctors trying to provide treatment as fast as possible.

- While you wait for help, don't administer cardiac aid such as "hands-only" CPR unless the person goes into cardiac arrest. A person having a stroke may be disoriented or have trouble moving, but CPR should be reserved for people who are unconscious and have no pulse. Otherwise, it could be harmful.

Sources: **1.** *Cardiopulmonary Resuscitation (CPR): First Aid,* by the Mayo Clinic, 2012, retrieved from http://www.mayoclinic.com/health/first-aid-cpr/FA00061. **2.** *Heart Attack First Aid,* by Medline Plus, 2011, retrieved from http://www.nlm.nih.gov. **3.** *How to Use an Automated External Defibrillator,* by the National Heart, Lung, and Blood Institute (n.d.), retrieved from http://www.nhlbi.nih.gov/health/dci/Diseases/aed/aed_use.html. **4.** *Stroke: Preventing and Treating 'Brain Attack,'* by Harvard Health Publications (n.d.). **5.** *Stroke Warning Signs and Symptoms,* by the American Stroke Association, 2012, http://www.strokeassociation.org/STROKEORG/WarningSigns/Stroke-

firefighters, and emergency medical technicians usually are trained and equipped to use a defibrillator.

If a person suddenly loses consciousness, failing to respond when asked if okay, tilt his or her head upright. If the person does not take a normal breath within 5 seconds, he or she may be experiencing a sudden cardiac arrest. If an AED is not available, the American Heart Association recommends that you call 911 and then begin "hands-only" CPR. The technique is simple, involving only pushing hard and fast in the center of the victim's chest until help arrives.

>> If you have 2 minutes to spare, you can learn "hands-only" CPR. Watch this video from the American Heart Association at http://handsonlycpr.org.

A person who survives a sudden cardiac arrest may have surgery to place an *implantable cardioverter defibrillator* (*ICD*), which is similar to a pacemaker, but transmits stronger electric pulses to help prevent further dangerous arrhythmias. For information on helping someone "on the scene" in a CVD emergency, see the **Special Feature** on page 297.

Congestive Heart Failure

In **congestive heart failure,** the heart can no longer pump enough blood to meet the body's needs. As a result, blood may pool—or become congested—in other areas of the body, such as the lungs, the abdomen, or the arms and legs. This pooled blood quickly becomes depleted of oxygen and nutrients, so the affected regions become damaged and dysfunctional. More than 6 million adults in the United States live with congestive heart failure.[24]

We noted earlier that the forms of CVD are interrelated, and indeed a common cause of congestive heart failure is CHD, which damages heart muscle, reducing its ability to beat strongly. Persistent tachycardia may also cause the heart to work too hard, slowly wearing it out. However, a landmark heart health study found that hypertension, which forces the heart to work harder than it should to pump blood, is the most common risk factor for congestive heart failure.[27]

A failing heart results in a failing circulation. The arms and legs may swell with fluid. Pooling of fluid in the lungs may make breathing difficult. The abdomen may swell, and the person may gain "water weight." Heart failure also typically causes exhaustion, loss of appetite, and an inability to concentrate.

A low-sodium diet, smoking cessation, and maintenance of a healthful weight are all essential in slowing the progress of congestive heart failure. The physician may prescribe diuretics and other medications to slow the heartbeat, dilate blood vessels, and reduce the total workload on the heart. Heart surgery may be necessary, either to open blocked coronary arteries or to insert a pacemaker or ICD.[28]

Stroke

As you've learned in this chapter, a blockage in an artery that feeds the heart can cause a heart attack. What would happen if similar damage affected an artery serving the brain? The answer is a **stroke** (also called a *cerebrovascular accident*), a medical emergency in which the blood supply to a part of the brain ceases. More than 6 million Americans—2.7%—have suffered a stroke.[29]

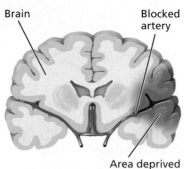

(a) Ischemic stroke **(b)** Hemorrhagic stroke

FIGURE 12.8 Two Types of Stroke. (a) In an ischemic stroke, a blocked artery damages brain tissue by depriving it of blood. (b) In a hemorrhagic stroke, a weakened artery leaks or ruptures, releasing blood into and damaging the brain tissue as well as depriving brain cells beyond the rupture.

Types of Stroke

Strokes can take either of two forms **(Figure 12.8)**.

Ischemic Stroke. The far more common form is **ischemic stroke,** in which either a cerebral artery or one of the carotid arteries that run through the neck into the brain becomes blocked. All brain tissues normally served by the blocked artery become starved of oxygen and nutrients.

Hemorrhagic Stroke. The term *hemorrhage* means uncontrolled bleeding. In **hemorrhagic stroke,** a weakened cerebral artery leaks or ruptures, spilling blood into brain tissue. The blood compresses and damages the brain cells in the area of the spill; moreover, the brain regions that would normally have been served by the broken vessel are deprived of blood. In some cases, the bleeding seeps into the compartment between the brain and the skull (called the subarachnoid space). The two most common causes of hemorrhagic stroke are uncontrolled hypertension and the presence of an *aneurysm,* a weak spot in an artery wall that may rupture.

Signs and Symptoms of an Impending Stroke

Brain cells deprived of blood quickly die. Thus, a person having a stroke may suddenly feel weak, numb, or paralyzed in the arm, leg, or face, especially on one side of the body. Vision may become blurry, and speech may become slurred. A sudden and severe headache is also common and may be accompanied by dizziness or vomiting. The person may suddenly become confused or experience delusions.

Some people at risk for stroke may experience a fleeting episode of a milder version of these symptoms days, weeks, or months before having a full stroke. Such a mini-stroke, known as a **transient ischemic attack,** or TIA, isn't always easy to recognize, but it is a clear warning sign of an impending stroke.

congestive heart failure A gradual loss of heart function.

stroke A medical emergency in which blood flow to or in the brain is impaired. Also called a *cerebrovascular accident* (*CVA*).

ischemic stroke A stroke caused by a blocked blood vessel.

hemorrhagic stroke A stroke caused by a leaking or ruptured blood vessel.

transient ischemic attack (TIA) A temporary episode of strokelike symptoms, indicative of high stroke risk.

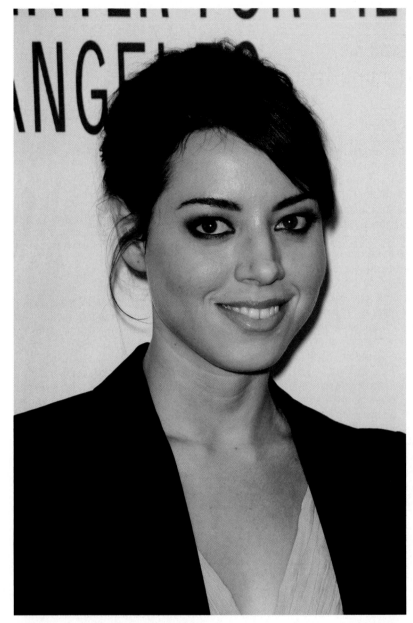

Being young doesn't mean you're immune from cardiovascular disease. Aubrey Plaza, one of the stars of TV's Parks and Recreation, suffered a stroke when she was only 20 years old.

Long-Term Effects of a Stroke

Prompt treatment can greatly reduce the long-term effects of a stroke. These include:

- Paralysis, especially on one side of the body
- Impaired speaking, swallowing, and chewing
- *Aphasia*, a difficulty in understanding and expressing ideas in spoken or written words
- Loss of memory, impaired decision-making, and personality changes
- Pain, cold, and other uncomfortable sensations

Rehabilitation efforts, including speech therapy and physical and occupational therapy, can help reduce some of these effects.

Clinical Management of a Stroke

Anyone showing signs of a stroke requires immediate medical attention to prevent or reduce brain damage. In an ischemic stroke, the goal of emergency treatment is to open the blocked cerebral artery and restore blood flow to that area of the brain. Believe it or not, aspirin is the best-proven immediate treatment for ischemic stroke. The patient may be given an injection of a clot-busting drug, or the physician may be able to thread a device into the brain that can grab and remove the clot.[30]

In a hemorrhagic stroke, aspirin is never given because it promotes bleeding. Instead, drugs are used to reduce the force of blood moving into the damaged area, to help control the bleeding, and to prevent seizures. Surgery can sometimes repair or isolate the ruptured vessel.[30]

Once a stroke patient is stabilized, rehabilitation can begin. This often requires admission to a special facility, where the patient works with a neurologist and speech and physical therapists.

Other Forms of Cardiovascular Disease

Less common types of CVD in the United States include the following:

- **Congenital heart disease.** About 9 in every 1,000 babies are born with some type of heart defect.[31] Some of the more frequent defects include holes in the walls that divide the chambers of the heart, abnormal narrowing of the coronary arteries, and malformations of the arteries that connect the heart and lungs. Most congenital heart defects can be treated with drugs or surgery.

- **Heart valve disorders.** Blood flows through your heart in only one direction, from atrium to ventricle, because the chambers of your heart are gated with valves. These flaps of connective tissue swing open and shut like one-way doors, allowing blood to pass from atrium to ventricle but preventing it from pooling or streaming backward. Congenital defects, infections, or heart disease can damage these. In some cases, a valve may let too little blood pass. In others, a valve may leak. Medications can ease some valve problems, whereas more serious malfunctions may require surgical repair.

- **Hypertrophic cardiomyopathy.** Up to half a million Americans have hypertrophic cardiomyopathy (HCM), a genetic disorder resulting in a thick, stiffened muscle wall that cannot pump enough blood during vigorous activity. Children with HCM are not allowed to play competitive sports because HCM can cause sudden death in an athlete.

- **Rheumatic heart disease.** A potentially fatal condition, rheumatic heart disease begins when a bacterial infection—caused by the same *Streptococcus* bacterium that causes strep throat—flares into rheumatic fever. Along with an elevated temperature, the illness causes inflammation of connective tissues throughout the body. Sometimes that damage includes the heart valves. Rheumatic heart disease is easily prevented by taking antibiotics in the early stages of a strep infection.

Risk Factors for Cardiovascular Disease

This section identifies the risk factors for CVD—including those you can't change and those you can. We've encountered many of them already in our discussion of type 2 diabetes. And as we'll see shortly, several of them are defining factors in cardiometabolic risk.

- **Your age.** Most cases of heart attack, sudden cardiac arrest, and stroke occur in people older than 65. You can't stop yourself from aging, but you can work to make sure every year of life is as healthy as possible.

- **Your sex.** Men face greater heart attack risks than women, and they tend to have heart attacks earlier in life. However, CVD is still the

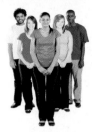

DIVERSITY & HEALTH

Gender Differences in Risk for Heart Disease

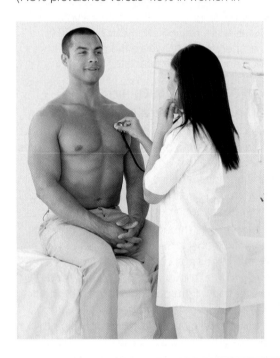

Although heart disease is the leading killer of both men and women in the United States, men typically develop it at greater rates than women (7.8% prevalence versus 4.6% in women in 2010)[1] and suffer cardiac crises about 10 years earlier than women.[2]

For many years, researchers theorized that these differences in rate and timing were due to lifestyle factors. Men have higher rates of smoking and alcohol abuse, for example. But they soon came to recognize that lifestyle factors alone couldn't explain the numbers. Something else had to be going on. Further research revealed that "something else" to be hormones.

The female reproductive hormone estrogen is produced in significant amounts by a woman's ovaries until she experiences menopause. While it's circulating in the bloodstream, estrogen appears to protect blood vessels against atherosclerosis.[3] This explains why women's risk of CVD increases greatly after menopause, when estrogen production plummets.

This doesn't mean, however, that young women should be any less vigilant about their heart health. Heart disease can begin as early as the teen years, and 80% of women ages 40 to 60 have at least one risk factor.[4] The bottom line? One in four men and one in four women will die of heart disease.[4,5] So both men and women can benefit from adopting heart-healthy behaviors as early in life as possible.

Critical-Thinking Questions

1. Men and women tend to gain and store weight in different ways. (See Chapter 6.) How might this influence men's higher risk for heart disease?

2. Whether you're male or female, how concerned are you about your risk for heart disease? How would you compare that with your concern about your risk for type 2 diabetes or cancer?

3. Risk factors for CVD include: obesity; a diet high in red meats, refined grains, and sweets; a low level of physical activity; smoking; drug abuse; and short sleep. How many of these risk factors—if any—apply to you? Does identifying these factors change your perception of your CVD risk? If so, how?

References: **1.** "Prevalence of Coronary Heart Disease—United States, 2006-2010," by the Centers for Disease Control and Prevention, October 14, 2011, *Morbidity and Mortality Weekly Report, 60*(40), pp. 1377–1381. **2.** *Heart Attack Risk Factors,* by the Mayo Foundation, November 17, 2011, http://www.mayoclinic.com/health/heart-attack/DS00094/DSECTION=risk-factors. **3.** "Estrogen Protection, Oxidized LDL, Endothelial Dysfunction and Vasorelaxation in Cardiovascular Disease: New Insights into a Complex Issue," by C. Packer, 2007, *Cardiovascular Research, 73*(1), pp. 6–7. **4.** *Lower Heart Disease Risk,* by the National Heart, Lung, and Blood Institute at the National Institutes of Health, January 22, 2013, http://www.nhlbi.nih.gov/educational/hearttruth/lower-risk/index.htm. **5.** *Men and Heart Disease Fact Sheet,* by the Centers for Disease Control and Prevention, October 18, 2012, http://www.cdc.gov/dhdsp/data_statistics/fact_sheets/fs_men_heart.htm.

top killer of women in the United States over the course of their lifetime, and women need to pay attention to CVD risks as well. The **Diversity & Health** box explores some of the factors behind gender differences in CVD rates.

- **Your genetic inheritance.** Children of parents with CVD are more likely to develop the condition. Race is also a risk factor. (See the **Diversity & Health** box on page 288.) But inheritance isn't destiny. By reducing the CVD risks you can control, you can help make sure that your genes don't equal your fate.

- **Your blood pressure.** At a doctor's visit or health fair, have your blood pressure measured. Hypertension in adults is defined as blood pressure equal to or greater than 140 over 90. For more detailed guidelines, see Table 12.1 on page 294.

- **Your blood lipids.** If you have abnormal levels of various lipids circulating in your bloodstream,

dyslipidemia Disorder characterized by abnormal levels of blood lipids, such as high LDL cholesterol or low HDL cholesterol.

low-density lipoprotein (LDL) A cholesterol-containing compound that, as it degrades, releases its cholesterol load into the bloodstream; often referred to as "bad cholesterol."

high-density lipoprotein (HDL) A cholesterol-containing compound that removes excess cholesterol from the bloodstream; often referred to as "good cholesterol."

a condition known as **dyslipidemia,** the health of your heart and blood vessels is at risk. A simple blood test can give you a variety of data about your blood lipid levels (**Table 12.2**). These include your total cholesterol score, the level of triglycerides circulating in your bloodstream, and your readings for two cholesterol-carrying protein compounds:

- LDL, short for **low-density lipoprotein,** is a molecule that packs a lot of cholesterol with very little protein. It's often dubbed "bad" cholesterol because excess LDLs degrade over time, releasing their cholesterol load into your bloodstream, where it can become trapped in injured blood vessels. A high LDL score means there's a lot of cholesterol "littering" your bloodstream, so it increases your risk for CVD.

- HDL, an abbreviation of **high-density lipoprotein,** is half protein with little

TABLE 12.2 Classification of Blood Lipid Levels for Adults

LDL Cholesterol	Classification
< 100	Optimal
100–129	Near optimal/above optimal
130–159	Borderline high
160–189	High
≥ 190	Very high

HDL Cholesterol	Classification
< 40	Low
≥ 60	Optimal

Total Cholesterol	Classification
< 200	Desirable
200–239	Borderline high
≥ 240	High

Triglycerides	Classification
< 150	Normal
150–199	Borderline high
200–499	High
≥ 500	Very high

Source: Data from the *Third Report of the Expert Panel on Detection, Evaluation, and Treatment of High Blood Cholesterol in Adults* (NIH Publication No. 05-3290), by the National Heart, Lung, and Blood Institute, 2005.

cholesterol. It's often called "good" cholesterol because it picks up free cholesterol in the bloodstream and transports it to your liver for recycling. You can think of HDL as your arteries' "housekeeper." A high HDL score means a lower risk for CVD.

- **Your blood glucose.** A blood glucose level of 110 mg/dL or higher increases your risk for CVD. Given that 110 is considered prediabetes, you don't have to have full-blown diabetes before your blood glucose level begins to increase your CVD risk.

- **Inflammatory markers.** As noted earlier, inflammation plays a key role in atherosclerosis. Physicians can detect inflammation in the body by measuring your blood level of a protein—called *C-reactive protein (CRP)*—produced by the liver during an inflammatory response. A high level of CRP (above 3.0 mg/L) indicates that inflammation is going on somewhere in the body, but not necessarily in the blood vessels. So it's not likely that a physician would order a CRP test unless you had other significant risk factors, such as hypertension and dyslipidemia.

- **Homocysteine.** The amino acid homocysteine can only be metabolized by the body when we consume adequate amounts of the B vitamins folate, B_6, and B_{12}. High levels of homocysteine in the blood are associated with an increased risk of MI and stroke.

- **Your weight.** Obesity increases the risk for CVD and death from CVD.[24] Several factors explain the link between obesity and CVD:
  - Obesity increases the total volume of blood circulating in the body as well as the total metabolic demand of body cells. Therefore, the cardiac workload is greater.

- The left ventricle of the heart grows excessively large in obese people, a condition called *left ventricular hypertrophy*, and this increases the risk for ventricular dysfunction.
- In obese people, fat cells can actually infiltrate and replace heart muscle, disturbing regions such as the sinus node where the heart's electrical impulses are generated.
- Fat cells—especially those stored in abdominal fat—manufacture and release into the bloodstream a variety of inflammatory chemicals.

- **Your diet.** The American Heart Association reports that a diet rich in fruits, legumes and other vegetables, whole grains, fish, and poultry was associated with a 28% reduction in CVD deaths, whereas a diet high in red meats, processed meats, refined grains, and sweets was associated with a 22% increase in CVD deaths.[24]

- **Your level of physical activity.** Exercise reduces blood sugar, increases HDL cholesterol, combats atherosclerosis, strengthens the heart muscle, and expends calories, helping you to maintain a healthful body weight.

- **Smoking.** Nicotine constricts the blood vessels, and carbon monoxide damages their walls, increasing their susceptibility to atherosclerosis. Smoking also increases blood pressure, increases the tendency for blood to clot, and decreases HDL cholesterol.

- **Drug abuse.** Researchers have found a connection between the abuse of prescription and illicit drugs and adverse cardiovascular effects, ranging from abnormal heart rate to heart attacks. For example, prescription stimulants can cause an irregular heatbeat and sudden heart failure, and marijuana increases blood pressure, quadrupling the risk of a heart attack within the first hour after use.[32]

- **Your emotions and level of stress.** Negative emotions like anger, depression, and anxiety can raise your CVD risk.[33] Researchers speculate that this might be due in part to the ways some people find to cope with these emotions—such as by overeating, smoking, or drinking too much alcohol. Another risk factor is stress: A 2013 study found that long-term, elevated cortisol levels increase the risk for CVD as much as traditional risk factors such as hypertension.[18]

- **Your sleep.** Short sleep increases your CVD risk. In one study adolescents with short sleep duration had excessive LDL cholesterol and poor HDL cholesterol.[34] Studies have also consistently linked short sleep with hypertension.[35]

- **Your income.** Research shows that lower-income adults have an increased rate of CVD. (See the **Diversity & Health** box on page 288.)

>> **What's your risk for a heart attack or stroke? Find out at** www.heart.org/gglRisk/locale/en_US/index.html?gtype=health.

Cardiometabolic Risk

Now that you've learned about diabetes and CVD, you're ready to tackle a concept that has recently emerged as a critical public health concern: cardiometabolic risk. For decades, researchers have noted that obesity and insulin resistance together promote a variety of serious metabolic abnormalities. They used the term

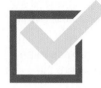

SELF-ASSESSMENT
What's Your Risk for a Heart Attack?

Circle your answers.

1. Do you smoke? Yes No

2. Is your blood pressure 140/90 mm Hg or higher, OR have you been told by your doctor that your blood pressure is too high? Yes No Don't Know

3. Has your doctor told you that your LDL ("bad") cholesterol is too high, OR that your total cholesterol level is 200 mg/dL or higher, OR that your HDL ("good") cholesterol is less than 40 mg/dL? Yes No Don't Know

4. Has your father or brother had a heart attack before age 55, OR has your mother or sister had one before age 65? Yes No Don't Know

5. Are you over 55 years old? Yes No

6. Do you have a BMI score of 25 or more? (See Figure 6.1 on page 129) Yes No Don't Know

7. Do you get less than a total of 30 minutes of moderate-intensity physical activity on most days? Yes No Not Sure

8. Has a doctor told you that you have angina (chest pains), OR have you had a heart attack? Yes No Don't Know

HOW TO INTERPRET YOUR SCORE

If you circled any of the "Yes" answers, you're at an increased risk of having a heart attack. If you circled "Don't Know" for any questions, ask your doctor for help in answering them.

To complete this Self-Assessment online, visit **MasteringHealth**™

Adapted from The Healthy Heart Handbook for Women, NIH Publication No. 07-2720, by the U.S. Department of Health and Human Services, National Heart, Lung, and Blood Institute (NHLBI), National Institutes of Health (NIH), 2007.

Cardiometabolic risk

Metabolic syndrome —
- Abdominal obesity (a waist circumference ≥ 40 inches for males and 35 inches for females)
- Elevated blood pressure (≥ 130/85 mm Hg)
- Elevated fasting blood glucose (≥ 110 mg/dL)
- Elevated blood triglycerides (> 150)
- Low HDL cholesterol (< 40)
- High LDL cholesterol (≥ 130)
- Smoking
- Inflammatory markers (notably CRP)
- Insulin resistance

FIGURE 12.9 Cardiometabolic Risk. These nine factors dramatically increase your risk of developing type 2 diabetes and cardiovascular disease.

---

metabolic syndrome to refer to this cluster of abnormalities, which includes, for example, high fasting blood glucose and low HDL cholesterol. More recently, researchers have come to recognize that these abnormalities increase a person's risk not only for type 2 diabetes, but also for CVD. As a result, many public health groups have expanded the concept of metabolic syndrome to include the risk factors traditionally associated with CVD, such as smoking. Their name for this expanded concept is cardiometabolic risk.[36]

In 2009, the Agency for Healthcare Research and Quality (AHRQ, part of the Department of Health and Human Services) published lengthy guidelines defining **cardiometabolic risk (CMR)** as a cluster of modifiable factors that identify individuals at increased risk for type 2 diabetes mellitus and cardiovascular disease.[37] CMR includes all five of the

metabolic syndrome A set of five unhealthy physical and metabolic conditions together linked to an increased risk for type 2 diabetes and other metabolic disease.

cardiometabolic risk (CMR) A cluster of nine modifiable factors that identify individuals at risk for type 2 diabetes and cardiovascular disease.

factors that make up the definition of metabolic syndrome, plus four other factors. These are identified in **Figure 12.9.**

Although the first factor—abdominal obesity—is particularly dangerous, obesity in general has become a "gold standard" for identifying people at high CMR. Men and women whose BMI is 30 or higher are at significantly increased risk of cardiometabolic disease and early death.[38]

The AHRQ recommends that all males have an initial CMR screening at age 35, and females at age 45. If you're obese, or if you have already been diagnosed with type 2 diabetes, hypertension, or dyslipidemia, you should have a CMR screening immediately, and annually. In addition, because depression is the most frequently cited psychological disorder associated with diabetes, you can anticipate that, if your physician finds any of the factors associated with CMR, he or she is likely to also screen you for depression.[37]

When college students are screened for CMR, studies show that one or more of the nine factors are already present in a significant percentage. For example, a 2012 study involving nearly 3,000 students found that 77% of males and 54% of females already had at least one risk factor, and nearly 10% of males and 3% of women met all criteria for metabolic syndrome.[39] A smaller 2012 study of college students yielded very similar data.[40]

Individuals found to be at CMR have a variety of clinical treatment options. However, lifestyle measures—discussed shortly—are essential.

Cancer

Although more people die of heart disease than cancer, few diseases evoke more fear. But recent developments in our understanding of cancer can also evoke another emotion—hope. Our ability to detect and treat cancer is improving rapidly, as is our understanding of how to prevent it.

To be sure, cancer remains a health priority for good reason. In a given year, about 1.6 million new cases of cancer will be diagnosed in the United States, and more than 580,000 people will die from the disease.[41] Cancer is the second leading cause of death in the United States. Statistics on cancer cases and deaths by body site are illustrated in **Table 12.3.**

Despite these disturbing figures, more people are surviving cancer than ever before. The five-year survival rate for cancer is now 68%, up from 49% 35 years ago.[41] However, significant health disparities persist in cancer rates, especially for African Americans, who are more likely to develop and die of cancer than any other ethnic group.[41] Eliminating this disparity is a key focus of national cancer prevention efforts.

To reduce your own risk for cancer, it helps to have a basic understanding of how the disease arises and—in some cases—spreads. You'll also need to know about risk factors, early detection, and warning signs to watch for. After that, we'll provide a quick look at some common cancers, and discuss treatment—and survival.

What Is Cancer?

Cancer is a group of diseases characterized by uncontrolled reproduction of abnormal cells and, in some cases, the spread of these cells to other sites in the body. These cells often don't start as abnormal, but for a variety of reasons, they undergo changes in their operating instructions that turn them into rogue agents of abnormal growth.

Understanding how this happens starts with a look at the body's genetic material, *DNA*. The structures and functions of just about every cell in the body are controlled by DNA because the precise sequence of parts of the DNA molecule tells the cell what proteins to build and how to build them. DNA enables cells to divide and replicate, ensuring that the body's tissues are as vital as possible. For instance, the cells lining your digestive tract are replaced every few days, and your skin cells are continually being shed and replaced. If you're injured, the cell replacement process speeds up to help you heal.

Genes are the basic units of your DNA that control this cell growth. They normally operate a bit like the accelerator and brakes on a car. If you need lots of new cells quickly, growth-related genes accelerate their production. Once enough new cells are in place, the same genes slow the process back down to normal. As you can imagine, if something damages these genes, they will no longer be able to regulate cell reproduction appropriately.

The genes that control cell reproduction can be damaged

---

cancer A group of diseases marked by the uncontrolled multiplication of abnormal cells.

carcinogen A substance known to trigger DNA mutations that can lead to cancer.

TABLE 12.3 Leading Sites of New Cancer Cases and Deaths, 2013 Estimates

	Estimated New Cases		Estimated Deaths	
Site		Incidence (% of all cases)	**Site**	Mortality (% of all cases)
Male			**Male**	
Prostate		238,590 (28%)	Lung and bronchus	87,260 (28%)
Lung and bronchus		118,080 (14%)	Prostate	29,720 (10%)
Colon and rectum		73,680 (9%)	Colon and rectum	26,300 (9%)
Urinary bladder		54,610 (6%)	Pancreas	19,480 (6%)
Melanoma of the skin		45,060 (5%)	Liver and intrahepatic bile duct	14,890 (5%)
Kidney and renal pelvis		40,430 (5%)	Leukemia	13,660 (4%)
Non-Hodgkin lymphoma		37,600 (4%)	Esophagus	12,220 (4%)
Oral cavity and pharynx		29,620 (3%)	Urinary bladder	10,820 (4%)
Leukemia		27,880 (3%)	Non-Hodgkin lymphoma	10,590 (3%)
Pancreas		22,740 (3%)	Kidney and renal pelvis	8,780 (3%)
All sites		854,790 (100%)	All sites	306,920 (100%)
Female			**Female**	
Breast		232,340 (29%)	Lung and bronchus	72,220 (26%)
Lung and bronchus		110,110 (14%)	Breast	39,620 (14%)
Colon and rectum		69,140 (9%)	Colon and rectum	24,530 (9%)
Uterine corpus		49,560 (6%)	Pancreas	18,980 (7%)
Thyroid		45,310 (6%)	Ovary	14,030 (5%)
Non-Hodgkin lymphoma		32,140 (4%)	Leukemia	10,060 (4%)
Melanoma of the skin		31,630 (4%)	Non-Hodgkin lymphoma	8,430 (3%)
Kidney and renal pelvis		24,720 (3%)	Uterine corpus	8,190 (3%)
Pancreas		22,480 (3%)	Liver and intrahepatic bile duct	6,780 (2%)
Ovary		22,240 (3%)	Brain and other nervous system	6,150 (2%)
All sites		805,500 (100%)	All sites	273,430 (100%)

Source: Data from *Cancer Facts & Figures, 2013,* by the American Cancer Society, 2013, p. 10.

by a variety of external hazards. These include the toxins in tobacco and tobacco smoke, alcohol, many chemicals used in industry, radiation (including from sunlight and tanning beds), and even certain viruses.[42] When we come into contact with such agents—whether by absorbing them via our skin, or breathing or ingesting them—they can cause dangerous *mutations,* or DNA changes, that can lead to cancer. These cancer-generating agents are known as **carcinogens.** Our body's defenses seek out cells with such mutations and repair the damage, cause the cells to self-destruct, or kill them. But some mutations are more severe than the body can fix, or the encounter with the carcinogen is so frequent that the body's defenses become overwhelmed. And, in some people, other features of their DNA actually diminish their body's ability to protect and repair its cells.

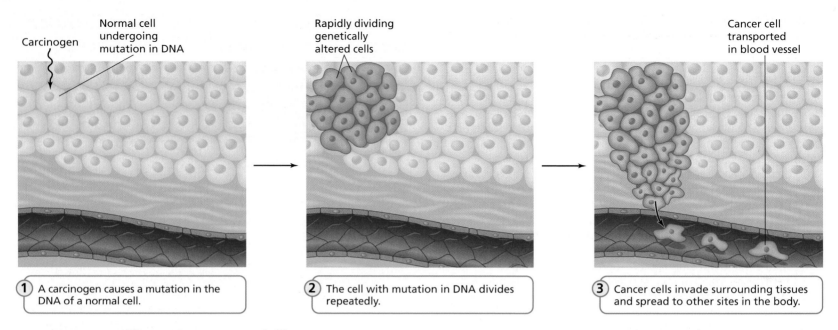

| Carcinogen — Normal cell undergoing mutation in DNA | Rapidly dividing genetically altered cells | Cancer cell transported in blood vessel |

① A carcinogen causes a mutation in the DNA of a normal cell.

② The cell with mutation in DNA divides repeatedly.

③ Cancer cells invade surrounding tissues and spread to other sites in the body.

FIGURE 12.10 Progression of Cancer.

Source: From Thompson, Janice; Manore, Melinda; and Vaughan, Linda. *The Science of Nutrition*, 3rd ed, p. 413. © 2014. Reprinted and electronically reproduced by permission of Pearson Education, Inc., Upper Saddle River, NJ.

If growth-control genes are irreparably damaged, they become cancer-causing **oncogenes,** issuing faulty orders for accelerated cell growth. As cells begin reproducing out of control, they form clusters of immature cells that serve no purpose. Their only function is to keep multiplying. Such clusters of cells eventually form clumps of abnormal tissue called **tumors.**

Not all tumors are cancerous. **Benign tumors** grow very slowly, do not invade surrounding tissues, and do not spread to other parts of the body. In contrast, **malignant tumors** are by definition cancerous **(Figure 12.10).** They invade surrounding tissue, and their cells can break away and enter the bloodstream or lymphatic system, where they circulate and find new places to take root. This aggressive spreading process, called **metastasis,** makes malignant tumors far more dangerous. When malignant cells have metastasized throughout the body, the cancer is far more challenging to treat.

It's important to note that, whereas cancer can spread throughout the body, it cannot be spread from person to person. Although certain cancer-associated viruses, such as HIV or hepatitis, are contagious, cancer itself is not.

Risk Factors for Cancer

Given the complex series of interactions involved in cancer, it's no surprise that many different factors can influence cancer risk. These include genetic and biological factors, lifestyle factors, environmental exposure to carcinogens, and exposure to infectious agents. To get a sense of your level of risk, complete the nearby **Self-Assessment.**

Genetic and Biological Factors

As you've learned, cancer is fundamentally a disease of the DNA. It involves not only the genes that

oncogene A mutated gene that encourages the uncontrolled cell division that results in cancer.

tumor An abnormal growth of tissue with no physiological function.

benign tumor A tumor that grows slowly, does not spread, and is not cancerous.

malignant tumor A tumor that grows aggressively, invades surrounding tissue, and can spread to other parts of the body; all cancers are malignant.

metastasis The process by which a malignant tumor spreads to other body sites.

become damaged in cancer, but other genes involved in preventing this damage.

Some types of cancer run in families or are more common in certain ethnic groups. These include breast, ovarian, colon, prostate, stomach, skin, and lung cancers. But researchers are learning that these cancers are rarely due to a "cancer-causing gene." Instead, in many cases, such as with breast and ovarian cancer, the inherited risk is more closely linked to weaker versions of genes that normally suppress tumor formation.[43] People who inherit a weaker version of a suppressor gene are more likely to develop cancer if they encounter carcinogens.

Cancer can also be related to biological factors, such as the body's hormones. This is especially true for women. The age at which a woman had her first period and entered menopause, along with whether she used hormonal birth control, or had children (and if so, at what age) all factor into her risk for breast cancer.

Lifestyle Factors

When you think about the vegetables you eat, do you picture a colorful salad or a bag of fries? How often do you exercise? Are your BMI and waist size within a healthful range? Do you smoke, or spend time with someone who does? Do you drink alcohol, and if so, how much?

The same basic lifestyle choices that are important in CMR also affect your risk of cancer. We identify healthy lifestyle choices later in this chapter.

Environmental Exposure to Carcinogens

Do you like to tan? Do you have a job that involves working with chemicals or radiation, or live in an area with high levels of air pollution? If so, you may be exposing your body—and your DNA—to carcinogens on a regular basis. Some of these risks are more a matter of personal choice and are easier

SELF-ASSESSMENT
Am I at Risk for Cancer?

Next to each statement, check the answer that applies to you.

1. I eat a variety of vegetables and fruits every day.
   ☐ Always   ☐ Sometimes   ☐ Never

2. I choose whole-grain foods (breads, pastas, and cereals), rather than foods made from refined grains. I also choose brown rice instead of white rice.
   ☐ Always   ☐ Sometimes   ☐ Never

3. I avoid excess dietary fat.
   ☐ Always   ☐ Sometimes   ☐ Never

4. I choose foods rich in omega-3 fatty acids, such as salmon, canned tuna, and other fatty fish.
   ☐ Always   ☐ Sometimes   ☐ Never

5. If I eat red meat, I choose lean cuts and eat smaller portions.
   ☐ Always   ☐ Sometimes   ☐ Never

6. I prepare meat, poultry, and fish by baking, broiling, or poaching rather than by frying, barbecuing, or grilling over a flame.
   ☐ Always   ☐ Sometimes   ☐ Never

7. I limit my intake of processed meats containing nitrates, such as bacon, ham, deli meats, and hot dogs.
   ☐ Always   ☐ Sometimes   ☐ Never

8. I get at least 150 minutes of moderate intensity or 75 minutes of vigorous intensity activity each week (or a combination of these), preferably spread throughout the week.
   ☐ Always   ☐ Sometimes   ☐ Never

9. I limit sedentary behavior such as sitting, watching TV, and other screen-based entertainment.
   ☐ Always   ☐ Sometimes   ☐ Never

10. I have maintained a healthy weight at all ages.
    ☐ Always   ☐ Sometimes   ☐ Never

11. I avoid tobacco in all its forms.
    ☐ Always   ☐ Sometimes   ☐ Never

12. I drink no more than one drink a day if I'm a woman or two drinks a day if I'm a man.
    ☐ Always   ☐ Sometimes   ☐ Never

13. I avoid intense sunlight, or when in the sun, I wear protective clothing and a UVA and UVB sunscreen.
    ☐ Always   ☐ Sometimes   ☐ Never

14. I am not exposed to environmental carcinogens (chemicals, radiation, airborne particles, air pollution, secondhand smoke, or pesticides) through work or at home.
    ☐ Always   ☐ Sometimes   ☐ Never

15. I have access to quality health care and receive regular examinations by a health-care provider.
    ☐ Always   ☐ Sometimes   ☐ Never

16. If I am a woman, I have been vaccinated against HPV.
    ☐ Yes   ☐ No

17. I have never been sexually active or I have always practiced safer sex to avoid exposure to STIs that can promote cancer.
    ☐ Yes   ☐ No

Totals: _____ Always   _____ Sometimes   _____ Never   _____ Yes   _____ No

HOW TO INTERPRET YOUR SCORE

For questions 1–15, the more "Always" the better. For questions 16–17, each "No" answer increases your risk. Focus on improving the behaviors for which you selected "No," "Never," or "Sometimes." Those answers indicate that these are factors that can contribute to your risk of cancer. The **Choosing to** **Change Worksheet** at the end of the chapter will assist you in improving these areas.

To complete this Self-Assessment online, visit MasteringHealth™

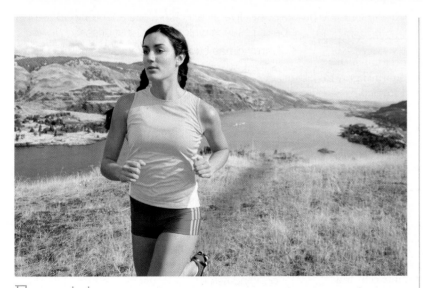

Exercising is one of the best things you can do to reduce your risk of cancer.

to control. For instance, you can opt to avoid sunbathing or visiting the tanning salon. But reducing your exposure to carcinogens in your workplace or neighborhood can be more challenging.

Many jobs involve working with chemicals or radiation, or produce airborne particles, such as wood dust from sanding, that are known carcinogens. Be sure you are aware of all safety procedures used at your workplace and follow them. State and federal laws lay out clear occupational safety requirements that companies must follow. If you devise your own summer job that requires you to work with chemicals—for instance, house painting, house cleaning, or landscaping—research the appropriate safety measures, such as wearing gloves and mask, and follow them!

>> **How safe is the environment at your summer job? Visit** www.osha.gov/SLTC/youth/summerjobs.

If you live in an area known for air pollution, you can start reducing your risks by paying attention to public service announcements identifying days when pollution levels are especially high and avoiding outdoor exercise during those times. If pollutants from nearby industry or a landfill or other waste site are a concern, or the safety of your public water supply is uncertain, consider getting involved in public pollution-reduction efforts. Many communities have environmental and health advocacy groups dedicated to reducing air, water, and land pollution.

Exposure to Infectious Agents

Certain infectious microorganisms are known carcinogens. Researchers theorize that they trigger cancer by causing persistent inflammation, suppressing a person's immune system, or stimulating cells into extended periods of growth. In the United States, some of the more common cancer-causing infectious agents include the following viruses:

- **Hepatitis B and C.** These forms of the hepatitis virus can lead to liver cancer.[41]

- **HIV.** This virus, in suppressing the immune system, can lead to certain types of cancer that are otherwise rare. These are called *opportunistic* cancers because they occur when reduced immune defenses give them the opportunity to develop.

- **HPV.** The human papillomavirus, or HPV, is usually transmitted through sexual contact. Nearly all women with cervical cancer have evidence of HPV, although not all cervical HPV infections turn into cancer. A vaccine is now available that increases immunity against certain strains of HPV associated with cervical cancer. You'll find more information on cervical cancer later in this chapter. HPV is also linked to a rise in cases of throat cancer, most likely due to transmission during oral sex.[41]

Detecting Cancer

Because cancer can occur in sites as varied as lungs, bones, and blood, no single test can detect all cancers. But an increasing variety of detection methods are allowing more cancers to be caught earlier, when they are easier to treat.

Some types of cancer can be found even before they cause any symptoms. Tests that "screen" large numbers of people to check for the presence of disease or conditions associated with disease are called *screening tests*. For instance, a colonoscopy is an examination of the colon (the large intestine) with a tiny camera. It allows a physician to find and remove precancerous growths called *polyps*. Screening tests are also used for many other types of cancer. Methods under development include screening tests that could analyze body fluids for signs of cancer-related DNA.

When cancer is suspected, either following the results of a screening test or because a patient has detected a suspicious mass, the physician may perform a **biopsy,** removing a small sample of the abnormal growth so that it can be studied for signs of cancer. In addition, lab tests of blood or other body fluids can check for the presence of substances called *tumor markers* that suggest cancer. Other detection methods rely on imaging technologies. These include ultrasound (US), magnetic resonance imaging (MRI), computed tomography (CT), and positron emission tomography (PET), each of which has advantages and disadvantages for different types of tissues.

You should also be aware of five general signs and symptoms that the American Cancer Society (ACS) identifies as common early indicators of cancer. Most often, these *are not due to cancer*.

biopsy A test for cancer in which a small sample of the abnormal growth is removed and studied.

carcinoma Cancer of tissues that line or cover the body.

sarcoma Cancer of muscle or connective tissues.

central nervous system cancer Cancer of the brain or spinal cord.

lymphoma Cancer of the lymphoid tissues.

myeloma Cancer arising in plasma cells, a type of immune cell, and invading the bone marrow.

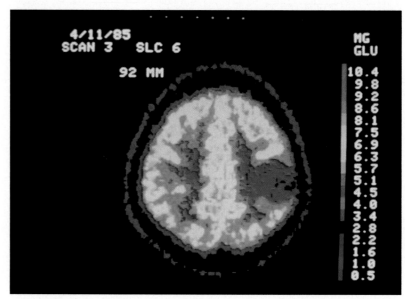

A PET scan of a cancerous growth in the brain. The cancer appears as the blue spot on the right.

However, if you notice any of them, and don't see an obvious reason for them, make an appointment with your doctor:[44]

- Unexplained weight loss
- Fever
- Fatigue
- Pain
- Skin changes, including darkened skin, yellowed skin and eyes (jaundice), reddened skin, itching, and excessive hair growth

Along with these general signs and symptoms, stay aware of changes in your health that may be due to specific cancers. For instance, a change in bowel habits is associated with colon cancer. Signs and symptoms of the most common types of cancer are identified ahead.

Types of Cancer

Cancers can be grouped into five broad categories according to the type of tissue in which the cancer arises:

- **Carcinomas** begin in the body's epithelial tissues, which include the skin and the tissues that line or cover internal organs. These are the most common sites for cancer, and cancers that occur here usually come in the form of solid tumors.

- **Sarcomas** start in the muscles, bones, fat, blood vessels, or other connective or supporting tissue. Sarcomas also take the form of solid tumors.

- **Central nervous system cancers** begin in the tissues of the brain and spinal cord. These form solid tumors and do damage both by directly altering nerve function and by growing large enough to interfere with the function of surrounding tissue.

- **Lymphomas** and **myelomas** involve different types of cells of the immune system.

Lymphomas form tumors that invade the lymphoid tissues (lymph nodes, spleen, and bone marrow), whereas myelomas invade the bone marrow.

- **Leukemias** start in the tissues that make your blood. This type of cancer does not cause solid tumors, instead filling the blood with abnormal blood cells.

Common Cancers in Men and Women

Although cancer can arise in hundreds of different sites in your body, some sites are far more prone to cancer than others. We'll start with a look at cancers that affect both men and women, and follow with a separate overview of common sex-specific cancers.

Skin Cancer

More than 2 million people develop skin cancer each year.[41] The vast majority of these cancers are treatable basal and squamous cell carcinomas, but about 76,000 are **malignant melanomas,** the most deadly form of skin cancer, which results in more than 9,000 deaths each year.[41]

Risk Factors. Risk factors for all forms of skin cancer include:[41]

- Fair skin and red or blonde hair.
- Skin that sunburns easily and does not tan easily.
- History of excessive sun exposure, including sunburns, or use of tanning beds.
- Past history of skin cancer.

In addition, malignant melanoma is more common in people who have a family history of melanoma or numerous (more than 50) moles.

What should you watch for? Less serious forms of skin cancer look like bumps, colored spots, or scaly patches on the skin. These may bleed, itch, or ooze. In contrast, melanoma may arise as a new mole or other skin lesion or changes to an existing one. When examining any mole, use the ABCD acronym shown in **Figure 12.11** to help you remember the signs to look for.[41] Some sources add a fifth letter, E, for

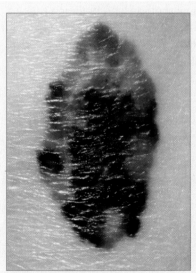

Asymmetry, where one side does not match the other.

Border irregularity, where edges are uneven or scalloped.

Color changes, where pigmentation is not uniform.

Diameter, where the size is more than 6 millimeters (about the size of a pea).

Evolving, where the appearance is changing in size, shape, or color over time.

FIGURE 12.11 Malignant Melanoma. This lesion shows the distinctive characteristics of malignant melanoma, the deadliest form of skin cancer.

STUDENT STORY

Surviving Cancer

"HI, MY NAME IS AMANDA. I'm 19. I was diagnosed with acute lymphocytic leukemia at the age of 13. I was on chemo for about 3 years, had two surgeries, and had to miss about 2 years of school. The surgeries affected me socially because I basically had plastic tubes in my chest, so it was hard to give people hugs. People didn't understand, you know, when they would try to hug me—I'd be like, 'Oh you can't hug me, I'm a little bit fragile right here.' I've been in remission since 2007. I go for blood tests all the time just to make sure it hasn't come back.

My mother had breast cancer and shortly after she was in remission, she was diagnosed with ovarian cancer. Also, my mother's mother died of breast cancer, and her sister, my great-aunt, died of leukemia. So we have a lot of cancer in the females in our family.

I go for mammograms fairly regularly. I would say at least once a year. I am pretty young to be getting mammograms but I probably should be going about twice a year because the frequency of cancer in my family is so high."

1. If you were friends with Amanda when she was undergoing cancer treatment, how could you have supported her?

2. Do you have a family history of cancer? If so, are you taking extra precautions such as scheduling regular cancer screenings?

evolving. That is, the lesion changes in size, shape, or color over the course of about a month. If you notice any of these skin changes, see your doctor as soon as possible.

If you have a family history of melanoma, many doctors recommend a yearly skin exam from a dermatologist. Otherwise, regular screenings are not necessary. But everyone's risk begins to increase at age 20, so it's a good idea to check your skin periodically for signs of change.

Reducing Your Risk. Especially for people with fair skin, lots of unprotected sun exposure equals higher risks. Avoid extended time in the sun without a hat, protective clothing, and/or high sun protection factor (SPF) sunscreen. Avoid tanning, which is linked to an increased risk of melanoma and other forms of skin cancer. Tanning beds are classified as carcinogenic.[41] They emit doses of ultraviolet (UV) radiation far more powerful than those that come from the sun, and are associated with a 75% increased risk of melanoma. In 2013, the FDA proposed new regulations that would require tanning beds to have labels warning consumers of their dangers. The FDA is also considering banning the use of tanning beds by consumers under age 18.[45]

Lung Cancer

With more than 228,000 new cases diagnosed each year, lung cancer is the third most

leukemia Cancer of blood-forming tissue.

malignant melanoma An especially aggressive form of skin cancer.

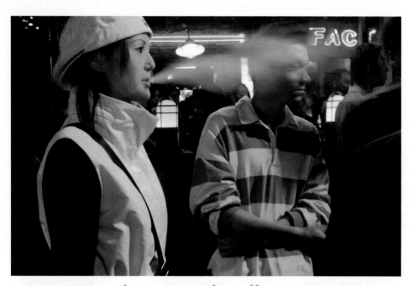

Lung cancer is the most deadly cancer in the United States, and smoking is its largest risk factor. Consider that before you light up.

common malignancy in the United States. Moreover, it accounts for nearly 160,000 deaths, which is more than 27% of all deaths from cancer.[41]

Risk Factors. Risk factors for lung cancer include:

- A history of smoking or being exposed to secondhand smoke. The longer you've smoked or been exposed to tobacco smoke, the higher your risk.
- Exposure to radon. In some areas, this naturally occurring radioactive gas exists in high concentrations in the soil and, over time, seeps into people's homes or water supplies. Radon is estimated to cause about 21,000 lung cancer deaths each year.[46]
- Exposure to other cancer-causing substances, such as asbestos or arsenic.
- Genetic factors.

What should you watch for? By the time any of the following symptoms have appeared, a case of lung cancer is usually fairly advanced:

- Spitting up blood-streaked mucus.
- Chest pain.
- A persistent cough.
- Recurrent attacks of pneumonia or bronchitis.

So far, this cancer has proven very difficult to detect early, and there are no established general screening guidelines. CT scans have been found effective at catching the disease early in people at high risk, but given the risks of radiation exposure due to CT scans as well as a high level of false positive results, the ACS recommends shared clinician-patient decision-making on a case-by-case basis.[41]

Reducing Your Risk. Smoking or regular exposure to second-hand smoke remain the single largest risk factors for lung cancer. If you smoke, get started on a plan to quit and, in the meantime, keep your smoke away from others. In addition, check your home for radon. According to the U.S. Environmental Protection Agency, nearly 1 in 15 U.S. homes has elevated radon levels.[46] You can purchase an inexpensive test kit to check the air in your home. You can also talk to campus officials about

radon testing in campus buildings, and ask your employer for test results from your workplace.

Colorectal Cancer

More than 102,000 cases of colon cancer and 40,000 cases of rectal cancer are diagnosed each year in the United States. These result in the deaths of over 50,000 people annually, making colorectal cancer the second leading cause of cancer death overall.[41]

Risk Factors. Risk factors for colorectal cancer include:

- A family history of colorectal cancer.
- A family history of polyps, or precancerous growths, in the colon or rectum.
- Being over the age of 50.
- Presence of an inflammatory bowel disorder, such as colitis or Crohn's disease.

What should you watch for? In its early stages, when it is easiest to treat, colorectal cancer often has no outward symptoms. As the cancer progresses, warning signs include bleeding from the rectum, blood in the stool, and changes in bowel habits.

Screening is recommended for everyone once they reach the age of 50, using methods that include:

- A yearly test that detects blood in the stool.
- Every 5 to 10 years, an internal imaging test that looks for polyps, such as a colonoscopy.
- For people at higher risk, such as those with a family history of colorectal cancer, doctors usually recommend a more frequent screening schedule.

Reducing Your Risk. The following measures may help to prevent colorectal cancer:

- Engaging in regular exercise.
- Consuming a diet rich in fiber and plant-based foods.
- Maintaining a healthy weight.
- Limiting alcohol consumption.
- Avoiding smoking.
- Following recommended screening guidelines because precancerous polyps can be removed during colonoscopy, and cancerous tumors can often be surgically removed if caught at earlier stages.

Pancreatic Cancer

Pancreatic cancer is one of the most deadly types of cancer. Most patients die within the first year of diagnosis, and just 6% survive for five years.[41] There are approximately 45,000 cases diagnosed each year, and over 38,000 deaths.[41] The poor prognosis (estimated outcome) is due in part to the fact that pancreatic cancer typically goes undetected until it has advanced beyond the point at which treatment can be effective.

Risk Factors. Risk factors for pancreatic cancer include:

- Smoking and use of smokeless tobacco.
- Obesity.
- Diabetes.
- Chronic pancreatitis (inflammation of the pancreas).
- Genetic factors.

Also, there is some evidence that eating a diet high in red or processed meats increases the risk for pancreatic cancer.

What should you watch for? Signs of pancreatic cancer rarely appear until the disease is advanced. These include:

- Abdominal discomfort and/or mid-back pain.
- Jaundice, or a yellowing of your skin and the whites of your eyes.
- Unexplained weight loss.

Currently, no standard screening guidelines exist for pancreatic cancer. Researchers are looking for ways to detect this cancer early and determine who would benefit most from screening.

Reducing Your Risk. Reduce your risk by following basic health guidelines, which include:

- Not using any form of tobacco.
- Maintaining a healthy weight.
- Eating a healthy diet and exercising regularly.

Oral Cancer

About 41,000 malignancies of the lips, tongue, mouth, and throat are diagnosed each year, and about 7,900 deaths result from oral cancers.[41]

Risk Factors. Risk factors include:

- Smoking and use of smokeless tobacco.
- Excessive drinking. Combining heavy drinking and smoking is linked to a 30-fold increased risk.[41]
- HPV infection.

What should you watch for? Symptoms include:

- A sore that doesn't heal **(Figure 12.12)**.
- Red or white patches that don't heal or go away.
- An unexplained lump or thickening in the mouth, throat, or neck.
- Ear pain.
- Coughing up blood.

Although there are no general screening guidelines, doctors and dentists usually make checking for oral cancer a routine part of any regular exam.

Reducing Your Risk. The best strategies are to avoid all types of tobacco products and excessive drinking and to use a dental dam or similar protection if engaging in oral sex.

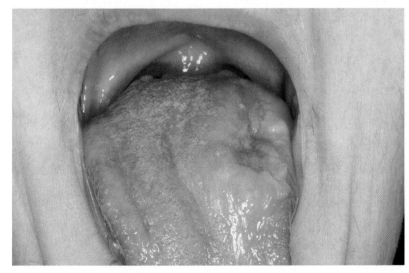

FIGURE 12.12 Oral Cancer.

Common Cancers in Men

Cancers affecting the male reproductive system include prostate cancer and testicular cancer. Although both are common, prostate cancer tends to occur in older men, whereas testicular cancer more commonly develops in younger men.

Prostate Cancer

The prostate is a gland in the male reproductive system that secretes a fluid that assists in the movement of sperm. It is located below the bladder. Prostate cancer is the most commonly diagnosed malignancy among men in the United States and the second most deadly. Over 238,000 cases are diagnosed each year, resulting in nearly 30,000 deaths.[41]

Risk Factors. Risk factors include:

- Age: 97% of cases occur in men over 50.
- Race. African American men are more likely to be diagnosed with prostate cancer and are more likely to have an aggressive form.
- Family history.
- Diet. A diet high in processed meats or dairy foods may increase risk.

What should you watch for? Detecting prostate cancer in its early stages can be difficult. Symptoms tend to develop in the disease's later stages, and may include:

- Difficulty urinating.
- The urge to urinate frequently.
- Blood in the urine.
- Pain or burning with urination.

Reducing Your Risk. There is no conclusive evidence of lifestyle changes that can lower your risk. Men over age 50 should speak with their health-care provider about whether or not it is advisable to have a prostate screening test (a PSA test). African American men should have this discussion at age 45.[41]

Testicular Cancer

Testicular cancer is one of the most common malignancies in young men. About 7,900 men are diagnosed with it each year, and about 370 will die from it.[41]

Risk Factors. The risk factors for testicular cancer include:

- Being a white male between the ages of 20 and 39.
- Having a family history of cancer.
- A history of an undescended testicle; that is, a testicle that did not descend from the abdomen into the scrotum before birth. The risk of cancer is increased for both testicles and remains whether or not the individual has had surgery to move the testicle into place.

Reducing Your Risk. Because researchers still haven't uncovered the cause of testicular cancer, the most effective preventions aren't yet clear. Testicular self-exams can aid in detection (see the **Spotlight** on page 310), but there is no definitive evidence that they lead to a reduction in deaths from testicular cancer, and the ACS has no recommendation regarding them. If you are concerned about testicular cancer or have a family history of it, consult your doctor for advice on what to do.

Common Cancers in Women

The most common cancers affecting the female reproductive system include breast cancer, ovarian cancer, and cervical and uterine cancers.

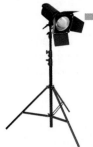

SPOTLIGHT
Testicular Self-Exam

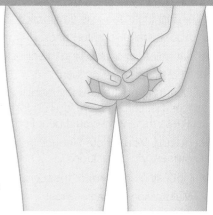

Some men are at increased risk for testicular cancer. These include men with an undescended testicle, previous testicular cancer, or a family member who has had this cancer. If you have such a risk, discuss it with your health-care provider and ask whether or not you should be performing regular testicular self-exam (TSE). Medical experts do not recommend doing regular

TSE if you are not in a high-risk group.

Here are instructions on how to perform TSE if you and your health-care provider decide that this is right for you:

If you choose to do TSE, timing is important. Perform the exam during or after a shower, when the skin of the scrotum is warm and relaxed. While standing:

- Feel your scrotal sac until you find one testicle.

- Hold the testicle with one hand while firmly but gently rolling the fingers of the other hand over the testicle as shown in the figure. Examine its entire surface.

- Repeat the procedure on the other testicle.

The epididymis of a normal testis feels like a small "bump" on the side of the testis. Normal testicles also contain blood vessels

and other structures. It's easy to confuse these with cancer. If you have any doubts, see a doctor.

Source: Adapted from *Testicular Self-Examination*, by the National Library of Medicine's MedlinePlus website, 2011. http://www.nlm.nih.gov.

Breast Cancer

With more than 230,000 new cases and 40,000 deaths each year, breast cancer is the most common cancer among women in the United States and the second leading cause of cancer death in women.[41] Although more women are surviving breast cancer, prevention, detection, and treatment remain a top health concern.

Risk Factors. Risk factors include:

- A family history of breast cancer, on either side of your family.
- Genetics. About 5–10% of cases of breast cancer occur in women with an abnormal variant of tumor suppressor genes identified as *BRCA1* and *BRCA2.* Normal versions of these genes appear to offer protection from cancer.
- Menstrual periods that started early and ended late in life.
- Use of hormonal medications, such as birth control pills or hormone replacement therapy.
- Being overweight or obese (for postmenopausal women).
- Never having children, or having your first child after age 30.
- Heavy, long-term smoking.
- Alcohol consumption.

What should you watch for? Symptoms usually include changes in breast tissue, such as:

- A lump or thickening in your breast or in the lymph nodes under your arm.
- Dimpling, skin distortion, or skin irritation.
- Unusual nipple appearance or discharge.

Reducing Your Risk. A healthy lifestyle—including maintaining a healthful weight, limiting alcohol use, and regularly exercising—is a great starting point for any woman who wants to reduce her risk. Women who breast-feed for several months may have added

protection, and women who do not use postmenopausal hormone therapy may also lower their risk.[41]

Women whose family histories put them at increased risk should talk to their doctors about what to do. A doctor may advocate mammograms or other screenings at an earlier age, or even genetic testing. Women at especially high risk may consider *chemoprevention* (the use of drugs to reduce cancer risk), or in the most extreme cases, surgical mastectomy to reduce their cancer risk.

The ACS recommends that women in their 20s and 30s have a clinical breast exam at least once every three years, and at least once a year once they are over 40. The ACS recommends annual mammograms for women aged 40 and older. Breast self-exams (BSE) are optional because they have both benefits and limitations.[47] Women are advised to talk with their health-care provider about whether or not to perform BSE. See the **Spotlight** on page 312 for instructions.

Ovarian Cancer

Over 22,000 women are diagnosed with ovarian cancer each year, and 14,000 die from it.[41] Ovarian cancer causes more deaths among women than any other cancer of the female reproductive system. Like pancreatic cancer, it is usually advanced before it is detected.

Risk Factors. Risk factors for ovarian cancer include:

- A family history of ovarian cancer or breast cancer.
- Mutations in the BRCA 1 or BRCA 2 genes.
- Age. Ovarian cancer most often develops in women after menopause.
- Never having children.
- Infection that leads to pelvic inflammatory disease.
- Obesity.
- Use of estrogen-only hormone replacement therapy.

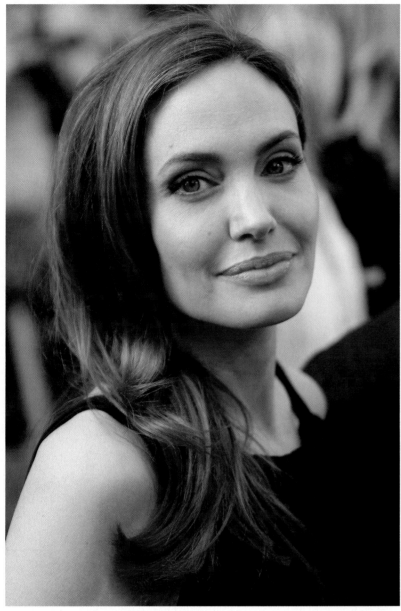

Angelina Jolie opted to have a preventive double mastectomy when she learned that she carries the BRCA1 gene, which increases her risk for breast and ovarian cancer.

Symptoms of ovarian cancer are nonspecific and mimic other common conditions, like bladder and digestive disorders, which can make diagnosis difficult. Women with ovarian cancer are more likely to have a feeling of abdominal pressure, swelling, or bloating; urination urgency; feeling full quickly after eating; and pelvic discomfort or pain.

Reducing Your Risk. Women between the ages of 35 to 40 who have gene mutations and a strong history of cancer may elect to have their ovaries removed. This, however, is a very important personal decision and the pros and cons should be discussed in depth with a physician.

Cervical and Uterine Cancers

About 80% of the approximately 62,000 cases of these cancers each year arise in the lining of the uterus, or endometrium.[41] The rest arise in the cervix, at the base of the uterus. Uterine cancer results in

approximately 8,000 deaths each year, and cervical cancer results in approximately 4,000 deaths.[41]

Risk Factors. The risk factors for endometrial cancer are factors that increase the woman's exposure to estrogen. These include obesity, estrogen-only hormonal replacement therapy, late menopause, and never having children. The cause of cervical cancer is persistent infection with certain strains of HPV.[41] Other risk factors include smoking and long-term use of oral contraceptives.

What should you watch for? Signs include unexplained vaginal bleeding or discharge. Cervical cancer can also cause pain during sex. However, in most cases, it develops silently. That's why a Pap test, performed during a woman's pelvic exam, is the most effective way to check for cervical cancer. This swab of the cervix is used to look for precancerous cell changes. An HPV DNA test, which detects the presence of HPV strains associated with cancer, is also available.

The ACS recommends the following screening schedule:[41]

- Have your first Pap test at age 21.
- Continue getting tested every three years through age 29. From ages 30 to 65, continue screening every five years using both the Pap test and the HPV test, or every three years if using the Pap test only. After age 65, if previous tests have been negative, screening may no longer be necessary.

Reducing Your Risk. Two vaccines, Gardasil and Cervarix, are available for the prevention of the most common types of HPV that cause cervical cancer. Gardasil is also protective against HPV associated with anal cancer and is recommended by the ACS for both males and females ages 9 through 26.[41] After age 26, talk to your doctor about vaccination.

The HPV vaccines do not protect against all carcinogenic strains, so it's also essential to practice safer sex. If you have male partners, use a condom.

Treating Cancer

Over many decades, cancer treatment has evolved into a variety of methods that attempt to remove or shrink malignant tumors and impede metastasis:[48]

- Surgery offers the greatest chance for cure, especially if performed before the cancer has metastasized.
- Chemotherapy is the use of potent drugs to kill cancer cells, slow their growth, or keep them from spreading. It can also be used to relieve pain and other symptoms caused by a tumor.
- Radiation therapy uses high-energy subatomic particles or waves to damage or destroy cancer cells.
- Targeted therapy uses drugs or other substances to precisely locate and attack cancer cells with less damage to surrounding, healthy tissues.
- Immunotherapy (also called biologic therapy) either stimulates the patient's immune system to increase its effectiveness against cancer cells, or directly administers immune system proteins.

Many other types of treatment, including heat, light, and stem cell transplants, are also used, and more are in development.

Change Yourself, Change Your World

If you're feeling discouraged about your chance of developing a chronic disease, notice that all nine CMR factors are modifiable—meaning they

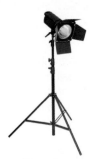

Breast Awareness and Self-Exam

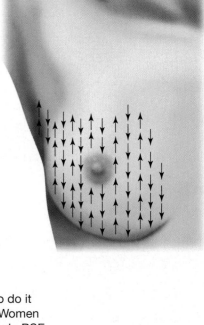

Experts agree that women should be aware of how their breasts normally look and feel. This is known as breast awareness. In contrast, there is no agreement about whether or not women should perform breast self-exam (BSE). This lack of consensus reflects uncertainty about what role BSE might play in finding breast cancer or saving lives. So a first step is to talk with your health-care provider about whether or not BSE is right for you.

If you choose to do BSE, timing is important. Most women's breasts are not as tender or lumpy about 3 to 5 days after their menstrual period begins, so this is a good time to examine them. If you've gone through menopause, do BSE on the same day of each month.

The following is a two-step approach including examination by touch and visual inspection. After you've become comfortable with BSE, have your health-care provider review your technique during your next routine exam.

**Step One:
Examination by Touch**

- Lie on your back. It is easier to feel the breast tissue if you are lying down.
- Place your right hand behind your head. With the middle fingertips of your left hand, gently yet firmly press down using small motions to examine the tissue of the right breast. Use a pattern like the one shown in the figure to make sure you're covering all of your breast tissue.
- Next, sit or stand. Palpate your armpit because breast tissue goes into that area.
- Gently squeeze the nipple, checking for discharge.
- Repeat the process on the left breast.

**Step Two:
Visual Inspection**
Stand in front of a mirror with your arms by your side. Look at your breasts both directly and in the mirror for:

- changes in skin texture, such as dimpling, puckering, indentations, or skin that looks like an orange peel.
- changes in the shape and contour of each breast.
- changes in the nipple, e.g., check to see if the nipple turns inward.

Do the same with your arms raised above your head.

Remember, it is acceptable for women to opt not to do BSE or to do it only occasionally. Women who choose not to do BSE should still know how their breasts normally look and feel and report any concerns to their health-care provider.

Source: Adapted from *Breast Self-Exam,* by the National Library of Medicine's MedlinePlus website, 2012. http://www.nlm.nih.gov.

---

are within your power to change! And many of the same healthy behaviors that reduce your CMR can reduce your risk for cancer as well. The sooner you start, the better for your body.

Personal Choices

Several large-scale research studies have identified proven steps you can take to reduce your risk for chronic disease. For example, two recent studies have shown that people who practice most of the following healthy lifestyle behaviors have a 65–70% reduced CMR.[49,50] If they sound familiar—they should! Although researchers link these behaviors specifically to CMR reduction, they're the same choices we've been advocating throughout this text to benefit every aspect of your life.

Don't Smoke

If you smoke, get the help you need to quit. Start with a visit to your campus health center. Do it *today.* As you've just learned, the ingredients in tobacco smoke constrict and irritate artery walls, trigger inflammation, promote atherosclerosis, and increase blood pressure. Moreover, smoking causes many types of cancer and is directly responsible for 80% to 90% of all lung cancer deaths. Overall, smoking causes one out of every five deaths that occurs in the United States each year.[51] (For more information on smoking cessation, see Chapter 8.)

Shed Any Extra Pounds

If you're overweight or obese, shedding even a few pounds can reduce your CMR. But remember to watch more than the number on the scale. Aim for a waist measurement of less than 40 inches if you are a man or less than 35 inches if you are a woman. And keep your BMI within the range for normal weight (18.5 to 24.9). We can't all hit an ideal weight or body shape and freeze ourselves there. But we can all work to stay within a weight range that is healthy and right for our body type.

Eat Right

To reduce your risk for chronic disease, choose meals built around fruits, legumes and other vegetables, and whole grains, with occasional fish and poultry. These meals provide vitamins and minerals, complex carbohydrates, essential fatty acids, lots of fiber, antioxidant phytochemicals, and low levels of sodium and saturated fat. Several studies support the wisdom of limiting consumption of red and processed meats to reduce your risk for both chronic disease and premature death.[52,53,54]

An eating plan that has consistently been found to reduce chronic disease risk is the Mediterranean diet. The foods that are basic to this plan include legumes and other vegetables, fruits, whole grains, nuts, olives, and olive oil, along with some cheese, yogurt, fish, poultry, eggs, and wine.

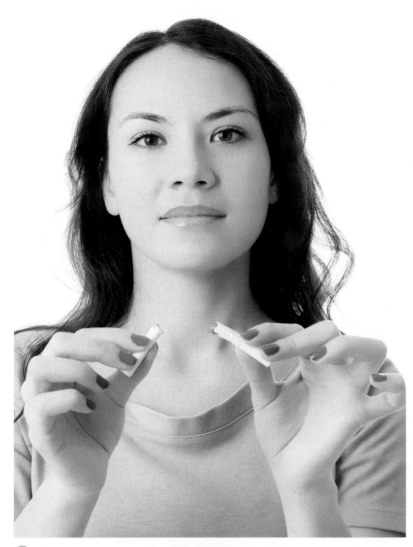

Quit. Not smoking is one of the best things you can do to reduce your cardiometabolic risk.

A large 2013 study specifically supported the health benefits of adopting a Mediterranean diet.[55] The **Practical Strategies** box on page 314 has specific suggestions for dietary changes that reduce the risk for chronic disease.

 Download a poster identifying the main elements and benefits of the Mediterranean diet at http://meddietexperience.weebly.com/mediterranean-diet-poster.html.

Get Moving

You've learned that obesity is a risk factor for diabetes, CVD, and many types of cancer. Physical activity burns calories and helps you control your weight. A study of obese adults found that those who followed a weight-loss diet and engaged in a program of physical activity lost more weight on average (24 pounds) than those who only followed the diet (18 pounds).[56] In addition, regular physical activity helps control blood glucose levels and strengthens the heart, resulting in a reduction in CMR.[57] Moreover, the ACS recommends a minimum of 30 minutes of moderate exercise 5 days a week to reduce the risk of cancer.[58] A recent review study suggests that exercise both reduces the risk of cancer and improves cancer prognosis by modulating chemical pathways involved in cancer progression.[59]

If you aren't exercising right now, aim for the ACS recommended minimum of 30 minutes of physical activity 5 days a week. If you already meet that level, start slowly increasing the intensity and duration of your workouts. Remember to balance cardiorespiratory fitness, or activities that build heart and lung capacity, with strength training. (For more information on physical activity, see Chapter 5.)

Limit Your Alcohol Intake

You know that heavy drinking is bad for your health overall. It is also bad for your cardiovascular health and increases your risk for many types of cancer. One study of college students found that those on their way to developing hypertension were also far more likely to drink heavily.[60] Another study associated heavy drinking in young adulthood with a significantly increased CMR later in life—even among those who had stopped drinking entirely by middle adulthood.[61] And public health organizations worldwide now classify alcoholic beverages as human carcinogens: A landmark analytical study of epidemiological data found that alcohol consumption, even at moderate levels (1.5 drinks per day or less) results in 3–4% of all U.S. cancer deaths.[62] Moreover, the latest evaluations by the World Health Organization, the World Cancer Research Fund, and the American Institute for Cancer Research support the conclusion that "there is no level of alcohol consumption for which cancer risk is null."[63]

Get Enough Sleep

We noted earlier that chronic short sleep is linked to high blood pressure and poor blood lipids.[34,35] Aim for 8 hours of sleep a night.

Maintain Dental Hygiene

Although a link between gum disease and CVD has been proposed for decades, a recent expert panel from the American Heart Association found no causative association distinct from that of risk factors common to both, such as smoking. However, the panel did find that the systemic inflammation common in gum disease has a short-term negative effect on blood vessel functioning, so daily brushing and flossing is still good advice.[64] Moreover, a dentist is often the first to spot signs of oral cancer, so don't skip your check-ups.

Manage Your Emotions

A large review study concluded that people who anger easily and are prone to hostility have a significantly increased risk for heart disease.[65] Moreover, the National Cancer Institute reports that, although psychological stress has not been shown to directly cause cancer, it can weaken the immune system.[66] So if you need help managing your anger or stress levels, get it. (See Chapter 2 for information on psychological resources.)

Reduce Environmental Risks

Many air, water, and land pollutants are carcinogenic. Find out what pollutants you might be exposed to, and take steps to reduce your risk. Remember that one of the most harmful pollutants is tobacco smoke, so if you live with a smoker, insist that he or she take it outside.

Offset Your Non-Modifiable Risk Factors

Do you know your family's history of diabetes, CVD, and cancer? If not, ask. Becoming aware of inherited risks is important because it allows you to discuss them with your health-care provider and to take steps, such as improving your diet and exercise habits, to reduce those risks.

Get Screened

Take advantage of visits to your primary health-care provider to have your blood glucose, blood pressure, and blood lipids measured, and to talk to your health-care provider about any recommended cancer

Practical Strategies

Making healthy diet choices can substantially reduce your chronic-disease risk. Here are a few suggestions:

- **Fill your plate with plants.** Eat meat less often and, when you do, keep the portion small and load your plate with vegetables. Avoid fatty and processed meats like pepperoni, bacon, sausage, low-grade ground beef, and luncheon meats. With fried or barbecued meats, remove any blackened regions because carcinogenic chemicals build up in these areas. Several times a week, replace meat entirely with plant-based protein choices such as beans, lentils, tofu, and tempeh.

- **Put some color in your diet.** All sorts of colorful fruits and vegetables, from apples and blueberries to black beans and sweet potatoes, contain phytochemicals associated with a reduced risk for chronic disease. You don't need to carry around a detailed list of foods to find them—just aim for a mix of colors.

- **Boost your consumption of omega-3 fatty acids.** Fatty fish such as salmon provides EPA and DHA, two omega-3 fatty acids known to reduce triglyceride levels, inflammation, and arterial plaque formation. The 2010 *Dietary Guidelines for Americans* suggests that you eat fish at least twice a week.

- **Replace high-fat dairy foods.** Choose nonfat or low-fat versions of milk, yogurt, cheese, and other dairy products, or choose soy milk or another milk alternative. Replace butter with *trans* fat–free margarine, peanut butter or another nut butter, and plant oils.

- **Fill up on fiber.** Fiber not only helps you feel full and eat less, but can help slow the release of glucose into your bloodstream as well as reduce arterial inflammation, blood pressure, and blood levels of LDL cholesterol. Whole grain breads and cereals and fresh fruits and vegetables are good sources.

- **Decrease your sodium intake.** Cut back on processed foods, which tend to contain a great deal of sodium. One serving of regular canned soup, for example, can contain almost half of a day's recommended allowance of sodium. Opt for fresh foods when possible, or choose low-sodium versions of prepared foods.

- **Eat yogurt.** Yogurt and other fermented dairy products contain *probiotics*, strains of bacteria beneficial to human health. By reducing blood vessel inflammation, for example, they reduce the formation of atherosclerotic plaque in arteries. Probiotics also create acids that disrupt the liver's production of cholesterol, and actually break down and consume cholesterol for food. Blend with fresh fruit for an even more nutritious treat.

- **Go organic.** Choose organic meats, eggs, dairy, and produce more often to reduce your overall exposure to pesticides, some of which are carcinogens. When you can't find organic produce, or it's just too pricey, scrub it under running water to reduce the pesticide level, then peel it if possible. Remove the outer leaves of lettuces. In addition, trim off the fatty parts of meats, where carcinogenic residues called dioxins build up.

- **What about alcohol?** A moderate alcohol intake—no more than two drinks per day for males and one drink per day for females—increases levels of HDL cholesterol while decreasing LDL cholesterol; it also reduces the risk of abnormal clot formation in the blood vessels. However, alcohol packs 7 calories per gram, more than either protein or carbohydrate, and calories from alcohol tend to be stored in the abdomen. Also, alcohol in any amount is a known human carcinogen. So go easy.

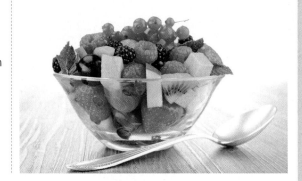

---

screenings. If you don't have a care provider, stop in at your campus health center and ask about the screenings you need.

Supporting a Friend with a Chronic Disease

If you're healthy, it can be tough to know how to support people you care about who may be struggling with diabetes, heart disease, or cancer. Whether they've just been diagnosed, or have been coping with the disease for a long time, it's likely that they most would like to have someone to talk to about their challenges, fears, and dreams. Someone like you. How do you listen with your heart? And what do you say in return? Here are some tips:[67,68]

- **Listen.** If your friend wants to talk, be a good listener. Don't rush in to fill the silence, which can help the person focus and can even be comforting. Listen not just to what is said, but to how it's said.

- **Learn.** Again, if your friend wants to talk, invite him or her to tell you more about the condition—how it affects life day to day, what treatments seem helpful, and what the frustrations might be. Discover what you could do to help your friend by asking these simple questions:

  1. What is the hardest thing about having this condition?

  2. What do I and your other friends do that makes things a little easier? What do we do that makes things harder?

  3. What can I do to help that I'm not doing now?

- **Follow through.** Whether it's accompanying your friend on a medical visit or going for a walk together, do your best to provide the help your friend asks for. Most importantly, tell your friend that you want to be there for him or her and that she or he is not alone.

- **Share feelings, not advice.** How does your friend's situation affect you? Do you feel as if you can't indulge in a pastry whenever your friend with diabetes is around, or that you can't talk about your dreams for the future because your friend has a life-threatening cancer diagnosis? Opening up about such feelings can help clear the air and allow you and your friend to support each other. However, try to avoid giving advice. Even if you've struggled with the same illness yourself, everyone's journey is different. Accept that your friend needs your presence, not your advice, and that's enough.

- **Know when to get help.** If your friend is clearly not sticking to the treatment plan—for instance, if he or she is refusing to take prescribed medication or keep medical appointments, smoking, abusing alcohol, or binge-eating—consider the behavior a cry for help, and encourage your friend to get it. For example, offer to go with your friend to your campus health services center.

Campus Advocacy

Throughout this text, we've identified ways to promote a healthier campus environment—everything from advocating for more healthful food choices in dining halls and neighborhood restaurants to lobbying for a tobacco-free campus. Here, we discuss a few more ways you can address the problems of diabetes, CVD, and cancer:

- Most campus health centers sponsor special health-screening events offering free or very low-cost blood pressure checks and other screenings. Volunteering to help at such events is a great way to learn more about chronic disease risks and to meet staff and students. At the very least, take advantage of such screenings whenever they're offered!

- Find out the location of the AEDs on your campus, including in campus housing and in classrooms, labs, and other buildings you regularly use. If anyone were to suffer a sudden cardiac arrest on campus, that information could very well enable you to save the person's life.

- Next time it's offered on your campus, register for training in CPR. Both the American Red Cross and the American Heart Association commonly offer certification classes, which usually are just a few hours long, and held on an evening or a Saturday at very low cost.

- Ask for the results of radon testing in your dorm and classroom buildings, and if you see pesticides being used on campus lawns and gardens, research and recommend natural alternatives.

- Consider getting a group of students together to sponsor a road race or "walk-a-thon" to raise money for the American Diabetes Association, American Heart Association, or American Cancer Society. Or keep it simple: next time your birthday comes around, ask family members and friends to make their gift a donation to a cancer organization of your choice.

- If you have type 1 diabetes, contact your campus chapter of the College Diabetes Network. This group can provide information, peer support, and many other resources to help make managing your diabetes a little easier.

- Help college students coping with cancer by supporting the work of the National Collegiate Cancer Foundation (NCCF). The NCCF was founded in 2005 by Dan Waeger, who was a 22-year-old MBA student when he was diagnosed with cancer. The mission of the NCCF is to provide services and support to young adults with cancer who are pursuing higher education throughout their treatment and beyond. Waeger passed away in 2009, but his example challenges all of us to make a difference in the world.[69]

>> **To get involved in the work of the NCCF, visit** www.collegiatecancer.org.

>> **Watch videos of real students discussing cardiovascular disease, diabetes, and cancer at** MasteringHealth™

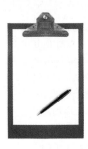

Choosing to Change Worksheet

To complete this worksheet online, visit MasteringHealth™

Remember that just four key behaviors can have a tremendous influence in increasing your risk for developing diabetes, cardiovascular disease, or cancer. They are (1) poor nutrition, (2) lack of physical activity, (3) tobacco use, and (4) excessive alcohol consumption.

Directions: Fill in your stage of change in Step 1 and complete Step 2 with your stage of change in mind. Then complete Steps 3, 4, or 5, depending on which ones apply to your stage of change.

Step 1: *Your Stage of Behavior Change.* Please check one of the following statements that best describes your readiness to reduce your chronic disease risk.

_____ I do not intend to reduce my chronic disease risk in the next six months. (Precontemplation)

_____ I might reduce my chronic disease risk in the next six months. (Contemplation)

_____ I am prepared to reduce my chronic disease risk in the next month. (Preparation)

_____ I have been reducing my chronic disease risk for less than six months. (Action)

_____ I have been reducing my chronic disease risk for more than six months. (Maintenance)

Step 2: *Recognizing Your Risk.* After reading through the chapter, what risk factors do you have for chronic disease? (Refer to pages 289–290, 299–301, and 304–306 to see all the risk factors, and remember the big four risk factors: poor nutrition, low physical activity, tobacco use, and alcohol use.) Next to each risk factor, indicate whether it is modifiable (you can change it) or not.

Risk Factor	Modifiable?

Step 3: *Precontemplation or Contemplation Stages.* What are some reasons to reduce your chronic disease risk factors?

_____

_____

Pick one or two of the **modifiable** risk factors from Step 2. What is holding you back from taking action on reducing your risk factors and how can you overcome these obstacles? Fill in the grid below.

Obstacle to Reducing Risk	How Can You Overcome It?

Step 4: *Preparation and Action Stages.* Some of the strategies for reducing your chronic disease risk from the chapter are:

- Don't smoke.
- Shed extra pounds.
- Eat right.
- Get moving (increase physical activity).
- Limit your alcohol intake.
- Get enough sleep.

- Maintain good oral hygiene.
- Practice safe sex.
- Wear sunscreen and avoid tanning beds.
- Get screened (monitor your blood pressure and blood lipids).

Select one recommendation that you feel highly confident in implementing and set a start date:_____

Set a **SMART goal** and write it down:_____
_____

Step 5: *Action and Maintenance Stages.* For one week, keep track of your progress in reducing your chronic disease risk. Evaluate your progress and explain whether or not you will modify your plan._____
_____

Chapter Summary

- Diabetes is a disorder in which blood glucose levels are consistently elevated above normal. It arises from problems with the body's production or use of insulin, a hormone secreted by the pancreas that assists the uptake of glucose by body cells.

- Type 1 diabetes develops when the body's own immune system destroys the beta cells in the pancreas that manufacture insulin. Type 2 diabetes develops when the body cells resist the effects of insulin. Other forms of diabetes include gestational diabetes and type 1.5.

- Poorly managed diabetes damages blood vessels throughout the body, leading to a variety of severe complications such as blindness, tissue death, and kidney failure.

- The cardiovascular system consists of the heart and blood vessels. It supplies the body with oxygen and nutrients and carries away wastes.

- The four most common forms of cardiovascular disease (CVD) are hypertension, coronary heart disease, congestive heart failure, and stroke. CVD is the top killer of men and women in the United States.

- Atherosclerosis is the development of plaque along the lining of an artery. It contributes to most forms of CVD.

- Hypertension is a blood pressure consistently higher than normal. It may produce no symptoms, but it greatly increases the risk for CVD.

- Coronary heart disease is characterized by atherosclerosis affecting a coronary artery. It can lead to angina (chest pain) and/or a heart attack or arrhythmia and sudden cardiac arrest.

- Congestive heart failure is an inability of the heart to pump blood effectively, causing blood to back up (congest) in the lungs or other body regions.

- Stroke is a blockage or rupture of a cerebral artery. Permanent brain damage or death can result.

- Cardiometabolic risk (CMR) is a cluster of nine modifiable factors—including obesity and smoking—that identify individuals at increased risk for type 2 diabetes and CVD.

- Cancer is the second most common cause of death in the United States. The term covers a wide group of diseases marked by uncontrolled growth of abnormal cells.

- Cancer begins when the DNA in body cells undergoes a mutation. As cells with mutated DNA multiply unchecked, a tumor forms. Malignant tumors begin to invade nearby tissues. Metastasis is the spread of cancer cells to sites distant from the original tumor.

- Skin cancer is the most common cancer, but only the least common form, malignant melanoma, tends to be invasive.

- Lung cancer is responsible for more than 150,000 deaths annually, more deaths than any other type of cancer. Colorectal cancer is the second most deadly overall, accounting for about 50,000 deaths annually.

- Although testicular cancer is the most common cancer in young males, prostate cancer is the most common cancer in men of all ages.

- A mutation in the BRCA1 or BRCA2 genes dramatically increases a woman's risk for breast cancer, the most common cancer in women, as well as for ovarian cancer. Together, breast and ovarian cancers are responsible for 20% of cancer deaths in women.

- Sexually transmitted infection with a carcinogenic strain of the human papillomavirus (HPV) is a direct cause of cervical cancer.

- Top strategies for reducing your risk for chronic disease include: Avoid all forms of tobacco; maintain a healthy weight; eat a nutritious diet; exercise regularly; limit consumption of alcohol; limit sun exposure; reduce your exposure to infection and toxic environmental chemicals; get adequate sleep; take care of your psychological health.

- Listening without an agenda, learning about your friend's situation, and following through on your offers to help are significant ways you can support a friend with a chronic disease.

GET CONNECTED

>> Visit the following websites for further information about the topics in this chapter:

- American Cancer Society
  www.cancer.org
- American Diabetes Association
  www.diabetes.org
- American Heart Association
  www.heart.org
- Centers for Disease Control and Prevention
  www.cdc.gov
- MedlinePlus
  www.nlm.nih.gov/medlineplus
- My Family Health Portrait, a tool from the U.S. Surgeon General
  https://familyhistory.hhs.gov/fhh-web/home.action

MOBILE TIPS!

Scan this QR code with your mobile device to access additional tips about diabetes, cardiovascular disease, and cancer. Or, via your mobile device, go to **http://chmobile.pearsoncmg.com** and navigate to Chapter 12.

- National Cancer Institute
  www.cancer.gov

Website links are subject to change. To access updated web links, please visit MasteringHealth™

TEST YOUR KNOWLEDGE

1. What percentage of deaths each year in the United States are due to chronic disease?
   a. 25%
   b. 50%
   c. 70%
   d. 90%

2. What is the cause of type 1 diabetes?
   a. eating a high-sugar diet
   b. the inability of body cells to respond to insulin properly
   c. the release of excessive amounts of insulin into the bloodstream
   d. immune system destruction of insulin-secreting cells in the pancreas

3. Among American adults, diabetes is the most common cause of
   a. kidney failure.
   b. blindness.
   c. nontraumatic lower limb amputations.
   d. all of the answers are correct.

4. Which form of CVD is known as a "silent killer"?
   a. hypertension
   b. coronary heart disease
   c. congestive heart failure
   d. stroke

5. Which of the following statements about cardiovascular disease is true?
   a. Atherosclerosis increases the risk for hypertension, coronary heart disease, congestive heart failure, and stroke.
   b. The best emergency treatment for a person experiencing the warning signs of myocardial infarction is to shock the heart using an automated external defibrillator (AED).
   c. A TIA is a warning sign of an impending heart attack.
   d. A high-sodium diet is essential for maintaining body fluid levels in patients with congestive heart failure.

6. Which of the following is one of the nine factors in cardio-metabolic risk?
   a. having a body mass index (BMI) greater than or equal to 25
   b. drinking more than two alcoholic beverages a day for males, and more than one for females
   c. smoking
   d. all of these are risk factors

7. Which of the following statements about cancer is true?
   a. Oncogenes are genes known to suppress the development of malignant tumors.
   b. Carcinogens are substances known to promote metastasis of malignant tumors.
   c. A malignant tumor is a tumor that has metastasized.
   d. Not all tumors are cancer.

8. The second most common cancer affecting both men and women is
   a. oral cancer.
   b. malignant melanoma.
   c. pancreatic cancer.
   d. colorectal cancer.

9. Which of the following behaviors has been shown to reduce your risk of developing a chronic disease?
   a. taking fiber supplements
   b. engaging in regular physical activity
   c. drinking alcohol in moderation
   d. all of these answers are correct

10. Which of the following actions is most appropriate for supporting a friend with a chronic disease?
   a. Bring your friend little gifts such as homemade cookies or an iTunes card to show you care.
   b. Share your feelings about how your friend's condition has affected you, but avoid giving advice.
   c. If your friend talks about the condition, listen for a short time, then try to change the subject to keep your friend's mind off it.
   d. Make plans for a trip or other event together to give your friend something to look forward to.

Get Critical

What happened

In the spring of 2012, even before its release, a documentary film called *Pink Ribbons, Inc.* was making waves in the United States and Canada. The film challenges an icon that has become, to millions of women across North America, nearly as sacred as the stars and stripes or the maple leaf flag. Known as the pink ribbon, it adorns cars, clothes, greeting cards, cosmetics, and even food items. Buy the yogurt with the pink ribbon on the label, and you'll be contributing to the cure.

Or will you? *Pink Ribbons, Inc.* contends that very little of your purchase price goes to breast cancer research, and reveals how, every October—designated "Breast Cancer Awareness Month"— the pink ribbon logo helps boost the sales of everything from soap to soup. Moreover, the film charges that many of the very products bearing the pink label, including national brands of cosmetics and food items, contain carcinogens. The film includes interviews with many breast cancer survivors who are outraged at having their ugly disease reduced to a pretty pink ribbon. In the words of one survivor, "It's almost as if our disease is being used for people to profit, and that's not okay."[1]

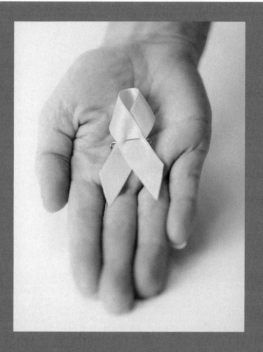

What do you think?

- Have you ever purchased a product with a pink ribbon on the label? If so, what motivated you? What assumptions did you have when you made the purchase?

- In the film, a women's health advocate expresses concern that the pink ribbon campaign attempts to normalize a horrifying abnormality. She proposes that it obscures the fact that, despite decades of funding for research, we still don't know what causes breast cancer, and we haven't found a cure. How do you feel about her remarks? Does the pink ribbon campaign normalize breast cancer, in your view, or distract women from the real issues—such as industrial toxins—that might be contributing to the disease?

Reference: **1.** Source: from *Pink Ribbons, Inc.* directed by Lea Pool. A production of the National Film Board of Canada (NFB), 2011.

CONSUMER HEALTH

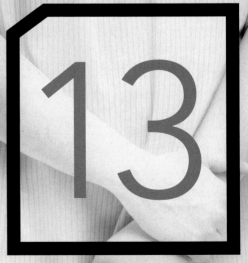

About **75% of Internet users** have sought **health** information **online**.[i]

About **49%** of U.S. adults take at least one prescription **medication** each month.[ii]

About **78%** of college students report using some type of **alternative medicine**, such as herbal remedies.[iii]

13

Learning Objectives

DESCRIBE different aspects of *self-care*.

KNOW when it's time to seek professional health care.

UNDERSTAND the basis of conventional medicine, how to choose a provider, and how to be a smart patient.

DESCRIBE the different types of complementary and alternative medicine, and how to evaluate them.

IDENTIFY multiple methods of paying for health care.

DISCUSS the genomic revolution and the future of personal health.

KNOW how to pull the knowledge in this chapter together into your personal plan for getting the care you need.

It's near the end of the semester, and you've been feeling physically run-down.

Things got worse this morning, when you woke up with a bad sore throat, a fever, and—most troubling—a skin rash. What should you do?

Maybe you'll go online and do a search on your symptoms to decide whether they are serious enough to seek professional help. You might take an over-the-counter medicine for the sore throat and fever, and ask a parent or friend for advice about the rash. If you decide to consult a doctor, things can quickly get complicated: What doctor should you see? How will you pay for the health care? What if you don't have health insurance?

These are all examples of questions related to **consumer health.** In the United States today, we have more tools and options for taking care of our health than ever before. The Internet holds an unprecedented amount of health information. We can purchase a wide range of over-the-counter drugs and medications. We can choose to seek care at a traditional hospital, at a drug store clinic, or at a campus health center. We can try alternative therapies like acupuncture or chiropractic, and select from a broad array of health-care professionals and insurance plans.

But this growing world of health choices also requires active and informed decision making. Increasingly, the burden is on you to research information, evaluate it, and make educated decisions that are best for you. You need to be a smarter health consumer than ever before. This chapter will help!

Choosing Self-Care

There are many things you can do on your own to stay healthy. As you've learned throughout this book, some of the most important health behaviors are preventive, promoting your overall wellness and reducing the likelihood that you will get sick in the first place. Maintaining basic wellness behaviors, learning how to critically evaluate health information (especially online), educating yourself about over-the-counter medications, using home health tests, and knowing when it's time to seek professional help are all examples of **self-care.**

Practicing Prevention

Prevention begins with the basic wellness behaviors you've learned about in this book, such as eating nutritiously, exercising, and refraining from unhealthful behaviors like smoking or excessive drinking. Regularly brushing your teeth and flossing, making sure you get enough sleep, keeping your stress level under control, and maintaining good relationships are additional aspects of self-care (**Figure 13.1** on page 322). Commonsense

consumer health An umbrella term encompassing topics related to the purchase and consumption of health-related products and services.

self-care Actions you take to keep yourself healthy.

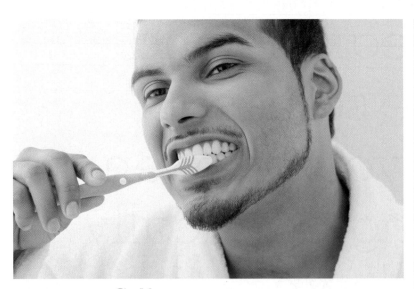

FIGURE 13.1 Self-care. Self-care includes basic wellness habits such as regularly brushing your teeth.

preventive behaviors—such as wearing a seat belt inside a car, wearing a helmet while riding a bike, or practicing safer sex—can protect you from serious injuries and illnesses. Similarly, the simple act of regularly washing your hands with soap and hot water can protect you from contracting infectious diseases. Prevention also means staying on top of regular health checks, including physicals and dental visits.

Finding Accurate Health Information

If you are living away from home for the first time, you have new responsibilities for making your own decisions about your care. Making any health-related decision intelligently starts with analyzing health information for yourself.

Evaluating Health Information and Tools

Using the Internet as a health resource has become so common that some health professionals joke that they've been replaced by

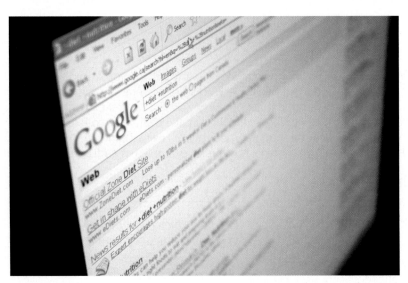

The Internet is increasingly the first place people turn for health information.

"Dr. Google." Yet going online doesn't necessarily mean that one knows what to do with the health information found there. One study of college students found that although they use the Internet more than any other health information source, they also find online information to be the least believable.[1]

As you may recall, in Chapter 1, we introduced some basic strategies for evaluating online information. (See **Media and Health: Evaluating Health Information in the Media** on page 11 of Chapter 1.) But the online world represents only one facet of all the health information you are likely to encounter each day. You may hear about scientific studies on news programs or see ads for health-related products in magazines. A friend might recommend a new health-related software program, or "app," for your phone. Regardless of where you find your health information, you will be able to evaluate it better if you get answers to a few basic questions:

- What is the source? Is the information provider a health expert, or a group of such professionals? What are the source's credentials?
- What does the source have at stake? Is the information provider relatively unbiased? Will anyone benefit financially from how the information is perceived or used? If you are using a mobile app, does it have a one-time cost, or ongoing fees?
- Is the information or tool supported by facts? Are those facts stated clearly, with supporting evidence to establish their credibility?
- Does the information or tool come with a "time stamp"? Does the site or app say when its underlying information was published or last updated, and is that date recent? If it relies on scientific studies, are those relatively recent or somewhat dated?
- Is the information presented in a balanced manner? Does it include and discuss other options or points of view, or pretend they don't exist?
- Does the information or tool offer something that sounds too good to be true? Achieving good health and wellness is a rewarding but ongoing process. Simplistic quick fixes may be of little actual substance.
- Does the site carry HONcode certification? The HONcode is a code of ethics for health and medical websites that guides site developers in setting up good-quality, objective, and transparent medical information. Sites with HONcode certification carry a HONcode label.

>> **For more information about the HONcode, visit** www.hon.ch/HONcode.

In addition to using these questions to evaluate health information in the news and other media, you can also watch for these "red flags":[2]

- The information is anonymous.
- There is a conflict of interest.
- The information is one-sided or biased.
- The information is outdated.
- There is a claim of a miracle or secret cure.
- No evidence is cited.
- The grammar is poor and words are misspelled.

Much of the health information and tools you'll find online or in the media claim to rely on scientific research studies. The Internet has made these studies more accessible than ever before, and you don't need to be a scientist to read them. Next, we'll look at how you can make sense of scientific findings.

Understanding Research Studies

Reliable health information is supported by **evidence-based medicine**—practices that are based on systematic, scientific study. The process that supports quality research is called the "scientific method" and includes the following steps: First, the researcher makes an observation that prompts one or more questions about the factor observed. The researcher then formulates an educated guess (or hypothesis) that attempts to answer one or more of the original questions and conducts an experiment to test that educated guess. The experiment generates data that either challenges the hypothesis or supports it. Scientists typically share the results of their experiments with other researchers in the form of published research studies.

Not all studies are equally reliable. To evaluate the validity and reliability of such studies, ask:

- Is the description of this research specific and detailed? Credible research claims should include who conducted the study and their credentials, the research institutions involved, the question the study was trying to answer, and the dates the research was conducted and/or published.

- Who published this research? Quality science is published in *peer-reviewed journals,* publications where experts screen and evaluate all submissions. Research findings are also sometimes presented at meetings of scientific societies.

- Who were the study participants? Was the research done on animals or people? Studies conducted on people usually have the greatest medical validity.

- How many people participated? The larger the pool of participants, the more significant the results. Specially significant studies often involve tens of thousands of people over several years.

- What were the profiles of the participants? How similar were they to you? The results of a health study of breast cancer prevention in 10,000 postmenopausal women may not be relevant if you are a woman in your 20s.

- Is the study the first of its kind? Scientific findings carry more weight if they have been replicated by other researchers.

- Do the people behind the study have any conflicts of interest? Credible studies disclose who paid for the research and whether the scientists involved have any financial or other interest in the outcome.

Credible health information sites highlight this type of scientific information.

Options for Self-Care

In addition to practicing prevention and finding good health information, self-care means being your own caregiver from time to time. In order to care for yourself well, you need to understand the basic principles of commonly used medical products. We discuss those next.

Evaluating Over-the-Counter Medications

In any given week, more than 80% of U.S. adults are taking at least one type of medication.[3] The most readily available are **over-the-counter (OTC) medications,** which do not require a doctor's

prescription. More than $17 billion worth of OTC drugs are sold in the United States each year.[4] The U.S. Food and Drug Administration (FDA) regulates both prescription and OTC medications. The FDA defines OTC medications as those that:[5]

- Have benefits outweighing their risks

- Have low potential for misuse

- Consumers can use for self-diagnosed conditions

- Can be adequately labeled

- Do not require consultation with health practitioners for safe and effective use of the product

About 74% of college students take at least one OTC drug a week, with pain relievers the most common.[6]

Many OTC drugs are effective and are often more affordable than prescription medications. One analysis showed that brand-name prescription drugs can cost over 10 times more than OTC medications.[7] But OTC medications can still carry risks and side effects. It is important not to exceed the recommended dosage, to use the medications for their intended purposes, and to talk to your doctor or pharmacist if you have any questions. (See **Consumer Corner: Using an Over-the-Counter Medication Safely** on page 324.)

 Medicines in My Home at www.accessdata.fda.gov/videos/cder/mimh/index.cfm **is an interactive presentation on how to choose and use OTC medications safely.**

Taking Home Health Tests

Gone are the days when the only health-measuring instrument kept at home was a thermometer. Via drugstores and websites, we now have access to a wide range of medical devices that enable us to assess our health at home (**Figure 13.2** on page 324). Some of the most common include:

- Pregnancy tests

- Blood pressure kits

- Fertility thermometers and apps

- Cholesterol tests

- Blood glucose monitors

- Colon cancer risk tests

- HIV tests (*Note: If you think you may have been exposed to HIV, consider taking the HIV test in a clinic or hospital setting where on-site counseling will be available. Taking this test at home is not ideal because there will be no medical professional present to advise you in the event that you have a positive result. In addition, some at-home HIV tests marketed online do not have FDA approval. Make sure any at-home HIV test you use is approved by the FDA.*)

When you take any kind of home health test, it is very important to follow the test instructions precisely. Not doing so can result in erroneous results. Also keep in mind that any number of external factors can also cause test results to be inaccurate. For example, a

evidence-based medicine Health-care policies and practices based on systematic, scientific study.

over-the-counter (OTC) medication A medication available for purchase without a prescription.

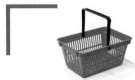
Using an Over-the-Counter Medication Safely

A typical OTC medication label looks like this:

Drug Facts

Active ingredient (in each tablet)	**Purpose**
Chlorpheniramine maleate 2 mg.....................................Antihistamine	

Uses temporarily relieves these symptoms due to hay fever or other upper respiratory allergies: ■ sneezing ■ runny nose ■ itchy, watery eyes ■ itchy throat

Warnings
Ask a doctor before use if you have
■ glaucoma ■ a breathing problem such as emphysema or chronic bronchitis
■ trouble urinating due to an enlarged prostate gland

Ask a doctor or pharmacist before use if you are taking tranquilizers or sedatives

When using this product
■ drowsiness may occur ■ avoid alcoholic drinks
■ alcohol, sedatives, and tranquilizers may increase drowsiness
■ be careful when driving a motor vehicle or operating machinery
■ excitability may occur, especially in children

If pregnant or breast-feeding, ask a health professional before use.
Keep out of reach of children. In case of overdose, get medical help or contact a Poison Control Center right away.

Directions

adults and children 12 years and over	take 2 tablets every 4 to 6 hours; not more than 12 tablets in 24 hours
children 6 years to under 12 years	take 1 tablet every 4 to 6 hours; not more than 6 tablets in 24 hours
children under 6 years	ask a doctor

Other Information ■ store at 20–25°C (68–77°F) ■ protect from excessive moisture

Inactive ingredients D&C yellow no. 10, lactose, magnesium stearate, microcrystalline cellulose, pregelatinized starch

---

When you're using an OTC medication, be sure to read the label carefully and note:

- What is its active ingredient? Do you have any allergies to this ingredient? Are you taking any other medications that may interfere with or combine poorly with this ingredient?

- What is the medication's intended purpose or use? Are you using the medication properly?

- What are the warnings accompanying this medication? Could this medication be harmful to you?

- What are this medication's side effects? If it causes drowsiness or sleepiness, think twice before putting yourself in a situation where it is important to be alert (such as driving a car).

- What is the correct dosage? Keep in mind that dosage amounts can vary depending on age and other factors.

- How should the medication be safely stored? Improperly storing a medication may compromise its effectiveness.

In addition, look for an expiration date to be sure you are not purchasing or using a medication past its time. Also, keep all medicines out of sight and reach of children.

Source for Drug Label: U.S. Department of Health and Human Services, The U.S. Food and Drug Administration. (2010). *The New Over-the-Counter Medicine Label: Take a Look.*

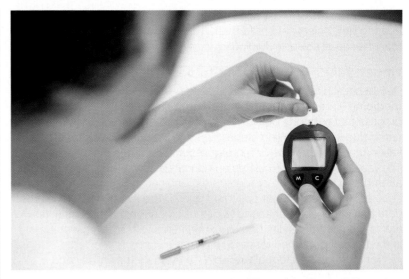

FIGURE 13.2 Home Health Tests Are Now Available for Everything From Fertility Testing to HIV Detection.

pregnancy test may yield a "negative" result if the woman takes the test too early in her pregnancy. Drinking copious amounts of fluid or taking prescription medications may also interfere with the accuracy of some home health tests. If your test results indicate that you have a medical issue, consult a doctor immediately to confirm the results.

Managing Chronic Conditions

If you have a chronic health condition, such as diabetes, allergies, or asthma, you'll often be responsible for providing your own routine care. Many people with diabetes, for example, have to monitor their blood glucose levels on a regular basis and use supplemental medication, such as insulin, to balance those levels out. People with severe allergies—such as to bee stings—need to carry a special injection kit they can use to stop a severe allergic reaction in case of an emergency.

But although the daily management of a chronic condition often falls to the individual, it is important to remember that this type of self-care is never your responsibility alone. Your health-care provider will work with you to develop your care plan. Sometimes, managing a chronic condition can feel isolating and even overwhelming. If you have a chronic condition, seek out regular emotional and medical support. If you know someone with a chronic condition, offer to help, and check in with them often.

When to See a Doctor

Smart self-care includes knowing when it's time to seek professional help. Many of us only call a doctor when we are extremely sick. However, preventive checkups and exams are also important.

Checkups and Preventive Care

By working with your health-care providers to get regular screenings and checkups, you can prevent problems or catch them early, when they are often far easier to treat. See **Table 13.1** for checkup and screening recommendations. Remember to schedule checkups for all aspects of your health, including oral health, vision, and vaccinations.

TABLE 13.1 Recommended Health Screenings

Preventive Service	Who Needs It	How Often	Comments
Blood pressure measurement	All adults	Every 2 years for those with normal blood pressure	Those with elevated blood pressure (over 120/80) need to be under medical care.
Cholesterol measurement	All adults	At least once every 5 years; more often if results indicate risk	
Pap test	All women starting at age 21	Between ages 21 and 29, at least every 3 years; between ages 30 and 65, every 5 years; for women over 65 who have had normal screenings for 10 years and are not at elevated risk, not necessary	
Mammogram	All women aged 50 to 75; women with a strong family history of the disease may start screenings earlier	Every 1 to 2 years	Other tests such as MRI may be suggested, depending on risk factors.
Colorectal cancer screening	Everyone aged 50 and over; earlier for those at higher risk, such as those with a family history of the disease	Occult blood test annually, sigmoidoscopy every 5 years; or colonoscopy every 10 years	
Prostate cancer screening	Men aged 50 and over	Digital rectal exam (DRE) yearly, prostate-specific antigen (PSA) on doctor's advice	Check with your doctor about PSA test.
Thyroid disease screening	Women aged 50 and older, those with high cholesterol, and those with other risk factors should discuss with their doctor	Check with your doctor	
General vision check	All adults	Every 2 years up to age 60; yearly thereafter	People at risk of vision damage or loss should consider starting yearly exams early in life.
Glaucoma screening	People at high risk, including those over 65 who are very nearsighted or diabetic, African Americans over age 40, and those with a family history of the disease	Talk with your vision care specialist	Many eye specialists advise screening all adults starting at age 40 or 50.
Dental checkup	All adults	Check with your dentist	Suggest checkup every 6 months.
Tetanus/diphtheria booster	All adults	Every 10 years	
Influenza vaccine	Everyone aged 65 and over; people at higher risk, such as those with chronic health conditions	Every year in autumn	
Pneumococcal vaccine	Everyone aged 6 months and over, especially people at higher risk for complications or those who live with or care for others who are at higher risk for complications	Every 5 years	
Rubella vaccine	All women of childbearing age	Once	Avoid during pregnancy.
Hepatitis B vaccine	All young adults, as well as adults at high risk	Check with your doctor	
Meningococcal vaccine (MCV4 or MPSV4)	Includes college freshmen living in a dorm; military recruits; people traveling to or residing in countries where the disease is common	At least once every 5 years, but more often if your results indicate risk	Of special concern to students living in high-density housing situations.
Skin and mole exam	All adults	Check with your doctor	Can be done as part of a regular checkup; those with a personal or family history of skin cancer may also consider regular checkups with a dermatologist.

Source: Based on: **1.** "The Wellness Guide to Preventive Care," from University of California, Berkeley website, 2008. **2.** *Vaccines and Preventable Diseases: Meningococcal Disease* by the Centers for Disease Control and Prevention, Vaccines and Immunizations website, 2012. **3.** *Recommended Eye Examination Frequency for Pediatric Patients and Adults*, from the American Optometric Association website. **4.** *New Screening Guidelines for Cervical Cancer*, from the American Cancer Society website, March 14, 2012.

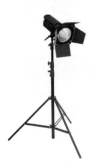

Should You Get Vaccinated?

By the time you are in college, you may think your days of needing vaccinations are behind you. Although it's true that most vaccines are administered during childhood, some are recommended for college-aged students and are worth considering. A few examples:

- If you live in a dorm or other high-density housing situation, consider obtaining a vaccine against *meningitis*, a very contagious illness that mimics symptoms of the flu and can be fatal.

National vaccine guidelines call for all freshmen living in dorms to receive this vaccine, but if you are past your freshman year and still living in a dorm with no vaccine protection, talk to your doctor or student health center.

- If you haven't had a tetanus booster shot in the last 10 years, now is the time. Vaccine guidelines for adults call for getting a "booster shot" to protect your immunity once a decade. If you can't remember when you last received such a shot, check with your pediatrician's office. You can usually receive a tetanus booster from your student health center.

- A vaccine is available that protects against human papillomavirus (HPV), a virus that can cause genital warts and cervical cancer. This vaccine is most often recommended for females in their preteen or early teen years, before they become sexually active, but is also recommended for girls and women aged 13–26. An HPV vaccine is also available for males and can protect against genital warts.

- Federal health officials now recommend that everyone over the age of six months receive a flu shot. This is especially important for certain groups, including pregnant women, health-care workers, and people with chronic health conditions such as asthma.

 For more information about vaccine recommendations for college students, visit the Centers for Disease Control's website at www.cdc.gov/vaccines/adults/rec-vac/college.html.

Health Problems Beyond Self-Care

Obviously, emergency situations require urgent care. Seek an emergency physician for yourself or someone else if any of the following situations arise:[8]

- Severe injuries, such as those sustained in a car accident
- Serious burns
- Sudden, severe pain anywhere
- Adverse reactions to a medication or an insect bite
- Other severe allergic reactions
- Heavy bleeding
- Difficulty breathing
- Signs of a heart attack (for details, see Chapter 12)
- Signs of a stroke (for details, see Chapter 12)
- Sudden worsening of a chronic health condition, such as diabetes or asthma

Keep in mind that the preceding list covers only some of the situations in which people need emergency care. Use your common sense in deciding when a situation requires urgent attention, and consult a health professional whenever you're not sure.

Outside of emergencies, it's not always easy to know when a medical condition warrants professional care. *The Merck Manual,* a reputable guide to common health issues, suggests seeking care if any of the following situations arise:[9]

- Vomiting or inability to keep fluids down, painful swallowing, coughing that lasts more than two or three weeks, earache, symptoms that last more than 7 days

- Black or bloody stools, or more than six to eight watery stools in children (symptomatic of dehydration)
- A feeling that food is stuck in the throat, development of or change in heartburn, especially during exercise, frequent heartburn, persistent or severe abdominal pain, persistent nausea
- Symptoms that prevent participation in usual activities; unexplained weight loss; dizziness; persistent fatigue; sweating, especially heavy or cold sweats
- Severe headache that peaks in intensity within seconds; memory loss or confusion; blurred or double vision; slurred speech; loss of balance or dizziness; seizures; numbness in the arms, face, or legs; nausea
- Rapid or galloping heartbeats (palpitations); chest pain
- Pain in the calves that worsens when walking; swelling in the ankles or legs
- No periods by age 16; sudden stopping of periods; a period that lasts much longer than normal or is excessively heavy; a sudden feeling of illness while using tampons; severe cramps
- Fever of 100.4°F (38°C) or above; a rash that is painful, involves swelling, or oozes
- Swelling or redness in or around an eye; problems with vision
- Moderate or severe abdominal pain; symptoms of dehydration; green, black, or bloody vomit

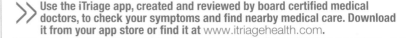 Use the iTriage app, created and reviewed by board certified medical doctors, to check your symptoms and find nearby medical care. Download it from your app store or find it at www.itriagehealth.com.

Conventional Medicine

Conventional medicine, also called *allopathic* or *Western medicine,* is the predominant type of care in the U.S. health system. Although conventional medicine includes many complex, fast-developing types of care, a few key features shape its foundation:

- The use of science and the *scientific method.* Evidence-based medicine, which you learned about earlier in this chapter, is just one example of how science underlies all aspects of conventional medicine.

- A focus on physical causes and symptoms. Conventional medicine looks for physical causes of illness, such as injuries or pathogens, and assumes that each illness leads to a set of discernible symptoms similar in most people who suffer from that condition.

- An emphasis on physical exams, such as X-rays or blood tests, and physical treatments, such as drugs or surgery, to treat the physical causes of disease.

- A focus on public health. By controlling the spread of the microscopic physical causes of disease through programs such as improved sanitation and vaccination, conventional medicine has vastly improved health and life expectancy in the last century.

Practicing conventional medicine requires many years of education and training and a professional license. Some of the most common types of practitioners of conventional medicine include:

- **Medical doctors,** or **M.D.s,** who can either serve as *general practitioners* or *specialists* who focus on a particular type of care.

- **Physician assistants,** or physician associates (**P.A.s**), are licensed health professionals who practice under the supervision of a physician and provide a broad range of care.

- **Dentists,** who hold either doctor of dental surgery (**D.D.S.**) or doctor of medical dentistry (**D.D.M.**) degrees and specialize in care of the teeth, gums, and mouth.

- **Optometrists,** or **O.D.s,** who examine the eyes and provide vision care.

- **Podiatrists,** or **D.P.M.s,** who specialize in care of and surgery for the feet.

- **Nurses,** who may hold an R.N. or other degrees, provide a wide range of health services in many types of health-care settings. They often provide detailed or extensive care in times of greater medical need, such as when a patient is recovering from surgery in the hospital.

- **Nurse practitioners,** R.N.s who have undergone additional training and can perform some of the duties and provide some of the care of a medical doctor **(Figure 13.3)**.

Where to Find Conventional Health Care

Conventional medicine was once offered primarily through doctor's offices and hospitals, but its

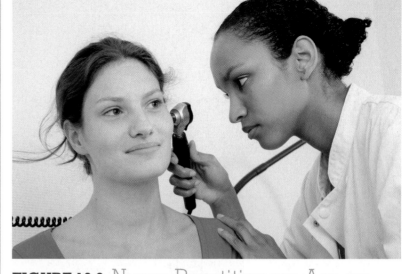

FIGURE 13.3 Nurse Practitioners Are an Example of Conventional Health-Care Providers.

conventional medicine Commonly called Western medicine, this system of care is based on the scientific method; the belief that diseases are caused by identifiable physical factors and have a characteristic set of symptoms; and the treatment of physical causes through drugs, surgery, or other interventions.

medical doctor (M.D.) A physician trained in conventional medicine, with many years of additional formal education and training and a professional license.

physician assistant (P.A.) A licensed health professional who practices under the supervision of a physician and provides a broad range of care.

dentist (D.D.S.) A conventional medicine practitioner who specializes in care of the teeth, gums, and mouth.

optometrist (O.D.) A licensed professional who provides vision care.

podiatrist (D.P.M.) A licensed professional who specializes in the care of the feet.

nurse A licensed professional who provides a wide range of health-care services and supports the work of medical doctors.

nurse practitioner Registered nurses who have undergone additional training and can perform some of the care provided by a medical doctor.

availability has since expanded to better meet the needs of patients. The following are examples of facilities that offer conventional care:

- **Student health centers** serve students on campus. Some focus on basic primary care and student health needs, such as minor illnesses and contraception. Others feature a wider range of care, including substance abuse counseling, vision care, pharmacy, and dental services. Few offer emergency services. On most campuses, student health centers are available to all enrolled students and most of the costs are covered by fees paid as part of student enrollment.

- **Primary care facilities** meet everyday medical needs, seeing patients for checkups, screenings, and minor ailments and providing referrals to more specialized care if needed. Costs are often covered by patient health insurance or a combination of insurance and patient payments.

- **Nonprofit clinics** provide primary care for free or at a reduced cost. They often focus on underserved communities and groups who would otherwise have little access to primary care.

- **Retail clinics,** also known as convenient care clinics, operate out of large stores and pharmacies (**Figure 13.4** on page 328). These clinics are designed to provide basic primary care in a timely manner for people who either don't have a primary care doctor, can't wait for an appointment at a primary care facility, and/or lack health insurance. Costs are lower than they would be at most traditional doctor's offices and are often paid directly by the patient or through insurance.

- **Urgent care centers** typically see patients with illnesses that need immediate attention but don't require the full resources of an

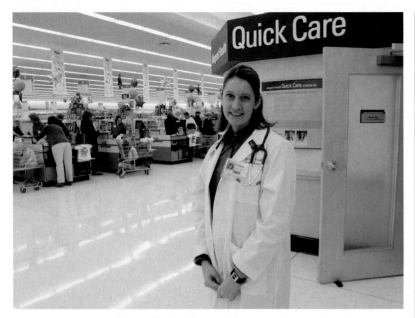

FIGURE 13.4 Health Services Are Sometimes Offered Through Large Retail Stores.

emergency department. These centers often see many patients on evenings and weekends, when primary care centers are closed. Although not as expensive as emergency departments, urgent care centers often charge a premium for their services, which can either be covered by insurance or paid directly by the patient.

Living Without Health Insurance

"MY NAME IS HOLLY. I am 45 years old. I was a single parent for about 12 years. I could not afford insurance for myself—it just wasn't in my budget. My kids always came first. If I got sick, I stayed at home and took care of myself. One time I had really bad abdominal pain and did not go to see the doctor because I didn't have any insurance. It got so bad that I couldn't stand up. I had to go to the emergency room and they did emergency surgery on me. My gall bladder had ruptured and the poison from that went through my system. I ended up being in the hospital for five days because of that. If I had gone to the doctor sooner, they would have caught it sooner. My doctor's bill ended up being a little over $12,000. That's a lot of money for a single mom."

1. Holly is a nontraditional-aged college student. What are some healthcare options that may be available to her despite her lack of health insurance?

- **Specialists centers** focus on specific categories of medicine, such as obstetrics, cardiac care, or cancer. Most patients access specialists through referrals from a primary care center. Specialty care is an important part of the medical system but can be quite costly to patients if not covered by insurance.
- **Hospitals** provide the highest level of care. Hospitals handle everything from emergencies to surgeries to complex screenings and cancer treatment. Patients can be seen on an *outpatient* basis, in which they visit the hospital but don't stay overnight, or on an *inpatient* basis, where care is provided for an extended period and overnight stays are included.

Choosing a Provider

If you are the age of a traditional college student, you probably haven't had much say in the past over who served as your healthcare provider, but at some point you will need to choose a primary care provider. Your primary care provider will see you for checkups and most screenings, answer your basic health questions, treat minor ailments, write prescriptions, and provide referrals for more complex health concerns.

To get started, check two resources—your insurance plan and your friends and family. If your health insurance limits the providers you can see, start with providers from the plan's list. Then ask your friends and family for their recommendations.

Once you have a list of providers to contact, start by calling their offices and ask a few questions of a nurse or other office staff:

- Is this provider accepting new patients? Some providers have a full roster and can't take any more patients into their practice.
- What insurance plans does this office accept?
- If a physician, is this doctor *board-certified,* meaning that he or she has undergone extra training after medical school to specialize in an area such as family practice?
- How does the office handle lab work? Is there a lab in-house or nearby, or will you have to travel to a different location for a procedure such as a blood test?
- Is this a group practice? If so, will you mostly see your provider or all the providers in the group? If so, how many of them are there and what are their specialties?
- Who will care for you if your provider is unavailable?
- Is this practice affiliated with any hospitals or specialty centers?

When you meet your provider in person, make sure that he or she listens to you, encourages you to ask questions, answers your questions completely, and treats you with respect. If you don't feel comfortable with a provider, shop around until you do.

Being a Smart Patient

Once you've chosen a provider, your visits will be more productive if you think of your provider as a partner. Your provider has the expertise to help you improve your health, but his or her work will be more effective if you are actively and constructively engaged in the process. Here are some suggestions from the American Academy of Family Physicians for how to get the most out of a medical appointment:

- *Talk* **to your provider.** Be sure to tell your care provider any past or current health issues or concerns, even if they are embarrassing. Many medical appointments are only 15 minutes long, so effective communication is key to letting your doctor treat you.

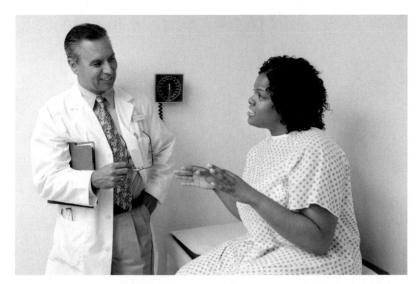

Ask your care provider questions to be sure you understand your care needs.

- **Ask questions.** Let your provider know if you don't understand something. If you need more time to discuss an issue, be vocal about it.
- **Take information home with you.** Take notes during your appointment, ask your provider for handouts, or ask the office to supply background or reference materials.
- **Follow up with your provider.** Follow the instructions you receive, such as getting additional tests or seeing a specialist. If you've been given a new medication and feel worse or have problems with the drug, let your provider know right away. If you took a test and haven't received the results, let your provider's office know.
- **Prevent medical errors through active communication.** Let your provider know all the medicines, supplements, and other substances you may be taking (including alcohol) to help prevent risky drug interactions. Be proactive about sharing information with all members of your medical team, especially if you have more than one caregiver. Make sure you understand the side effects of any medication you are prescribed. If you are being discharged from care, make sure you understand any follow-up treatments to be done at home.[10]

Handling Prescription Medications Properly

Prescription medications, which can only be obtained legally by receiving a prescription, or written order, from a health-care provider, cover a vast range of therapies, including everything from heart medication and painkillers to breathing aids and antibiotics. These medicines are typically more potent than OTC drugs—and also carry greater risks. Because prescription medications are powerful, it is especially important to use them properly. Unfortunately, some college students don't always follow the directions for taking prescription medications. In one recent survey, almost 13% of college students said they had taken a prescription medication not prescribed to them.[11]

Of special concern are prescription opioid painkillers. The rates of use and abuse of these medications have skyrocketed in recent years. In 2010, the amount of prescription painkillers such as oxycodone and codeine sold to pharmacies, hospitals, and doctors' offices was four times larger than in 1999.[12] According to federal health estimates, enough prescription painkillers were prescribed in 2010 to medicate every American adult around the clock for a month.[12]

The growing use of these opioid painkillers has caused huge increases in their misuse. Prescription painkillers often wind up in the hands of people have become addicted, or who were not prescribed them. The medications are especially dangerous when mixed with other prescription drugs, such as sleep aids or anti-anxiety medicines.[13] Because of this dangerous brew, prescription drugs are now the leading cause of drug overdose deaths in the United States.[14] Federal health officials calculate that for every prescription painkiller overdose death, there are 10 hospital admissions for abuse, 32 emergency department visits for misuse or abuse, 130 people who abuse these drugs or are dependent on them, and 825 people who take them for nonmedical reasons.[13] Men are more likely to die from prescription painkiller overdoses, with more than 10,000 male fatalities in 2010.[15] But deaths among women are now climbing at a faster rate than among men, with about 18 women now dying every day of a prescription painkiller overdose in the United States.[15]

To take prescription painkillers and other prescription drugs safely, be sure to do the following:[12]

- Use prescription drugs only as directed by a health care provider. Don't take prescription medications that are not prescribed to you.
- Be sure you are the only one to use your prescription drugs. Don't share or sell them.
- Never take larger or more frequent doses of your medications, particularly prescription painkillers, to try to get faster or more powerful effects.
- Store prescription painkillers in a secure place and dispose of them properly. For suggestions on medication disposal, see **www.fda .gov/ForConsumers/ConsumerUpdates/ucm101653.htm**.
- Get help for substance abuse problems if needed.

Complementary and Alternative Medicine (CAM)

Conventional medicine can be very effective, but it has its limits. Conventional medicine's focus on physical ailments after they arise may sometimes overlook preventive steps and care that could have warded off illness. Some people are interested in health practices that take a broader, more holistic approach, looking beyond the body to include the mind and spirit as well.

complementary and alternative medicine (CAM) Health practices and traditions not typically part of conventional Western medicine, either used alone (alternative medicine) or in conjunction with conventional medicine (complementary medicine).

These interests have led to the growth of **complementary and alternative medicine (CAM).** The term *alternative medicine* is used to refer to those practices and traditions not typically part of conventional Western medicine, including everything from herbal remedies and meditation to chiropractors and traditional Chinese medicine. *Complementary medicine,* also sometimes referred to as *integrative medicine,* refers to care combining conventional and alternative medicine. Many of us routinely practice complementary medicine without

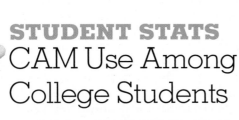
CAM Use Among College Students

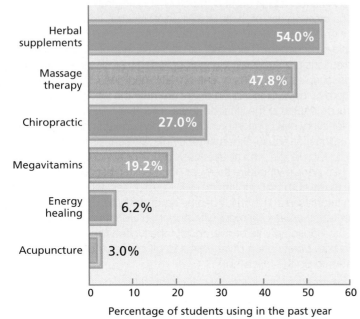

	Percentage
Herbal supplements	54.0%
Massage therapy	47.8%
Chiropractic	27.0%
Megavitamins	19.2%
Energy healing	6.2%
Acupuncture	3.0%

Percentage of students using in the past year

Data from "Coping Styles and Self-Regulation Predict Complementary and Alternative Medicine and Herbal Supplement Use Among College Students," by R. A. LaCaille & N. J. Kuvaas, 2011, *Psychology, Health & Medicine, 16*(3).

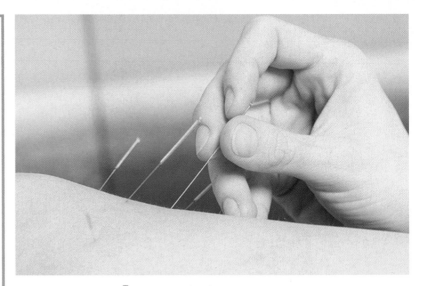

FIGURE 13.5 Acupuncture. A type of traditional Chinese medicine, acupuncture is an example of alternative health care.

- **Manipulative and body-based practices** are based on physical manipulation of the body, and typically involve therapies such as chiropractic medicine or massage.
- **Energy therapies** involve interaction with energy fields. These include biofield therapies, believed by practitioners to surround the body, and bio-electromagnetic–based therapies involving the alternative use of electromagnetic fields.

For a more detailed look at some of the better-known CAM practices, please see **Table 13.2** on page 331.

Evaluating Complementary and Alternative Therapies

As you can see in **Table 13.2,** the effectiveness of many CAM therapies is still being studied, and research is inconclusive for many of these practices. If you are considering a CAM therapy, either on your own or through a practitioner, NCCAM offers the following suggestions:[17]

- Be an informed consumer. Find out what the scientific evidence is about any therapy's safety and effectiveness.
- Be aware that individuals respond differently to treatments, whether conventional or CAM. How a person might respond to a CAM therapy depends on many things, including the person's state of health, how the therapy is used, or the person's belief in the therapy.
- Keep in mind that "natural" does not necessarily mean "safe." (Think of mushrooms that grow in the wild: some are safe to eat, whereas others are not.)
- Learn about factors that affect safety. For a CAM therapy that is administered by a practitioner, these factors include the training, skill, and experience of the practitioner. For a CAM product such as a dietary supplement, the specific ingredients and the quality of the manufacturing process are important factors.
- Tell all your health-care providers about any CAM practices you use. This will help ensure coordinated and safe care.

realizing it, perhaps trying an herbal remedy to treat a cold but seeing a traditional doctor for a serious injury. For a glimpse at how many college students use CAM, see the **Student Stats** box above.

Alternative medicine has become such a common part of our approach to health that federal health officials now discuss and study it in a scientific way, and many states now require some CAM practitioners to be licensed. The National Center for Complementary and Alternative Medicine (NCCAM) groups CAM into five major domains:[16]

- **Whole medical systems** are built on theories and systems encompassing the totality of a person's health. These systems have typically evolved apart from and earlier than conventional Western medicine. Traditional Chinese medicine is a prime example **(Figure 13.5)**.
- **Mind–body medicine** uses techniques designed to boost the mind's capacity to affect the body. Some of these techniques are now considered part of Western medicine, such as patient support groups. Others, such as prayer or meditation, are still considered CAM.
- **Natural products** rely on substances found in nature, such as vitamins and herbs. These practices focus on using plant-derived medicines called botanicals, dietary supplements, and sometimes even beneficial microbes such as priobiotics to treat disorders ranging from the common cold to serious conditions such as depression and cancer. But just because these therapies are "natural" does not make them safe. As with any medication, natural remedies may have side effects or dangerous interactions with other medicines, especially when taken in large amounts. For more information on using supplements safely, see Chapter 4.

TABLE 13.2 Common Types of Complementary and Alternative Medicine

Practice	Description	Common Use	Risks	Scientific Evaluation
Acupuncture	This ancient system revolves around the concept of the free flow of qi (pronounced chee), or energy, through the body. Illness is believed to occur when qi is blocked or disrupted. Practitioners restore and rebalance qi not only to treat illness but prevent it and increase overall energy.	Thin needles are inserted at key qi points in the body to balance or restore energy flow. A related technique, acupressure, uses firm touch at key energy points. In addition to being a common part of overall traditional Chinese care, acupuncture has also been used in Western settings for everything from pain relief to reducing nausea during cancer treatment.	Acupuncture appears to have relatively few side effects, although problems can arise when needles are not used or sterilized correctly.	Acupuncture appears to be effective in treating chronic pain, in treating women's health disorders such as PMS or painful periods, and in easing side effects of cancer care.[1]
Homeopathy	Homeopathy is based on the assumption that "like cures like." That is, a substance that produces symptoms or illness is thought to cure or alleviate symptoms of that same illness, if administered in very diluted quantities.	Homeopathy is used in an attempt to treat common health problems such as nausea, sinus infections, and fever.	Given the very diluted levels at which homeopathic substances are usually used, few side effects have been reported.	A large analysis of more than 100 homeopathy studies found that the practice offered no significant effect.[2]
Naturopathy	Naturopathy incorporates traditional therapies and techniques from all over the world, from herbs to dietary changes and exercise, with an emphasis on supporting health rather than treating disease.	Naturopathy is especially popular with some people interested in an overall health approach that promotes wellness and prevents illness.	Some treatments, such as herbs, can have drug interactions and other side effects.	According to NCCAM, scientific studies of the effectiveness of naturopathy are still preliminary.[3]
Ayurveda	One of the world's oldest medical systems, Ayurveda originated in India. It aims to integrate and balance the body, mind, and spirit to help prevent illness and promote wellness.	Ayurvedic medicine uses a variety of products and techniques to cleanse the body and restore balance. People who use Ayurveda, either on its own or in conjunction with conventional medicine, often choose it in the belief that it will help cleanse their body of harmful substances and energies and help restore vitality and overall health.	Some of the herbal and dietary substances, along with other practices meant to cleanse the digestive tract, can have drug interactions if used with conventional medicine, as well as other side effects. One NCCAM study of Ayurvedic medications found that some contained toxins such as mercury or lead.[4]	According to NCCAM, scientific studies of the effectiveness of Ayurveda are still preliminary and more research is needed.[4]
Natural products	These approaches focus on using herbs, other plant-derived medicines called *botanicals,* and dietary supplements to treat various conditions.	Botanicals, herbs, and supplements are used in an attempt to treat conditions ranging from the common cold to serious conditions such as depression and cancer. *Echinacea,* or coneflower, for example, is popularly used to treat colds and upper respiratory infections.	This group of alternative therapies is among the most risky, as these substances have the potential for harm if taken in high doses or for long periods of time, or if they interact badly with conventional drugs. For example, one botanical, *ephedra,* is now banned in the United States because of its harmful side effects.	Studies have found that these therapies have limited usefulness at best. But researchers also caution that most such studies are still preliminary and more research is needed.[5]
Mind–body medicine	Mind–body medicines rely on the connection between the mental and physical realms and seek to create a more positive interaction between the two. Guided imagery, yoga, and meditation are popular forms of mind–body medicine.	Mind–body techniques are used to help prevent illness by reducing factors such as stress, and to help treat disorders such as depression, anxiety, and insomnia. These therapies are also sometimes used to support cancer patients by reducing patient anxiety, isolation, and stress.	Most mind–body therapies are considered relatively safe, although more strenuous forms, such as very active yoga, carry some risk of injury.	Some studies show some benefit, but most scientists caution that research is still preliminary. One study of the efficacy of meditation as a treatment for a variety of illnesses found some benefit, but cautioned that more research remains to be done.[6]
Manipulative therapies	Remedies that focus on moving, stretching, or re-aligning sections of the body. These therapies focus on restoring overall wellness by correcting parts of the body that are out of alignment.	These techniques are often used to treat stiffness and pain. Chiropractic medicine, which focuses on structure and connections of joints and muscles, is an especially popular form.	Any intense physical manipulation of the body, especially of the spine, can be very dangerous, especially if a practitioner lacks training.	When administered correctly, chiropractic medicine has been shown to be effective for joint and bone pain, such as low back pain.[7]
Energy therapies	These forms of treatment focus on fields of energy originating within the body (biofields) or from external sources (electromagnetic fields). Changing or increasing the flow of the fields of energy, practitioners say, can have a variety of health benefits. Qigong, a movement-based component of traditional Chinese medicine, and magnet therapy are examples of energy treatments.	Energy fields are used for a variety of reasons, including stress reduction, pain relief, and improvement of cardiac health.	Risks appear to be relatively minor.	Most of the research done to date is either preliminary or inconclusive. One large analysis of the efficacy of qigong in reducing high blood pressure, for example, found some encouraging evidence, but cautioned that further study is needed.[8]

Source: Data from: **1.** "The Status and Future of Acupuncture Clinical Research," by J. Park, K. Linde, E. Manheimer, A. Molsberger, K. Sherman, C. Smith, J. Sung, A. Vickers, & R. Schnyer, 2008, *The Journal of Complementary and Alternative Medicine, 14*(7). **2.** "Are the Clinical Effects of Homoeopathy Placebo Effects? Comparative Study of Placebo-Controlled Trials of Homoeopathy and Allopathy," by A. Shang, K. Huwiler-Müntener, L. Nartey, P. Juni, S. Dörig, J. Sterne, D. Pewsner, & M. Egger, 2005, *Lancet, 366.* **3.** *Backgrounder: An Introduction to Naturopathy,* from the National Center for Complementary and Alternative Medicine website, May 2009. **4.** *Backgrounder: Ayurvedic Medicine: An Introduction,* by the National Center for Complementary and Alternative Medicine website, May 2009. **5.** *Backgrounder: Herbs at a Glance,* from the National Center for Complementary and Alternative Medicine website, May 2009. **6.** "Systematic Review of the Efficacy of Meditation Techniques as Treatments for Mental Illness," by A. Arias, K. Steinberg, A. Banga, & R. Trestman, 2006, *The Journal of Alternative and Complementary Medicine, 12*(8). **7.** "Diagnosis and Treatment of Low Back Pain: A Joint Clinical Practice Guideline from the American College of Physicians and the American Pain Society," by R. Chou, A, Qaseem, V. Snow, D. Casey, J. Cross, P. Shekelle, & D. Owens, from *Annals of Internal Medicine, 147.* **8.** "Qigong for Hypertension: A Systematic Review of Randomized Clinical Trials," by M. Lee, R. Pittler, M. Guo, & E. Ernst, 2007, *Journal of Hypertension, 25*(8), pp. 1525–1532.

If you are considering using a CAM practitioner, the following guidelines, adapted from NCCAM, may help:[18]

- Speak with your primary health-care provider(s) regarding the therapy in which you are interested. Ask if they have a recommendation for the type of CAM practitioner you are seeking.
- Make a list of CAM practitioners and gather information about each before making your first visit. Ask basic questions about their credentials and practice. Where did they receive their training? What licenses or certifications do they have? How much will the treatment cost? How many treatments will be required to derive a benefit?
- Check with your insurer to see if the cost of therapy will be covered.
- After you select a practitioner, make a list of questions to ask at your first visit.
- Come to the first visit prepared to answer questions about your health history, as well as prescription medicines, vitamins, and other supplements you may take.
- Assess your first visit and decide whether the practitioner is right for you. Did you feel comfortable with the practitioner? Could the practitioner answer your questions? Does the treatment plan seem reasonable and acceptable to you?

Paying for Health Care

In the United States, we are surrounded by highly advanced medical care—at a steep price. Our system is the most expensive in the world, spending more per person than any other country and spending the most on health as a percentage of gross domestic product.[19] According to the nonprofit National Coalition on Health Care, health spending reached nearly $2.6 trillion in 2010, or almost $8,402 per person, and costs for all of us continue to rise each year.[20] In 2011, the average annual cost for family insurance coverage obtained through work reached $15,073, a 113% increase from the $7,061 cost a decade earlier. In addition, each family's share of those costs soared as well, with families picking up $4,129 of that price tag, compared with $1,787 in 2001.[21] A set of new health-care reforms called the Affordable Care Act, implemented in 2014, is predicted to cause a spike in some health care costs.[20] (We'll discuss the Affordable Care Act and what it means for you in more detail later in this chapter.)

As a student, you likely have access to basic care through your student health center, with costs covered by fees you pay as part of student enrollment. You may still be on your family's insurance plan, or your campus may offer a free or low-cost health insurance plan for students. According to one federal study released in 2008, about 80% of college students had some type of health insurance.[22] No matter your coverage, it's important to understand what you need to pay for out of your own pocket.

Discount Programs

Does your student health center cover the cost of your prescriptions? If not, does it offer a program with nearby pharmacies that lets you fill your prescriptions at a reduced price? If so, you are taking part in a **health discount program.** These programs are increasingly offered by employers

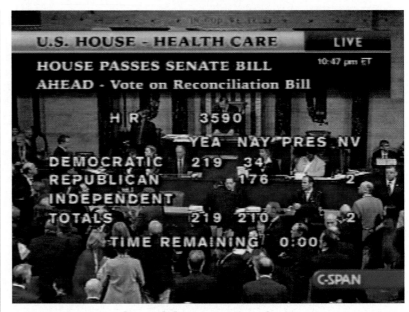

The passage of health-care reform in 2010 was a historical and controversial event.

and large institutions that want to provide some level of assistance with medical costs but don't want to pay for full insurance. Discount programs typically offer prices from 5% to 25% lower than average, although some programs for students may provide deeper discounts.

Health Insurance

At its essence, **health insurance** is your buffer against medical costs.

A health insurance policy is a contract between an insurance company and an individual or group, in which the insurer agrees to cover a defined set of medical costs if the insured party pays a defined price. Insurers either pay your health-care providers directly, or reimburse you for covered health-care expenses, although almost all plans limit the types of care covered. Although many plans cover primary care, for example, they may offer little or no coverage for services such as mental health services, substance abuse programs, or physical therapy. Alternative medicine is rarely covered. Many plans also restrict which doctors you can see and may place rules on seeing specialists. A few plans may refuse or limit your coverage if you already have an illness, or a **pre-existing condition,** although this restriction is being phased out because of national health-care reforms. Under the Affordable Care Act, people with pre-existing medical issues cannot be denied health insurance.

When it comes to paying for health insurance, there are several concepts you should understand: premiums, co-pays, and deductibles. A **premium** is the amount you pay an insurance company for an insurance policy. Premiums are usually charged monthly, and the amount of a premium depends on the level of health insurance benefits offered, your age, any pre-existing conditions you may have, certain lifestyle habits (such as smoking), and even your sex. A **co-pay** (co-payment) is a flat fee charged at the time of a

---

health discount program A system of health discounts given to members of groups, such as employees of a particular company or students attending a particular college.

health insurance A contract between an insurance company and a group or individual who pays a fee to have some or all health costs covered by the insurer.

pre-existing condition A health issue that existed prior to application to or enrollment in an insurance plan, which insurers sometimes use to restrict care or set the price paid for insurance.

premium The amount you pay an insurance company for an insurance policy, usually monthly.

co-pay A flat fee charged at the time of a medical service or when receiving a medication.

---

medical service or when receiving a medication. Co-pays are set at the time an insurance policy is offered, so before committing to an insurance policy, check the co-pay amount, which should be explicitly stated in the policy. Co-pays can vary widely with an insurance policy and are usually set higher when the premium is lower. A **deductible** is the total amount of out-of-pocket health-care expenses that a patient must pay before the health insurance begins to cover health-care costs. For example, if the deductible for your health insurance is $3,000, and you are in an accident that causes $20,000 in health-care costs, you must pay $3,000 out of pocket before your health insurance kicks in for the remainder of the bill. Deductibles are reset each year. As with co-pays, the amount of your deductible will be explicitly stated in the insurance policy before you sign it, and deductibles are usually set higher when the premium for the policy is lower.

Insurance plans come in many forms. Some are created for groups, such as collections of people who work at the same company. Others are created for individuals who buy their insurance straight from an insurance company. Common types of policies available to individuals and groups include *managed-care plans, public programs,* and *fee-for-service plans.*

 Not sure what to look for in a health insurance policy? Consumer Reports can help: www.consumerreports.org/cro/2012/09/your-health-insurance-buying-guide/index.htm.

Managed-Care Plans

Managed-care plans offer you lower costs but also less choice. In a managed-care plan, insurers have contracts with particular doctors, hospitals, and other health-care providers, and you must often limit your visits to these caregivers or face additional expense. Most people with employer-based insurance are in one of three types of managed-care plans:

- **HMOs,** or **health maintenance organizations,** restrict choice the most but also usually cost the consumer the least, requiring that all care be funneled through and managed by the primary care provider.

- **PPOs,** or **preferred provider organizations,** offer more choice by letting the consumer see a wider range of providers without a referral but also usually carry a higher cost to the consumer.

- **POSs,** or **point-of-service plans,** offer some HMO members greater flexibility by letting them see outside physicians for an additional fee.

Managed-care plans can also be purchased on the individual insurance market. But this coverage can cost thousands of dollars a year.

---

deductible The total amount of out-of-pocket health-care expenses that a patient must pay before health insurance begins to cover health-care costs.

managed-care plan A type of health insurance in which the insurer contracts with a defined group of health providers, which the consumer must use or face higher out-of-pocket costs.

health maintenance organization (HMO) A type of managed care in which most health care is funneled through and must be approved by the primary care doctor.

preferred provider organization (PPO) A type of managed care in which the consumer is encouraged to stay within an approved network of providers but has more choice over who is seen when.

point-of-service (POS) plan A type of managed care that lets HMO consumers see a broader list of providers for an additional fee.

Medicaid A joint federal-state public insurance program that covers low-income individuals and families.

Medicare A federal public insurance program that covers people with long-term disabilities and anyone 65 or older.

fee-for-service plan A type of health insurance in which you choose your providers, and you and your insurer divide the costs of care.

mini-med plan A type of managed-care plan, sold individually to younger people, which carries lower costs but does not cover many services.

health savings account (HSA) A consumer-controlled account that comes attached to a high-deductible health insurance plan and covers the costs of the deductible and other health-related expenses approved by the federal government.

flexible spending account (FSA) A consumer-controlled account, usually offered through employers, that uses pre-tax dollars to cover approved health-related purchases.

Public Programs

Public health insurance programs provide government-sponsored coverage for individuals and families who could otherwise not afford health coverage. These plans usually operate in a way similar to managed care, funneling services through primary care clinics whenever possible. Common types of public insurance include **Medicaid,** usually offered to low-income individuals and families through joint state-federal sponsorship; **Medicare,** a federal program that covers many health costs for all Americans who have certain disabilities or are age 65 or older; and state and local children's health programs.

Fee-for-Service Plans

Fee-for-service plans allow you to use any medical provider you choose and then submit a bill to your insurance company, which pays part of it, leaving you to cover the rest.

One type of fee-for-service plan is a *high-deductible* or *catastrophic* plan, which carries lower fees up front but only provides coverage after a person has paid a high deductible. In addition, many insurers have started offering a special version to younger people who may be out of college and find themselves without health insurance. These so-called **mini-med plans** often come at a more affordable monthly price than other types of individual coverage and pay for some health basics, such as primary care and trips to the emergency department. But they often don't cover other types of care, such as prenatal care and childbirth. If you are considering a mini-med plan, make sure you understand what the plan doesn't cover and see whether its limits fit your life for the next few years before you buy.

Health Insurance and the Affordable Care Act

Major national reforms known as the Affordable Care Act should make it easier for many people to afford health insurance. Beginning in 2014, states and the federal government will create "health exchanges," in which people who don't have insurance can shop for individual policies at competitive rates. See the **Special Feature: What the Affordable Care Act Means for You.**

Health Savings Accounts and Flexible Spending Accounts

Special savings accounts can help you maximize your health dollars. Two of the most common are **health savings accounts,** or **HSAs,** and medical **flexible spending accounts,** or **FSAs.**

what the
Affordable Care Act
means for you

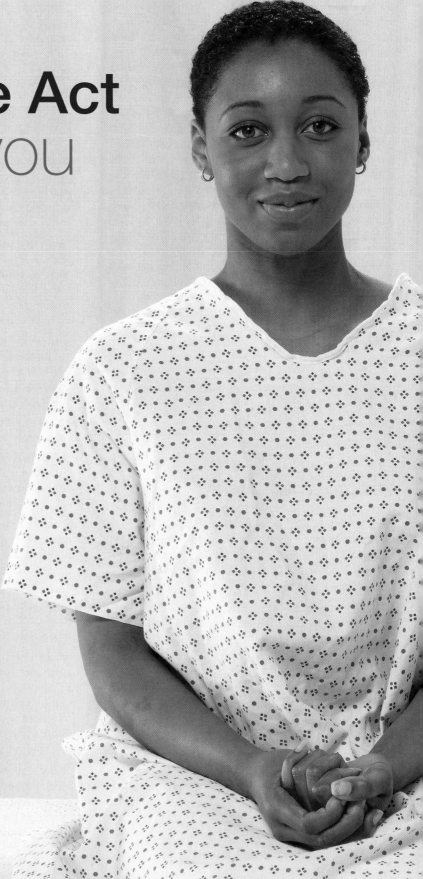

In 2012, health insurance made big headlines as the Supreme Court upheld as constitutional key provisions of the Affordable Care Act, which was designed to increase health-care access for millions of Americans. Some elements of the Affordable Care Act face delays in some states. However, many of the reforms are already in place and can make a real difference to students and young people. Here are some highlights:

- **A new requirement that many Americans be insured or pay a penalty.** This feature of the law, known as the "individual mandate," requires Americans to have at least minimal health insurance to cover emergencies and serious conditions. The penalty for not having coverage is planned to be fully in place by 2016.

- **New health insurance "exchanges."** In order to help Americans afford the cost of the insurance being required by the individual mandate, these insurance marketplaces are intended to create large pools of insured individuals and small businesses, enabling them to compare health plans and enroll at a lower cost than possible if they sought insurance independently. Individuals and small companies have typically faced higher prices and other restrictions in the insurance market, and the exchanges are intended to reduce disparities and improve access to affordable coverage. Exchanges are already available in some states, and more states will likely participate in time.

- **Better protections for people with pre-existing conditions.** Children and adults insured through private insurance plans, such as those offered through an employer, cannot be denied coverage because of pre-existing conditions.

- **Get sick, stay insured.** Health plans cannot cut off coverage if a person becomes sick, a practice known as rescission.

- **No lifetime limits.** Insurers can no longer place a lifetime cap on the insurance benefits you receive.

- **For young people, the magic number is 26.** You can now stay on a parent's insurance plan until your 26th birthday, if your parent so chooses.

- **Guaranteed coverage for women's health.** Certain preventive health services for women, including FDA-approved contraceptives, cervical cancer and HIV screenings, mammograms, and well-woman checkups, must now be offered to women in newly created health plans without any out-of-pocket cost. Under the new health-care law, women will also be shielded from having to pay more for insurance than men.

>> **Learn more about the Affordable Care Act, including details about how the reforms affect you,** at www.healthcare.gov.

Sources: *Taking Health Care into Your Own Hands,* by HealthCare.gov (publication date not available), retrieved from www.healthcare.gov; **and** *Affordable Health Care for America: Key Provisions That Take Effect Immediately,* from the Office of Speaker Nancy Pelosi, May 3, 2010, retrieved from http://docs.house.gov/energycommerce/IMMEDIATE_PROVISIONS.pdf; **and** *Healthcare.gov, Learn, All Topics,* by HealthCare.gov (publication date not available), retrieved from www.healthcare.gov.

Waiting for Health Coverage

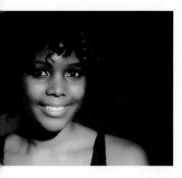

HSAs can be offered through an employer, or individuals can set them up through a bank, insurance company, or other trustee. HSAs were developed for people with high-deductible health insurance plans as a way to give them a tax benefit on savings accounts designated for medical costs. HSA funds can be used to cover medical expenses that are approved by the federal government, such as medical visits and prescriptions costs. An estimated 4.5 million people in the United States use this form of savings-related health coverage.[23]

FSAs, offered through employers, allow employees to save pre-tax dollars to cover certain medical and health expenses. Unlike an HSA, you do not need a particular type of insurance plan to use an FSA. To withdraw money from your FSA to pay for health-related expenses, you must show receipts to prove that you spent the funds for allowed medical or health purposes. You also must use the funds in your FSA within the same year as you contribute them, or you will lose them.

Students and Health Insurance

Most college students have some form of health insurance. But the ways students are insured varies widely and is changing under the Affordable Care Act. Meanwhile, a significant percentage—about 20%, or 1.7 million students—have been uninsured, according to a federal analysis:[22]

- About 67% of students have insurance through a family member's employer. This means that someone in the family, most likely a parent, has insurance through work and includes the student in that coverage. Under the Affordable Care Act passed in 2010, a young person can stay on a parent's insurance policy until age 26. In the past, many policies stopped covering dependents when they reached their early 20s, at which age many students became uninsured.

- About 7% of students have insurance through another type of commercial policy, such as a student insurance plan offered by a college or university. More than half of all colleges now offer student health plans. Costs for this coverage vary widely, ranging anywhere from $30 to $2,400 a year, with most plans costing less than $1,000 a year. Many of these plans make use of the campus health center—some don't cover primary care, for example, if the student health center already provides this care. In 2011 and 2012, federal health-care regulators began developing rules to ensure that students insured under these types of plans receive the same protections as other Americans under the Affordable Care Act.[24]

- About 6% of students are covered by public insurance programs, such as Medicaid, for low-income individuals and families, or Medicare, for students with long-term disabilities. Recipients may also receive some care through their student health centers.

- About 20% of students have no health insurance. Among 18- to 23-year-olds, those aged 22 and older are more likely to be uninsured. Students of color are far more likely to be uninsured than white students, with Latinos more likely to be uninsured than any other group. Students reporting lower family incomes were also more likely to be without coverage.

See **Practical Strategies: Tips for Affordable Health Care** for ideas about how to find health care that won't put you in debt.

What Happens When I Graduate?

When it's time to get your diploma, find out what happens to your health insurance. Students going straight to graduate school or a job offering health insurance may have little or no gap in their coverage. But if you face going without coverage for any length of time, you'll need to take steps to protect yourself.

If you have insurance through your parents, that coverage can continue until you reach the age of 26. If you have health insurance through your school, that coverage often ends around the time of your graduation. If you are covered through a public program, your insurance is less likely to be tied to your student status, but find out for sure.

When your coverage ends, you'll likely have options to extend it, but at a high price. College and university policies can often be extended, but the cost will likely be at least double the cost of the original premium. For example, if your campus policy cost $1,200 per year, you'd pay at least $2,400 per year for the extension. You may be able to extend your coverage under your family or campus policy through a program called *COBRA*, but such policies often cost at least $300 or more a month, for a yearly bill of $3,600 or more.

You may also choose a policy on the individual insurance market. For younger people who are less likely to get sick, these are often more affordable options than programs such as COBRA, usually carrying premiums of about $100 to $200 a month. Many of these policies, however, currently offer the type of "mini-med" coverage described earlier in this chapter. Many types of services probably won't be included. Make sure you understand the limits of your policy, and purchase one that gives you as much flexibility and coverage as possible. A new option is to purchase a comprehensive individual policy through the Health Insurance Marketplace created by the Affordable

Practical Strategies

Tips for Affordable Health Care

No form of health-care coverage will pay for every penny of your health-care costs. To help ensure you don't wind up with medical bills that you can't afford, keep these strategies in mind:

- If you have your own insurance, make sure you understand the basic limits of the policy. How much do you have to pay in deductibles? What other out-of-pocket payments or "co-payments" are you responsible for? Does your insurance restrict your care geographically? Does it have a separate prescription plan? What services or providers are excluded? Does it stop covering you when you reach a certain age? What are the rules on visiting a hospital in an emergency? Make sure you keep a current copy of your insurance card, which you'll need to show medical providers when you receive care.

- Learn about what services are offered at your college's student health center. If a service isn't provided, ask about discount programs the center may have with other providers. Student health centers may have discount arrangements with local pharmacies, dentists, and other types of health providers.

- Avoid heading to the emergency department or calling an ambulance unless you truly require emergency attention. Although emergency

departments are required to treat all patients who enter their doors seeking help (even patients with minor illnesses who don't have insurance), the care they provide is expensive, and you'll be billed directly. For less serious ailments, you can often receive the care you need at a much lower price from a community or retail clinic.

- Take care of your health preventively, which will help reduce the amount and cost of medical care you may need.

Care Act. If you live in a state that participates in the Health Insurance Marketplace, you can receive insurance through your state-run marketplace. If your state does not participate, you can purchase it through a federal marketplace.

 For information about the new state and federal Health Insurance Marketplaces, including costs, coverage comparisons, how to apply, and whether your state runs a marketplace, go to: www.healthcare.gov/health-insurance-marketplace.

"Personalized Medicine" and the Future of Consumer Health

New medical advances against major diseases such as cancer are made each year. In the coming years, however, few advances will have as much potential to fundamentally reshape how you think about your health as personal **genomics.** Defined broadly as the study of the human **genome** (the biological code that "builds" a human being), genomics once seemed largely confined to science fiction. But with the decoding of the human genome completed in 2003, our understanding of this "code of life" has made it possible for us to examine our own genomes and understand some of the information they hold about our health. The goal of this effort is **personalized medicine,** or health care based on the idea that because your individual DNA is unique, your health is as well, and your care and treatments should be tailored to you at the genomic level.

A Short Course in Genetics and Genomics

Genomics sounds complex—and it is—but to get a basic understanding of your own genome, you only need to know a few key concepts:

- **DNA** (deoxyribonucleic acid) is the material that carries the biological instructions that "build" us. These instructions are *genetic,* meaning that they are inherited from our parents and ancestors. For example, your DNA is genetic information because you inherited it from your mother and father, who passed their DNA on to you when you were conceived. If you have a genetic disorder, it means you have a health condition passed on in the DNA you inherited from someone in your family.

- **Genes** are packets of DNA that carry the code for specific building blocks in your body.

genomics The study of genomes and their effects on health and development.

genome The complete genetic code of an organism.

personalized medicine Health care based on the idea that because your individual DNA is unique, your health is as well, and your care and treatments should be tailored to you.

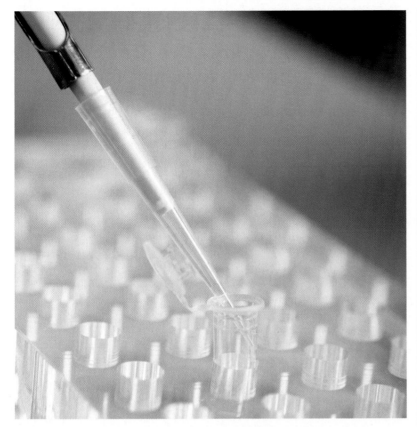

Advances in genomics are resulting in high-tech options for personalized health care.

- **Chromosomes** are packets of genes and supporting DNA that make up your genome.
- **Your genome** is your entire collection of DNA, coiled in a tight double spiral. Copies of your genome are found in almost every cell in your body. Although all human beings share mostly the same DNA, everyone's genome contains a few unique differences, or *genetic variants.* Your variants make you distinct in many ways, including in some of the ways your health may develop.
- **Your genome is not your destiny.** Although DNA is powerful, it is not the only factor that determines who you are or how healthy you may be. Environment and behavior choices are also powerful forces that can shape your health.

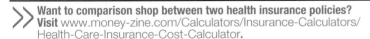
Want to comparison shop between two health insurance policies? Visit www.money-zine.com/Calculators/Insurance-Calculators/ Health-Care-Insurance-Cost-Calculator.

Uses of Genomic Information

As our understanding of the human genome evolves, this information is rapidly transforming health care. In the past, health has often been discussed in terms of "one size fits all" or "one size fits many." But genomic information increasingly enables people, either on their own or through their care providers, to find approaches more likely to work for them on an individual basis. Here are some of the ways genomic understanding is reshaping health.

Family Health Histories
Public health officials now encourage everyone in the United States to create a basic **family health history,** or a record of health conditions that have appeared in a family over time. Health histories used to be reserved for families with rare genetic conditions, such as the blood clotting disorder hemophilia. Now, however, genomic research has revealed that many common health conditions, such as type 2 diabetes, high cholesterol, and heart disease, have a genetic component. Creating a family health history enables you and your relatives to look for patterns of illness that might indicate genetic risk.

 You can find information on creating a family health history at www.hhs .gov/familyhistory.

Single-Gene Testing
If you or your care provider thinks you are at risk for a genetic illness, you may opt to have genetic testing, or analysis of a certain gene or section of a particular chromosome. Such *single-gene testing* can tell you whether you carry DNA variants known to be linked to particular health conditions. Some women with particular family backgrounds, for example, choose to be tested for breast cancer–related variants in genes called *BRCA1* and *BRCA2.* If they find that they are at increased genetic risk, they may opt for medical treatments that reduce their risk.

These tests are powerful, but they are also expensive and emotionally complex. Most such genetic testing is usually conducted with the help and support of a *genetic counselor,* a medical professional who helps patients understand genetic testing, assess their own feelings and beliefs about such testing, decide whether they want testing, and determine how they will respond to the results.

Whole-Genome Scanning and Sequencing
Other genetic technologies analyze your whole genome at once and see what it says about your risk for a variety of health conditions. In some cases, this form of testing only looks at specific points on your genome, a process called **whole-genome scanning.** Scientists can also decode and spell out every point on your genome, a process called **genome sequencing.** Scanning is simpler and cheaper, for now. However, sequencing has the potential to be more powerful, and costs are coming down rapidly as technologies improve.

If you find yourself thinking about any form of DNA testing, consider speaking with a genetic counselor first to help you find options that are right for you. These health-care professionals are experts in explaining genetic options and helping people sort through personal values as they consider genetic testing or personalized medicine.

DNA Tests and Medical Choices
In addition to providing information about risks for certain illnesses, DNA information can sometimes help us decide how to treat them. Each of us, for example, carries DNA variants that affect how our bodies process certain medications. The study of this DNA–drug interaction, called **pharmacogenomics,** has already changed the way some doctors prescribe certain blood thinners and other medications. In the case of some

family health history A detailed record of health issues in one's family that presents a picture of shared health risks.

whole-genome scanning A form of genetic testing that looks for variants throughout a person's genome.

genome sequencing The full decoding and readout of an entire genome.

pharmacogenomics The use of DNA information to choose medications and make prescribing decisions.

cancers, doctors can now analyze the DNA of tumors to determine which drugs might best treat them.

Ethical, Social, and Legal Implications of Genomic Advances

Genomic advances can enable you to take a more personal approach to your health. But for many, it also raises doubts and fears. What about privacy? Will others use your genetic information to discriminate against you, or to justify higher insurance premiums?

These questions are already shaping new laws designed to help build a lifetime of better health in the genomic era. In 2008, U.S. lawmakers enacted the *Genetic Information Nondiscrimination Act,* or *GINA.* This law strengthens the privacy of personal DNA information and prohibits genetic discrimination in health insurance and employment.

Still, other questions remain. Should genetic discrimination also be barred in other types of insurance, such as disability insurance? How widely should personal DNA information be shared? Will DNA knowledge make people feel more empowered about their health, or more hopeless? These and other important questions will continue to drive discussion, regulation, and personal decisions as the genomic era unfolds.

Change Yourself, Change Your World

"Be a smart patient? My own best health-care advocate? I'm just trying to get through this term!" The idea of being an active health consumer may feel a little daunting, but paying attention to just a few basic steps on a regular basis will go a long way.

Personal Choices

Investing a little time in these five areas will pay off, now and in the long run:

- **Practice prevention.** Use the information you've gained from this course and this book to build and maintain wellness. Take the **Self-Assessment** to see if you're practicing prevention enough.
- **Make informed choices.** Spend time learning about any new health option. If you don't have the information you need, ask. Make sure you get all the details.
- **Find the right care before you need it.** Don't wait until you are sick to find a doctor. Learn about care providers on campus and in your community. That knowledge will make everything easier when you do need care.
- **Know when you need help.** When you have the busy schedule of a student, it's easy to push health issues aside for later. But waiting can mean complications. Taking an hour to visit the student health center might make the difference between resting for a day or two and losing a bigger chunk of time to illness.
- **Know how you'll pay.** Few surprises can be as bad as a big medical bill that you didn't expect. Before you get sick, understand your health insurance, what it covers, and what costs it leaves in your hands. If you have an HSA or FSA, stay on top of your balance.

Campus Advocacy

You don't have to wait for federal health-care reform to help your fellow students get the care they need. Across the country, groups of students are working to bring insurance reform and more affordable coverage to their campuses.

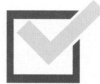
At Tufts University in Massachusetts, for example, students formed the Students Health Organizing Coalition (SHOC) in 2008 to help address the needs of their peers with little or no insurance coverage and sizable amounts of medical debt. The group first met with campus officials, and then expanded its reach to state regulators and legislators, demanding insurance reform.

SHOC's work led to a state report that exposed larger profit margins for student insurers, even if they offered less coverage than other types of health insurance. The state of Massachusetts then decided to offer improved insurance coverage to state residents at most state schools. SHOC representatives later testified on a panel before the U.S. Senate as federal lawmakers considered student insurance reform.

To help improve insurance coverage for students on your campus, start by asking friends and classmates about their insurance experiences. Host a roundtable discussion, or set up an online forum where fellow students can post their stories. You are likely to find that many of your fellow students face insurance dilemmas. Once you know the nature of such issues on your campus, you and other concerned students can speak with your campus administrators and health center about possible changes that help get everyone on your campus the coverage—and health care—they need.

>> **Watch videos of real students discussing consumer health** at MasteringHealth™

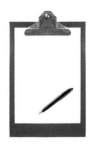

Choosing to Change Worksheet

To complete this worksheet online, visit MasteringHealth™

It's easy not to worry about preventive care or health insurance until you get sick or injured. But a little planning can reduce your risk of illness and protect you if or when you need medical care.

Directions: Fill in your stage of change in Part I and complete the rest of the part with your stage of change in mind. Regardless of your stage of change, everyone should complete Part II.

Part I: Becoming Proactive About Preventive Care

Step 1. *Your Stage of Behavior Change.* Check one of the following statements that best describes your readiness to be proactive about your health care.

_____ I do not plan to take part in preventive care in the next six months. (Precontemplation)

_____ I might take part in preventive care in the next six months. (Contemplation)

_____ I am prepared to begin taking part in preventive care in the next month. (Preparation)

_____ I have been taking part in preventive care for less than six months. (Action)

_____ I have been taking part in preventive care for six months or longer. (Maintenance)

Step 2. *Response to Self-Assessment.* Complete the Self-Assessment on page 338.

1. Which questions did you answer "No" to? Based on this Self-Assessment, what can you do to be more proactive about your preventive care?

_____

_____

_____

2. What concerns or obstacles, if any, do you have about the preventive care behaviors described in this chapter? Write down who you could contact to ask questions about your concerns or how you could overcome these obstacles.

Example: I am concerned that having an eye exam will cost a lot of money. I could visit the campus health center to see if there are any low-cost programs for optometrist visits.

_____

_____

_____

Part II: Scheduling Preventive Care Appointments

Use this worksheet to start becoming more proactive about your health.

	Past Behavior	Future Behavior
Physical exam	When was the last time you had a physical exam?	When will you schedule your next exam?
Gynecological exam with Pap test (for females)	When was the last time you had a gynecological exam?	When will you schedule your next exam?
Dental care	When was the last time you visited a dentist?	When will you schedule your next exam?
Vision care	When was the last time you had a general vision exam?	When will you schedule your next exam?
Protection from influenza	When was the last time you received an influenza vaccination?	If it's been over a year since your last vaccination, when will you schedule your next one?
Health insurance	Do you have health insurance?	If you do not have health insurance, when will you investigate the options available to you?

Chapter Summary

- Our health system is increasingly one in which individuals have an abundance of choices, but also the responsibility of researching information, critically evaluating it, and making educated decisions.

- *Self-care* includes maintaining basic wellness habits, evaluating health information critically, using over-the-counter medications properly, using home health tests properly, and knowing when it is time to see a doctor.

- Preventive care, such as periodic screenings and checkups, can help prevent health problems or catch them early when they are often easier to treat.

- *Conventional medicine* is characterized by a focus on the physical aspects and treatment of disease; the presence of discernible, defined symptoms; the maintenance of public health; and the use of scientific evidence and the scientific method.

- Conventional care is now available from a wide variety of facilities and providers, ranging from hospitals to student health centers to retail clinics.

- When choosing a health-care provider, find out whether he or she is covered by your insurance plan, and ask friends and family for recommendations. When you meet a care provider in person, make sure he or she listens to you, answers your questions completely, and treats you with respect. Be vocal and honest with your provider about all aspects of your health.

- Prescription medications are now the number one cause of overdose deaths in the United States. It is very important to handle prescription medications as directed.

- *Complementary and alternative medicine* (CAM) encompasses therapies and practices outside those of conventional medicine. CAM practices often look beyond the physical aspects of disease to issues that connect mind, body, and spirit.

- Examples of CAM include traditional Chinese medicine, natural products such as herbs and botanicals, mind–body therapies, manipulative therapies, and energy therapies.

- CAM is popular, but many CAM practices have not been proven safe or effective. Research any CAM therapy or provider before starting care, and make sure both your CAM and conventional practitioners know the full range of care you are receiving as well as your health history and habits to make sure you are being treated safely.

- Options for paying for health care include discount health programs, health insurance, health savings accounts, and flexible spending accounts.

- Health insurance policies come in many forms, including managed-care plans, fee-for-service plans, and public plans.

- *Genomics* is the study of the human genome. Genomic research is spurring the development of personalized health care based on an individual's DNA.

- Examples of genomic applications in health care include prenatal testing, single-gene testing, whole-genome scanning, and genome sequencing.

GET CONNECTED

>> Visit the following websites for further information about topics in this chapter:

- The Medical Library Association's Top 100 List: Health Websites You Can Trust
  http://caphis.mlanet.org/consumer/index.html

- Evaluating Online Sources of Health Information (from the National Cancer Institute, part of the National Institutes of Health)
  www.cancer.gov/cancertopics/cancerlibrary/health-info-online

- Agency for Healthcare Research and Quality (AHRQ)
  www.ahrq.gov

- National Center for Complementary and Alternative Medicine
  http://nccam.nih.gov

- The Human Genome Project
  web.ornl.gov/sci/techresources/Human_Genome/home.shtml

MOBILE TIPS!

Scan this QR code with your mobile device to access additional tips about consumer health. Or, via your mobile device, go to **http://chmobile.pearsoncmg.com** and navigate to Chapter 13.

Website links are subject to change. To access updated web links, please visit MasteringHealth™

TEST YOUR KNOWLEDGE

1. What is NOT an example of preventive care?
   a. eating nutritiously
   b. wearing a seat belt
   c. scheduling regular physicals
   d. taking cold medicine correctly

2. What are the typical characteristics of credible health-related research?
   a. publication in a peer-reviewed journal
   b. a large pool of study participants
   c. results that have been replicated by other scientists
   d. all of these answers.

3. You should seek emergency care for all of the following, EXCEPT
   a. cold symptoms.
   b. difficulty breathing.
   c. sudden, severe pain.
   d. adverse reactions to a medication or insect bite.

4. Which of the following is NOT considered a practitioner of conventional medicine?
   a. medical doctors
   b. acupuncturists
   c. nurse practitioners
   d. dentists

5. Being a smart patient includes
   a. being honest and vocal with your doctor.
   b. asking questions when you don't understand something.
   c. following the instructions you receive from your doctor.
   d. all of these answers.

6. What is chiropractic an example of?
   a. alternative medicine
   b. conventional medicine
   c. energy therapy
   d. naturopathy

7. Which of the following is characteristic of managed-care health insurance plans?
   a. The more flexibility you want, the more the insurance will cost.
   b. They don't cover medication.
   c. There are no out-of-pocket fees associated with them.
   d. They offer no flexibility for medical care outside of the plan's approved providers.

8. Under the Affordable Care Act, children can stay on their parents' insurance plans until what maximum age?
   a. 18
   b. 21
   c. 26
   d. 30

9. Analyzing a certain gene to assess the risk of developing a genetic disease is an example of
   a. whole-genome sequencing.
   b. single-gene testing.
   c. genomics.
   d. genetic variation.

10. The study of DNA–drug interaction is called
    a. pharmacogenomics.
    b. single-gene testing.
    c. alternative medicine.
    d. carrier testing.

Get Critical

What happened

The whole human genome was sequenced for the first time in 2003 by the Human Genome Project. Funded by the U.S. and international governments and foundations, it cost about $2.7 billion to sequence.[1] Since then, costs to sequence a human genome have dropped dramatically.

Today, private citizens can purchase commercial genetic sequencing for as little as a few thousand dollars, which can search for the presence of over 1,800 disease genes.[2] These genes may increase the risk of diseases, such as certain cancers, heart disease, some neurological disorders, and even autism.[3] People use the results not only to guide their own care, but also during family planning to identify any genetic risks they may pass on to a child.

Although assessment of your whole genome holds promise, this form of testing remains controversial. Proponents say that broad genome assessment is now ready for widespread use and can provide more effective preventive measures and pharmaceutical treatment. Critics counter that our understanding of health-related genetic risks is still too new, and even if a genetic mutation is detected, it's often unclear how aggressively doctors should react to the discovery.[4]

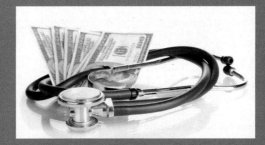

What do you think?

- If you discovered that you carried a genetic mutation related to an increased risk of disease, would it change how you lived your life?

- Would you want health insurance companies to know about your increased risk?

- If you found out about an increased disease risk while you were planning to have a family, would it change your plans? If you already had children and you discovered that you had a genetic risk for a disease that may or may not have been passed on to them, what and when would you tell your children about their own possible risk?

References: **1.** *The Human Genome Project: Frequently Asked Questions,* by the National Human Genome Research Institute, Newsroom, 2010. www.genome.gov. **2.** *NIH Fact Sheet: Human Genome Project,* by the National Institutes of Health, 2013, www.nih.gov. **3.** "Detection of Clinically Relevant Genetic Variants in Autism Spectrum Disorder by Whole-Genome Sequencing," by Y. Jiang, R. K. C. Yuen, X. Jin, M. Wang, N. Chen, X. Wu, . . . S. W. Scherer, 2013, *The American Journal of Human Genetics,* published online ahead of print issue. **4.** "Should Healthy People Have Their Genomes Sequenced At This Time?" by A. J. Butte & R. Green, February 15, 2013, *The Wall Street Journal.*

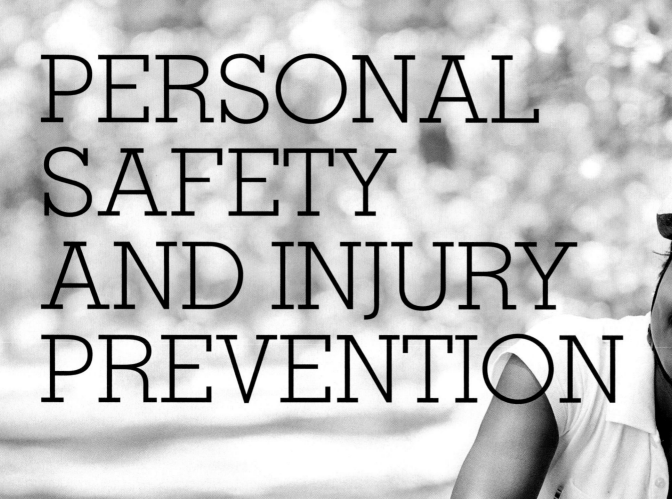

PERSONAL SAFETY AND INJURY PREVENTION

Nearly **72%** of teen and young adult (aged 15–24) **deaths** are caused by **injuries**.[i]

Each year, at least 3,000 Americans die because of car crashes involving **distracted driving**.[ii]

1 in 4 women has been the victim of **severe physical violence** by an intimate partner.[iii]

14

Learning Objectives

NAME the most common unintentional injuries and contributing factors.

DISCUSS ways you can reduce your risk of motor vehicle accidents.

IDENTIFY five steps for staying safe while walking and cycling.

DISCUSS contributing factors and prevention strategies for residential, recreational, and occupational injuries.

IDENTIFY trends in the incidence of violent crime in the United States and common contributing factors.

DISCUSS violence within communities, including school and campus violence.

DEFINE and **DESCRIBE** intimate partner violence, including the factors that keep victims in abusive relationships.

IDENTIFY types of sexual violence and strategies for preventing it.

EXPLAIN how you can help improve campus safety.

Stay out of trouble!

Did your parents ever shout this warning as you headed out the door? And if so, what did it mean to you? Driving within the speed limit? Staying sober at parties? In this chapter, we use the term **personal safety** to describe anything people do to stay out of trouble. Specifically, it's the practice of making decisions and taking actions that reduce your risk of injury and death.

Injuries are the number-one killer of Americans between the ages of 1 and 44.[1] They cause more deaths among people in this age group than all types of diseases—cancer, heart disease, infections, etc.—put together. What's more, injuries cost our economy over 400 billion dollars each year.[2] The good news is that a handful of simple choices can help you significantly reduce your injury risk.

Injuries fall into two main categories. An **unintentional injury** is any bodily damage not deliberately inflicted. Common examples are injuries sustained in motor vehicle accidents, falls, and fires. **Intentional injuries,** on the other hand, are purposefully inflicted through physical or sexual violence. Note that self-inflicted injuries and suicide are considered intentional injuries.

Overview of Unintentional Injuries

Unintentional injuries, or those that occur without intent to cause harm, send more than 29 million people to emergency departments in the United States each year.[3] In 2011, they caused over 122,000 deaths among Americans of all ages.[1] The National Safety Council (NSC) ranks the leading causes of unintentional injury death as follows:[4]

- Motor vehicle accidents caused over 34,000 deaths in 2011, making them the primary cause of unintentional deaths.[1]
- Unintentional poisonings, including drug overdose, rank a close second, killing about 33,000 Americans annually.[5]
- Falls, choking, drowning, and fires are other common causes of unintentional injury deaths. Together they account for more than 37,000 deaths each year.[5]

We tend to think of unintentional injuries as *accidents*, happening by chance. However, they typically involve one or more contributing factors such as intoxication, fatigue, and distraction. For this reason, many are considered preventable. Although every type of unintentional injury has unique circumstances, as a group they share these risk factors:

- **Substance abuse.** Heavy alcohol consumption or other substance abuse increases the risk of unintentional injuries. Alcohol is a factor in 60% of fatal burn injuries and drownings and 40% of fatal motor vehicle accidents and falls.[6]
- **Sex.** Males account for almost two-thirds of the deaths attributed to unintentional injuries.[5]
- **Age.** Compared with other age groups, young people (aged 15 to 29) account for the largest proportion of overall injury death.[1]
- **Environmental factors.** Factors such as heavy traffic or poor weather can increase risk of automobile, motorcycle, bicycle, or recreational injury.
- **Divided attention.** Performing any type of potentially dangerous activity without completely focusing on the task at hand increases the risk of injury.

Motor Vehicle Accidents

On average each year, more than 2 million people in the United States are injured in a motor vehicle accident (MVA); in 2011, more than 34,000 died.[1] Nearly one-quarter of all deaths among people

personal safety The practice of making decisions and taking actions that reduce your risk of injury and death.

unintentional injury (accidents) Bodily damage that is not deliberately caused.

intentional injury Physical harm that is purposefully inflicted through violence.

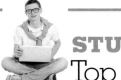

STUDENT STATS
Top Five Causes of Death in the United States Among People Aged 15–24

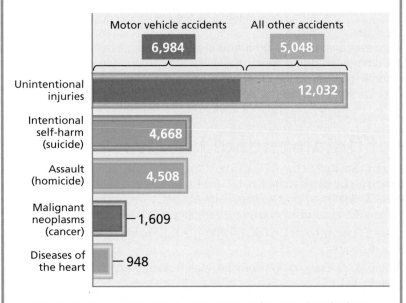

	Motor vehicle accidents	All other accidents
	6,984	5,048
Unintentional injuries		12,032
Intentional self-harm (suicide)	4,668	
Assault (homicide)	4,508	
Malignant neoplasms (cancer)	— 1,609	
Diseases of the heart	— 948	

Data from *Deaths: Preliminary Data for 2011*, by D. L. Hoyert & J. Xu, October 10, 2012, *National Vital Statistics Reports, 61*(6), Hyattsville, MD: National Center for Health Statistics, retrieved from http://www.cdc.gov/nchs/data/nvsr/nvsr61/nvsr61_06.pdf.

between the ages of 15 and 24 are due to MVAs.[1] No other single cause of death claims more young lives.

What Factors Increase the Risk for Motor Vehicle Accidents?

The National Safety Council identifies the following as key factors contributing to MVAs.[4]

Distracted Driving

Talking on your phone, sending a text message, or fiddling with your stereo while you drive dramatically increases your chance of an MVA. Consider these statistics:

- In 2011, 3,331 people were killed in MVAs involving distracted driving.[7] These crashes represent nearly 10% of all fatal MVAs that year.[1] More than 20% of them involved cell phone use.[4]

- The risk of getting into a car accident that causes injury goes up fourfold when a driver is speaking on a cell phone.[7] A recent national study found that speaking on a hands-free cell phone, with no manual contact, does not increase crash risk; however, the same study noted that interfaces often require drivers to manipulate their phones in order to place and end calls and when voice recognition from remote devices fails.[8] Moreover, another national study challenged the claim that drivers are safe as long as their hands are on the wheel

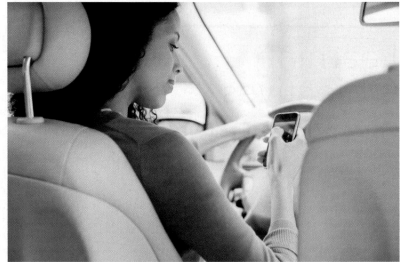

 Texting while driving is incredibly dangerous.

and their eyes on the road. It found that talking hands-free places a high "cognitive burden" on drivers that causes them to miss visual cues and have slowed reaction times.[9] Thus, controversy remains over the level of distraction posed by use of hands-free devices.

- The risk of an MVA is 23 times higher when texting while driving.[7] Texting takes a driver's eyes off the road for an average of 4.6 seconds, the equivalent at 55 mph of driving the length of a football field blindfolded.[7] And some drivers videotaped while texting had their eyes off the road for nearly half a minute.[8] It's hardly surprising, then, that texting while driving has been outlawed in 41 states and the District of Columbia.[10] Prosecutions for vehicular homicide for texting-while-driving fatality cases are becoming more common.

Despite the dangers of distracted driving, a 2011 study found that a startling 91% of college students admit to texting while driving.[11] Another study found that 92% of college students read text messages while driving and that 70% even initiate messages while driving.[12]

>> **Try the** *New York Times* **game that tests how distracted you become while trying to text message while driving:** www.nytimes.com/interactive/2009/07/19/technology/20090719-driving-game.html?_r=0.

Impaired Driving

Alcohol-impaired driving is responsible for about one-third of all highway fatalities each year in the United States and driving with a blood alcohol concentration (BAC) of 0.08% or higher is illegal in all 50 states.[13] But drinking even a small amount of alcohol impairs your vision, motor skills, judgment, and alertness. That's why, in 2013, the National Transportation Safety Board recommended that states adopt a new, lower BAC limit of 0.05%. (For more on alcohol-impaired driving, see Chapter 8.) Illicit drugs, sleep medications, pain medications, antianxiety medications, and even over-the-counter cold remedies can also reduce driving skills. A total of 18 states have strict laws that forbid any presence of a prohibited substance in the blood of drivers.[14]

Research studies have consistently found that drowsiness is a factor in about 1 out of 6 fatal MVAs.[15] Fatigue slows your reaction time and reduces your attention level, ability to process information, and the accuracy of your short-term memory, all of which impair your driving. As of 2013, New Jersey was the only state with a law specifically

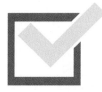

SELF-ASSESSMENT

Are You an Aggressive Driver?

Do you have aggressive habits that could threaten your safety or the safety of others on the road? Circle Yes or No for each question.

Do you . . .

1. Overtake other vehicles **only** on the left?　Yes　No

2. Avoid blocking passing lanes?　Yes　No

3. Yield to faster traffic by moving to the right?　Yes　No

4. Keep to the right as much as possible on narrow streets and at intersections?　Yes　No

5. Maintain appropriate distance when following other vehicles, bicyclists, or motorcyclists?　Yes　No

6. Provide appropriate distance when cutting in after passing a vehicle?　Yes　No

7. Use headlights in cloudy, raining, or low-light conditions?　Yes　No

8. Yield to pedestrians?　Yes　No

9. Come to a complete stop at stop signs or before a right turn at a red light?　Yes　No

10. Stop for red traffic lights?　Yes　No

11. Approach intersections and pedestrians at slow speeds to show your intention and ability to stop?　Yes　No

12. Follow right-of-way rules at four-way stops?　Yes　No

13. Drive below posted speed limits when conditions warrant?　Yes　No

14. Drive at slower speeds in construction zones?　Yes　No

15. Maintain speeds appropriate for conditions?　Yes　No

16. Use turn signals for turns and lane changes?　Yes　No

17. Make eye contact and signal intentions where needed?　Yes　No

18. Acknowledge intentions of others?　Yes　No

19. Use your horn sparingly around pedestrians, at night, around hospitals, and at other times?　Yes　No

20. Avoid unnecessary use of high-beam headlights?　Yes　No

21. Yield and move to the right for emergency vehicles?　Yes　No

22. Refrain from flashing headlights to signal a desire to pass?　Yes　No

23. Drive trucks at posted speeds, in the proper lanes, using nonaggressive lane changing?　Yes　No

24. Make slow, deliberate U-turns?　Yes　No

25. Maintain proper speeds around roadway crashes?　Yes　No

26. Avoid returning inappropriate gestures?　Yes　No

27. Avoid challenging other drivers?　Yes　No

28. Try to get out of the way of aggressive drivers?　Yes　No

29. Refrain from momentarily using High Occupancy Vehicle (HOV) lanes to pass vehicles?　Yes　No

30. Focus on driving and avoid distracting activities (e.g., smoking, use of a cell phone, reading, shaving)?　Yes　No

31. Avoid driving when drowsy?　Yes　No

32. Avoid blocking the right-hand turn lane?　Yes　No

33. Avoid taking more than one parking space?　Yes　No

34. Avoid parking in a disabled space (if you are not disabled)?　Yes　No

35. Avoid letting your door hit the car parked next to you?　Yes　No

36. Avoid using the cell phone while driving?　Yes　No

37. Avoid stopping in the road to talk with a pedestrian or other driver?　Yes　No

38. Avoid inflicting loud music on neighboring cars?　Yes　No

HOW TO INTERPRET YOUR SCORE

0–3 "No" answers: Excellent
4–7 "No" answers: Good

8–11 "No" answers: Fair
12–38 "No" answers: Poor

To complete this Self-Assessment online, visit MasteringHealth™

Adapted from Are You an Aggressive Driver or a Smooth Operator? from the New Jersey Office of the Attorney General, Division of Highway Traffic Safety website. Copyright © New Jersey Office of the Attorney General. Reprinted with permission.

prohibiting driving while drowsy; however, at least four other states have introduced legislation to make drowsy driving a punishable offense.[16]

 Watch a video on the dangers of drowsy driving at www.youtube.com/watch?v=JwCnJZyU70M.

Skipping Seat Belts

Almost all states require that drivers and passengers use seat belts and, if they are young children, child safety seats. Yet about 15% of vehicle occupants don't consistently use these proven lifesavers.[4] Seat belt use is lowest among people between the ages of 16 and 24; however, college students do better than their peers. In a national survey, less than 5% stated that they don't wear a seat belt consistently—or ever.[17]

Some people fail to buckle up in the belief that airbags provide sufficient crash protection, but seat belts are the single most effective prevention against injury or death in a car crash.[18] One benefit of seat belts is that they prevent you from being thrown from the car—an event that is five times more deadly than if you remain in the car during an accident.[19]

Speeding and Other Forms of Aggressive Driving

Aggressive driving is the operation of a motor vehicle in a manner that endangers people or property.[20] Examples of aggressive driving include speeding, driving too quickly for road conditions, tailgating, failing to

yield the right-of-way, cutting off other vehicles, and abruptly or improperly changing lanes. Aggressive driving is estimated to be a factor in more than 55% of fatal car crashes.[4]

Speeding—driving at a rate above the posted speed limit—reduces the amount of time you have to react to conditions in the road in front of you, increases the distance needed to stop in an emergency, and reduces the effectiveness of safety devices like seat belts and airbags. On an average day, 32 drivers are killed in speed-related accidents.[4]

How Can You Reduce Your Risk for Motor Vehicle Accidents?

Your first line of defense is prevention. Don't get behind the wheel if you've been drinking—even a small amount—or using any other drugs. Pick a designated driver, use your campus's SafeRides program, or call a cab. Never get in a car with a driver who is impaired.

Don't drive if you haven't had adequate sleep. You might not feel sleepy but many drivers in drowsy-driving MVAs report that they did not feel sleepy before they nodded off.

Don't set off if you haven't allowed enough time for your trip. If you can't get where you want to go by the time you want to get there, stay home, call, and reschedule.

Among people between the ages of 15 and 24, nothing claims more lives than **motor vehicle accidents**. To reduce your risk:

CHOOSE THIS.

NOT THAT.

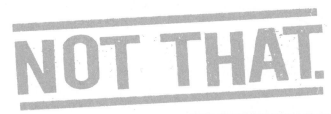

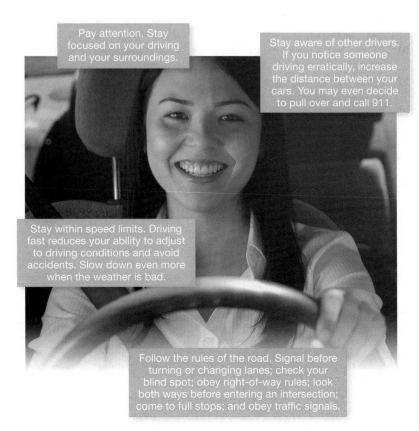

Pay attention. Stay focused on your driving and your surroundings.

Stay aware of other drivers. If you notice someone driving erratically, increase the distance between your cars. You may even decide to pull over and call 911.

Stay within speed limits. Driving fast reduces your ability to adjust to driving conditions and avoid accidents. Slow down even more when the weather is bad.

Follow the rules of the road. Signal before turning or changing lanes; check your blind spot; obey right-of-way rules; look both ways before entering an intersection; come to full stops; and obey traffic signals.

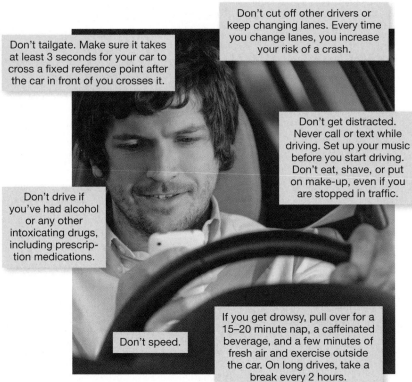

Don't tailgate. Make sure it takes at least 3 seconds for your car to cross a fixed reference point after the car in front of you crosses it.

Don't cut off other drivers or keep changing lanes. Every time you change lanes, you increase your risk of a crash.

Don't get distracted. Never call or text while driving. Set up your music before you start driving. Don't eat, shave, or put on make-up, even if you are stopped in traffic.

Don't drive if you've had alcohol or any other intoxicating drugs, including prescription medications.

Don't speed.

If you get drowsy, pull over for a 15–20 minute nap, a caffeinated beverage, and a few minutes of fresh air and exercise outside the car. On long drives, take a break every 2 hours.

Attentive and Defensive Driving:

The great majority of motor vehicle accidents could be prevented by attentive, defensive driving.

Distracted, Impaired, or Aggressive Driving:

Distracted, impaired, and aggressive driving are factors in a majority of fatal motor vehicle accidents. Avoiding these behaviors dramatically reduces your risk.

Before you set off, buckle up. It only takes a second. And in most states, it's the law.

> The National Safety Council offers courses in defensive driving. Find out more at www.nsc.org.

Once you get on the road, drive defensively, not aggressively. See the **Choose This, Not That** above for specific strategies.

If you're considering buying a new or used car, make sure it has all recommended safety features, such as airbags, antilock brakes, and electronic stability control. Before you get behind the wheel, make sure you have enough gas to get where you're going and that your oil and windshield-washer fluid levels are adequate. Check the air pressure in

your tires and check that your wipers and your headlights—both high and low beams—are in working order.

Other Traffic Injuries

Accidents while walking, jogging, or cycling on roadways can also cause injuries, one of the more common of which is **traumatic brain injury (TBI).** TBI is caused when the head is jolted or hit or when an object pierces the skull, resulting in a sudden injury that damages the brain. Although many TBI patients recover quickly, a significant number face a lifetime of disability and some die. Each year, about 1.7 million Americans sustain a TBI.[21] Spinal cord injuries, fractures, and internal injuries are also common in MVAs involving pedestrians and cyclists.

Accidents Involving Pedestrians and Cyclists

In 2010, over 4,200 pedestrians were killed in traffic accidents and 70,000 were injured.[22] Nearly half of these accidents involved alcohol and the majority occurred in the evening or at night. Thus, it's important to wear reflective clothing whenever you go out for an evening walk or run. Unlike cyclists, pedestrians should always travel on the side of the road opposite the direction of traffic so that you're facing oncoming vehicles, and wherever there are sidewalks, use them.

Overall, the number of MVA injuries and fatalities, although still significant, has been declining—except among motorcycle riders. Between 2002 and 2011, the annual number of motorcycle injuries increased by 25%, and fatalities increased by 41%.[23] In 2011 about 81,000 motorcycle riders and passengers were injured and over 4,600 died.[23] Motorcyclists are about six times more likely than those riding in a car to die in a crash.[23] In 2011, 30% of fatally injured motorcyclists had a BAC level of .08 or higher. Even though 37% of all motorcyclist fatalities could be prevented if riders were wearing a helmet, only 20 states require helmet use by all motorcyclists.[23]

Bikes may not pack the force or speed of a car or motorcycle but riding one still carries risks. In 2011, 48,000 Americans were injured cycling and 677 died.[24]

Although cars need to make room on the road for bikes, bike riders are responsible for road safety as well. Cyclists are required to travel in the same direction as the flow of vehicular traffic, and obey all traffic signs, signals, and lane markings.[24]

In 21 states, children and teens are required by law to wear a helmet while riding a bike; however, in all 50 states, helmets are optional for adults.[25] In a national survey, 67% of college students who ride a bike said they only sometimes, rarely, or never wear a bike helmet.[17]

Safety Tips for Pedestrians and Cyclists

The likelihood of being in an accident can be reduced if you follow these simple guidelines.

- **Follow the rules of the road.** When on foot, cross in designated crosswalks and travel against the flow of traffic. When cycling, don't cut through lanes of traffic, run lights, or blow through stop signs. Ride with the flow of traffic.

- **Stay visible.** Don't assume that drivers can see you. Avoid cycling in a car's blind spot or passing quickly. Whether walking or cycling, wear brightly colored clothing on your upper body. At night, make sure your clothes, helmet, and/or bike are outfitted with reflectors.

- **Keep your eyes on the road.** Bicyclists are considered vehicle operators and should avoid distraction. Pedestrians need to pay attention as well: Looking down to use your cell phone while crossing a busy street puts you at the mercy of drivers.

- **Wear a helmet every time you ride.** Wearing a helmet is the single most effective way to prevent TBI resulting from a bicycle crash.[24] Wear a helmet every time you ride. For more information on choosing the right bike helmet, see the **Consumer Corner**.

- **Don't drink and ride.** Nearly a quarter of cyclists killed in bike accidents are found to have blood alcohol concentrations at or above legal limits.[24] Impaired cyclists face the same increased risks of an accident as impaired drivers.

---

traumatic brain injury (TBI)
An injury that disrupts normal functioning of the brain, caused by a jolt or blow to the brain or a penetrating head wound.

Car Accident

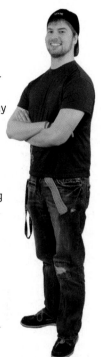

"HI, MY NAME IS CALEB. When I was 16 years old, I got in my very first car accident. I've been in other car accidents since then, but this was by far the worst. I was in a rush one day, and I was going through an intersection that I thought was a four-way stop and just stopped at the stop sign, didn't really look either way and continued going. Well, it turns out it was a two-way stop and there was a guy going about 40 miles an hour, and all I heard was just the blare of his horn. Within an instant the guy hit me. I was able to keep control of the car and I was wearing my seat belt, so I wasn't hurt at all, but my back left passenger door was just obliterated. The window was shattered out. The door was dented in beyond repair. I know if I hadn't been wearing my seat belt, any number of injuries could have happened."

1. What personal and environmental factors increased Caleb's risk of getting into a car accident?

2. What could Caleb have done to prevent that car accident from occurring?

Residential, Occupational, and Recreational Injuries

A surprising number of accidents and injuries occur at home, at work, or during recreational activities. A few basic precautions will help keep you safe.

Unintentional Poisoning

Every day, about 87 people in the United States die from unintentional poisoning and another 2,200 are treated at the hospital.[26] We all know that certain toxic substances, such as cleaning products, solvents, and pesticides, are hazardous. However, more than 90% of unintentional poisoning deaths each year are due to drugs.[26] In 2010, prescription opioid painkillers—such as oxycodone (OxyContin) and hydrocodone (Vicodin)—were responsible for 43% of these deaths.[27] These drugs are highly addictive. When taken in excess, they suppress breathing, sometimes to a degree that is fatal. They are also associated with an increased risk for heart attack.[28]

If you think you or someone you are with has been poisoned, call the National Poison Control Center at 1-800-222-1222. To avoid poisonings, store all potential poisons in their original bottles and keep them in a locked closet or upper cabinet out of the reach of children. Follow the label directions carefully. Never share or sell your prescriptions.

Choking and Suffocation

When a choking person's airway becomes blocked, oxygen can't reach the lungs. Permanent brain damage can occur within 6 minutes.[29]

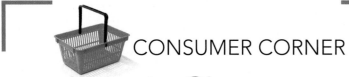

CONSUMER CORNER

How to Choose a Bike Helmet

You've gone into a sporting goods store to buy a new bike helmet and find yourself with dozens to choose from, ranging in price from $40 to more than $200. Where to start? Among bike helmets, a higher price does not necessarily equal greater safety. More expensive helmets may be tailored for specialty riders. If you aren't aspiring to be an expert road racer or mountain biker, you may not want to look at expensive specialty helmets.

Instead, you'll only need to focus on the core elements of a quality helmet—the strap, the foam liner, and the hard plastic outer shell. These make sure the helmet protects you by staying on in a crash, absorbing the shock of an impact, and providing a barrier between your head and a hard surface. Select a few helmets and try them on, paying attention to the following:

- **Size.** You need a fit that is snug but not so tight that the helmet is uncomfortable or rides up. When strapped on, the helmet shouldn't move more than an inch in any direction, and you shouldn't be able to get it off without unbuckling it no matter how you try. If your head shape is hard to fit, ask

a salesperson for help with extra padding or straps.

- **Sits straight.** The helmet should sit straight on your head, not tilted back or forward. If you have long hair that you often wear back, consider a helmet with a "ponytail port" so that your ponytail doesn't push your helmet forward.

- **Straps.** Avoid thin straps. Look instead for a set that fits snugly under your chin, with a "V" on either side that meets under your ears. Make sure the buckle is strong and doesn't pop open easily.

- **Sticker.** Helmets sold in the United States must meet safety standards set by the Consumer Product Safety Commission, and carry a CPSC sticker inside. If a helmet doesn't have one, give it a pass.

If you get in a crash, replace your helmet, even if it looks fine. The accident could have caused structural damage that you can't see but that could cause the helmet to fail in another accident. If something on your helmet breaks, don't try to fix it. Invest in a new one. In a crash, you can't count on those repairs to provide the protection you need.

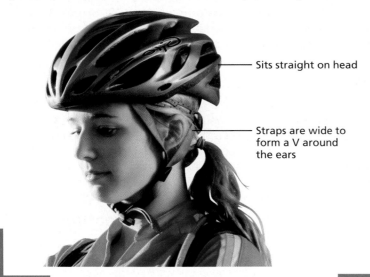

Sits straight on head

Straps are wide to form a V around the ears

Among young children, hot dogs cause the most food-related choking deaths, firmly and completely blocking the airway.[30] Grapes, cheese cubes and cheese "sticks," nuts, candies, and popcorn are other common "choking foods." If you're feeding young children, avoid all choking foods and cut other firm foods into small, thin pieces. Non-foods such as coins, buttons, and toys can be dangerous as well. Of all children's products, latex balloons cause the highest number of choking deaths.[30]

In adults, eating too fast, without chewing food properly, is the most common factor in choking. Consumption of even a small amount of alcohol increases the risk. Moreover, choking on vomited material is a significant danger for anyone who has lost consciousness after binge drinking. Never leave the person alone to "sleep it off": If he or she can't be roused, get emergency medical care.

If you're dining with someone who begins coughing forcefully and can speak, leave the person alone because a strong cough can dislodge the food. If the person grabs at his or her throat (the universal sign of choking) and cannot cough forcefully or speak, public health experts recommend following these steps:

- First, try back blows. Stand behind the person and lean him or her forward onto your non-dominant hand **(Figure 14.1a).** With the heel of your dominant hand, strike the person's upper back between the shoulder blades. This will often propel the food out of the person's mouth. If the first back blow is not successful, try up to four more, pausing between each to see if the blockage has cleared.

- If the person is still choking, try abdominal thrusts. Still standing behind the person, wrap your arms around his or her waist **(Figure 14.1b).** Place your clenched fist just above the navel. With your other hand, grab the fist and pull up and in toward you. Stop to see if the blockage has cleared. If not, give up to four more abdominal thrusts.

- If the person's airway is still blocked and you are the only rescuer, stop and call 911. If someone else is present, have that person call 911 while you continue cycles of back blows and abdominal thrusts.

You can take a class in basic emergency assistance from your local American Red Cross chapter or campus health center.

Drowning and Other Water Injuries

Drowning causes an average of 10 deaths a day, not including drownings due to boating accidents.[31] Two of these deaths are among children age 14 or younger. Children can die in less than five minutes in natural bodies of water, swimming pools, bathtubs, hot tubs, buckets, and even toilets. To protect them when they are around water, keep them within arms' reach at all times.

Drowning is also the second leading cause of unintentional injury death (after MVAs) among young people aged 10 to 19.[32] Among teens and adults, most drownings occur in natural water settings like lakes, oceans, or rivers. Consumption of alcohol is a factor in 60% of drowning deaths.[6]

The Centers for Disease Control and Prevention (CDC) offers the following water safety tips:

- Take swimming lessons! Also consider enrolling in a CPR (cardiopulmonary resuscitation) course.

- Swim with a companion, never alone. Whenever possible, swim at beaches that have a lifeguard on duty.

- Never drink alcohol when you are swimming or boating.

- Never dive or jump into an unknown body of water.

- Obey posted signs warning of unsafe swimming conditions.

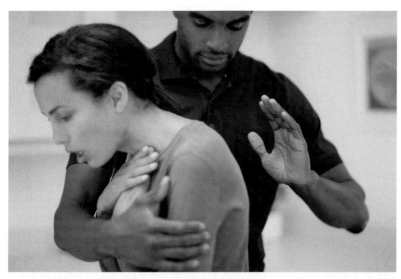

(a) Back blows

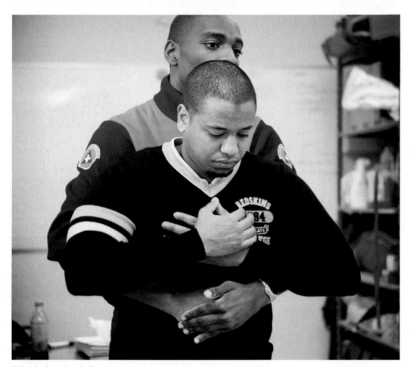

(b) Abdominal thrusts

FIGURE 14.1 How to Help Someone Who Is Conscious but Choking.

- Know the signs of a rip current: water that is choppy, discolored, foamy, or filled with debris and moving in a channel away from shore. Don't go into such waters. If you are caught in a rip current, swim parallel to shore. Swim toward shore only once you're free of the current.
- Always wear a personal flotation device (life jacket) when riding in a boat or participating in other water sports like jet skiing or waterskiing.

Fire Injuries

About 85% of all fire deaths occur in the home.[33] In 2010, fires claimed the lives of more than 2,600 people—not including firefighters. Most victims die from inhalation of smoke and toxic gases rather than from burns. The primary cause of fire-related deaths is smoking but other common causes of residential fires include candles, cooking, malfunctioning or improperly used heaters, and arson. Alcohol plays a role in about 60% of fatal burn injuries.[6]

Between January 2000 and January 2013, 82 fatal fires occurred on college campuses or in nearby off-campus housing, claiming 119 lives.[34] So next time you're tempted to complain about the fire drills in your classroom building or dorm, remember that they save lives.

Fire safety isn't difficult if you plan ahead. Every home should have a smoke detector on every level and every dorm room should have its own smoke detector. Smoke detectors should be tested monthly and the batteries replaced twice a year.

In campus fires, cooking causes more fatalities than smoking, so whenever you're using the stove or oven, don't leave it unattended. Candles should be in steady holders away from curtains and other linens and should be put out before you leave the area. Don't overload electrical outlets and make sure extension cords are used properly. If you use a portable space heater, keep it at least 3 feet away from anything flammable and never leave it unattended. If you smoke indoors, put out your cigarettes in ashtrays and never smoke in bed.

Make sure you know at least two escape routes from your dorm room or apartment and participate in fire drills. Practicing in advance will help you in the chaos of a real fire.

What should you do if you see a fire or smoke, or hear a fire alarm? The U.S. Fire Administration advises that you first feel the door for heat:[34]

- **If the door is hot**, fire may be on the other side. In that case, stay in the room, open a window, and scream for help.

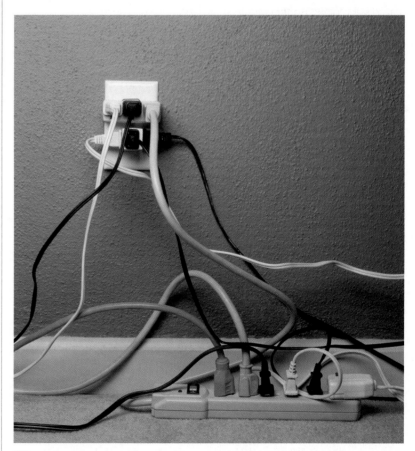

Fires can be started by overloading outlets with too many cords.

- **If the door isn't hot,** leave the room and head for your planned exit. As you do . . .
- **Get down and stay low.** Smoke rises, so crouching and crawling will enable you to move underneath the smoke so you can see better, reduce smoke inhalation, and get out more quickly. If your planned exit is blocked, exit by your alternate route.

>> Print out a copy of the U.S. Fire Administration's Get Out and Stay Alive brochure for college students at www.usfa.fema.gov/downloads/pdf/publications/fa-280.pdf.

Work-Related Injuries

Almost 3 million workers in the United States were injured on the job in 2011 and about 4,700 died.[35] If you work at a job where safety equipment is provided, use it! Goggles, masks, gloves, and other devices take only a few moments to put on and provide invaluable protection. Learn and follow all safety measures required in your workplace and if you aren't sure what they are, ask. Employers are required to provide necessary safety equipment, establish safety procedures, and provide training on both to all employees.

Even workers in offices, hospitals, and retail stores experience significant numbers of injuries each year, most often repetitive strain injuries and back injuries. Both of these types of injuries are also very common among college students, so let's take a closer look.

Repetitive Strain Injuries

Performing the same movements over and over, even slight movements with your hands and fingers, can injure and inflame your joints, connective tissues, and nerves. These **repetitive strain injuries,** or **RSIs,** can lead to pain, swelling, numbness, loss of motion, and even permanent nerve damage. For example, an RSI called **carpal tunnel syndrome (CTS)** is characterized by pain in the thumb, fingers, palm, wrist, and forearm. It can develop when you're constantly typing, texting, or otherwise flexing your hand and wrist. This causes the tendons within the carpal tunnel of your wrist to swell and press on a nearby nerve. Recent studies have linked excessive texting to the development of many RSIs, including CTS as well as tendinitis of the thumb (called Blackberry thumb).[36] To avoid RSIs, take frequent rest breaks from repetitive hand movements. If you experience symptoms, apply an ice pack to the affected area for about 15 minutes once every hour. See the **Practical Strategies** on the next page for more tips on how to work safely at your computer.

repetitive strain injury (RSI) An injury that damages joints, nerves, or connective tissue caused by repeated motions that put strain on one part of the body.

carpal tunnel syndrome (CTS) A repetitive strain injury of the hand or wrist, often linked to computer keyboard use or other types of repetitive motion.

>> For illustrations of carpal tunnel syndrome and more information about the condition, visit www.ncbi.nlm.nih.gov/pubmedhealth/PMH0001469.

>> For a video of seated stretches you can do while working at your computer, check out www.mayoclinic.com/health/lower-back-stretches/MM00711.

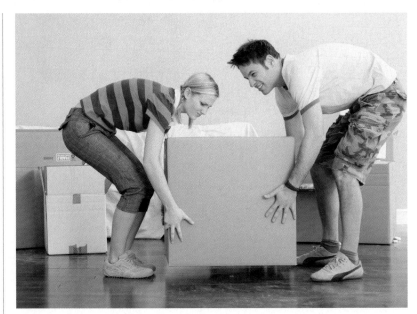

(a) The wrong way to lift

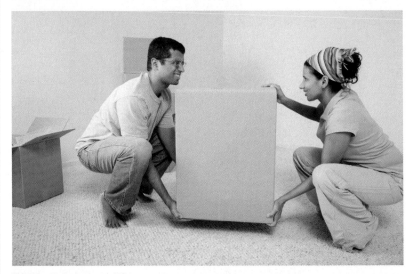

(b) The right way to lift

FIGURE 14.2 Proper Lifting. Rather than **(a)** bending over the object to be lifted, **(b)** stand near it and then bend your knees and hips. Bring the object as close as possible to your body, then hold onto it as you rise.

Back Injuries

Lifting heavy objects is a leading cause of injury. If you've got a heavy box or other object to pick up and carry, check out the instructions for lifting in **Figure 14.2.** Once you've lifted the item, keep it close to your body by holding your elbows close to your body. This helps keep strain off your spine. Don't twist your spine while carrying the load; if you need to change directions, change your foot placement. To release the object, lower it down by bending your knees, not your back.

If you suffer from back pain, your backpack might be to blame. How do you know? Pack it, and then put it on your bathroom scale. If it weighs more than 15% of your body weight, lighten the load. Here are some more tips:

- Use a pack with wide, padded straps.
- Place the heaviest items in the main compartment closest to your back.

Practical Strategies

Preventing RSI When Working on a Computer

Knowing how to set up your computer for optimal posture can help you avoid RSI.

- Keep your neck in a neutral position by using a laptop stand, monitor risers, books, or packages of paper to raise the top of the screen to about eye level.

- Angle the screen to avoid bending your head forward.

- Use a document holder to position documents you are typing from vertically, rather than bending your head to look at them.

- Allow for good hand and wrist posture by placing your keyboard and mouse on an adjustable keyboard tray that can be moved up or down. Keyboard and mouse should be positioned slightly at or below elbow height. If a laptop is your main computer, set up a work station with a regular-size external keyboard and mouse attached to it.

- When typing, don't bend and twist your hand to reach awkward key combinations. If you need to hit multiple keys at once, use a separate hand for each key, rather than contorting your hand to reach both keys with the same set of fingers.

- Keep your wrists straight. Don't rest your palms on the keyboard so that your hands are angled up from your wrists. Your wrists should be straight and your fingers should reach down slightly to find the keys.

- Use a chair that supports a comfortable upright or slightly reclined posture. Prop your feet up to maintain a comfortable trunk-thigh angle, if needed.

- Position the screen at a right angle to windows to reduce glare. Use a desk lamp or laptop light that plugs into a USB port for extra light, if needed.

- Clean your screen frequently with computer-safe antistatic cleaning material. Dust on the screen can make it difficult to read and increase eyestrain.

- Stop and stretch every 30 to 45 minutes.

- When carrying a laptop, use a wheeled case or a backpack with wide, padded straps, rather than a bag that places all the weight on one shoulder.

Source: Based on Ergonomic Tips for Laptop Users, by U.C. Berkeley's Ergonomics Program for Faculty and Staff from the University Health Services Tang Center at Berkeley website, 2007.

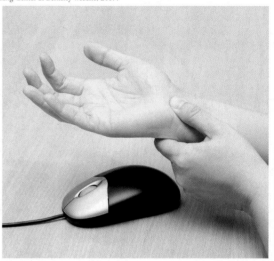

- Use proper lifting technique to put on your backpack (see Figure 14.2). Never bend over and sling your backpack onto one shoulder.

- When you've got it on properly, your pack should rest evenly between your shoulders against your upper back (**Figure 14.3** on page 352). The shoulder straps should be snug so that the pack doesn't hang below your waist.

- Exercise regularly. Maintaining your fitness will reduce your risk for back injury.

Overview of Intentional Injuries and Violence

Recall that intentional injuries are purposefully inflicted through **violence,** the use of force—threatened or actual—with the intent of causing harm. Violence is a serious health concern, especially for young people. In 2011, nonfatal injuries caused by violence accounted for more than 600,000 hospital emergency department visits from people between the ages of 15 and 24.[37]

The Federal Bureau of Investigation (FBI) defines **violent crime** as one of four offenses involving force or the threat of force: murder and non-negligent manslaughter, forcible rape, robbery, and aggravated assault. Although levels of violent crime in the United States have fluctuated in recent years, the overall number of violent crimes has dropped in the last two decades (**Figure 14.4** on page 352).[38] Still, in 2011, more than 1.2 million violent crimes were committed in the United States—nearly 3,300 a day.[38] Of these attacks:

- About 62% were aggravated assault, or an attack intended to cause serious injury, often involving a weapon.

- About 29% were robberies, or the taking of or attempt to take anything of value from a person by violence and/or by putting the victim in fear.

- Almost 7% were forcible rapes.

- Just over 1% were murders.

Many attacks have underpinnings in complex webs of personal, family, community, and social factors, including:

- **Sex.** Most violent crime is committed by men. Of more than 530,000 arrests for murder, rape, robbery, and assault in 2011, over 80% of those taken into custody were males. Men are also more often victims—more than 77% of all murder victims in the United States in 2011 were male.[38] See **Diversity & Health: Injuries and Violence: Special Concerns for Young Men** on page 353 for some possible reasons men are at higher risk than women.

- **Age.** Teens and young adults experience the highest rate of violent crime.

> **violence** Use of physical force—threatened or actual—with the intent of causing harm.
>
> **violent crime** One of four offenses involving force or the threat of force: murder and non-negligent manslaughter, forcible rape, robbery, and aggravated assault.

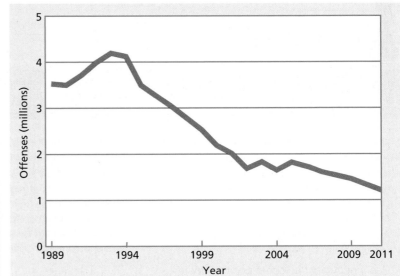

FIGURE 14.4 Violent Crime Rates Over the Last 20 Years. The serious violent crimes included are murder, rape, robbery, and aggravated assault. Rates include estimates for crimes not reported to the police.

Source: Data from "Four Measures of Serious Violent Crime" in *Key Facts at a Glance* by the Bureau of Justice Statistics, 2012. Retrieved from http://bjs.ojp.usdoj.gov/content/glance/cv2.cfm.

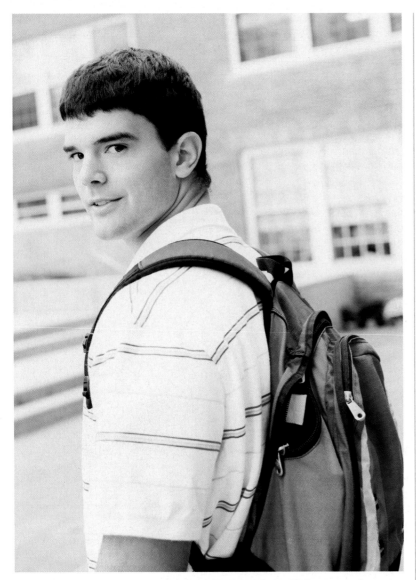

FIGURE 14.3 The Right Way to Wear a Backpack.

- **Guns.** The United States continues to have a high murder rate compared with other industrialized countries and many experts link this phenomenon to the easy availability of firearms. In 2011, about 68% of the nation's murders, 41% of robberies, and 21% of aggravated assaults were committed with the use of a gun.[38]
- **Poverty.** Communities that are distressed, with poor housing, high unemployment, and limited community services, often have higher rates of violence, especially among young people. Rates of violent crime also tend to be higher among disadvantaged socioeconomic groups. For example, African Americans are more likely to live in poverty than Caucasian Americans and are more likely to commit murder and to become murder victims.[38]
- **Interpersonal relationships.** Many crime victims know their attackers. About 22% of murders in 2011 occurred within families. Women are especially vulnerable to criminal acts at the hands of an acquaintance, friend, intimate partner, family member, or spouse.[39]
- **Drugs and alcohol.** Substances that disrupt judgment and impair your ability to control your emotions consistently emerge as a factor

in violence. Alcohol is a factor in about 60% of homicides and 50% of sexual assaults.[6] Every year, nearly 800,000 college students reported being physically or sexually assaulted by another student who'd been drinking.[40] The use of illicit drugs is also a factor in many types of crime.

- **Childhood environment.** Researchers have consistently noted that children raised in violent surroundings are more likely to grow up to be violent adults.[41]
- **Violence in the media.** From TV shows, movies, video games, and song lyrics, most children and teenagers are exposed to thousands of violent messages each year. Although most researchers agree that violence in the media contributes to an increased level of aggressive behavior and a perception that violence is normal, the strength of this association is still unclear. We explore this issue in the **Media and Violence** box on page 354.
- **Personal and cultural beliefs.** Some individuals hold values or religious beliefs that sanction violence.
- **Stress.** Think about the last time you were under a great deal of stress and how you were quicker to anger than you might have been otherwise. People who are consistently under stress are more likely to react violently.

Violence Within Communities

Although even one violent crime is too many, our society has been making progress in reducing this threat to our communities. At the end of this chapter, we'll discuss ways you can get involved in these efforts.

Assault

Assault, a physical attack or threat of attack on another person, is one of the leading categories of violent crime. **Aggravated assault** is an

aggravated assault An attack intended to cause serious physical harm, often involving a weapon.

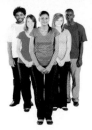

Injuries and Violence: Special Concerns for Young Men

Two of the biggest risk factors for injury and death due to accidents or violence are things none of us can control: age and sex. If you are young and male, your risk for traumatic injury and death is higher than that of women or any other age group. For example, males between the ages of 20 and 24 have the highest rate of non-fatal assault injuries, more than 50% higher than the rate for females of the same age.[1] Males of the same age also experience the highest rate of homicide deaths, more than six times higher than that of females.[1] Males also account for about 62% of alcohol-related emergency department visits in the 18–20 age group.[2] Sexual assault is one of the few situations where women are in

more danger, but for most other types of violence and injuries, young men are at higher risk.

The reasons for these higher risks are widely debated among researchers. Some suggest that the influence of the male hormone testosterone leads to more aggression, anger, and risk taking. Some point to gender roles that encourage men, especially young men, to be tough, aggressive, risk taking, or confrontational. Males also have higher rates of substance use and abuse, and higher rates of participation in sports like football and hockey where injuries are common. Moreover, men are more likely to work in hazardous occupations and experience five times as many injury-related workplace fatalities as females.[3] Often, a mix of these factors puts young men in harm's way.

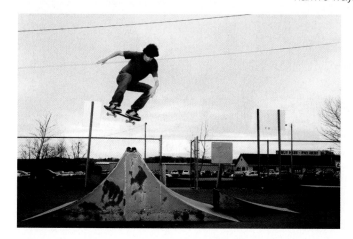

Reducing the risk of injury doesn't mean taking all the fun out of your life. Instead, experts suggest to channel your energies in ways less likely to get you hurt or killed. Here are just a few suggestions:

- Your car is no place for an adrenaline rush. Find thrills in sports, video games, or anywhere but behind the wheel.

- Watch how much you drink. As discussed throughout this chapter, alcohol is a significant risk factor for unintentional and intentional injuries and deaths. Whether you

are the aggressor or the victim, you don't want to wind up a drinking-related statistic. (For more information on alcohol and its effects, see Chapter 8.)

- Anger can't help you solve problems. It's natural to get angry, but anger can quickly escalate a conflict into violence. Learning to manage anger and find other ways to resolve problems is one of the manliest things you can do. (For more information about managing anger and stress, see Chapters 2 and 3.)

Critical-Thinking Questions

1. This box identifies several factors that might contribute to males' higher risk for trauma. What others can you think of?

2. Can you propose any factors that might be protective for females; that is, factors that might reduce their risk?

3. Think of an incident among your own family members, friends, or high school or college classmates in which one or more males suffered traumatic injury. Identify the specific factors involved (e.g., alcohol, anger, etc.).

References: **1.** *Youth Violence: National Statistics,* by the Centers for Disease Control and Prevention, 2013, http://www.cdc.gov/violenceprevention/youthviolence/stats_at_a_glance/nfa_age-sex.html. **2.** *News Release: SAMHSA Reports on Hospital Emergency Department Visits Involving Underage Alcohol Use,* by the Substance Abuse & Mental Health Services Administration, 2010, http://www.samhsa.gov/newsroom/advisories/1008065452.aspx. **3.** *Occupational Health: Comparative Quantification of Health Risks,* by M. Concha-Barrientos, D. I. Nelson, T. Driscoll, N. K. Steenland, L. Punnett, L. M. Fingerhut, . . . C. Corvalan, 2013. Geneva: World Health Organization, http://www.who.int/occupational_health/publications/quantification/en.

assault committed with the intent to cause severe injury, often involving a weapon. Although just over 750,000 aggravated assaults were committed in 2011, this number represents a decline of more than 15% from 2002.[38] More effective prevention programs and tougher law enforcement appear to have helped reduce the number of assaults.

Murder

Murder is the willful (not negligent) killing of another person. The FBI includes in this category non-negligent manslaughter, which is the willful killing of another "without malice aforethought"—in other words, without having previously planned to do so.

Murder is the third leading cause of death in the United States among people between the ages of 15 and 24, after unintentional injuries and suicides. Among all age groups nationwide, 14,612 people were murdered in 2011. This was a 10% decrease

murder The act of intentionally and unjustifiably killing another person.

from 2002.[38] As noted earlier, the great majority of murder victims and perpetrators are male. Two-thirds of murders involve firearms.[38] Mass murders, such as the murder of 14 people at a Colorado movie theatre in the summer of 2012 or the murder of 26 people at an elementary school in Newtown, Connecticut, in December 2012, often involve assault rifles, weapons that were developed for military and law enforcement use.

School and Campus Violence

When two students went on a murderous rampage at Columbine High School in 1999, many Americans began to fear that going to school amounted to putting one's life at risk. Subsequent incidents, such as the Newtown, Connecticut, shooting just mentioned, have reinforced this fear. Yet despite these high-profile tragedies, overall levels of school violence have dropped in the

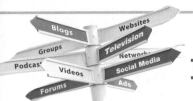

media and VIOLENCE

Does the Media Encourage Violent Crime— or the Fear of Violent Crime?

Over the past two decades, public health experts have become increasingly concerned about the violent content in TV shows, films, video games, and other media to which children, adolescents, and adults are exposed. Both controlled experiments and studies tracking populations from childhood through early adulthood have shown a correlation between exposure to violent media, increased aggression and desensitization to violence, and subsequent increased risk of engaging in violent crime.[1,2]

At first glance, the evidence seems substantial. However, attempts to demonstrate that exposure to media violence directly causes violent behavior in the real world have not succeeded. For example, a recent review of six decades of studies of the role of violent TV programming on crime rates concluded that, in contrast to many other factors that may influence individuals' tendency to engage in violent crime, such as strained family relationships, poverty, inadequate education, discrimination, and low level of opportunity, the media may be viewed as a scapegoat.[3]

At the same time, several recent studies have supported a link between high exposure to non-fictional crime-related media and an increased *fear* of crime.[4-6] These studies have found that, even though the actual rate of crime has been declining dramatically for many years, media coverage of crime has not declined. Indeed, the pervasiveness of crime-related TV news programs, documentaries, and reality shows has increased. A high level of exposure to crime-saturated news greatly increases people's perception of their own vulnerability to crime and their concern about crime. As one study concluded, the more often people watch non-fictional crime programming, the more fearful they become of criminal victimization.[4]

You might want to bear this in mind the next time your local TV news program reports a robbery at a nearby convenience store. Instead of panicking, remind yourself that the very fact that it's unusual is what makes it news.

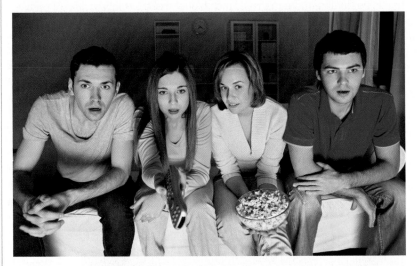

Does watching violence increase violence?

Critical-Thinking Questions

1. Why might policy-makers use the media as a "scapegoat" for explaining violent behavior?

2. Even if you don't usually watch your community's evening TV news program, tune in tonight. Use the stopwatch app on your cell phone to keep track of the minutes of programming devoted to crime. Does this seem excessive to you? Why or why not?

3. Are you afraid of becoming the victim of crime? If so, do you believe that your fears are reasonable? What factors in your life increase your risk? What factors are protective?

References: **1.** *Fact Sheet: Media Violence,* by C. Lomonaco, T. Kim, & L. Ottaviano, 2010, Southern California Academic Center of Excellence on Youth Violence Prevention, University of California, Riverside, http://stopyouthviolence.ucr.edu/factsheets/FACTSHEET%20MediaViolenceRevisedSpring2010.pdf. **2.** Robertson, L.A., McAnally, H.M., and Hancox, R.J. (2013, February 18). "Childhood and Adolescent Television Viewing and Antisocial Behavior in Early Adulthood." *Pediatrics.* DOI: 10.1542/peds.2012-1582. **3.** "Violent Crime on American Television: A Critical Interpretation of Empirical Studies," by A. Hetsroni, 2012, *Sociology Mind, 2*(2), 141–147. **4.** "Watching the Detectives: Crime Programming, Fear of Crime, and Attitudes About the Criminal Justice System," by L. A. Kort-Butler, 2011, *The Sociological Quarterly,* 52, 36–55. **5.** "The Impact of Media on Fear of Crime Among University Students: A Cross-National Comparison," by S. A. Kohm, C. A. Waid-Lindberg, M. Weinrath, & T. O'Connor Shelley, 2012. *Canadian Journal of Criminology and Criminal Justice,* 54, 67–100. **6.** *Violence: Comparing Reporting and Reality,* by S. Tiegreen & E. Newman, 2009, Dart Center for Journalism and Trauma, retrieved from http://dartcenter.org/content/violence-comparing-reporting-and-reality.

past decade. Moreover, a national analysis found that students are much more likely to be seriously hurt or killed off campus than while at school. During the 2009–2010 school year, for example, there were 19 homicides of school-aged children within American schools but 1,396 homicides of school-aged children within their homes and communities.[42]

In 2007, a student at Virginia Tech killed 32 others and himself. In response to the tragedy, U.S. colleges and universities have developed new emergency response plans and procedures, upgraded communication systems, and implemented new safety techniques and services. At the same time, some are finding their policies in conflict with state laws; 28 states allow students to carry a concealed weapon on a college campus.

Another common problem on college campuses is **hazing,** a set of initiation rituals for fraternities, sports teams, or other groups. Hazing rituals typically involve humiliation, isolation, alcohol consumption, sleep deprivation, or physical or sexual abuse. Peer pressure or other power dynamics induce those being hazed to participate in high-risk activities that they wouldn't perform otherwise. Surveys suggest that more than half of college students involved in fraternities, clubs, teams, and similar organizations experience hazing.[43] According to one expert on hazings, a total of 27 deaths were attributed to hazing in the decade between 2002 and 2011. Alcohol poisoning and aggravated assault are usually the causes of death.[44]

All U.S. colleges and universities are required to disclose statistics about the crimes reported on and near their campuses. The legislation that mandates this disclosure is the Jeanne Clery Act, named after the Lehigh University student who, in 1986, was raped and murdered in her dorm room when dormitory security doors were propped open, allowing a perpetrator to enter. Unfortunately, many campus crimes still go unreported, with victims often too embarrassed, ashamed, or afraid to step forward. Reporting a crime is the first step toward addressing the problem and making a campus safer for everyone.

>> **The Clery Center advocates for victims of campus crime. Contact them at** http://clerycenter.org.

Hate Crimes

Certain crimes are fueled by bias against another person's or group's race or ethnicity, religion, national origin, sexual orientation, or disability. Any acts—whether physical assaults or vandalism against property—due to such prejudice have been classified as **hate crimes.** More than 6,200 incidents involving such offenses were reported to the FBI in 2011. Of these,

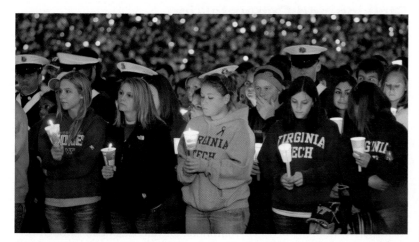

The Virginia Tech shootings in 2007 prompted colleges to reevaluate their safety and alert procedures.

almost half were driven by bias against the victim's race, whereas sexual orientation bias was involved in just over 20% of hate crimes.[45] Almost 10% of these hate crimes occurred in schools or on college campuses.[45]

Terrorism

Terrorism is premeditated, politically motivated violence against nonmilitary people by subnational groups or clandestine agents, usually in an effort to influence a larger audience. The effects of terrorism are experienced on many levels: It can destroy property and injure or kill individuals, disrupt the patterns of daily life in a community, and cultivate widespread fear.

Since 2001, the year in which more than 3,000 Americans died in the September 11 attacks, the numbers of deaths and injuries due to terrorism in the United States have dropped greatly. However, the bombing in April 2013 at the Boston Marathon confirms that stringent security measures are still critical.

The government agency responsible for defending the nation against terrorist threats is the Department of Homeland Security, which was created in response to the terrorist attacks in 2001. Other agencies, such as the FBI, the Central Intelligence Agency (CIA), the U.S. military, and state and local law enforcement also guard against terrorism. Ongoing efforts work not just to disarm, catch, or kill terrorists, but to discredit their tactics, diminish the perception of threats, and reduce their abilities to win public support and new recruits.

These efforts matter both on U.S. soil and abroad. In 2011, more than 10,000 terrorist attacks occurred in 70 countries, causing over 12,500 deaths.[46] However, this represents a nearly 29% decline in attacks since 2007.[46]

Violence Within Relationships

We all desire relationships that are grounded in mutual support, respect, and affection, but sometimes we find ourselves in relationships characterized by abuse. In a phenomenon known as **domestic violence,** one or more members of a household experience physical, psychological, or sexual harm from another member. When the abuse is perpetrated by a current or former partner or spouse, it is known as **intimate partner violence (IPV).** Forms of IPV include physical and emotional abuse, and sexual violence, such as rape, when it occurs between intimate partners. We discuss sexual violence later in this chapter.

Intimate Partner Violence

Victims of intimate partner violence can be married or not married, heterosexual, gay or lesbian, living together, separated, or dating. Many cases go

hazing Initiation rituals to enter a fraternity or other group that can be humiliating, hazardous, or physically or emotionally abusive, regardless of the person's willingness to participate.

hate crime A crime fueled by bias against another person's or group's race or ethnicity, religion, national origin, sexual orientation, or disability.

terrorism Premeditated, politically motivated violence against noncombatant individuals, usually as a means of influence.

domestic violence An abusive situation in which a family member physically, psychologically, or sexually abuses one or more other family members.

intimate partner violence (IPV) An abusive situation in which one member of a couple or intimate relationship may physically, psychologically, or sexually abuse the other.

Abusive Relationship

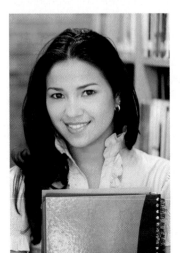

"HI, I'M JENNY. I was dating a guy for a few months who I really liked and everything seemed great at first, but he slowly started to get more and more controlling. First he didn't want to go out with my friends, then after a while he didn't want *me* to go out with my friends. He got really jealous any time he saw me talking to another guy and he started making me check in with him every day to let him know my schedule. He even checked my cell phone to see who I was talking to. One day we got into a fight about it and he grabbed me and pushed me into a wall. I got really scared and left immediately. I broke up with him by text and I've avoided him ever since."

1. What could have happened if Jenny had stayed with her abusive boyfriend?

2. What else could Jenny have done in response to her boyfriend's behavior along with breaking up with him?

3. Was Jenny right to break up with him with a text or should she have met up with him to explain?

Some people who find themselves the victim of an episode of abuse end the relationship and leave immediately. But other victims stay and may find themselves subject to further and more severe abuse. This situation is referred to as *the cycle of violence*:

- **Tension building.** A phase in which relatively minor abuse occurs and the victim responds by trying to please the abuser and avoid provoking another attack.

- **Acute battering.** A phase in which the abuser lashes out more forcefully, no matter how accommodating or conciliatory the victim has been.

- **Remorse.** A phase in which the abuser may feel shock and denial over the abuse and swear it will never happen again. Over time, however, the tensions and need for control that started the cycle resurface, and abuse starts anew, often more seriously than before.

Victims stay in abusive relationships for a variety of reasons. Some are financially dependent on their partners or have children and don't want to break up their family. Some come from belief systems or cultures that forbid family separation or divorce. Some may still love their abuser. Others may lack the self-confidence to take action or don't know where to go. Some may be afraid of what their partner might do to them if they try to leave.

A variety of organizations provide counseling and shelter to victims of IPV. One annual survey of domestic violence groups found that on a given day, more than 64,000 adults and children received shelter or other types of support related to IPV.[50] More than 10,000 others seeking such help had to be turned away for lack of adequate resources.

IPV persists, in part, because of a broad lack of understanding of how and why it occurs. In one survey of college students, more than half agreed with IPV myths such as that some instances are caused by women picking physical fights with their partners, or that most women can get out of an abusive relationship if they really want to.[51] College men taking the survey were more likely to agree with these myths than college women.

 For an interview from CNN that explores the myths surrounding sexual assault, watch www.cnn.com/video/data/2.0/video/living/2011/04/06/rape.and.sex.abuse.myths.hln.html.

For one woman's story about the cycle of abuse and what kept her from leaving her abuser, listen here: www.npr.org/2013/05/31/175617775/why-don-t-domestic-violence-victims-leave.

unreported so the exact scope of this problem is hard to pin down. The CDC estimates that 12 million Americans experience IPV each year.[47] Women are disproportionately affected:[47, 48]

- 1 in 4 women has been the victim of severe physical violence by an intimate partner versus 1 in 7 men.

- Nearly 1 in 5 women has been raped versus 1 in 71 men.

- Women make up 70% of all deaths due to IPV versus 30% for men.

At its core, abuse in an intimate relationship arises from the abuser's need for control. This is thought to be related at least in part to a phenomenon called "anxious attachment": People who experience a high level of anxiety when forming and maintaining attachments have a high need to control their relationships. One way males do this is by identifying with rigid gender stereotypes. When a woman violates her partner's expectations of submission and dependence, the man may resort to violence to manage the perceived threat to his masculinity.[49]

The effort at control may take the form of emotional or physical abuse. Emotional abuse includes comments and actions that try to erode the other person's confidence, independence, and sense of self-worth, such as keeping a partner from contacting family or friends, or from getting a job. Physical abuse includes any type of physical assault or use of physical restraint. In most cases, emotional abuse accompanies physical abuse in a relationship.

Stalking and Cyberstalking

Stalking is a pattern of harassment or threats directed at a specific person that is intended to cause intimidation and fear, often through repeated, unwanted contact. Stalking may also take the form of contact through digital and online communications, a phenomenon called *cyberstalking*. Although both traditional stalkers and cyberstalkers are motivated by an obsession with having power and control over their victims, cyberstalkers are more likely to avoid detection, using tactics such as creating a variety of screen names at different sites to maintain their anonymity.

Common stalking behaviors include:

- Making unwanted phone calls

- Sending unwanted letters, emails, or text messages

stalking A pattern of harassment and threats directed at a specific person that is intended to cause intimidation and fear, often through repeated, unwanted contact.

- Following or spying
- Showing up at places where the victim would be, with no legitimate reason
- Waiting for the victim, with no legitimate reason
- Leaving unwanted items or presents for the victim
- Posting information or spreading rumors about the victim online, in a public place, or by word of mouth

According to a national survey, more than 5 million women are stalked each year in the United States.[47] Women were about three times as likely to be stalked as men, and men make up the majority of stalkers. Overall, 1 in 6 women has been stalked in her lifetime, versus 1 in 19 men.[48] Stalking and cyberstalking occur more frequently among college students than in the general population: In two recent surveys of college students, 5% and 12% reported that they had experienced stalking.[17, 52] However, researchers have estimated the true prevalence at more than 40% of students.[52, 53] Self-reported estimates are thought to be too low because many, if not most, incidents go unreported, in part because the victim doesn't recognize the behavior as stalking.[52, 54]

College students also experience unique consequences of stalking victimization. In addition to the psychological distress felt by victims generally, they're at risk for academic consequences, including lower grades, additional time needed to graduate, and dropping out.[52]

If you are being stalked, don't try to reason with your stalker. Stalking is not rational behavior. Instead, start by letting the stalker know that the attention is unwelcome. Have someone else deliver this message for you—this thwarts the stalker's goal of trying to force contact with you. Avoid being alone as much as possible, vary your routines, and stop posting information about your location on social media sites. Also avoid revealing your whereabouts through GPS locator apps. Keep a record of all contacts with the stalker. Get a new phone number, but leave the old one active. Ask a friend to screen and keep a record of calls to the old number. If the stalker persists, get help from your resident advisor, campus health center, campus security, or law enforcement.

Addressing Violence Within Relationships

If you find yourself attracted to someone, is there any way to tell—before you get in too deep—if the person has the potential for violence? Although there's no such thing as an IPV profile, the CDC has gathered a list of risk factors. They include:[55]

- Low self-esteem
- Low academic achievement
- A history of aggressive or delinquent behavior
- A history of having been abused as a child
- Alcohol or other substance abuse
- Anger and hostility
- Depression and social isolation
- Belief in strict gender roles
- Desire for power and control

What if you're already in a relationship that's causing you to feel unsafe, or you've experienced one or more episodes of IPV? What if you're frightened by something you see in the relationship of a friend? Don't wait for things to "get better": Contact your student health center or the National Domestic Violence Hotline at 1-800-799-SAFE (7233) or at TTY ("text telephone" for the hearing impaired) 1-800-787-3224, or visit **www.thehotline.org**.

Sexual Violence

Although no standard definition of the term has emerged, **sexual violence** encompasses several forms of nonconsensual sexual activity, including noncontact sexual abuse, such as voyeurism or verbal harassment, unwanted touching, attempted but uncompleted sex acts, and completed sex acts. The common factor in all of these is the lack of consent of the victim, either because he or she refused consent, or was threatened, coerced, intoxicated, underage, developmentally disabled, or otherwise legally incapable of either giving or refusing consent. Sexual violence is often referred to as sexual assault.

Risk Factors for Sexual Violence

Factors that increase the risk for sexual violence include:

- **Hostility toward women.** Men who report hostility toward or low opinions of women are more likely to show higher levels of sexual aggression.
- **Shared tolerance of sexual violence.** Membership in a fraternity or other male-only social group that holds attitudes tolerant of sexual violence—such as "Some women ask for it"—increases the likelihood that a man will engage in sexual violence.[56]
- **Low self-control.** Many studies point to low self-control as a personal characteristic of sexual offenders. This factor is thought to be especially potent when combined with membership in a male-only social group with attitudes tolerant of sexual violence.[57] In a sense, the man relinquishes control to the group ideology.
- **Substance abuse.** In one study of college students, about 15% of men reported having used some form of alcohol-related coercion to obtain sex.[57] According to the Core Institute, the nation's largest database of statistics on alcohol and other drug use on campus, nearly 78% of sexual assaults on campus involve alcohol or other drug use.[58]
- **"No" isn't always heard as "No."** Some men have problems understanding a woman's sexual refusals. Less direct refusals, such as "I don't think it's a good idea," may be misinterpreted as agreeing to sex.[59]

Sexual Harassment

Unwanted language or contact of a sexual nature that occurs in school or workplace settings is considered **sexual harassment** when it explicitly or implicitly affects a person's job or academic situation, work or school performance, or creates an intimidating, hostile, or offensive environment. Sexual harassment is a form of discrimination that violates the federal Civil Rights Act of 1964.

According to the U.S. Equal Employment Opportunity Commission, sexual harassment can occur in a variety of circumstances, including but not limited to the following.

- The victim and the harasser may be a woman or man and the two parties do not have to be of the opposite sex. In 2011, of the 11,364 charges of sexual harassment filed in the United States, just over 16% were filed by males.[60]

sexual violence Any form of nonconsensual sexual activity.

sexual harassment Unwelcome language or contact of a sexual nature that explicitly or implicitly affects academic or employment situations, unreasonably interferes with work or school performance, or creates an intimidating, hostile, or offensive work or school environment.

- The harasser can be the victim's supervisor (or teacher), an agent of the employer (or school), a coworker (or fellow student), or a nonemployee (or nonstudent).
- The victim does not have to be the person harassed but can be anyone affected by the offensive conduct.
- Harassment may occur even if the victim suffers no economic injury or stays on the job or at school.[61]

On campus, sexual harassment can take the form of everything from a student making sexually explicit remarks that make others uncomfortable to a professor demanding sexual favors from a student in exchange for a better grade. In one survey of college students, 62% of all students (male and female) reported having been sexually harassed while enrolled in school. About 80% of those harassed said their harasser was a student or former student. Among college males, 51% admitted to having sexually harassed someone, and about 22% said they had done so more than once. Only 10% of those harassed said they had reported the incident to a campus official.[62]

If you are being harassed, the first step is to confront your harasser. In person or in writing, tell the harasser to stop and state that you consider the actions to be sexual harassment. If direct communication has no effect, keep a record of all harassing contacts and behavior and report the problem to campus or workplace supervisors. They are required by law to investigate.

Rape

Rape is a form of sexual violence involving oral, anal, or vaginal penetration using force, threats, or taking advantage of circumstances that make a person incapable of consenting to sex. Any sexual activity with a person younger than the legally defined "age of consent" is also considered a form of rape called **statutory rape,** regardless of whether any coercion or force was involved.

The FBI refers to the crime of rape as *forcible rape* and defines it more narrowly as "the carnal knowledge of a female forcibly and against her will." In 2011, FBI records showed that over 83,000 women in the United States were forcibly raped.[38] However, because males also experience rape, many rapes go unreported. And because definitions of what constitute rape vary, estimates of the actual incidence of rape in the United States are much higher. As noted earlier, a large-scale national survey found that about 1 in 5 women and 1 in 71 men in the United States report having been raped at some point in their lives.[47] The same survey found that more than 1 million women had been raped the previous year. Among female victims, 79% of rapes occur before age 25. In one survey of college women, almost 20% said they'd been sexually assaulted during their undergraduate years.[57]

Rape and other forms of campus crime are especially common during the first few weeks of a new school year, a period referred to as the "red zone" when parental involvement abruptly ends and students are in new situations, often among people they've just met. As noted earlier, nearly 78% of sexual assaults on campus involve the use of alcohol or other drugs, which is especially common at parties and other social events early in a new academic year.[58]

Date Rape

Of rapes documented among college students, many take the form of **date (acquaintance) rape.**

---

rape Nonconsensual oral, anal, or vaginal penetration by body parts or objects, using force, threats of bodily harm, or taking advantage of circumstances that make a person incapable of consenting to sex.

statutory rape Any sexual activity with a person younger than the legally defined "age of consent," regardless of whether any coercion or force was involved.

date (acquaintance) rape Coerced, forceful, or threatening sexual activity in which the victim knows the attacker.

date rape drugs Drugs used to assist in a sexual assault, often given to the victim without his or her knowledge or consent.

This form of coerced sexual activity, in which the victim knows the attacker, can have a severe long-term emotional impact because the victim is assaulted by someone who was trusted. Many cases go unreported. Drinking and drug use are factors, and in some instances the victim is unknowingly given a drug to facilitate rape.

Date Rape Drugs

Drugs used to assist in a sexual assault, or **date rape drugs,** are powerful, dangerous, and difficult to detect once they've been slipped into a drink. They can make a victim weak or confused or cause loss of consciousness—as well as make it difficult for the victim to remember later what happened while he or she was drugged. Under federal law, convicted rapists who use a date rape drug to incapacitate a victim automatically have 20 years added to their sentences.

Reducing the Risk of Date Rape

Preventing date rape requires joint efforts. To avoid becoming a victim:

- When dating someone you don't know well, stay in public or go out in a group. Arrange for your own transportation; don't rely on your date for transport.
- Watch out for coercive behavior. If your date tries to pressure you into activities you'd rather avoid, such as drinking heavily, you may face similar pressures for sex as well.
- Trust your instincts. If you feel uncomfortable with someone, leave.
- Stay sober. Drinking makes it harder for you to communicate clearly and set limits about sex.
- Don't accept drinks, including nonalcoholic ones, from other people. If you're at a club, even if someone offers to buy you a drink, go up to the bar yourself and watch as the bartender prepares it. Keep your drink with you at all times. If you've left it unattended, pour it out. And don't drink from a punch bowl or other open container.
- Be assertive and direct with both your words and your actions. If you are being pressured for sex and don't want to participate, say "No!" or "Stop it!" loudly. If the pressure persists or worsens, tell the other person that he or she is attempting rape. Yell, make a scene, and run away.

To avoid becoming an assailant:

- Accept that "No" means "No." Even if you think the person's flirtatious manner might mean "Yes," pay attention to the words, and back off.
- Someone who is intoxicated cannot legally consent to sex. Again, sex with someone who is drunk or under the influence of drugs is rape.
- Drinking and drugs make it harder for you to communicate clearly and set limits about sex, too.
- Remember what being together offers—and what it doesn't. It offers both of you a chance to get to know each other better in a social setting. It is not an automatic ticket to sex. You both have the right to set limits and refuse any level of sexual activity.

Defending Yourself Against Rape

What if you've followed all the precautions but still find yourself in a threatening situation? Experts suggest that, unless the assailant is carrying a weapon, immediate action on your part can be effective. Some potential victims think and talk their way out of an attack. For instance, you might say that you have genital herpes

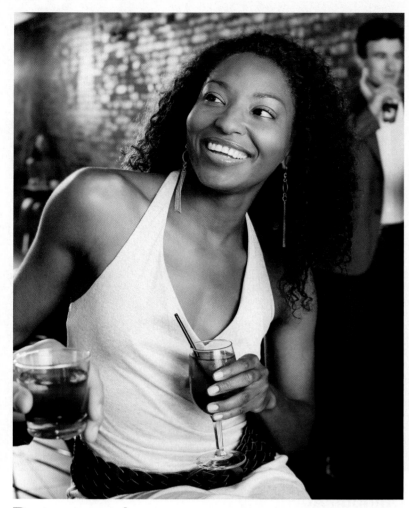

Date rape drugs can be difficult to detect once added to drinks.

or are HIV-positive, or that your father is a local police officer. You can also try crying hysterically, acting as if you're having a mental breakdown, or repeatedly yelling "Fire!" as loud as you can.

If you can't get away, fighting may increase your risk for injury but it will also decrease the chance that the rape attempt will succeed. Rather than wasting your energy flailing about, strike for the attacker's most vulnerable areas: eyes, ears, temples, base of skull, windpipe (Adam's apple), spine, groin, and knees. Because thigh muscles are far more powerful than arm muscles, kicking can be more effective than hitting. Some self-defense experts advise dropping to the floor. This gives you a firm base from which to strike with your legs and can confuse an assailant used to upper-body fighting, giving you an extra second to roll out of reach and run.

Again, if your attacker is armed, you may endanger your life by fighting. Every situation is different, so use your best judgment. Choosing not to resist does not equal consent.

> **Just Yell Fire is an award-winning video series teaching women practical self-defense. View the college version here:** www.justyellfire.com/movie .php?video=JYF_Campus_Life#content.

If You Are Raped or Sexually Assaulted

If you are raped or otherwise sexually assaulted, remember that you are not to blame. Sexual violence occurs because the attacker is hostile, not because of something you've said, done, or worn. It is a violent crime and sex happens to be the weapon.

After an assault, go to a place where you feel safe and call someone you trust. Write down as many facts about the attack as you can remember. Try not to change your clothes or clean up; you'll destroy physical evidence that may be helpful if you report the attack to the police. Instead, go to a hospital to be treated for any injuries you've received and screened for sexually transmitted infections. If female, you can be monitored for pregnancy and you may be offered emergency contraception. Physical evidence can be collected at that time while you decide whether to report the attack. When you seek medical care, ask for referrals to a counselor who can help you deal with the many emotional and psychological challenges that can arise after a sexual assault.

The decision to report a rape or sexual assault can be difficult. You may be reluctant to talk about the attack publicly. A classic study from the U.S. Department of Justice of sexual victimization among college students identified several barriers to reporting a sexual assault, including shame, guilt, and embarrassment; concerns about confidentiality; fear of reprisal from the assailant; fear of being treated with hostility by law enforcement officials; and concerns about not having sufficient evidence and not being believed.[63] Moreover, a year-long investigation of sexual assault on college campuses by the Center for Public Integrity revealed that, even when found guilty, perpetrators rarely face tough punishments such as expulsion and criminal proceedings, whereas many victims feel so traumatized that they drop out of school.[64]

Reporting the crime, however, may help restore your sense of power and control. Sexual assailants tend to repeat their behavior. By reporting a sexual assault, you may prevent another attack in the future.

Effects of Sexual Violence

Sexual violence has immediate and long-term consequences on physical, psychological, and social health.[48] Victims are often physically injured, suffering cuts, bruises, or even fractures, head trauma, or internal bleeding. Many develop sexually transmitted infections. In the following days and weeks, victims often experience flashbacks, panic attacks, and sleep problems. Over time, they may develop low self-esteem, depression, eating disorders, and post-traumatic stress disorder. Their risk of suicide increases. They may try to cope with their trauma by drinking, using illicit drugs, or engaging in risky sex.[48] They may also have a decreased capacity to form intimate bonds with partners.

Change Yourself, Change Your World

By taking some basic injury-prevention precautions, knowing how to support a friend who has experienced violence, and encouraging others to look for nonviolent ways to resolve conflicts, you can help keep yourself from becoming a statistic and build a safer campus and community.

Personal Choices

Fires, falls, crimes, and abusive relationships unfortunately do occur on college campuses. For general tips on how to reduce your personal risk for unintentional and intentional injury on campus, see the **Special Feature** box on the next page. You can help make your whole campus safer by:

- **Knowing your campus safety rules and resources.** Learn what they are and share that information with others.
- **Challenging social pressures that encourage violence.** You may encounter acquaintances or groups that encourage domination of others, hostility to outsiders, binge drinking, or sexual aggression. Don't play along.

10 Tips for CAMPUS SAFETY

1 Program numbers for campus safety services into your cell phone, because most 911 calls from cell phones go to highway safety dispatchers, not local police. Also program in the direct line for the local police department. Sign up for email alerts from your campus safety services as well.

2 Whether you live in a dorm, group house, or apartment, know where the smoke detectors are and make sure they are working. Know where the emergency exits are and what your fire escape plan is, with two ways out.

3 To reduce your risk for falls, keep entryways, stairways, and hallways well-lit and free of clutter. Don't stand on chairs, beds, or shelves to change ceiling lights or swat an insect above your reach.

Instead, use a proper footstool or short ladder.

4 Drink in moderation, if at all. Alcohol is a factor in fires, falls, drownings, and many other injury situations as well as in aggravated assaults, rapes, and other campus crimes.

5 Keep your valuables hidden. That's not always easy to do in a small dorm room, but it should still be possible to keep money, ATM cards, jewelry, and other valuables out of plain sight.

6 Protect your financial and personal data, too. If you make purchases online using your credit card, don't use a shared computer. If you own a smartphone, password-protect it. Also, make sure you know how to remotely lock it and erase

personal data. If it's lost or stolen, you'll need to act fast.

7 Keep your doors locked when you're home and when you're out, and don't loan out your keys. Never prop open access doors or let strangers in. If someone has arrived to visit another occupant, they can get the person they are visiting to let them in.

8 Don't travel alone after dark. Take a shuttle, go with a friend, or use the security escorts available on many campuses.

9 Give friends or family your schedule of classes, work, and other activities.

10 Know your surroundings and trust your instincts. If something doesn't seem right, get help by calling campus security.

Source: Based on Seven Tips for Campus Safety, from Clery Center for Security on Campus, Inc. website, 2008; College Student Safety Tips, from Livesecure.org, 2009; College Safety Tips—Campus Safety Tips, from Collegesafe.com, 2003.

- **Reporting crime.** If you see or hear about a crime, let campus security or police know.

Helping a Friend

The U.S. Department of Health and Human Services offers the following suggestions for helping a friend who's being abused:[65]

- Assuming you're somewhere private, ask your friend to tell you about what she or he has been going through. Listen. Don't interrupt.

- Tell your friend you're concerned about her or his safety. Try to help your friend to see that what's going on isn't right and that she or he can do something about it and has your support.

- Offer specific assistance. For instance, offer to accompany your friend to your campus health center. Or invite your friend to stay at your place while she or he figures out what to do.

- Stay involved. If your friend decides to leave the relationship, she or he may need your help working through feelings of sadness, anxiety, or regret. If your friend decides to stay, although it might be hard for you to understand, remind your friend that you're there no matter what.

To support a friend who has been sexually assaulted—or who believes that she or he was assaulted while intoxicated—the most helpful thing you can do is to listen. Give your friend time to explain what happened and explore what she or he wants to do next. Offer to accompany your friend to the campus health center or security office or to call the police or an advocacy agency in the community. Stay with your friend as long as you're needed. In the days and weeks that follow, continue to listen as your friend "processes" what's happened. Avoid suggesting that the incident was in any way your friend's fault. Even if substance abuse was involved, your friend was a victim of crime and was in no way to blame.

Campus Advocacy

Although it's easy to feel overwhelmed by issues of campus safety, the good news is that there are many ways you can help. Here are just a few:

- Students Against Violence Everywhere (SAVE) has more than 2,000 chapters in schools and colleges nationwide. SAVE works to promote personal safety and reduce violent crime and victimization. Chapters typically meet one or two evenings per month to organize service projects and awareness campaigns. For more information, check out **www.nationalsave.org**.

- Join Students Active for Ending Rape (SAFER), the American Association of University Women's student group dedicated to fighting sexual assault on campus. Download the AAUW-SAFER Campus Sexual Assault Program in a Box from **www.aauw.org/resource/campus-sexual-assault-program-in-a-box** to get started.

- Men often feel as if their gender automatically makes them responsible for the problem of violence and excludes them from becoming part of the solution. Not so. A national organization called Men Can Stop Rape shifts the responsibility for violence prevention toward men by promoting healthy, nonviolent masculinity and engaging men as allies in proactive solutions to end violence against women. This organization is operating right now on college campuses across the nation. Find out more about its Campus Men of Strength Clubs at **www.mencanstoprape.org/The-Campus-Men-of-Strength-Club**.

>> **Watch videos of real students discussing personal safety at** MasteringHealth™.

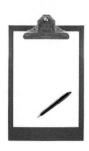

Choosing to Change Worksheet

To complete this worksheet online, visit MasteringHealth™

Part I. Understanding Your Risk from Aggressive Driving

Complete the "Are You an Aggressive Driver?" Self-Assessment on page 345 and list each of your aggressive habits.

_____

_____

Part II. Avoiding Aggressive Driving

Directions: Fill in your stage of change in Step 1 and complete Steps 2, 3, or 4, depending on which one applies to your stage of change.

Step 1: _Your Stage of Behavior Change._ Please check one of the following statements that best describe your readiness to make your driving safer.

_____ I do not intend to improve my driving in the next six months. (Precontemplation)

_____ I am contemplating improving my driving in the next six months. (Contemplation)

_____ I am planning on improving my driving in the next month. (Preparation)

_____ I have been improving my driving for less than six months. (Action)

_____ I have been improving my driving for six months or longer. (Maintenance)

Step 2: _Precontemplation and Contemplation Stages._ Consider what you can do to make your driving less aggressive. What are the advantages of adopting these behaviors to increase driving safety? (List at least three.)

1. _____

2. _____

3. _____

What are some things that might get in the way of your efforts to implement these behaviors? (List at least two.)

1. _____

2. _____

What ideas do you have to overcome these obstacles?

_____

_____

Step 3: _Preparation._ How do you expect to benefit from increased driving safety?

_____

_____

List a **SMART goal** for improving your driving.

_____

Step 4: _Action and Maintenance._ In what ways have you benefited from adopting these behaviors and actions?

_____

_____

What motivates you the most to continue practicing these behaviors and why?

_____

_____

Chapter Summary

- Injuries are the leading cause of death among Americans between the ages of 1 and 44.
- One of the most significant risk factors for injuries is substance abuse.
- Motor vehicle accidents claim more lives among Americans aged 15 to 24 than any other single cause of death.
- Distracted driving, impaired driving, poor use of safety features, speeding, and other forms of aggressive driving are risk factors for MVAs.
- Motorcyclists are about six times more likely than those riding in a car to die in a crash. Bicycle injuries cause several hundred deaths each year. In both cases, failure to wear a helmet increases the risk for disability and death.
- Every day, about 87 Americans die from unintentional poisoning. Many of these deaths are due to overdose of legal and illicit drugs.
- In adults, eating too fast, without chewing food properly, is the most common factor in choking. Back blows and abdominal thrusts can save the life of someone who is choking.
- Drowning is the second leading cause of unintentional injury death in people aged 10 to 19. Consumption of alcohol is a factor in 60% of drowning deaths.
- On campus, cooking, careless handling of lit cigarettes or candles, and improper use of space heaters and electrical devices are the causes of most fires. Alcohol plays a role in about 60% of fire fatalities.
- Both repetitive strain injuries and back injuries are common among college students. Take frequent breaks from typing and texting and lighten the load in your backpack.
- Violence is a leading cause of death and injury among young people, especially young men. Violent crimes include murder, forcible rape, robbery, and aggravated assault.
- The rate of violent crime in the United States has been declining for many years.

- Murder is the third leading cause of death in the United States among people between the ages of 15 and 24.
- Hazing is a set of initiation rituals involving humiliation, isolation, alcohol consumption, sleep deprivation, or physical or sexual abuse. A form of violence, it can result in serious illness, injury, or death.
- Intimate partner violence is experienced by more than 12 million Americans each year. It includes psychological abuse as well as physical and sexual assault. Victims stay in abusive relationships for a variety of reasons.
- Stalking is a pattern of harassment or threats directed at a specific person that is intended to cause intimidation and fear. It includes cyberstalking, in which the stalker uses digital and online communications. More than 5 million American women experience stalking each year.
- Sexual assault is a common problem on college campuses. Drinking and drug use are factors in more than three-fourths of these assaults. Low self-control, membership in a male-only social group that shares attitudes tolerant of sexual assault, and hostility toward women are other common factors in campus sexual assault.
- You can greatly reduce your risk for rape by staying sober, attending social gatherings with one or more friends, and communicating your choices firmly and clearly. If you find yourself in a threatening situation, unless the assailant is carrying a weapon, you may be able to talk, act, run, scream, and/or fight your way out of it.
- Declining rates of violent crime show that prevention works, including personal steps such as knowing and respecting campus safety rules, staying sober, encouraging a culture of respect, refusing to remain silent if you witness any aggressive act, and reporting crime. You can help support a friend experiencing violence by listening without judgment and encouraging practical actions such as using campus resources.

GET CONNECTED

>> Visit the following websites for further information about the topics in this chapter:

- National Center for Injury Prevention and Control
  www.cdc.gov/injury/index.html
- National Safety Council
  www.nsc.org
- American Association of Poison Control Centers
  www.aapcc.org
- Injury Prevention Web
  www.injuryprevention.org
- Motorcycle Safety Foundation
  www.msf-usa.org
- National Domestic Violence Hotline
  www.thehotline.org

MOBILE TIPS!

Scan this QR code with your mobile device to access additional tips about reducing your risk for intentional and unintentional injuries. Or, via your mobile device, go to **http://chmobile.pearsoncmg.com** and navigate to Chapter 14.

- Rape, Abuse, & Incest National Network (RAINN)
  www.rainn.org
- No Woman Left Behind
  www.facebook.com/NWLBCampaign

Website links are subject to change. To access updated web links, please visit MasteringHealth™

TEST YOUR KNOWLEDGE

1. Which of the following causes more deaths in the United States?
   a. motor vehicle accidents
   b. violence, such as a fight or a gunshot
   c. drowning
   d. unintentional poisoning

2. Of the following behaviors, which is a contributing factor in the greatest number of motor vehicle accidents?
   a. feeling drowsy
   b. texting
   c. talking on your hands-free cell phone
   d. aggressive driving

3. Safety experts advise that pedestrians reduce their risk of injury by
   a. wearing a helmet.
   b. walking with the flow of the traffic.
   c. wearing brightly colored clothing.
   d. waiting until they are within a crosswalk to use their cell phone.

4. Which of the following statements about unintentional injuries is true?
   a. Drowning is the second leading cause of unintentional injury death among people aged 10 to 19.
   b. Overdoses of prescription opioid painkillers now account for more than 40% of all unintentional drug overdose deaths.
   c. Alcohol consumption is a common contributing factor in choking deaths, drownings, and fatal fires.
   d. All of these answers are true.

5. In the United States, violent crime
   a. has increased every year since 1980.
   b. is more common in schools than off campus.
   c. occurs more frequently in regions that are economically distressed.
   d. is more commonly committed by men but women are more often the victims.

6. Which of the following is a common cause of death in hazing incidents?
   a. drowning
   b. alcohol poisoning
   c. aggravated assault
   d. alcohol poisoning AND aggravated assault

7. Which of the following statements about intimate partner violence is true?
   a. Nearly 6 million Americans experience IPV yearly.
   b. Intimate partner violence can be physical, psychological, or sexual.
   c. Stalking and cyberstalking are forms of intimate partner violence.
   d. All of these answers are true.

8. Date rape
   a. is more likely if one or both people on a date have been drinking.
   b. doesn't carry the same legal penalties as stranger rape.
   c. is legally known as statutory rape.
   d. All of these answers are true.

9. Sexual harassment
   a. occurs in both schools and workplaces.
   b. by definition involves loss of employment or academic standing.
   c. affects about twice as many women as men.
   d. applies only to the two people involved, not to anyone else.

10. Which of the following is likely to be the most helpful strategy for supporting a friend experiencing intimate partner violence?
    a. Encourage your friend to break off the relationship.
    b. Tell your friend that you are concerned about her or his safety.
    c. Try to convince your friend to report the incident to the police.
    d. Discuss how her or his actions contributed to the incident.

Get Critical

What happened

- Shortly after midnight on April 21, 2013, two freshmen at Virginia State University drowned in the Appomattox River. They had been participating in an initiation ritual to gain membership in a social club called the Men of Honor, which required them to cross the river, despite darkness and strong currents. Four men were arrested and charged with manslaughter.

- On November 19, 2011, a member of Florida A&M University's marching band was beaten, kicked, and suffocated to death in a hazing incident that took place on a bus after a football game. A dozen students were charged with manslaughter.

- In the early morning hours of February 25, 2011, a Cornell University sophomore was found dead in the library of his fraternity house. He had been kidnapped, forced to drink vodka until he passed out, and then left alone on the sofa to "sleep it off." Three students were charged with manslaughter but were acquitted. The fraternity was disbanded and fined $12,000.

What do you think?

- In response to the death at Cornell, fraternity members argued that the victim had participated in the hazing voluntarily and thus was responsible for the outcome. Do you agree? Why or why not?

- Young people—especially college freshmen—are thought to be especially vulnerable to hazing because, having just left their family's authority and immediate social support, they seek replacements in the campus group. What other factors might contribute to students' willingness to participate?

- Florida A&M University now requires all students to sign a pledge not to engage in hazing (either as a "hazer" or "hazee") before they can sign up for classes. Cornell University forbids "pledging" (the performance of humiliating or potentially harmful acts as a condition of membership) at their fraternities and sororities. Do you think these actions will make a difference? How else might campus social organizations qualify members?

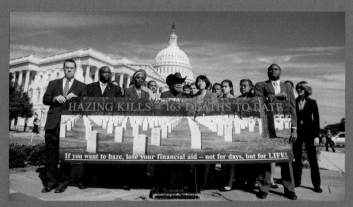

A protest against hazing after the FAMU hazing death.

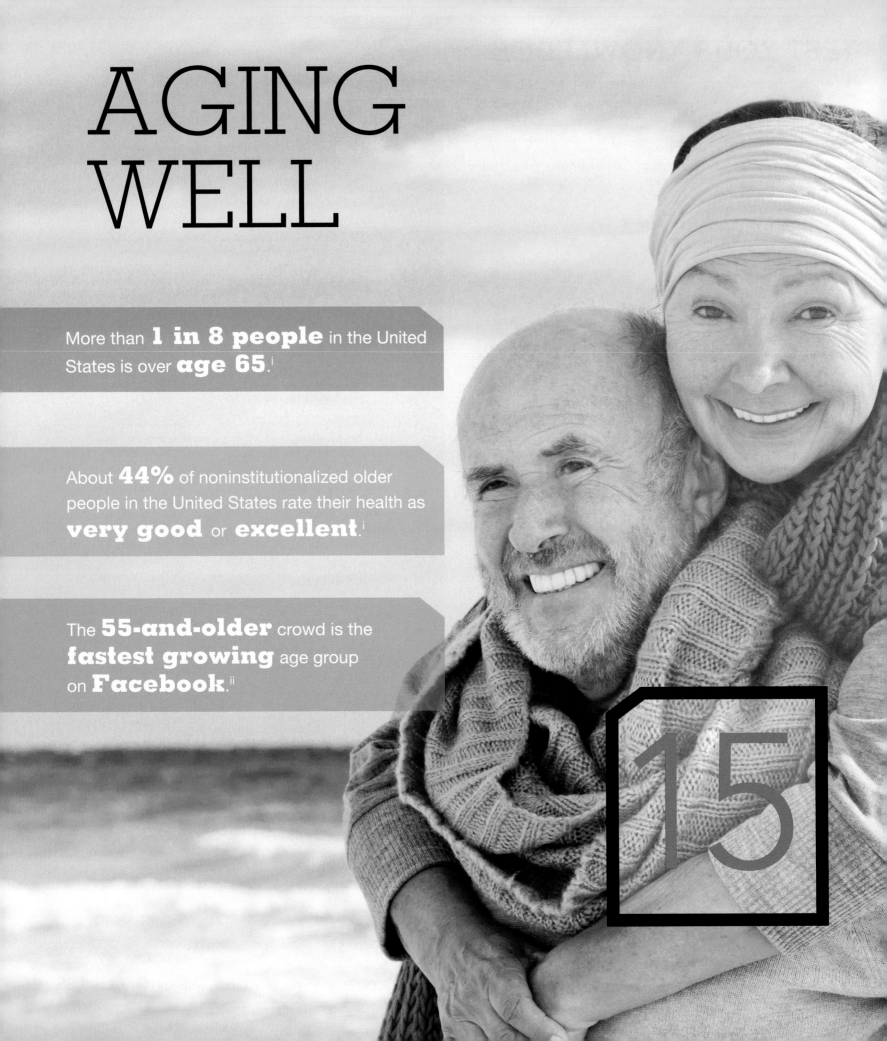

AGING WELL

More than **1 in 8 people** in the United States is over **age 65**.[i]

About **44%** of noninstitutionalized older people in the United States rate their health as **very good** or **excellent**.[i]

The **55-and-older** crowd is the **fastest growing** age group on **Facebook**.[ii]

15

Learning Objectives

DISCUSS how life expectancy in the United States has increased in the past century.

DESCRIBE the physical and psychosocial changes that typically accompany aging.

IDENTIFY at least five key strategies for aging successfully.

LIST four definitions of death and **EXPLAIN** how people develop a concept of death.

COMPARE and contrast the available options when planning for the end of life.

DISCUSS care of the body and planning a service after death.

IDENTIFY the stages of grief and the potential effects of grief on health.

EXPLAIN how to start aging well right now and how to support someone with a terminal diagnosis or someone who is grieving.

Aging brings many gifts:

a stronger sense of who you are and what you value; greater power to make your way in the world; and a broader range of experiences that, in turn, can expand your appreciation for others and deepen your compassion. But aging also brings challenges. Your body starts to show the wear and tear of time. Loved ones die. And you face the task of defining for yourself what is a good life, and a good death.

This chapter can help increase your awareness of the gifts of aging, and prepare you for its challenges. Whatever your age, the information here is relevant for you simply because aging and dying are part of the human experience. What's more, the healthy choices you make today will help you to age with vitality. And, finally, understanding end-of-life issues can help you cope with the death of loved ones and clarify your thoughts and feelings about your own passing.

As with other aspects of health, aging is as social as it is personal. We'll start by looking at how America, as a whole, is growing older.

Aging in the United States

The United States is in the midst of a longevity revolution.[1] Between 2000 and 2011, the population of older Americans (aged 65 and above) increased more than 18%. Currently, more than one in eight Americans is over the age of 65. And people reaching the age of 65 have an average life expectancy of an additional 19.2 years. By the year 2060, an estimated 92 million people in the United States will fall within this age category **(Figure 15.1)**.[1] In another significant shift from the past, older Americans are becoming more racially and ethnically diverse. In 2000, about 83% of older adults in the United States were Caucasians. By 2030, that figure will fall to about 72%, with Hispanics, African Americans, and Asian Americans representing growing segments of the older population.[1]

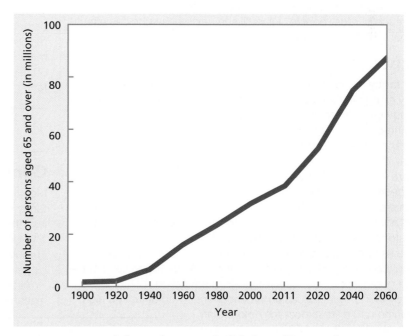

FIGURE 15.1 Number of Older People in the U.S. Population, 1900–2060.

Source: Data from *A Profile of Older Americans: 2012*, page 3, from the Administration on Aging, website, 2013.

> ## " The healthy choices you make today will help you to age with vitality."

Trends in Health and Health Care

As the number of older people in the United States grows, key aspects of aging—health and wellness—are changing:

- More older people are giving a positive report on their overall health. The number of people aged 65 to 74 rating their own health as only fair or poor has fallen from almost 28% in 1993 to below 25% in 2010.[2] Older African Americans, Native Americans, and Hispanics are less likely to rate their own health as excellent or good than are Asian Americans or Caucasians.[1]

- At the same time, most older Americans have at least one chronic health condition. More than 70% have hypertension, for example, and 20% have diabetes.[1] But major contributors to poor health among older people are also preventable or reversible. Fewer than half of older Americans report engaging in regular leisure-time physical activity and about 28% are obese.[1]

- Older Americans use more health care than any other age group. In addition to their health-insurance coverage under the federal Medicare program, their out-of-pocket spending on health care averages over $4,700 annually.[1] It's clear, then, that improving the health of older people must be a priority if we're to curb our nation's increasing health-care spending.

The keys to avoiding chronic disease as you age—a balanced diet, regular exercise, and avoidance of tobacco and alcohol abuse—lie within the reach of most people. As we'll see next, these choices affect not only how well, but also how long you can expect to live.

Life Expectancy

Life expectancy in the United States has climbed steadily over the last century along with improved nutrition, the growing availability of vaccines, advances in treatments such as surgery and medications, and public health campaigns, such as those that discourage smoking. Life expectancy for a person born in the United States in 2011 is now projected at 78.7 years.[3]

Still, there is room for further improvement. Some of the leading causes of death, such as heart disease, stroke, and type 2 diabetes, can be prevented or moderated by maintaining a healthful weight, exercising, and not smoking. Some researchers are concerned that America's high rate of obesity has already reduced U.S. life expectancy by at least five years and could reduce it even further in coming decades.[4]

Troubling disparities in life expectancy also exist among racial groups and among populations with different levels of education. For example, a 2012 study found that Caucasian American men with at least a high school diploma had a life expectancy more than 14 years greater than that of African American men who did not complete high school. For women, the comparable gap was more than 10 years.[5]

Christopher J. L. Murray, a professor of global health at the University of Washington, describes the

life expectancy The length of time a person can expect to live, usually measured in years.

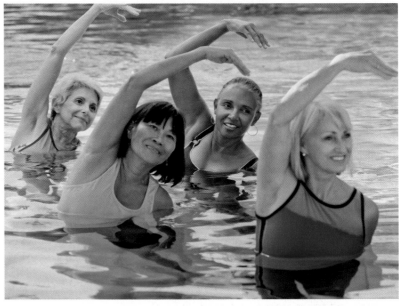

Women in the United States have a life expectancy almost five years longer than men's.

United States as a country of "eight Americas" in terms of longevity, distinguishing between these eight groups using a variety of racial, ethnic, economic, and geographic factors. According to this analysis, Asian Americans can expect to live the longest—almost 85 years. On the other end of the spectrum, African Americans living in the rural South can expect to live about 71 years.[6]

 Watch a short video from the University of Washington identifying factors driving the eight Americas at www.youtube.com/watch?v=YdfQ87LgyV0.

You might think that the United States is a world leader in life expectancy, but that's far from true. In the Central Intelligence Agency's ranking of the 221 countries of the world, the United States comes in at number 50, with the top 32 countries experiencing a life expectancy of 80 years or more. In Monaco, the world leader, the average life expectancy is almost 90 years.[7]

 Although nothing can predict how long you'll live, you can calculate your life expectancy based on your health, habits, and lifestyle at www.longevitycentres.com/tools-agecalculator.html.

Gender and Longevity

Men, in general, cannot expect to live as long as women. Life expectancy for U.S. males now stands at about 76.3 years, almost 5 years less than women, who have a life expectancy of about 81.1 years.[3] This gender-based longevity gap is not unique to the United States. Throughout the developed world, women tend to live several years longer than men.[8]

Although the factors contributing to this gap are still under study, research has identified a few, including:

- **Delayed cardiovascular risks.** Women tend to develop cardiovascular disease in their 70s and 80s, about 20 years later than men.

- **Sex chromosomes.** Human beings have one pair of sex chromosomes, which determine—along with many other traits—whether you are male or female. Women have two X chromosomes. Men have one X chromosome and one Y. The X chromosome is larger than the Y chromosome and holds many more genes, some of which perform important functions. Thus, women have a backup set of these genes, allowing their genomes to choose the best of the pair.

- **Fewer risk-taking behaviors.** Men are much more likely than women to die from unintentional injuries, such as car crashes, or intentional injuries caused by violence.
- **Lower rate of smoking.** Although the difference in the rate of smoking among males and females is narrowing, 21.6% of men are current smokers, versus 16.5% of women. Smoking and other forms of tobacco use are the single greatest preventable cause of death in the United States.[9]
- **More effective health management techniques.** Women are more likely to visit their health care provider regularly, including for preventive care.[10]

What Happens As You Age?

When they hear the term *aging*, most people think of biological aging—the physical changes that begin at birth and continue until death. But aging is also psychosocial, encompassing changes in cognition, memory, and mood as well as changes in relationships, career, and income.

Physical Changes

Have you ever heard the saying that, from the moment we're born, we begin to die? That's not physiologically true because throughout childhood and adolescence, our cells are multiplying and our tissues and organs are growing. But at a certain point, cells reach their limit of replication. Telomeres, regions of DNA at the ends of our chromosomes, begin to shorten, until eventually the DNA can't be copied again and the cell dies. As more and more cells die, our tissues degrade. We age. As you read the following discussion of the physical changes characteristic of aging (**Figure 15.2**), bear in mind that you can delay and even reduce some of them. We'll explore how later in this chapter.

Changes in Body Composition

With aging, decreased production of certain hormones leads to a gradual decline in muscle tissue and a corresponding increase in body fat. At the same time, body fat shifts from subcutaneous stores, just below the skin, to deeper stores, such as around the liver and other organs. This shift coincides with an increased cardiometabolic risk. However, a healthful diet and an active lifestyle can reduce this loss of lean tissue and gain in fat.

Hearing Loss

Losing the ability to hear clearly is a common sign of aging, but that doesn't make the change any easier to accept. Age-related hearing loss, called **presbycusis,** usually arises from damage to microscopic hair cells in the inner ear. Loss of the ability to hear conversation can cause the person to feel confused and frustrated and to withdraw from social contact.

Any hearing loss should be tested and treated. A variety of devices, such as hearing aids or phone

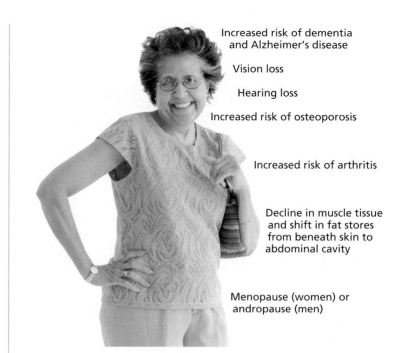

Increased risk of dementia and Alzheimer's disease

Vision loss

Hearing loss

Increased risk of osteoporosis

Increased risk of arthritis

Decline in muscle tissue and shift in fat stores from beneath skin to abdominal cavity

Menopause (women) or andropause (men)

FIGURE 15.2 Physical Changes Due to Aging.

presbycusis Age-related hearing loss, which usually develops gradually, often due to damage to or changes in the inner ear.

presbyopia Age-related decline in the ability to focus on objects up close, especially in low light.

cataracts An age-related vision disorder marked by clouding of the lens of the eye.

glaucoma An age-related vision disorder arising from an increase in internal eye pressure that damages the optic nerve and reduces peripheral vision.

age-related macular degeneration (AMD) An age-related vision disorder caused by deterioration of the macula that reduces central vision.

amplifiers, may help. In severe cases, surgery may restore some hearing. When you are still young, do all you can to protect your hearing. (For a refresher on basic hearing safety, see Chapter 17.)

Vision Loss

Vision usually declines with age. By their mid-40s, many people have developed **presbyopia,** a gradual decline in the ability to focus on objects up close, especially in low light. This vision disorder can be addressed by wearing reading glasses when looking at objects at close range.

By age 80, more than half of all Americans develop **cataracts,** a clouding of the lens of the eye that dims vision (**Figure 15.3a**).[11] This condition can be addressed successfully through surgery.

Glaucoma develops when fluid builds up in one or both eyes, increasing internal pressure and damaging the optic nerve, typically causing a loss of peripheral vision (**Figure 15.3b**). Over 2 million Americans are thought to have glaucoma, and it is the second leading cause of blindness (after diabetic retinopathy). The condition can be detected through an eye exam and is treated through medication, laser therapy, or surgery.[12]

Age-related macular degeneration (AMD) impairs the center of a person's vision rather than the periphery (**Figure 15.3c**). The disorder arises when the *macula,* a region of tissue at the center of the retina, deteriorates. It is somewhat common, affecting about 1.5% of Americans. Although no one knows the precise cause, smoking increases the risk. The condition can be detected through an eye exam but is difficult to treat. Surgery or light therapy may help some patients. A study from the National Eye Institute indicates that taking a specific formulation of antioxidant vitamins and minerals may be able to slow the progression of the disease.[13]

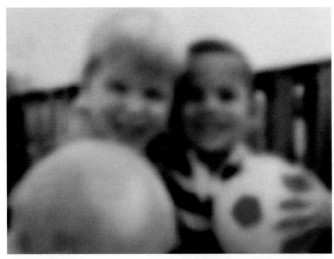

(a) Cataract

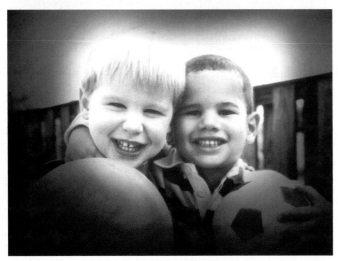

(b) Glaucoma

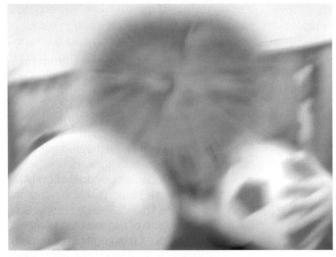

(c) Age-related macular degeneration

FIGURE 15.3 Vision Problems Common to Aging.

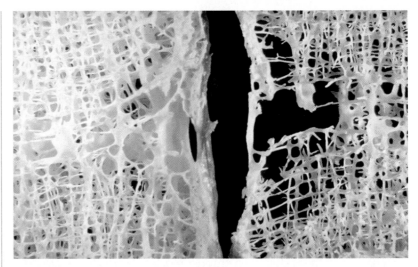

FIGURE 15.4 Effects of Osteoporosis on the Vertebrae of the Spine. Vertebral bone tissue of a person with osteoporosis (right), and of a healthy person (left).

Chronic Diseases

Aging increases your risk of many chronic diseases. Rates of cardiovascular disease, type 2 diabetes, and some cancers all rise significantly after age 65. (For a discussion of these major chronic diseases and how to address them, see Chapter 12.) Two chronic bone disorders associated with aging are arthritis and osteoporosis.

Arthritis. More than 50 million adults in the United States—about 22%—have some form of **arthritis.**[14] The most common form is *osteoarthritis,* a type that often arises with age. In people with osteoarthritis, cartilage wears away in the hands and weight-bearing joints of the body, such as the knees, hips, and ankles. Osteoarthritis often arises from a mix of genetic factors and damaging force, such as injury, repetitive motion, or excessive body weight. Although there is no cure for osteoarthritis, rest, physical therapy, and medication can all help.

Osteoporosis. As you can see in **Figure 15.4**, **osteoporosis** is a disease characterized by excessively porous bones that are fragile and brittle and therefore fracture easily. Approximately 2 million fractures each year are due to osteoporosis.[15] Osteoporosis arises when bone density decreases with age, and it is one of the leading disabling conditions among older people in the United States.[16]

Although 20% of people with osteoporosis are men, osteoporosis is more common in women for several reasons. Females have an absolute bone density lower than that of males. Women weigh less, on average, than men of the same height, and, therefore, women's bones experience less of the weight-bearing stress that prompts bone building. Also, the female reproductive hormone estrogen helps maintain bone mass, and after menopause, estrogen declines. Finally, women live an average of five years longer

arthritis Inflammation of one or more joints in the body, resulting in pain, swelling, and limited movement.

osteoporosis A disease characterized by low bone mass and deterioration of bone tissue, leading to fragile bones and an increased risk of fractures.

than men, and because bone loss increases with age, osteoporosis is more likely to show up in women.

Some risk factors for osteoporosis, such as sex, age, and family history, can't be changed. But other risk factors are within your control. Smoking, excessive alcohol consumption, a sedentary lifestyle, underweight, and a diet low in calcium and vitamin D all increase the risk.

Menopause

Menopause, or the permanent cessation of a woman's menstrual cycle and fertile years, is a normal, natural process, not an illness. But the hormonal changes that trigger menopause may cause temporary physical discomfort as well as increase a woman's risk for cardiovascular disease and osteoporosis. For these reasons, some women turn to health remedies to address the effects of menopause.

Technically, menopause begins one year after a woman's last menstrual period. In the United States, that usually occurs in a woman's early 50s, but menopause-related changes often begin several years earlier. In *perimenopause,* women may notice changes in their periods, find they are more likely to build up stores of abdominal fat, have trouble sleeping, or start experiencing some of the classic symptoms of menopause, such as mood swings, vaginal dryness, bursts of perspiration known as hot flashes, and night sweats. These symptoms usually arise from the natural decline of reproductive hormones. Once a woman is 12 months past her last period, her ovaries produce much less estrogen and no progesterone and no longer release eggs. The years that follow menopause are referred to as *postmenopause*.

After decades of the monthly hassles that having a period brings, some women welcome menopause. This is especially true if a woman experiences relatively few menopausal symptoms and side effects. For others, the process brings more mixed feelings. Some women may mourn the loss of their fertility, feel less feminine, or equate menopause with old age. Some may experience extremely uncomfortable or even debilitating physical or psychological symptoms. In these cases, treatments may include:

- **Psychotherapy to help combat fears surrounding menopause.** For instance, the end of menstruation doesn't mean that a woman is facing death: The average woman lives about 30 years after menopause.
- **Hormone therapy (HT).** Administration of synthetic reproductive hormones, referred to as *hormone therapy*, increases bone density and is an effective short-term treatment for hot flashes and other menopausal symptoms. However, HT can also increase the risk for certain chronic diseases. Thus, women considering it should discuss the risks and benefits with their physician.[17]
- **Vaginal estrogen.** This topical medication relieves vaginal dryness and discomfort.
- **Bone-building medications.** These nonhormonal drugs, known as bisphosphonates, are prescribed to prevent or decrease postmenopausal bone loss. However, they are associated with some potentially serious side effects, so again, women should discuss the risks and benefits with their physician.[18]

>> **The Office of Dietary Supplements provides information on good food sources for calcium:** http://ods.od.nih.gov/factsheets/Calcium-HealthProfessional.

- **Antidepressants.** Some antidepressants may help with hot flashes or the mood swings surrounding menopause.

Many women also have success with self-care measures, including:

- **Avoiding hot flash triggers.** Some women find that certain factors, such as spicy food, hot beverages, or sleeping quarters that are too warm, worsen the number and intensity of hot flashes.
- **Quitting cigarettes.** Smoking increases hot flashes and brings on earlier menopause.
- **Exercising regularly.** Exercise not only reduces the risk of post-menopausal health concerns such as osteoporosis and heart disease, but helps control weight and promotes healthful sleep.

Specific physical activity recommendations for older adults are discussed shortly.

Andropause

Levels of the male reproductive hormone testosterone begin to decline gradually around age 30. By about age 70, testosterone levels can have dropped by as much as half of what they were in young adulthood. This decline, and the physical and emotional changes that accompany it, are generally referred to as **andropause,** or *male menopause*. Men who experience andropause may report any of the following:[19]

- Changes in sexual functioning, including reduced desire, erectile dysfunction, and infertility
- Physical changes, including increased level of body fat and decreased muscle mass and strength
- Disturbed sleep, including insomnia or hypersomnia
- Emotional disturbances, such as depression and difficulty concentrating

Of course, any of these signs and symptoms could be due to factors other than declining testosterone levels. Thus, it's important that men experiencing them have a comprehensive clinical evaluation. The number of prescriptions for synthetic testosterone, which has been shown to improve muscle mass and strength, has tripled since the year 2001.[20] However, researchers estimate that at least one-quarter of prescriptions are written without testing the patient's blood testosterone level to be sure a deficiency exists. This concerns experts because testosterone therapy can thicken the blood, and some studies suggest that, for men who have hypertension, unhealthful blood lipids, or high blood glucose, testosterone supplementation can increase the risk for heart attack and stroke.[21] One thing we do know is that a program of medically supervised regular physical activity, including strength training, can preserve muscle mass and strength, reduce levels of body fat, promote healthful sleep, and relieve depression.

Sexuality

An active sex life is usually associated with the young, but older people are far from out of the game. As people age, sexual desire and activity may ebb and flow, but sexuality remains an important aspect of life. Just over half (53%) of all people aged 65 to 74 remain sexually active.[22] Sex in older adulthood carries the same risk for sexually transmitted infections (STIs) as in youth, and a recent global research study suggests that the incidence of STIs among older adults is increasing worldwide. The study authors suggest that **ageism** might be partially to blame for this rise; that is, public health agencies deny older adults' sexual identity and, therefore, leave them out of safer-sex public service campaigns.[22]

menopause The permanent end of a woman's menstrual cycle and reproductive capacity.

andropause Period marked by a decline in the male reproductive hormone testosterone and its resultant physical and emotional effects; also referred to as *male menopause*.

ageism Prejudice or discrimination against older adults.

Changes Affecting Cognition and Memory

Normal age-related changes in brain anatomy and function usually prompt some degree of cognitive decline.[23] Examples include greater difficulty in multitasking, remembering names of people and places, and learning new information quickly. However, significant memory loss and confusion are not a routine aspect of aging. In fact, many people become wiser with age because their decades of accumulated experiences help them solve new problems. Moreover, many cognitive skills can be boosted through "brain fitness" activities, which are discussed later in this chapter.

Some older adults, however, do experience true degenerative neurological disorders. These include various forms of dementia, the most severe form of which is Alzheimer's disease.

Dementia. A broad term for a decline in brain functioning, **dementia** may arise at any point in life but is much more common in people over the age of 80. Genetics, a history of a stroke, cirrhosis of the liver, malnutrition, exposure to toxins, and other factors may play a role.

Although there is no guaranteed path to preventing dementia, healthful behaviors may make a difference. Researchers are currently investigating the role of body weight, diet, exercise, and participation in socially and intellectually stimulating activities in preventing all forms of age-related dementia, including the most common form—Alzheimer's disease.[24]

Alzheimer's Disease. Few age-related illnesses are more feared than this progressive, fatal brain disorder. In **Alzheimer's disease (AD),** nerve cells in the brain are found to be filled with abnormal collections of proteins. These impair functioning and cause nerve cells to disconnect from one another **(Figure 15.5)**. Thus, their ability to transmit messages is lost. Eventually, the affected nerve cells die. As the disorder progresses, entire regions of brain tissue atrophy (shrink), and brain mass is lost.

The damage may begin as many as 10 to 20 years before any problems become evident. Eventually, however, the disease steals memory, concentration, and the ability to perform most daily tasks. In normal age-related memory loss, the person typically forgets only certain details of an event. In AD, all memory of an event vanishes: For example,

a person may watch a favorite television program, and a few minutes after it ends ask when the program is going to begin. Gradually, AD also affects mood and personality, in some cases leaving the person depressed, highly anxious, combative, and even delusional.

» **To view a video showing what happens to the brain in AD, go to** www.nia.nih.gov/alzheimers/alzheimers-disease-video.

One in eight older Americans—more than 5 million adults—has AD. This number is expected to escalate in the coming decades as more people live longer.[25] Leading risk factors include:[24]

- **Age.** Most cases of AD occur in people older than 60. This version of the condition, known as *late-onset Alzheimer's,* is the most common. A rare form of the disease, known as *early-onset Alzheimer's,* can begin in a person's 30s or 40s.

- **Genetics and family history.** If AD runs in your family, you are at increased risk for developing the disease yourself. With the help of affected families, researchers have located several genes associated with an increased risk for each type of AD.

- **Poor health.** A growing body of research indicates that vascular health and the body's ability to move blood through the brain plays a role in the disease. Factors that harm the cardiovascular system, such as hypertension, low HDL ("good cholesterol"), insulin resistance, and obesity, also increase the risk. Poor physical health overall is a significant risk factor for cognitive decline in older adults.[26] Poor psychological health also takes a toll: Having depression nearly doubles the risk of developing AD later in life.[27]

- **Lifestyle factors.** A sedentary lifestyle, poor diet, and low levels of intellectual stimulation and social engagement are all associated with an increased incidence of cognitive decline.

There are currently no treatments that alter the underlying course of AD, although several prescription medications may slow the cognitive decline. There are also no proven prevention strategies. However, maintaining a healthful body weight and keeping physically, socially, and intellectually active might reduce your risk. Eating a diet rich in fruits, vegetables (especially cruciferous and green leafy vegetables), whole grains, and healthy plant oils may be particularly beneficial, especially when combined with regular physical activity.[24]

» **Alanna Shaikh is a public health expert who has a family history of Alzheimer's disease. She shares her "plan for getting Alzheimer's" here:** www.ted.com/talks/alanna_shaikh_how_i_m_preparing_to_get_alzheimer_s.html.

Psychosocial Changes

As a college student, you are probably experiencing some powerful psychosocial changes. You may recently have moved from another town or state, leaving behind family members and friends. And you may already be planning for your post-college career or graduate school. If you think about the challenges that such shifts represent for you, you can begin to imagine how challenging similar changes can be in the lives of older adults.

Family Changes

After spending 18 years raising their children, day in and day

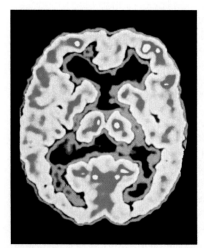

(a) Healthy brain

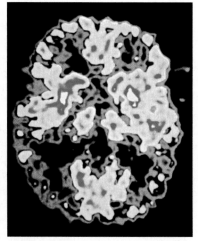

(b) Brain with Alzheimer's disease

FIGURE 15.5 Brain Activity and Alzheimer's Disease. Reds and yellows indicate high activity in tissues; blues and greens represent lower activity in tissues.

dementia A decline in brain function.

Alzheimer's disease (AD) A progressive, fatal form of age-related dementia.

out, older adults may welcome their newfound freedom as their kids head off to college or join a spouse in a distant state. Yet it's common for parents of adult children to struggle with feelings of loss and to question their worth. This so-called *empty nest syndrome* challenges older adults to rethink not only their day-to-day responsibilities, but also how they define their identities.

The empty nest syndrome also challenges couples. Older people who've raised children together will suddenly find themselves spending more time alone than they have in years and will probably need to get to know each other again as individuals. Some couples, once their children have left home, find that the bonds that connected them as individuals have frayed, and they may separate. Others find that their connection is stronger than ever, and enjoy the extra time they have together.

At the same time that they are adjusting to their own aging, many older adults begin taking on significant caregiving tasks for very elderly parents. They may find themselves spending many hours each week taking them to medical appointments, shopping for them, and making a variety of arrangements for their care. This change in family dynamics can be highly stressful, but it can also give older adults and their elderly parents precious opportunities to share memories and feelings, resolve conflicts, and affirm their love and caring.

Changes in Residence

Eighty-one percent of older Americans are homeowners, and 19% are renters; however, the size and type of dwelling that older adults own or rent often changes.[1] Empty nesters may discover that the four-bedroom house in which they raised their family now feels too large, or the maintenance too burdensome. It's not uncommon, then, for older adults to move to a smaller home. Some move in with a son or daughter and may help with housework and caring for their grandchildren. In 2011, 2 million older adults lived with grandchildren, and one-fourth of these were their grandchildren's primary caregivers.[1] About 2.7% live in residential communities for older adults, where some form of support service is provided to residents.

Currently, about 3.6% of older adults live in institutional settings such as nursing homes. New—and often less costly—options for older adults with health constraints are medical cottages, also known as "granny pods." These are small, affordable dwellings that can be installed in a family's backyard, giving both older adults and their children a measure of privacy, while maintaining close proximity. The units are equipped with special adaptations for older residents, such as soft flooring to prevent fractures if the resident falls, track lighting leading from bedroom to bathroom, hand rails, and call devices should the resident need assistance.

At the same time, many older adults are embracing a concept called *aging in place*, which the U.S. Centers for Disease Control and Prevention defines as the ability to live in one's own home and community safely, independently, and comfortably regardless of age, income, or ability level.[28] The National Aging in Place Council is a group of professional service providers, from elder specialists to financial planners to home and landscape contractors, whose aim is to support older adults who wish to live independently in their homes.

Changes in Employment

Although retirement is meant to bring freedom from work, some seniors may find themselves unsure of who they are if they aren't attached to a profession. Many seniors find that using their professional skills to volunteer provides an easier transition from the professional world to retirement. And many—18.5% in 2012—continue to work past age 65.[1]

Handling Aging

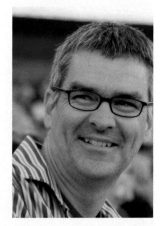

"HI, MY NAME IS STEPHEN. After having dropped out of college decades ago, I'm finally coming back to school and taking night classes to get my B.A. I'm 47, and a lot of my classmates are 20, 30 years younger than me. Compared to my first time in college, it's true that I'm not as athletic as I was, I have a few more aches and pains, and it's harder to keep weight off than when I was 20, but nowadays, I'm much more invested in my classes and I feel sharper than ever. Sometimes I feel like an old guy compared to my classmates, but then I think of my mom who's 73 and as active as ever. I guess we have good genes in our family that keep us young."

1. Stephen says he feels sharper than ever. Why do you think that is?

2. Why is it harder for Stephen to keep weight off now compared with when he was 20?

3. Do you think Stephen is right that "good genes" are keeping him young? What else will keep him healthy and aging well? Which do you think is most important, genes or lifestyle factors?

Economic Changes

Retirement may bring more free time—but reduced work translates into reduced income. Older adults who have no employer pension or retirement savings and find themselves living on their Social Security income may discover that they must reduce their spending, sometimes drastically, even as certain costs, such as medical expenses, may be rising. Unfortunately, 43% of single older adults and 22% of couples rely on Social Security benefits for 90–100% of their total income. In 2010, the most recent year for which there is data, the average monthly Social Security benefit was just over $1,300 for men and $1,000 for women.[29] If you had to survive solely on Social Security benefits, could you do it?

Clearly, personal retirement savings are critical—but people in the United States are notoriously poor at funding their retirement accounts. A recent analysis of federal data found that the average American household headed by a person with a 401(k) employer-based retirement plan had less than one-quarter of the amount in the fund that would be needed—along with their Social Security and any pension funds—to maintain their standard of living in retirement.[30]

As a result of these factors, the traditional view of retirement as a time of leisure has changed. Increased life expectancy means that people will need an income longer. As noted earlier, over 18% of Americans now work at least part-time past age 65.

>> **Want a rough estimate of your Social Security retirement benefits? Check out** www.socialsecurity.gov/estimator.

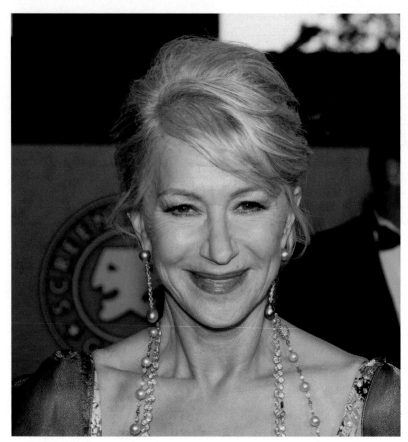

Helen Mirren, at age 69, is at a high point in her career.

Mood Changes

In 2012, only 2% of older Americans reported experiencing psychological distress in the past 30 days.[1] Nevertheless, retirement, reduced income, chronic pain, functional limitations, and the death of loved ones are significant psychological challenges, and rates of depression and suicide are relatively high among older adults. Whereas the suicide rate is about 11 per 100,000 in the general population, about 14 of every 100,000 people aged 65 and older die by suicide. Caucasian men aged 85 and older are most likely to take their own lives, with a rate of nearly 50 suicides per 100,000 persons in that age group.[31]

If an older relative or friend talks about feeling sad or hopeless, listen carefully and offer to help him or her find care. Many hospitals and senior centers offer support groups and mental health services designed for older adults. Above all, spend time with your loved one. Showing older adults that they are important to you can help them reject feelings of abandonment.

Substance Abuse and Polypharmacy

Despite the perception that substance abuse is an issue only for adolescents and young adults, it is a serious and growing health concern for older adults.[32] A 2011 federal study estimated that 5.8% of Americans aged 50 and older had used illicit drugs in the past year. The drugs most commonly abused are marijuana and prescription drugs, including prescription narcotics.[32]

Alcohol abuse is also a common problem among older adults. Approximately 40% of older Americans consume alcohol; however, precise statistics on alcohol abuse are difficult to gather.[33]

polypharmacy Simultaneous use of several prescription medications that can interact in dangerous ways.

We do know that older adults are more sensitive to alcohol's effects because they metabolize alcohol more slowly than younger people. As a result, alcohol stays in their bodies longer. Also, as we age, our body fluid level declines. Thus, older adults have a higher percentage of alcohol in their blood than younger people after drinking the same amount.[33] Alcohol can also reduce the actions of some medications and increase the effects of others. Medication and alcohol interactions can even be fatal.

Another medication-related concern for older adults is **polypharmacy,** the use of several drugs that can interact in dangerous ways.[34] On average, individuals aged 65 to 69 take nearly 14 prescription medications a year. Polypharmacy is responsible for up to 28% of hospital admissions and is the fifth leading cause of death in the United States.[34]

What Contributes to Successful Aging?

Although it might be difficult to imagine yourself as a senior citizen, you are aging! And the behaviors you establish right now can help you do it successfully. That's because, although genetic factors do appear to play some role in how long and how well a person lives, about 70% of life expectancy appears to be due to lifestyle choices and other non-genetic influences.[35] As discussed in the nearby **Diversity & Health** box, longevity researchers are trying to identify the specific behaviors that enable people in certain communities around the world to enjoy a longer lifespan and better quality of life. One habit that comes up consistently in such research is exercise.

Physical Activity

Regular physical activity is one of the most beneficial things you can do for your health at any point in life. Consistent exercise greatly reduces your chronic disease risk and slows many of the physical aspects of aging, such as decreased bone density and muscle mass and increased body fat. It also helps relieve the pain of joint conditions, such as arthritis, and eases mental health concerns, such as anxiety and depression.

Moreover, physical activity has been shown to boost *adult neurogenesis*—the generation of new neurons in certain regions of the brain, giving older adults some protection against cognitive decline.[36, 37] The National Institute on Aging reports that higher levels of physical activity are associated with a reduced risk of dementia. Even moderate exercise, such as brisk walking, has been shown to increase nerve cell activity in key parts of the brain and improve cognitive functioning.[24, 37]

It's never too late to enjoy the benefits of exercise. For people who are 65 years of age or older, are generally fit, and have no limiting health conditions, public health experts recommend at least:

- Two hours and 30 minutes of moderate-intensity aerobic activity, such as brisk walking, each week AND muscle-strengthening activities that work all major muscle groups at least 2 days a week, OR
- One hour and 15 minutes of vigorous-intensity aerobic activity, such as jogging, every week AND muscle-strengthening activities that work all major muscle groups at least 2 days a week, OR
- An equivalent mix of moderate- and vigorous-intensity aerobic activity AND muscle-strengthening activities that work all major muscle groups at least 2 days a week.[38]

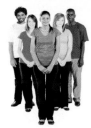

DIVERSITY & HEALTH

Aging in the Blue Zones

Athlete, explorer, and educator Dan Buettner teamed up with medical researchers, longevity experts, anthropologists, and National Geographic to identify communities around the world where people lived better and longer. People living in these so-called *Blue Zones* reach age 100 at rates 10 times greater than the United States average. The Blue Zone communities include:

- Okinawa, Japan
- Nuoro Province, Sardinia, Italy
- Ikaria, Greece
- Nicoyan Peninsula, Costa Rica
- A community of 9,000 Seventh Day Adventists in Loma Linda, California

The Blue Zone researchers identified nine factors common to all five of these communities. They are:

1. **Engagement in spontaneous physical activity.** Rather than spending an hour a day at a gym, the world's longest-lived people

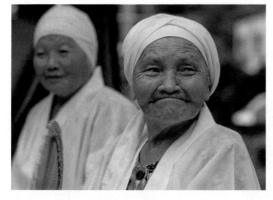

Okinawans have some of the longest life expectancies in the world.

move without thinking about it. They walk, garden, and do much of their housework without mechanical appliances.

2. **Sense of purpose.** The Blue Zone researchers found that knowing "why you wake up in the morning" increases life expectancy by up to seven years.

3. **Stress management.** Although people in the Blue Zones experience stress just like anyone else, they engage in practices that help them to shed that stress. The techniques differ—Okinawans take a few moments each day to remember their ancestors, whereas Sardinians enjoy happy hour—but the results are increased quality and length of life.

4. **Amount and timing of meals.** Long-lived people tend to eat until they're no longer hungry, but not until they feel full. They also eat their smallest and last meal in the late afternoon or early evening.

5. **Content of meals.** Beans are the cornerstone of most Blue Zone diets. A small portion of meat is eaten on average only about once a week.

6. **Wine.** People in all Blue Zones (except Adventists) drink 1–2 glasses of alcohol (typically wine) per day, usually with friends at meals.

7. **Membership in a spiritual community.** Most centenarians belong to some type of spiritual community. The Blue Zone research associates this habit with an additional 4 to 14 years of life expectancy.

8. **Maintenance of family ties.** Blue Zone families keep aging parents and grandparents nearby or in the home and invest in their children with time and love.

9. **Maintenance of social ties.** The world's longest-lived people participate in social circles that support healthy behaviors.

Researchers from the New England Centenarian Study at Boston University identify some of the same factors as important in longevity. However, they include a few more observations: Few centenarians are obese. A substantial smoking history is rare. And many centenarian women gave birth to a child after age 35. The researchers found that a woman who has a child after age 40 has a fourfold increased probability of living to 100.

> ### Critical-Thinking Questions
>
> 1. Of the twelve total factors identified in the two studies, which six would you rank as the most critical to longevity? Explain the reasons behind your choices.
>
> 2. Why do you think being able to identify your sense of purpose might be important to your quality of life and longevity? Take a few moments to write down your own sense of "why you wake up in the morning."
>
> 3. Do your social ties "support healthy behaviors"? If so, in what ways? If not, what actions could you take to forge social ties that better support your health?

Sources: The Blue Zones, 2nd ed., by D. Buettner, 2012, Washington, DC: National Geographic Society, http://www.bluezones.com/about/; and *The New England Centenarian Study*, July 29, 2012, Boston University School of Medicine, http://www.bumc.bu.edu/centenarian/overview.

For a refresher on physical activity, including aerobic exercise, muscle-strengthening fitness, and overall types and intensities of exercise, see Chapter 5.

Good Nutrition

A healthful diet can extend your productive years and reduce your risk of chronic disease. In addition to the essentials of good nutrition important for people of all ages, nutritional guidelines recommend that older adults:[39]

- Get enough calcium and vitamins D and B_{12} from foods and/or supplements.

- Limit sodium intake to 1,500 milligrams per day to help control blood pressure.
- Make colorful, high-fiber fruits and vegetables half of each day's diet. The National Institute on Aging reports that several studies have associated higher vegetable consumption with lower levels of cognitive decline.[24]
- Choose whole grain breads, cereals, rice, and pasta.
- Choose mostly plant-based sources of protein, such as tofu, beans, and nuts, with fish, poultry, lean meats, eggs, and low-fat dairy less often.

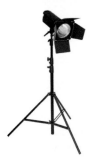
Exercise: The Life Preserver

Want to live longer? Work out more.

Numerous studies show that fitness, especially higher levels of cardiorespiratory fitness, is among the best predictors of longevity.[1] Research reveals that people with higher levels of physical activity face a risk of death one-quarter of that of older adults with low levels of physical activity, even after excluding older adults with chronic disease.[2] Another study found that people between the ages of 70 and 88 were more likely to live longer if they either continued an existing exercise program or started a new one.[3]

The Centers for Disease Control and Prevention (CDC) advises at least 30 minutes of cardiorespiratory activities, such as brisk walking, biking, or running, at least five days a week (or 150 minutes total per week).[4] But strength training matters, too: The CDC advises twice weekly sessions. Both flexibility and balance are critical to reduce the risk for falls, and the CDC recommends stretches, tai chi, yoga, or similar exercises a few minutes a day, most days of the week.

At any age, we all need a regular mix of these types of activities. (For an overview of fitness and exercise options, see Chapter 5.)

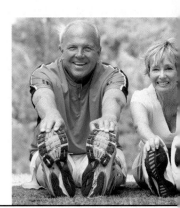

References: **1.** "Exercise and Longevity," by V. Gremeaux, M. Gayda, R. Lepers, P. Sosner, M. Juneau, & A. Nigam, 2012, *Maturitas, 73*(4), 312–317. **2.** "Total Daily Physical Activity and Longevity in Old Age," by A. S. Buchman, L. Yu, P. A. Boyle, R. C. Shah, & D. A. Bennett, 2012, *Archives of Internal Medicine, 172*(5), 444–446. **3.** "Physical Activity, Function, and Longevity Among the Very Old," by J. Stessman, R. Hammerman-Rozenberg, A. Cohen, E. Ein-Mor, & J. Jacobs, 2009, *Archives of Internal Medicine, 169*, pp. 1476–1483. **4.** "How Much Physical Activity Do Older Adults Need?" by Centers for Disease Control and Prevention, 2011, available at http://www.cdc.gov/physicalactivity/everyone/guidelines/olderadults.html.

- Drink plenty of water to help prevent constipation.
- Limit alcohol intake to no more than one drink per day for women and two drinks per day for men.

In 2011, the Center for Aging at Tufts University released a version of the United States Department of Agriculture's MyPlate modified for older adults (see **Figure 15.6**).

Weight Management

As we mentioned earlier in this chapter, almost a third of older adults are obese and therefore at increased risk for cardiovascular disease, type 2 diabetes, many forms of cancer, sleep apnea, and arthritis. Obesity is also increasingly linked to a greater risk of cognitive impairment as a person ages.[24]

As you know, obesity develops as a consequence of an imbalance between energy intake (in food and beverages) and energy expenditure (in metabolism and physical activity). Stress is also a factor. The good news is, if you establish health habits that enable you to manage your weight now, you'll find it easier to maintain those habits—and your healthful weight—as you age. (For a review of how to maintain a healthful weight, see Chapter 6.)

Avoiding Tobacco

When feeling sad, stressed, or unwell, resist the temptation to reach for a cigarette. About 9% of older Americans smoke.[40] Yet smokers have a risk of death from any cause that is three times higher than that of people who never smoked, and their life expectancy is 10 years lower.[41] Smoking has also been linked to chronic diseases, reduced lung function, premature balding, and wrinkles. Moreover, a 2012 study found that smoking actually erodes regions of brain tissue, resulting in significantly impaired cognition over people who have never smoked, and a 2013 study found that nonsmokers exposed to secondhand smoke experience similar harm.[42, 43] If you smoke, now is the time to quit.

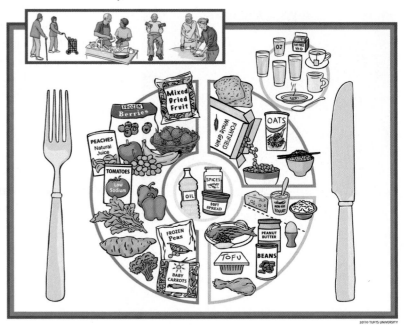

MyPlate for Older Adults

FIGURE 15.6 MyPlate for Older Adults. The icon illustrates the importance of fruits and vegetables, whole grains, and plant-based proteins such as tofu and beans. It also includes several examples of liquids, including soup, to encourage adequate hydration, and flavoring foods with spices instead of salt for reduced sodium intake. The plate is accompanied by icons depicting regular physical activity.

Source: Tufts University. © 2012, Tufts University. For details about the MyPlate for older adults, please see http://nutrition.tufts.edu/research/myplate-older-adults.

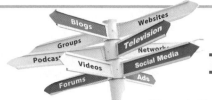

media and AGING

Do High-Tech Games Boost the Brain?

Americans intent on warding off age-related declines in memory and cognition are increasingly turning to high-tech "brain fitness" products, including DVDs, Internet programs, video games, and apps played on hand-held devices. Advertisements for such products claim they can help consumers prevent memory loss, boost concentration, reasoning, and problem-solving, and even reverse cognitive decline, but what's the evidence for such claims?

Overall, few brain fitness apps and similar products have been scientifically tested and fewer still have had their findings reported in peer-reviewed journals.[1] And the studies that have been published have had inconclusive results. For example, a recent study of an Internet game designed to improve cognitive function found it effective in boosting the specific cognitive tasks the game drilled; however, the researchers found no transfer of improvements to tasks that had not been drilled, even when they were closely related.[2] Another study of a Nintendo concentration game found that the study participants did experience a transfer of improvements in "processing speed" and "executive function" (such as ability to manage time and switch focus to achieve goals) but attention and overall cognitive status did not improve.[3]

The bottom line? Larger and more rigorous studies are required to determine the effectiveness of high-tech brain-fitness games. For now, however, the widely held belief that commercially available high-tech brain games lead to improvements in general cognitive function lacks scientific evidence.[2]

References: **1.** "Exercising the Brain to Avoid Cognitive Decline," by W. E. Reichman, A. J. Fiocco, & N. S. Rose, 2010. *Aging Health, 6*(5), 565–584. **2.** "Putting Brain Training to the Test," by A. M. Owen, A. Hampshire, J. A. Grahn, R. Stenton, S. Dajani, A. S. Burns, . . . C. G. Ballard, 2010, *Nature, 465*(7299), 775–778. **3.** "Brain Training Game Improves Executive Functions and Processing Speed in the Elderly: A Randomized Controlled Trial," by R. Nouchi, Y. Taki, H. Takeuchi, H. Hashizume, Y. Akitsuki, Y. Shigemune, . . . R. Kawashima, 2012, *PLoS One, 7*(1), e29676. doi: 10.1371/journal.pone.0029676. Epub 2012 Jan 11.

Mental Exercise

Just as exercise can maintain or restore your physical fitness, a daily "brain workout" can contribute to a state known as **brain fitness.** One study found that people who participate regularly in brain-engaging activities such as completing crossword puzzles, reading books, playing a musical instrument, singing in a chorus, or going to a museum experienced a risk of dementia that was nearly half that of people who did not engage in such activities.[24] Moreover, people who have a full social network and participate in many social activities tend to have less cognitive decline and a lower dementia risk than those who are more isolated.[24]

The key to beneficial activities lies in their interactivity. Any pastime that makes you think and requires that you connect with ideas, nature, or other people helps preserve thought and function. Staying connected through email, social networking sites, blogs, and Skype can also help. Interest among consumers in maintaining cognitive ability has led to the development of a new "brain games" industry. See the

brain fitness A person's ability to meet the cognitive requirements and demands of daily life, such as problem-solving and memory recall.

Media and Aging box to find out whether or not these games confer the benefits they claim.

Stress Management

Beginning today, challenge yourself to recognize signs of excessive stress in your life, and address them. Be sure to get enough sleep on a regular basis. Limit your consumption of alcohol, and eat right. Regular exercise is essential: A recent study found that aerobic exercise such as running stimulates the production and maintenance of brain cells that produce the neurotransmitter GABA, which exerts a calming effect in stressful situations.[44] It's also important to maintain a healthy network of personal relationships and friends who can serve as a sounding board and help you find your way through life's challenges. For a refresher on stress and stress management techniques, see Chapter 3.

Understanding Death and Dying

When was the last time you contemplated death? Or sat down with a friend or family member and talked about it? Not the death of a specific person, but the concept of death itself—your knowledge of the

>> **Want to see how fast you can match squeaks, squawks, and croaking sounds to the animals that make them? Or decipher encrypted quotations? Have fun playing the American Association of Retired Persons' Brain Games at** http://games.aarp.org.

dying process, your beliefs about an afterlife, and even your fears? If you've rarely given death and dying much thought, you might find the following discussion helpful.

What Is Death?

Historically, a person was pronounced dead if he or she had stopped breathing and had no heartbeat. But because of advances in medical technologies that artificially sustain physiological functions, clinicians now recognize several definitions of death.

- **Brain death** is the cessation of brain activity as indicated by various medical devices and diagnostic criteria.
- **Functional death** is the end of all vital organ functions, including heartbeat, breathing, and blood flow.
- **Cellular death** is the end of all vital functions at the cellular level, such as cellular respiration and other metabolic processes.
- **Clinical death** is a medical determination that life has ceased and is often defined by medical criteria that focus on a combination of functional and neurological factors.

These physiological definitions of death give us a shared standard for identifying death of the body. However, your larger ideas about death are influenced by your age, life experiences, and the values and beliefs you cherish.

How Do We Develop Our Concepts of Death and Dying?

Our concepts of death and dying are influenced by our developmental stage as well as sociocultural factors.

Stage of Development

Most young children are unaware of death's permanence. They may realize that some absence occurs with death but consider it just a

Death is an inevitable part of life.

brain death The cessation of brain activity as indicated by various medical devices and diagnostic criteria.

functional death The end of all vital physiological functions, including heartbeat, breathing, and blood flow.

cellular death The end of all vital functions at the cellular level, such as cellular respiration and other metabolic processes.

clinical death A medical determination that life has ceased according to medical criteria that often combine aspects of functional and neurological factors.

near-death experience (NDE) A profound psychological event usually occurring in a person close to death and marked by a characteristic pattern of perceptions and common features such as movement through space and perception of light.

passing phase. In kids' cartoons, characters get knocked off cliffs, hit by anvils, and run over by speeding cars. Yet they always bounce back. This resiliency echoes children's beliefs about the temporary nature of death.

Over time, personal experiences teach us that death is irreversible and permanent. A beloved grandparent passes on, and with each family celebration they don't attend, we realize that they really aren't coming back. We also begin gradually to understand that death is universal—that it happens to all living things and arises from both concrete externals, such as a car accident, and internal causes such as organ failure.[45] A classic review of nearly 100 studies of the concept of death in children suggests that a mature understanding of death typically evolves by approximately age 7.[45] However, it may take us a lifetime to come to terms with that understanding.

Through adolescence and even into young adulthood, most of us avoid fully acknowledging to ourselves that we will someday die. Although such denial of death may feel life-affirming, it can actually be life-threatening if it causes you to skip the seat belt or bring alcohol on a boating trip. Unintentional injuries represent the single largest cause of death of people aged 1 to 44.

Moreover, youth doesn't always mean perfect health. Young adults who get surprised by a high blood pressure or blood glucose reading at a routine checkup often realize that their body doesn't work the way it once did, and that these changes will continue to present challenges as the years add up. Most people are eventually presented with ample reminders that their body is aging and that, some day, death will come.

Sociocultural Factors

Our concepts of death and dying are also shaped by the families, communities, and societies in which we live. Indeed, Glennys Howarth, a leading author and researcher in death and dying, describes dying as a social relationship, involving a complex network of interactions among the dying person, loved ones, care providers, and many others.[46] Gender is an undeniable influence: The different ways in which men and women experience their roles, expectations, and socialization in turn affect their concept of death and their experiences of illness, dying, and bereavement.[47]

The beliefs and values with which we were raised or that we adopt as adults also significantly influence our concept of death. If we examine cultural celebrations such as the Mexican festival known as the Day of the Dead (Día de los Muertos) or Memorial Day in the United States, we find clues to a culture's beliefs about death and an afterlife, including the importance of honoring those who have gone before us. Of course many people turn to philosophical, religious, or spiritual teachings and practices to help them come to terms with death. Many strive more earnestly to live their values, dedicating themselves to social causes or environmental stewardship as they contemplate the legacy they would like to leave behind.

Over the past 30 years, increasing publicity about **near-death experiences (NDEs)** has also influenced our understanding of death and dying. NDEs are profound psychological and transcendental events that in many cases involve a sensation of leaving the body and

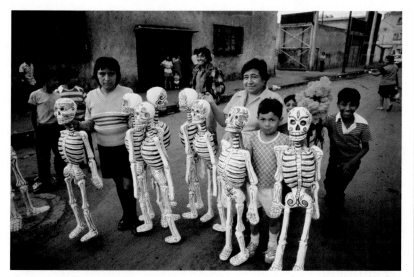

Día de los Muertos, a holiday begun in Mexico, helps those who celebrate it remember friends and family members who have died.

encountering an infinitely loving presence, often perceived as light. The International Association for Near-Death Studies reports that hearing about NDEs can be comforting to people who are seriously or terminally ill as well as those grieving the loss of a loved one.[48]

>> Watch a video of a young woman recounting her NDE at http://iands.org/audiovisuals/youtube-videos/426-held-by-white-light.html.

Planning for the End of Life

Although it may seem premature to "plan ahead" for death if you're in your late teens or 20s, doing so shows wisdom and concern for loved ones. Especially when an acute illness or accident makes death sudden and unexpected, family members are required to make numerous decisions in the midst of shock and grief. Your preparation can make these steps less distressing.

Complete Advance Directives

Advance directives are legal documents allowing a person to specify personal treatment preferences in case of a medical crisis. Without these documents, it can be difficult for loved ones and care providers to make important decisions on a person's behalf, and actions may be taken that the person would not have agreed with. Several types of advance directives are in common use, although they vary from state to state:

- **Health-care proxy.** A *health-care proxy* gives someone else—typically a relative or trusted friend—the power to make health decisions on your behalf, should you become unable to do so. Also called a *durable power of attorney for health care,* this document usually authorizes a person to have access to medical records and make a wide range of decisions, including deciding about treatments, including starting or continuing life support. Specific powers authorized to proxies vary according to state law.

- **Living will.** A *living will,* or *health-care directive,* states your wishes for medical treatment near the

advance directives Formal documents that state a person's preferences regarding medical treatment and medical crisis management.

end of life. As with health-care proxies, living wills are governed by state law; however, the documents usually prompt you to specify the extent of medical treatment you wish, your preferred provider, and how much discretion you give to your health-care proxy.

>> You can find your state's advance directive form online at www.caringinfo.org/i4a/pages/index.cfm?pageid=3289.

- **Do not resuscitate (DNR) order.** A *Do Not Resuscitate (DNR) order* instructs health-care providers not to try to restart a person's heart or lungs if heartbeat or breathing stops. DNR orders must be co-signed by a physician and placed in a person's medical chart.

Consider Organ Donation

If you are at least 18 years old, you can choose to become an organ/tissue donor. To do so, you can fill out and carry a donor card, enroll while signing up for your driver's license, or state your desire to donate as part of your state's advance directive form. When an organ donor dies, one or more of his or her organs and tissues may be donated to patients awaiting a transplant. Since the first successful kidney transplant was performed in Boston in 1954, medical and surgical techniques have advanced dramatically, and transplantation of the kidney, liver, lung, heart, pancreas, intestines, and corneas of the eyes is now routine.[49]

In 2012, there were more than 114,000 people in the United States on the waiting list to receive an organ transplant. About 79 people receive a transplant each day—but another 18 die waiting for one.[50]

>> Not sure how to get started planning for the end of life, whether for yourself or with a loved one? Visit The Conversation Project at http://theconversationproject.org.

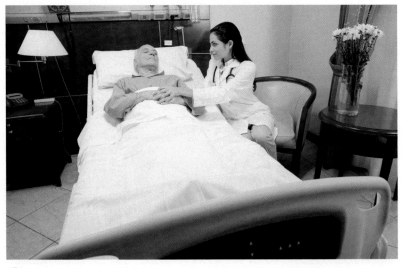

Caring for someone at the end of life can be done in a home, hospital, or hospice.

Write a Will

If you were to die, what would you want to have happen to your money? Your possessions? If you have them, your children, or even your pets? You probably have preferences, but without a will, it may be difficult to have them carried out.

A **will,** a legally binding document expressing your intention of what should be done with your property after death, is the best way to plan for the distribution of your **estate,** or money, property, and other possessions. It also allows you to name your *executor*, the person who makes sure your wishes are carried out, select a guardian for your children, and specify any funeral arrangements you wish. During your life, your will can be changed or replaced at any time. If you die **intestate,** or without a will or similar document, your state's laws will determine who receives your property. Those guidelines may or may not match your personal wishes.

Despite the clarity that wills provide, more than half of United States adults don't have one.[51]

Research Your Options for End-of-Life Care

If you or someone in your family were diagnosed with a **terminal illness,** what would be the best setting for providing care? Answering that question often requires consideration of a mix of personal preferences, family concerns, and medical needs. Three common settings for end-of-life care include the dying person's home, a hospital or nursing home, or a hospice facility. In any of these settings, the type of care most often given to people with a terminal illness is **palliative care.** The goal of palliative care is to relieve pain and suffering, rather than to prolong life or cure the disease. Although it is often given along with treatment-based care—for instance, the administration of pain medication to a person recovering from heart surgery would be classified as palliative care—for people at the end of life, it seeks to provide as much comfort as possible, rather than to prolong life.[52]

Home Care

When surveyed, most older Americans say they would prefer to die at home, yet only about one-quarter actually do.[53] This duality reflects the difficulties of providing end-of-life care in a home setting. Professional caregivers may be needed to provide intravenous pain medications, nutrition, or fluids, for example, or to perform any number of other types of highly skilled tasks. If the quality of a person's final days is being eroded by a lack of access to care, it may be best to consider a move to a professional care facility.

Hospital-Based Care

About one-third of older Americans die in hospitals.[53] Although these facilities have traditionally focused on treating and curing illness and sustaining life, they are increasingly offering the dying hospital-based palliative care, sometimes in dedicated palliative care units or facilities.

Hospice Care

About 1.5 million Americans receive **hospice** care each year, with most major insurance companies covering these services.[54] In 2010, more than 40% of U.S. deaths were under the care of a hospice program. The goal of hospice care is to provide the best possible quality of life for the dying and their families, usually within the last six months of a person's life, rather than to cure or treat disease. Thus, pain management, physical comfort, and emotional and spiritual counseling for both the patient and family members form the core of hospice care. Hospice patients with complex palliative care needs typically reside in hospice facilities. In most cases, however, hospice services are provided at home.[55]

Clarify Your Beliefs and Values

What if you had terminal cancer and decided you were ready to choose hospice care—but your family members were opposed? Or what if your condition were so painful that you longed to commit suicide? Such situations often arise at the end of life, requiring complex ethical deliberations. Here we discuss just three of the most contentious end-of-life issues.

Rational Suicide

Rational suicide is the deliberate hastening of his or her own death by a rational person who is terminally ill. Whereas some terminally ill patients end their lives by deliberately overdosing on medications, starving themselves, or taking other measures independently, many seek their physician's assistance to hasten their death. Such *physician-assisted suicide* is legally known as *physician aid in dying (PAD)* and is allowed in four states: Oregon, Washington, and Vermont by law, and Montana by

will A legally binding document stating what should be done with a person's property after death.

estate A person's personal holdings, including money, property, and other possessions.

intestate Dying without leaving a legal will.

terminal illness An irreversible condition that will result in death in the near future.

palliative care Type of care that focuses on reducing pain and suffering and caring for the whole person, rather than prolonging life or curing disease.

hospice A home-care program or facility that focuses exclusively on the dying and their loved ones, with a goal of providing comfort rather than facilitating a cure.

rational suicide Action taken deliberately by a reasoned, terminally ill patient to hasten his or her own death.

a Supreme Court ruling in 2010 that effectively legalized the practice. In PAD, the physician provides the medical means for a terminally ill patient to commit suicide but does not administer the medication. In contrast, administration of the lethal medication by the health-care provider is called active *euthanasia*, a word of Greek origin meaning "good death." Active euthanasia is illegal throughout the United States.

>> Watch the trailer for the award-winning 2011 documentary on PAD, *How to Die in Oregon*, **at** www.howtodieinoregon.com/trailer.html.

Passive Euthanasia

We rarely think about it this way, but the millions of Americans who use insulin or any other essential medication, who wear a pacemaker, or who undergo regular kidney dialysis are "on life support." Advances in medical technology can even keep patients alive when their lungs will never again be able to function independently. In the United States, mentally competent adult patients have the right to refuse any and all forms of medical care, even when, in the opinion of the health-care provider, refusing treatment will bring about their death.

A decision against life-sustaining intervention is referred to as **passive euthanasia.** Although it can be distressing for health-care providers and family members even when a competent, conscious adult refuses treatment, other medical situations can present true ethical dilemmas. For example, what happens when a person falls into a *persistent vegetative state,* in which they are deeply unconscious, would not survive without life support, and have no reasonable hope of improvement? If the patient hasn't stated life-support preferences beforehand, the decision whether to start or continue life support can be wrenching for loved ones. Or what if a conscious but combative patient in an advanced stage of AD refuses to eat or drink? Should feedings and fluids be administered by tube? Or consider an infant with a disorder that causes great suffering and, even with constant medical treatment, is uniformly fatal by age 2. If the infant were to develop an acute and potentially fatal infection, should the infection be treated, or should it be allowed to "take its course"? In the United States, 100% of hospitals with more than 400 beds and well over 80% of hospitals overall have a mechanism for addressing issues of medical ethics, such as an ethics board or committee, and many also have chaplains and other spiritual caregivers to help family members make such decisions.[56]

After a Death

When a loved one dies, the living face many immediate demands. Legal documents, such as a certificate of death, must be signed. Relatives, friends, and colleagues must be notified. Arrangements must be made for burial or cremation and usually for some form of memorial service. An obituary is typically submitted to the press. Final bills must be paid. And amid all this work, overwhelming feelings of grief may leave survivors unable to focus on the tasks at hand and in need of significant support. Here, we discuss the major tasks that immediately follow death and the grief that typically accompanies them.

Autopsy

Approximately 10% of U.S. deaths are followed by an **autopsy** (also known as a postmortem examination or obduction), which is a medical examination of a corpse. It is performed primarily to determine the cause of death, but may also be performed to

passive euthanasia Failure to begin or to maintain an intervention that is necessary to sustain a patient's life.

autopsy Medical examination of a corpse.

determine if the death resulted from an accidental injury, homicide, or suicide, or was from natural causes.[57]

All suspicious deaths are investigated by a medical examiner. A physician can also request an autopsy with consent of next-of-kin. In some cases, family members arrange for an autopsy—and pay for it—when they suspect that the death was due to malpractice. After tests are concluded, the findings are summarized in a report that often but not always includes a cause of death.

Care of the Body

In decades past, family members typically bathed and dressed the body of the dead in a final act of love and respect before a simple burial. Although many families now relinquish these tasks to professional funeral homes, others still choose to maintain such care within the family. In fact, many religions encourage care of the body as an essential spiritual practice.

By law, bodies can be buried or cremated. Some religions require that a body be buried, and many individuals value having the remains of their loved one buried in a cemetery they can visit regularly. An emerging trend is the choice of a "green burial," in which a body is simply wrapped in cloth and placed in the ground. In many states, laws permit burying a body on the family's property as long as it is outside the village, town, or city limits.[58] Cremation, incineration of a body, uses extremely high heat to reduce the corpse to fragments of bone, which are then pulverized. The resulting 4 to 6 pounds of bone "ash" can then be scattered, buried, or preserved in a memorial urn or box. There is no environmental or health risk from cremated remains.

Planning a Service

After death, our loved ones leave behind not only material remains but also the legacy of their lifetime. To comfort the survivors, many choose to hold one or more formal services such as the following:

- **Wake.** The traditional wake (sometimes called the "viewing") was a period of hours to days during which loved ones gathered in the home of the deceased to clean, dress, and watch over the body, pray, and support the bereaved. The word *wake* is derived from an ancient root meaning "to watch." Today, a wake may be held in a funeral home, church, or chapel, and may include a brief religious service, opportunities for individual prayer, and time for offering condolences. Food may be served.

- **Funeral.** To accompany the burial or cremation rites, some families choose to hold a funeral, usually a traditional religious service in which prayers are said for the deceased and the person's life is remembered by loved ones and friends. Music, poems, and a formal eulogy may be offered. The burial of the body or scattering of the ashes may be held immediately after the service.

- **Memorial service.** Although memorial services often include prayers and music of a spiritual nature, they typically involve less religious ritual than a funeral. Over time, the concept of a memorial service has evolved from a somber remembrance to a joyful celebration of the person's life, full of personal reminiscences, poems, songs, photos, and often a slide show or video. Food is typically a part of such services, and some even include dancing. It is not uncommon for people with a terminal illness to plan and pay in advance for their own memorial service.

Grieving

"HI, I'M MICHELLE.
When I was in high school, my uncle was killed in a car accident. It was a big shock to my family because he was still young and we weren't expecting it. I felt like a big part of what I had to do after it happened was support my mom and aunt, both of whom were really upset. Everyone felt so sad because we never had a chance to say good-bye. After the funeral, though, we all told stories and shared how he touched our lives. That made me feel a little better, and to this day I still try to talk about him and remember his spirit."

1. What types of things might Michelle have done to support her mom and aunt as they grieved for her uncle?

2. Why do you think telling stories about her uncle made Michelle feel better? What other types of things do people do to remember someone who's passed away?

3. What stage of grief do you think Michelle is in now?

Experiencing Grief

Every one of the approximately 2.5 million deaths in the United States each year touches the lives of those left behind. Their grief can last for months or even years.

Stages of Grief

Grieving the loss of a loved one is a deeply personal experience that is different for everyone. Still, grief experts have noted that many who grieve experience one or more of the following stages:[59]

- Disbelief, especially if a death is sudden or unexpected
- Yearning, reflecting the desire to have the person back in your life in a vibrant, vital way
- Anger, directed at everything from the death itself to the events surrounding the person's passing
- Depression, a persistent sadness that pervades daily life as the reality of the person's passing sets in
- Acceptance, blending together the joys of the person's life and the changes following his or her loss into a new perspective that reflects the totality of the experience

Each person works through these stages in his or her own way, and some experiences of grief can be more complex than others. If a loved one has lived a long life and died after an illness, it may be easier to find peace with the death. If a person dies at a young age, commits suicide, or is a victim of a fatal injury or other unexpected, traumatic event, grief may be much more complex, intense, and long-lasting. Loved ones experiencing such *complicated grief* may benefit from the assistance of a grief counselor, therapist, or support group attended by others who have had a similar loss.

Grief in Children

Children show their grief in many different ways. They may cry, get angry, become depressed, have trouble sleeping, regress in their behavior, or appear unconcerned about the loss. Typically, children need reassurance that they are not to blame for the loved one's death, that they are not vulnerable to the same injury or illness, and that they will be cared for. Moreover, a child's grief may continue for longer than it might in an adult.[60] Children may need to work through their grief in each of their developmental stages; for example, graduating from high school may prompt a renewed sense of the loss—and a renewed anguish—in a teen whose mother died many years earlier.

Effects of Grief on Health

Death of a close family member is widely acknowledged as one of the top stressors that a human being can experience. People grieving a death may suffer such severe stress that it becomes a risk to their own health. For example, many studies over the past 50 years have found a significant reduction in life expectancy in the first six months after the death of a spouse, with some studies citing a 40% increased risk of death during this period.[61] The effects of grief on health may include any of the following symptoms or conditions:

- External symptoms, such as digestive upset, changes in eating habits, headaches, fatigue, weakness, vague pain, and disturbed sleep
- Cardiac symptoms, such as higher blood pressure or irregular heartbeat
- Psychosocial symptoms, such as increased drinking, depression, suicidal thoughts, feelings of guilt, isolation from others, and significant spiritual conflict

Change Yourself, Change Your World

This chapter has of necessity included discussion of many unwelcome changes beyond your control. So let's look at things you *can* do to age with grace, to support loved ones as they face the end of life, and to cope with grief.

Personal Choices

If you find yourself feeling discouraged when thinking about the inevitable challenges of aging, bear in mind that aging is not a disease, but a normal, potentially vibrant and enriching stage of life. One key for aging well is to maintain six smart behaviors that slow the process down. A landmark study of aging from Harvard University followed more than 800 people for over five decades to determine the factors that best predict successful aging.[62] The results were surprising: Genetic and biological factors, such as the longevity of our parents or our cholesterol level, were not as important as these six lifestyle choices. Three of these are physical, and we mentioned them earlier in this chapter:

- Avoid tobacco, especially cigarettes.
- Maintain a healthful weight.
- Get regular exercise.
  The other three are a little less obvious:
- Develop successful coping skills (the ability to make the best of a bad situation).

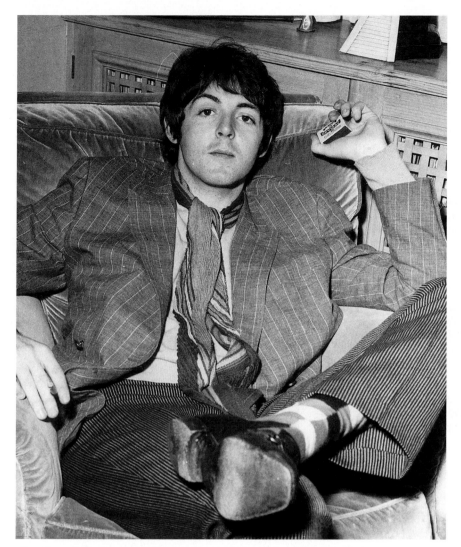
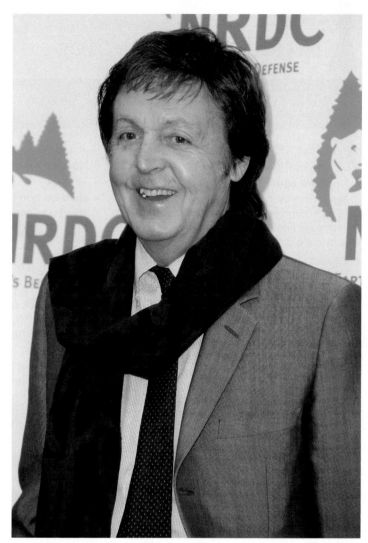

Aging happens to everyone (Beatle Paul McCartney in the 1960s and today). What you do today affects your quality of life as you get older.

• Maintain strong social relationships.
• Pursue education throughout every life stage.

If these behaviors already characterize your life, congratulations! But if you're struggling with one or two, such as managing your weight, or coping with stress, don't despair. Review the chapters in this book that discuss your particular challenge. If the practical strategies provided don't seem to be working, seek help from health-care professionals promptly, without waiting for the problem or behavior to reach a crisis stage.

Supporting a Loved One Who Is Dying

People's response to a terminal diagnosis is as unique as they are; still, certain reactions are more common than others. In her groundbreaking book *On Death and Dying*, psychiatrist Elisabeth Kübler-Ross, who worked with terminally ill patients in a Chicago hospital, proposed that individuals facing imminent death cycle back and forth through five overlapping and sometimes simultaneous states. You may notice that these are similar to the stages we identified for someone grieving the loss of a loved one, and, indeed, Kübler-Ross's work has influenced grief research. The states are:[63]

• *Denial*, in which patients refuse to accept the validity of the diagnosis
• *Anger*, which may be directed at the diagnosis, the physician, family members, themselves, or God
• *Bargaining*, in which patients try to avoid or delay death in exchange for repentance or service to others
• *Depression*, which can be brief or prolonged, and may be marked by withdrawal from loved ones
• *Acceptance*, a stage in which patients stop rejecting or fighting the diagnosis, may be introspective but not withdrawn, and may seek out time with loved ones, especially in order to make peace before death

When Kübler-Ross's work was published in 1969, it was the first comprehensive study of the psychology of the dying. In the decades since, many other researchers have refined and expanded our understanding of the experience. A consensus has emerged from this research that there is no "standard" way to experience dying and no prescribed method of supporting the dying person.

Practical Strategies

Coping with Grief

If you've lost a loved one, the following suggestions may help you cope:

- **Connect with others.** Draw friends and family members close. Share your memories of your loved one and your feelings about your loss. Find and talk to others who have also lost a loved one.

- **Expect—and allow yourself to feel—a range of emotions.** Don't tell yourself how to feel or let others tell you how you should feel.

- **Be patient with yourself.** Accept that grieving and healing take time.

- **Take care of yourself: Eat nourishing foods, engage in physical activity, and get enough sleep.** If your grief hampers your appetite, try having small, healthful meals and snacks throughout the day. Resist the urge to eat only those foods that comfort you.

- **For now, maintain your routine.** Avoid making dramatic changes in your life, such as transferring to a different school, at least for the first several months after the loss.

- **Hold on and let go.** Allow yourself to treasure your memories of your loved one, but try to let go of your memories of times when things went wrong, especially when you said or did things you now regret. Forgiving yourself is an important step toward healing.

- **Avoid quick fixes.** Substances such as drugs, alcohol, or over-the-counter sleep aids can be harmful, slow your recovery, and may actually cause new problems.

- **Be prepared for special days.** Holidays, your loved one's birthday, and the anniversary of his or her death are all times when strong feelings may come surging back. Plan in advance how and with whom you want to spend these days.

- **When you feel ready, create.** Work through your feelings in a poem, short story, or essay, or write an imaginary letter to your loved one. Record your words, accompany them with a slide show, and send a link to mutual family members and friends. Or paint a picture, plant a tree, run a marathon, or organize a benefit to commemorate your loved one.

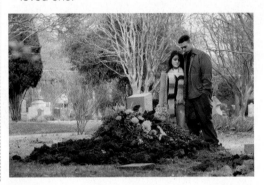

Sources: Based on *Coping with the Loss of a Loved One,* from the American Cancer Society website, 2009; and *End of Life,* from the Mayo Clinic website, 2010; and *Grief and Grieving – Home Treatment,* from the WebMD website, 2009.

If someone you love is diagnosed with a terminal illness, you may have several weeks or months to be with the person as he or she prepares for the end of life. You may welcome this opportunity to comfort and help, yet not know exactly how. Dr. Ira Byock, a palliative care specialist, advises that you and your loved one share one or more conversations in which you say "the four things that matter most." These are:[64]

- Please forgive me.
- I forgive you.
- I love you.
- Thank you.

When we ask and grant forgiveness, confirm our love, and thank our loved one for the gift of his or her presence in our lives, we leave nothing unsaid. We are prepared to say goodbye.

Supporting a Loved One Who Is Grieving

When people are grieving a loss, social support is key. They may need a hug or someone to listen. They might appreciate your taking on tasks such as handling phone calls and visits so that they can spend time alone. Or they might want to step away from their grief and join you in an activity that they find life-affirming.

Ongoing contact is also important. If a close family member has died, the first few days afterward require almost constant support of loved ones and friends. But your support continues to be important in the weeks and months that follow, especially on occasions such as holidays and the one-year anniversary of the person's death. When talking with the person, mention the deceased if it feels natural to do so. Although sharing philosophical or spiritual views of death can be comforting, avoid insisting on your own views of death or the possibility of an afterlife. Avoid clichés, and above all, avoid saying that you know how the person feels. You don't, even if you have suffered a very similar loss. Despite these cautions, don't be afraid to try to help. You won't go wrong as long as you let your own love for the grieving person lead the way.

The above advice applies as well when the grief is your own. That is, you, too, need practical assistance, social support, and the freedom to choose a break from your grief or time alone. For specific ideas, see the **Practical Strategies: Coping with Grief.**

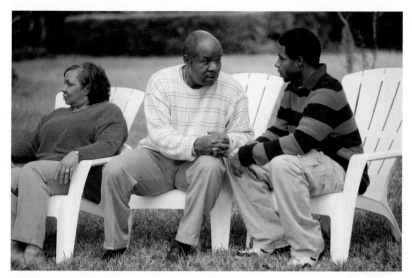

Talking openly with a loved one about death can be difficult, yet rewarding, for both of you.

Campus Advocacy

Are you a college student of traditional age? If so, it might be tough to imagine what it's like to be one of the 16% of undergraduates over age 35.[65] Attending college at an older age puts different stresses on students, from fitting in with younger students to juggling multiple roles to combating age-based stereotypes. Many older adults feel especially overwhelmed by their unfamiliarity with high-tech devices and software compared with their tech-savvy younger classmates.

How can you help? Reach out. Find out about older students' lives, why they enrolled in college, what came before this, and what they hope to achieve. If you notice someone struggling with any aspect of college life, whether registering for courses or downloading an assignment, offer to help. If they accept, avoid doing the task for them. Instead, take them through the process step by step. Maybe most importantly, just let them know *you* know they belong.

Whether older or younger, many college students experience the loss of a loved one. If you're one of them, don't try to cope alone. Visit your campus health services center, and ask about grief counseling. Or check out the National Students of AMF (supporting one another and **A**ctively **M**oving **F**orward). This nonprofit organization connects and empowers college students grieving the illness or death of a loved one to support one another. Its chapters have helped over 2,000 students on 170 college campuses nationwide. In addition, chapters work to raise awareness about the needs of grieving college students and host national grief support programs and events. Find them online at **www .studentsofamf.org.**

>> **Watch videos of real students discussing aging and death at** MasteringHealth™

Choosing to Change Worksheet

To complete this worksheet online, visit MasteringHealth™

As you've learned in this chapter, many of the health behaviors you choose today affect not only your life expectancy, but also your quality of life as an older adult. A recent study concluded that smoking, alcohol consumption, poor nutrition, and inactivity can age your body up to 12 years![66] The good news, according to the researchers, is that "modest but achievable adjustments to lifestyle behaviors are likely to have a considerable impact." So, healthy behaviors you adopt today will significantly impact your health and quality of life tomorrow!

Directions: Fill out Part I. Assess your stage of behavior change in Part II then fill out the remaining steps that apply to your stage of change.

Part I. Assess Your Behaviors

The study found that the following behaviors positively impact health as people age:

- Not smoking
- Eating 3 or more servings of fruits and vegetables each day
- Getting 2 or more hours of "leisure-time physical activity" per week
- Drinking no more than 7 alcoholic drinks per week for women or 10.5 per week for men

Consider these four behaviors. Which are you currently participating in?

_____

_____

Which of the above behaviors are you not participating in? What do you think is keeping you from participating in these behaviors?

_____

_____

_____

Part II. Take Action

Step 1. *Your Stage of Behavior Change.* Regarding the positive behaviors listed in Part I, indicate what stage of change you are in.

_____ I am not currently adhering to all of those behaviors and I do not intend to improve my behaviors in the next six months. (Precontemplation)

_____ I am not currently adhering to all of those behaviors but I might improve my behaviors in the next six months. (Contemplation)

_____ I am not currently adhering to all of those behaviors but I am prepared to improve my behaviors in the next month. (Preparation)

_____ I do adhere to all of those behaviors but I have been practicing them for less than six months. (Action)

_____ I do adhere to all of those behaviors and I have been practicing them for more than six months. (Maintenance)

Step 2. *Precontemplation and Contemplation Stages.* Even if you're not ready to make a change, describe what you might do differently so that you can adhere to the beneficial behaviors shown in Part I.

Example: I will take salsa dancing lessons at the student recreation center starting next week. Because I enjoy dancing, this will be a leisure-time physical activity that I will be motivated to do and that I can do for a lifetime.

_____

_____

_____

Step 3. *Preparation Stage.* How do you expect to benefit from adopting these behaviors?

_____

_____

Which of these reasons is most important to you, and why?

_____

_____

Write down your specific **SMART goal,** with a timeline, for adopting behaviors that will help you age well.

_____

_____

_____

Step 4. *Action and Maintenance Stages.* What is your **goal** for practicing these beneficial behaviors? In what ways have you benefited from adopting these behaviors?

_____

_____

What motivates you the most to continue practicing these behaviors and why?

_____

_____

_____

How easy are these behaviors to maintain? Is it truly a habit or do you need to expend some effort to do it?

_____

_____

_____

Step 5. *All Stages of Change.* What obstacles might get in your way to practicing these behaviors long-term? How can you address them?

Obstacle:	How to Address:

Chapter Summary

- The United States is heading toward a "longevity revolution," with life expectancy increasing and a growing percentage of the population falling into older age brackets.

- Women tend to live at least five years longer than men, and life expectancy also correlates closely with a person's racial or ethnic background, income, and region of residence. Negative behaviors such as smoking, alcohol abuse, and failing to participate in regular physical activity also reduce life expectancy.

- Aging brings many physical changes, such as declines in vision and hearing. Hormonal changes cause women to experience menopause, and some men to experience andropause. Chronic diseases, including arthritis and osteoporosis, become more common.

- Some older adults experience impairments in cognition and memory. The more mild form of this condition is referred to as age-related dementia. The more severe, progressive, and fatal form is Alzheimer's disease.

- Aging also brings psychosocial changes. These might include shifts in family dynamics, a change of residence, retirement, reduced finances, and an increased risk of depression and substance abuse as the aging person is challenged to adapt to the changing circumstances.

- Key steps in healthy aging include engaging in regular physical activity, consuming a nutritious diet, maintaining a healthful weight, avoiding smoking and other forms of substance abuse, challenging your mind, and reducing stress. Put these healthy habits in place when you are young.

- Death is often defined by the cessation of heartbeat, breathing, and other vital functions but may also be defined by other factors, such as the end of discernible brain-wave activity.
- Our concept of death evolves as we mature from childhood to adulthood and is influenced by our life experiences as well as our beliefs, values, and aspects of our culture.
- Numerous planning aids can help a person think through end-of-life issues ahead of time, state preferences, and make plans. These include advance directives for health, wills, and registration opportunities for organ/tissue donation.
- Options for end-of-life care include home care, hospital-based care, and hospice care in a hospice facility or in the person's home. In any setting, palliative care is a key aspect of care for the dying. The goal of palliative care is to decrease pain and suffering rather than to prolong the person's life.
- Rational suicide (including physician aid in dying) is the subject of ongoing debate.

- After a death, a person's body may be subject to autopsy, a medical examination that may or may not lead to identification of the cause of death.
- By law, a body must be buried or cremated. In either case, family members may also choose to remember their loved one by holding a wake, funeral, and/or memorial service.
- Grieving is a natural part of and reaction to death, and those experiencing grief, especially complicated grief, need the support of friends and loved ones through the long process of coming to terms with their loss. Children experience grief differently from adults, but no matter their age, people experiencing grief often suffer physical and psychological effects.
- Although people who are dying experience their situation in unique ways, some common responses have been identified, including stages of denial, anger, bargaining, depression, and acceptance. You can support the person by asking for and offering forgiveness, confirming your love, and thanking the person for his or her presence in your life.
- You can support someone who is grieving in practical ways as well as by simply being present.

GET CONNECTED

>> Visit the following websites for further information about the topics in this chapter:

- Administration on Aging
  www.aoa.gov
- Alzheimer's Association
  www.alz.org
- American Association of Retired Persons (AARP)
  www.aarp.org
- Caring Connections
  www.caringinfo.org
- National Institutes of Health Senior Health
  http://nihseniorhealth.gov

MOBILE TIPS!
Scan this QR code with your mobile device to access additional tips on aging well. Or, via your mobile device, go to **http://chmobile .pearsoncmg.com** and navigate to Chapter 15.

- RealAge Health Calculators and Assessments
  www.realage.com

Website links are subject to change. To access updated web links, please visit MasteringHealth™

TEST YOUR KNOWLEDGE

1. What is the life expectancy for someone born in 2011 in the United States?
   a. about 68 years
   b. about 78 years
   c. about 88 years
   d. about 98 years

2. Which of the following statements about older adult health is true?
   a. About one-fourth of Americans aged 65 to 74 rate their health as good or excellent.
   b. Almost 15% of older Americans are obese.
   c. The United States is ranked among the top 10 countries in the world in life expectancy.
   d. None of these answers are true.

3. Which of the following accurately characterizes arthritis?
   a. Arthritis is caused by loss of bone density.
   b. Arthritis damages your ligaments.

   c. Arthritis typically affects the hands and weight-bearing joints.
   d. Arthritis happens to everyone when they get older.

4. Alzheimer's disease
   a. impedes transmission of messages in the brain.
   b. impairs short-term memory.
   c. reduces length of life.
   d. All of these answers are true.

5. What can people who smoke cigarettes expect?
   a. to experience reduced quality of life as they age
   b. to experience greater cognitive decline than people who have never smoked
   c. to die younger than those who have never smoked
   d. all of these things

6. When a patient's heart stops beating, this is an example of
   a. clinical death.
   b. cellular death.
   c. functional death.
   d. brain death.

7. What is the goal of palliative care?
   a. to prolong life
   b. to relieve pain and suffering
   c. to prevent further deterioration in the patient's condition
   d. to cure disease

8. Which of the following statements is true?
   a. An autopsy is performed after nearly all deaths in the United States.
   b. A wake is traditionally held one or more days prior to burial of the body.
   c. Food is usually part of a funeral service.
   d. All of these statements are true.

9. Grief experts have noted that people who are grieving
   a. have a reduction in life expectancy.
   b. are at high risk for post-traumatic stress disorder.
   c. almost inevitably experience both intense anger and debilitating depression.
   d. need assistance from a psychotherapist or grief counselor.

10. Researchers have identified six factors that most strongly predict successful aging, which include:
   a. avoiding alcohol abuse.
   b. having healthful blood lipids, such as high HDL cholesterol.
   c. pursuing education through every life stage.
   d. having long-lived parents.

Get Critical

What happened

In May 2013, the Vermont House of Representatives overwhelmingly passed legislation allowing physician-aid-in-dying (PAD), which the Vermont governor promptly signed into law. But PAD ballot initiatives and legislative attempts have failed in many other states, and the practice remains deeply controversial.

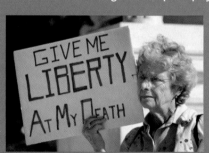

Some professional groups, such as the American Medical Association, take the position that doctors should never help hasten the end of life. A primary argument against PAD is that it would violate the Hippocratic oath, which requires physicians to "First, do no harm." Opponents argue that PAD could encourage physicians, patients, or family members to accept death prematurely. Physicians can and do make mistakes, both when diagnosing disease and when estimating patient survival time, and even in cases of terminal cancer, patients do sometimes recover spontaneously. Moreover, it might facilitate suicides among patients who are not terminally ill.

In contrast, some patient advocacy groups argue that the Hippocratic oath compels a physician to cease prolonging a terminally ill patient's suffering and provide a comfortable death. They argue that PAD spares patients unnecessary harm, allows patients to die with self-determination and dignity, reduces end-of-life health-care costs, and facilitates organ donation. They also point to cases in which, without access to PAD, terminally ill patients have committed suicide independently, sometimes in horrifying ways, causing themselves and their loved ones needless anguish.

What do you think?

- In 2011, there were 71 known deaths among patients receiving PAD in Oregon. This corresponds to approximately 2 deaths per 1,000 Oregon deaths. Over the previous 10 years, the average number of PAD deaths annually in Oregon was 51.[1] In your view, does this data support the position of PAD opponents or advocates? Why?

- If your state had a ballot initiative to allow PAD, would you support it? Why or why not?

- Currently, terminally ill, mentally competent patients requesting PAD must undergo a 15-day waiting period and an evaluation by a second physician before receiving the medication. But by late 2016, those restrictions will end in Vermont, and PAD will be a private matter between a patient and physician. If you support PAD overall, would you continue to support it if there were no requirement for a waiting period and second opinion?

Reference: 1. *Oregon's Death with Dignity Act—2012*, by Oregon Public Health Division, Oregon Health Authority, 2013, retrieved from http://public.health.oregon.gov/ProviderPartnerResources/EvaluationResearch/DeathwithDignityAct/Documents/year15.pdf.

Test Your Knowledge Answers

Chapter 1:
1. c **2.** d **3.** b **4.** b **5.** c **6.** d **7.** b **8.** b
9. a **10.** a

Chapter 2:
1. d **2.** b **3.** b **4.** c **5.** d **6.** a **7.** c **8.** d
9. c **10.** a

Chapter 3:
1. a **2.** b **3.** a **4.** c **5.** d **6.** b **7.** b **8.** a
9. d **10.** a

Chapter 4:
1. a **2.** c **3.** a **4.** b **5.** b **6.** c **7.** b **8.** c
9. d **10.** a

Chapter 5:
1. d **2.** d **3.** c **4.** c **5.** b **6.** d **7.** b **8.** a
9. c **10.** a

Chapter 6:
1. d **2.** c **3.** b **4.** a **5.** a **6.** b **7.** d **8.** d
9. a **10.** c

Chapter 7:
1. b **2.** b **3.** c **4.** a **5.** d **6.** a **7.** d **8.** d
9. b **10.** c

Chapter 8:
1. a **2.** d **3.** a **4.** b **5.** d **6.** c **7.** b **8.** b
9. c **10.** c

Chapter 9:
1. d **2.** b **3.** b **4.** d **5.** d **6.** b **7.** c **8.** d
9. a **10.** b

Chapter 10:
1. c **2.** a **3.** b **4.** a **5.** b **6.** b **7.** d **8.** c
9. c **10.** d

Chapter 11:
1. b **2.** b **3.** d **4.** a **5.** b **6.** a **7.** a **8.** d
9. d **10.** c

Chapter 12:
1. c **2.** d **3.** d **4.** a **5.** a **6.** c **7.** d **8.** d
9. b **10.** b

Chapter 13:
1. d **2.** d **3.** a **4.** b **5.** d **6.** a **7.** a **8.** c
9. b **10.** a

Chapter 14:
1. a **2.** d **3.** c **4.** d **5.** c **6.** d **7.** b **8.** a
9. a **10.** b

Chapter 15:
1. b **2.** d **3.** c **4.** d **5.** d **6.** c **7.** b **8.** b
9. a **10.** c

Chapter 16 (electronic chapter):
1. c **2.** b **3.** a **4.** b **5.** d **6.** c **7.** d **8.** a
9. d **10.** b

Chapter 17 (electronic chapter):
1. d **2.** c **3.** b **4.** a **5.** b **6.** c **7.** a **8.** d
9. b **10.** c

Credits

Photo Credits

Cover: Roberto Westbrook/Blend Images/Getty Images; **Inside Front Cover:** Joana Lopes/Shutterstock; hxdbzxy/Shutterstock; **Visual Walkthrough, p. 1:** sheff/Shutterstock; **Visual Walkthrough, p. 2:** Rido/Shutterstock; **Visual Walkthrough, p. 4:** Ljupco Smokovski/Shutterstock; **Visual Walkthrough, p. 6:** Stock Avalanche/Shutterstock; **Visual Walkthrough, p. 8:** nikola-master/Shutterstock

Chapter 1 opener: Andresr/Shutterstock; **p. 3:** Tyler Olson/Shutterstock; **p. 4:** John Dawson/Pearson; **p. 5:** Deyan Georgiev/Fotolia; **p. 6, top:** michaeljung/Shutterstock; **p. 6, bottom:** Tetra Images/SuperStock; **p. 7:** sheff/Shutterstock **p. 8:** Friedrich Stark/Alamy; **p. 9:** Fancy/Alamy Images; **p. 10, top:** Visions of America/SuperStock; **p. 10, bottom:** AF archive/Alamy; **p. 11, top:** Ryan DeBerardinis/Shutterstock; **p. 11, bottom:** ollyy/Shutterstock; **p. 12:** Ghislain & Marie David de Lossy/Cultura Creative/Alamy; **p. 14, left:** John Dawson/Pearson; **p. 14-1st from top:** Katrina Brown/Shutterstock; **p. 14-2nd from top:** Monkey Business Images/Shutterstock; **p. 14-3rd from top:** Tom Mareschal/Alamy; **p. 14-4th from top:** Lissandra/Shutterstock; **p. 15:** Supri Suharjoto/Shutterstock; **p. 16:** Helen King/Lithium/AGE Fotostock; **p. 17, bottom:** Maridav/Shutterstock; **p. 17, top:** Marco Prati/Shutterstock; **p. 22:** Kevin Mazur/WireImage/Getty Images

Chapter 2 opener: Paul Bradbury/OJO Images/Getty Images; **p. 25:** Glowimages Glow Images/Newscom; **p. 26, bottom:** Hill Street Studios/Blend Images/Alamy; **p. 27:** ZUMA Wire Service/Alamy; **p. 28:** Pacificcoastnews/Newscom; **p. 29:** Darren Greenwood/Design Pics Inc./Alamy; **p. 32, bottom:** Tom Wang/Shutterstock; **p. 33, left:** Radius Images/Alamy; **p. 33, right:** Pearson; **p. 34, bottom:** Stephen VanHorn/Shutterstock; **p. 35:** Stockbroker/MBI/Alamy; **p. 36, top:** Wiktoria Pawlak/Shutterstock; **p. 36, bottom:** Marjorie Kamys Cotera/Bob Daemmrich Photography/Alamy; **p. 38:** Pearson/John Dawson; **p. 40, top:** paffy/Shutterstock; **p. 40, bottom:** Super 7 Photo/Alamy; **p. 41, bottom:** Sigrid Olsson/Altopress/Newscom; **p. 42, bottom:** Jeff Greenberg/Alamy; **p. 43:** Gwoeii/Shutterstock; **p. 47:** AP Photo/Paul Sakuma

Chapter 3 opener: Ilya Bushuev/Vetta/Getty Images; **p. 50:** hektoR/Shutterstock; **p. 51, left:** Igor Kovalchuk/Shutterstock; **p. 51, right:** niderlander/Shutterstock; **p. 52:** Pearson; **p. 53, top:** Cristovao/Shutterstock; **p. 53, bottom:** Stockbyte/Getty Images; **p. 55, bottom:** Samuel Borges Photography/Shutterstock; **p. 57, right:** Minerva Studio/Shutterstock; **p. 59:** Malyugin/Shutterstock; **p. 60, bottom:** Artpose Adam Borkowski/Shutterstock; **p. 61:** Stockbyte/Getty Images; **p. 62, bottom:** PhotoAlto/Alamy; **p. 63:** Adrian Sherratt/Alamy; **p. 64, left:** Kenneth Man/Shutterstock; **p. 64, right:** runzelkorn/Shutterstock; **p. 65:** Robert Kneschke/Shutterstock; **p. 69:** Martin Zabala/ZUMApress/Newscom

Chapter 4 opener: Phil Date/Shutterstock; **p. 72:** Tom Grill/Corbis; **p. 74, bottom left:** Barry Gregg/Corbis; **p. 74, right:** Feng Yu/Shutterstock; **p. 75:** Fotocrisis/Shutterstock; **p. 76, bottom left:** sarsmis/Fotolia; **p. 76, right:** Gustavo Caballero/Getty Images; **p. 78, bottom:** Regien Paassen/Shutterstock; **p. 78- top 1st:** Barry Gregg/Corbis; **p. 78- top 2nd:** Barry Gregg/Corbis; **p. 78- top 3rd:** Barry Gregg/Corbis; **p. 78- top 4th:** Barry Gregg/Corbis; **p. 78- top 5th:** Barry Gregg/Corbis; **p. 78- top 6th:** Barry Gregg/Corbis; **p. 78- top 7th:** Barry Gregg/Corbis; **p. 79- bottom 1st:** Barry Gregg/Corbis; **p. 79- bottom 2nd:** Barry Gregg/Corbis; **p. 79- bottom 3rd:** Barry Gregg/Keepsake/Corbis; **p. 79- bottom 4th:** Barry Gregg/Corbis; **p. 79- bottom 5th:** Morgan Lane Photography/Shutterstock; **p. 79- top 1st:** Barry Gregg/Corbis; **p. 79- top 2nd:** Barry Gregg/Corbis; **p. 79- top 3rd:** Barry Gregg/Corbis; **p. 79- top 4th:** Barry Gregg/Corbis; **p. 79- top 5th:** Barry Gregg/Corbis; **p. 79- top 6th:** Barry Gregg/Corbis; **p. 80, right:** Lana Langlois/Shutterstock; **p. 81, bottom left:** Markus Mainka/Shutterstock; **p. 82, left:** bonchan/Shutterstock; **p. 82, right:** Pixelbliss/Fotolia; **p. 84, left:** Jesse Kunerth/Alamy; **p. 84, right:** Kati Molin/Shutterstock; **p. 86- right 1st:** Pearson; **p. 86- right 2nd:** Pearson; **p. 86- right 3rd:** Pearson; **p. 86- right 4th:** Pearson; **p. 86- right 5th:** Pearson; **p. 87:** USDA; **p. 88, bkgd:** Evgeni_S/Shutterstock; **p. 88, left:** andersphoto/Shutterstock; **p. 88, right:** Morten Degn/Shutterstock; **p. 89- top 1st:** Pearson; **p. 89- top 2nd:** Pearson; **p. 89- top 3rd:** Pearson; **p. 89- top 4th:** Pearson; **p. 89- top 5th:** Pearson; **p. 89- top 6th:** Pearson; **p. 89, bottom:** Pearson; **p. 91, bottom:** Bernabea Amalia Mendez/Shutterstock; **p. 92:** ksena32/Fotolia; **p. 93, bottom:** Taylor S. Kennedy/National Geographic Image Collection/Alamy; **p. 95, bottom:** Adam Gault/Photodisc/Getty Images; **p. 98:** AP Photo/PRNewsFoto/MilkPEP

Chapter 5 opener: Erik Isakson/Getty Images; **p. 101, bottom:** ranplett/E+/Getty Images; **p. 102, right:** Blue Jean Images/Alamy; **p. 103:** Westend61/Newscom; **p. 104:** djma/Fotolia; **p. 105, left:** Maksim Šmeljov/Fotolia; **p. 105, center:** Doug Menuez/Photodisc/Getty Images; **p. 105, right:** Stockbyte/Getty Images; **p. 106:** Pearson; **p. 107, right:** blue jean images/Getty Images; **p. 108-1st:** Pearson; **p. 108-2nd:** Pearson; **p. 108-3rd:** Pearson; **p. 108-4th:** Pearson; **p. 108-5th:** Pearson; **p. 108-6th:** Pearson; **p. 108-7th:** Pearson; **p. 109-1st:** Pearson; **p. 109-2nd:** Pearson; **p. 109-3rd:** Pearson; **p. 109-4th:** Pearson; **p. 109-5th:** Pearson; **p. 109-6th:** Pearson; **p. 109-7th:** Pearson; **p. 109-8th:** Pearson; **p. 109-9th:** Pearson; **p. 110, bottom:** Image Source/Getty Images; **p. 112-1st:** Pearson/Elena Dorfman; **p. 112-2nd:** Pearson; **p. 112-3rd:** Pearson; **p. 112-4th:** Pearson; **p. 112-5th:** Pearson; **p. 112-6th:** Pearson; **p. 112-7th:** Pearson; **p. 113-1st:** Pearson; **p. 113-2nd:** Pearson/Elena Dorfman; **p. 113-3rd:** Pearson/Elena Dorfman; **p. 113-5th:** Pearson/Elena Dorfman; **p. 113-6th:** Pearson/Elena Dorfman; **p. 116:** Walter Lockwood/Corbis; **p. 117, right:** MJTH/Shutterstock; **p. 118, bottom:** Kim Reinick/Shutterstock; **p. 119, left:** bonninturina/Fotolia; **p. 119, right:** yamannar/Shutterstock; **p. 120, bottom:** Hans Gutknecht/ZUMA Press/Newscom; **p. 121:** Pearson; **p. 124:** Getty Images.com

Chapter 6 opener: PhotoAlto/Odilon Dimier/Getty Images; **p. 128, right:** Vince Bucci/AP Images; **p. 130:** George Doyle/Stockbyte/Getty Images; **p. 131:** FREDERIC J. BROWN/AFP/Getty Images/Newscom; **p. 133:** ACE STOCK LIMITED/Alamy; **p. 135, bottom:** LUIS ACOSTA/AFP/Getty Images; **p. 136:** Pearson; **p. 137, top left:** Pearson; **p. 137, top right:** Pearson; **p. 137, center left:** Pearson; **p. 137, center right:** Pearson; **p. 137, bottom left:** Pearson; **p. 137, bottom right:** Pearson; **p. 137-4th:** Pearson/Elena Dorfman; **p. 140, right:** Jacek Chabraszewski/Fotolia; **p. 141:** OLJ Studio/Shutterstock; **p. 142, left:** Samuel Borges Photography/Shutterstock; **p. 142, right:** amanaimagesRF/Getty Images; **p. 144:** Alexander Raths/Fotolia; **p. 145:** Hisayoshi Osawa/Taxi Japan/Getty Images; **p. 147:** Pearson; **p. 151:** ZUMA Press, Inc./Alamy

Chapter 7 opener: JJAVA/Fotolia; **p. 154, bottom:** Design Pics Inc./Alamy; **p. 155, bottom:** Blend Images/Alamy; **p. 155, center:** Konstantin Sutyagin/Fotolia; **p. 158:** Joy Scheller iPhoto Inc./Newscom; **p. 159:** Rommel Canlas/Shutterstock; **p. 160, left:** J Marshall - Tribaleye Images/Alamy; **p. 160, right:** AJPhoto/Science Source; **p. 161:** Studio Pookini; **p. 162:** Multnomah County Sheriff/Splash/Newscom; **p. 163:** Nico Hermann/Westend61/Newscom; **p. 164:** Tom Wagner/Alamy; **p. 165, top:** Discovod/Shutterstock; **p. 165, center:** Peter Kim/Shutterstock;

Glossary

12-step programs Addiction recovery self-help programs based on the principles of Alcoholics Anonymous.

A

abortion A medical or surgical procedure used to terminate a pregnancy.

absorption The process by which alcohol passes from the stomach or small intestine into the bloodstream.

abstinence The avoidance of sexual intercourse.

acceptance and commitment therapy (ACT) An outgrowth of cognitive-behavioral therapy that increases patients' ability to engage in values-based, positive behaviors while experiencing difficult thoughts, emotions, or sensations.

accessory glands Glands (seminal vesicles, prostate gland, and Cowper's gland) that lubricate the reproductive system and nourish sperm.

acid rain* A phenomenon in which airborne pollutants are transformed by chemical processes into acidic compounds, then mix with rain, snow, or fog and are deposited on Earth.

acquired immunity The body's ability to quickly identify and attack a pathogen that it recognizes from previous exposure. In some cases acquired immunity leads to lifelong protection against the same infection.

active stretching A type of static stretching where you gently apply force to your body to create a stretch.

addiction A chronic, progressive disease of brain reward, motivation, memory, and related circuitry characterized by uncontrollable craving for a substance or behavior despite both negative consequences and diminishment or loss of pleasure associated with the activity.

advance directives Formal documents that state a person's preferences regarding medical treatment and medical crisis management.

advocacy Working independently or with others to directly improve aspects of the social or physical environment, or to change policies or legislation.

aerobic exercise Prolonged physical activity that raises the heart rate and works the large muscle groups.

age-related macular degeneration (AMD) An age-related vision disorder caused by deterioration of the macula that reduces central vision.

ageism Prejudice or discrimination against older adults.

aggravated assault An attack intended to cause serious physical harm, often involving a weapon.

Air Quality Index (AQI)* An index for measuring daily air quality according to a list of federal air criteria, published by city or region.

alcohol abuse Drinking alcohol to excess, either regularly or on individual occasions, resulting in disruption of work, school, or home life and causing interpersonal, social, or legal problems.

alcohol intoxication The state of physical and/or mental impairment brought on by excessive alcohol consumption (in legal terms, a BAC of 0.08% or greater).

alcohol poisoning Dangerously high level of alcohol consumption, resulting in depression of the central nervous system, slowed breathing and heart rate, and compromised gag reflex.

alcoholism (alcohol dependence) A physical dependence on alcohol to the extent that stopping drinking brings on withdrawal symptoms.

allergies Abnormal immune system reactions to substances that are otherwise harmless.

allostatic overload The wear and tear the body experiences as the result of continuous or repeated demands of allostasis.

altruism The practice of helping and giving to others out of genuine concern for their well-being.

Alzheimer's disease (AD) A progressive, fatal form of age-related dementia.

amenorrhea Cessation of menstrual periods.

amino acids Nitrogen-containing compounds that are the building blocks of proteins.

amniotic fluid Fluid that surrounds the developing fetus that aids in temperature regulation and allows the baby to move freely.

amphetamines Central nervous system stimulants that are chemically similar to the natural stimulants adrenaline and noradrenaline.

anaerobic exercise Short, intense exercise that causes an oxygen deficit in the muscles.

anal intercourse Intercourse characterized by the insertion of the penis into a partner's anus and rectum.

anaphylactic shock A result of anaphylaxis where the release of histamine and other chemicals into the body leads to a drop in blood pressure, tightening of airways, and possible unconsciousness and even death.

andropause Period marked by a decline in the male reproductive hormone testosterone and its resultant physical and emotional effects; also referred to as *male menopause.*

angina pectoris Chest pain due to coronary heart disease.

anorexia nervosa Mental disorder characterized by extremely low body weight, body image distortion, severe calorie restriction, and an obsessive fear of gaining weight.

antibiotic resistance When a bacterium is able to overcome the effects of an antibiotic through a random mutation, or change in the bacterium's genetic code.

antibodies Proteins released by B cells that bind tightly to infectious agents and mark them for destruction.

antigen Tiny regions on the surface of an infectious agent that can be detected by B cells and T cells.

antioxidants Compounds in food that help protect the body from harmful molecules called free radicals.

anxiety disorders A category of mental disorders characterized by persistent feelings of fear, dread, and worry.

Apgar score A measurement of how well a newborn tolerated the stresses of birth as well as how well he or she is adapting to the new environment.

appetite The psychological response to the sight, smell, thought, or taste of food that prompts or postpones eating.

arable* Suitable for cultivation of crops.

arrhythmia Any irregularity in the heart's rhythm.

arteries Vessels that transport blood away from the heart, delivering oxygen-rich blood to the body periphery and oxygen-poor blood to the lungs.

arthritis Inflammation of one or more joints in the body, resulting in pain, swelling, and limited movement.

assertiveness The ability to clearly express your needs and wants to others in an appropriate way.

assortative mating The tendency to be attracted to people who are similar to us.

asthma A chronic pulmonary disease in which the air passages become inflamed, making breathing difficult and causing shortness of breath, wheezing, coughing, and chest tightness.

atherosclerosis Condition characterized by narrowing of the arteries because of inflammation, scarring, and the buildup of fatty deposits.

atria The two upper chambers of the heart that receive blood from the body periphery and lungs.

attachment theory The theory that the patterns of attachment in our earliest relationships with others form the template for attachment in later relationships.

attention deficit hyperactivity disorder (ADHD) A type of attention disorder characterized by inattention, hyperactive behavior, fidgeting, and a tendency toward impulsive behavior.

attention disorders A category of mental disorders characterized by problems with mental focus.

autonomy The capacity to make informed, un-coerced decisions.

autopsy Medical examination of a corpse.

B

bacteria (singular *bacterium*) Single-celled microorganisms that invade a host and reproduce inside. Harmful bacteria release toxic enzymes and chemicals.

ballistic stretching Performing rhythmic bouncing movements in a stretch to increase the intensity of the stretch.

balloon angioplasty An arterial treatment that uses a small balloon to flatten plaque deposits against the arterial wall.

barbiturates Types of central nervous system depressants often prescribed to induce sleep.

bariatric surgery Weight-loss surgery using various procedures to modify the stomach or other sections of the gastrointestinal tract in order to reduce calorie intake or absorption.

basal metabolic rate (BMR) The rate at which the body expends energy for only the basic functioning of vital organs.

bath salts Any of a group of drugs containing a synthetic compound similar to cathione, an amphetamine-like stimulant.

behavior change A sustained change in a habit or pattern of behavior that affects health.

behavior therapy A type of therapy that focuses on changing a patient's behavior and thereby achieving psychological health.

behavioral addiction A form of addiction involving a compulsion to engage in an activity such as gambling, sex, or shopping rather than a compulsion to use a substance.

benign tumor A tumor that grows slowly, does not spread, and is not cancerous.

benzodiazepines Medications commonly prescribed to treat anxiety and panic attacks.

binge drinking A pattern of drinking alcohol that results in a blood alcohol concentration of 0.08 or above (about five or more alcoholic drinks within 2 hours for men, or four or more alcoholic drinks within 2 hours for women).

binge eating The rapid consumption of an excessive amount of food.

bioaccumulation* The process by which substances increase in concentration in the fat tissues of living organisms as the organisms take in contaminated air, water, or food.

biomagnification* The process by which certain contaminants become more concentrated in animal tissue as they move up the food chain.

biomonitoring* Analysis of blood, urine, tissues, and so forth to measure chemical exposure in humans.

biopsy A test for cancer in which a small sample of the abnormal growth is removed and studied.

bipolar disorder (manic-depressive disorder) A mental disorder characterized by occurrences of abnormally elevated mood (or mania), often alternating with depressive episodes, with periods of normal mood in between.

birth control pills Pills containing combinations of hormones that prevent pregnancy when taken regularly as directed.

bisexuals People who are attracted to partners of both the same and the opposite sex.

blood alcohol concentration (BAC) The amount of alcohol present in blood, measured in grams of alcohol per deciliter of blood.

blood pressure The force of the blood moving against the arterial walls.

body burden* The amount of a chemical stored in the body at a given time, especially a potential toxin in the body as the result of environmental exposure.

body composition The relative proportions of the body's lean tissue and fat tissue.

body dysmorphic disorder Mental disorder characterized by obsessive thoughts about a perceived flaw in appearance.

body image A person's perceptions, feelings, and critiques of his or her own body.

body mass index (BMI) A numerical measurement, calculated from height and weight measurements, that provides an indicator of health risk categories.

bradycardia A slow arrhythmia.

brain death The cessation of brain activity as indicated by various medical devices and diagnostic criteria.

brain fitness A person's ability to meet the cognitive requirements and demands of daily life, such as problem-solving and memory recall.

bulimia nervosa Mental disorder characterized by episodes of binge eating followed by a purge behavior such as vomiting, laxative abuse, or extreme exercise.

burnout Phenomenon in which increased feelings of stress and decreased feelings of accomplishment lead to frustration, exhaustion, lack of motivation, and disengagement.

C

caffeine A widely used stimulant found in coffee, tea, soft drinks, chocolate, and some medicines.

calorie Common term for *kilocalorie*. The amount of energy required to raise the temperature of 1 kilogram of water by 1 degree Celsius.

cancer A group of diseases marked by the uncontrolled multiplication of abnormal cells.

capillaries The smallest blood vessels, delivering blood and nutrients to individual cells and picking up wastes.

carbohydrates A macronutrient class composed of carbon, hydrogen, and oxygen, that is the body's universal energy source.

carbon monoxide A gas that inhibits the delivery of oxygen to the body's vital organs.

carcinogen A substance known to trigger DNA mutations that can lead to cancer.

carcinogenic Cancer-causing.

carcinoma Cancer of tissues that line or cover the body.

cardiometabolic risk (CMR) A cluster of nine modifiable factors that identify individuals at risk for type 2 diabetes and cardiovascular disease.

cardiorespiratory fitness The ability of your heart and lungs to effectively deliver oxygen to your muscles during prolonged physical activity.

cardiovascular disease (CVD) Diseases of the heart or blood vessels.

carpal tunnel syndrome (CTS) A repetitive strain injury of the hand or wrist, often linked to computer keyboard use or other types of repetitive motion.

carrier A person infected with a pathogen who does not show symptoms but who is infectious.

carrying capacity* The number of organisms of one species that an environment can support indefinitely.

cataracts An age-related vision disorder marked by clouding of the lens of the eye.

cellular death The end of all vital functions at the cellular level, such as cellular respiration and other metabolic processes.

central nervous system cancer Cancer of the brain or spinal cord.

cesarean section (C-section) A surgical procedure involving the incision of a woman's abdominal and uterine walls in order to deliver the baby.

chain of infection Group of factors necessary for the spread of infection.

childbearing age The age range at which a woman can become pregnant, often defined as between 15 and 44 years old.

cholesterol An animal sterol found in the fatty part of animal-based foods such as meat and whole milk.

chronic bronchitis Inflammation of the main airways in the lungs that continues for at least three months.

chronic disease A disease that comes on gradually and lasts a long time; many chronic diseases can be managed but resist a complete cure.

chronic obstructive pulmonary disease (COPD) A category of diseases that includes emphysema, chronic bronchitis, and asthma.

chronic stress syndrome Collection of symptoms resulting from the long-term effects of prolonged exposure to the body's physiological stress responses.

circadian rhythm* Pattern of physical, emotional, and behavioral changes that follows a roughly 24-hour cycle in accordance with the hours of darkness and light in the individual's environment.

circumcision The surgical removal of the foreskin.

climate change* A change in the state of the climate that can be identified by changes in the average and/or variability of its properties that persist for an extended period.

clinical death A medical determination that life has ceased according to medical criteria that often combine aspects of functional and neurological factors.

clitoris An organ composed of spongy tissue and nerve endings that is very sensitive to sexual stimulation.

club drugs Illicit substances, including MDMA (ecstasy), GHB, and many others that are commonly used at nightclubs and parties.

cocaine A potent and addictive stimulant derived from leaves of the coca shrub.

cognitive-behavioral therapy (CBT) A form of psychotherapy that emphasizes the role of thinking (cognition) in how we feel and what we do.

cohabitation The state of living together in the same household; usually refers to unmarried couples.

complementary and alternative medicine (CAM) Health practices and traditions not typically part of conventional Western medicine, either used alone (alternative medicine) or in conjunction with conventional medicine (complementary medicine).

complex carbohydrates Contain chains of multiple sugar molecules; commonly called *starches* but also come in two non-starch forms: *glycogen* and *fiber.*

conception The fertilization of a female egg with male sperm.

condom (male condom) A thin sheath typically made of latex, polyurethane, or lambskin that is unrolled over the erect penis prior to vaginal penetration.

conflict avoidance The active avoidance of discussing concerns, annoyances, and conflict with another person.

conflict escalation Increasing conflict to a more confrontational, painful, or otherwise less comfortable level.

conflict resolution Resolving a conflict in a manner that both people can accept and that minimizes future occurrences of the conflict.

congestive heart failure A gradual loss of heart function.

consumer health An umbrella term encompassing topics related to the purchase and consumption of health-related products and services.

continuation rate The percentage of couples who continue to practice a given form of birth control.

contraception Any method used to prevent pregnancy.

contraceptive sponge A flexible foam disk containing spermicide that is inserted in the vagina prior to sex.

co-pay A flat fee charged at the time of a medical service or when receiving a medication.

conventional medicine Commonly called Western medicine, this system of care is based on the principles of the scientific method; the belief that diseases are caused by identifiable physical factors and have a characteristic set of symptoms; and the treatment of physical causes through drugs, surgery, or other physical interventions.

coronary artery bypass grafting (CABG) A procedure to build new pathways for blood to flow around areas of arterial blockage.

coronary heart disease (CHD) (coronary artery disease) Disease characterized by atherosclerosis of the arteries that feed the heart; angina; and reduced blood supply to the myocardium.

cortisol Adrenal gland hormone that is secreted at higher levels during the stress response.

counter-conditioning A behavior-change technique in which the individual learns to substitute a healthful or neutral behavior for an unwanted behavior triggered by a cue beyond his or her control.

cramp An involuntary contracted muscle that does not relax, resulting in localized intense pain.

cue control A behavior-change technique in which the individual learns to change the stimuli that provoked the lapse.

cunnilingus Oral stimulation of the vulva or clitoris.

D

danger zone Range of temperatures between 40° and 140° Fahrenheit at which bacteria responsible for foodborne illness thrive.

date (acquaintance) rape Coerced, forceful, or threatening sexual activity in which the victim knows the attacker.

date rape drugs Drugs used to assist in a sexual assault, often given to the victim without his or her knowledge or consent.

decibel* The unit of measurement used to express sound intensity.

deductible The total amount of out-of-pocket health-care expenses that a patient must pay before health insurance begins to cover health-care costs.

dementia A decline in brain function.

dentist (D.D.S.) A conventional medicine practitioner who specializes in care of the teeth, gums, and mouth.

dependence The state of being mentally attached to and/or physically needing a drug.

depressants Substances that depress the activity of the central nervous system and include barbiturates, benzodiazepines, and alcohol.

depressive disorder A mental disorder usually characterized by profound, persistent sadness or loss of interest that interferes with daily life and normal functioning.

determinants of health The range of personal, social, economic, and environmental factors that influence health status.

diabetes mellitus A group of diseases in which the body does not make or use insulin properly, resulting in elevated blood glucose.

diaphragm A flexible silicone cup filled with spermicide and inserted in the vagina prior to sex to prevent pregnancy.

diet The food you regularly consume.

Dietary Reference Intakes (DRIs) A set of energy and nutrient recommendations for supporting good health.

dietary supplements Products taken by mouth that include ingredients such as vitamins, minerals, amino acids, or herbs intended to supplement the diet.

dilation and evacuation (D&E) A multistep method of surgical abortion that may be used in pregnancies that have progressed beyond 12 weeks.

disease An alteration in body structure or biochemistry that is significant enough to cause the body's regulatory mechanisms to fail. Symptoms may or may not be present.

disordered eating A range of unhealthful eating behaviors used to deal with emotional issues that does not warrant a diagnosis of a specific eating disorder.

dissociative drug A medication that distorts perceptions of sight and sound and produces feelings of detachment from the environment and self.

distress Stress resulting from negative stressors.

domestic partnership A legal arrangement in which a couple lives together in a long-term committed relationship and receives some, but not all, of the rights of married couples.

domestic violence An abusive situation in which a family member physically, psychologically, or sexually abuses one or more other family members.

dopamine A neurotransmitter that stimulates feelings of pleasure.

drug abuse The use (most often the excessive use) of any legal or illegal drug in a way that is detrimental to your health.

drug misuse The inappropriate use of a legal drug, either for a reason for which it was not medically intended, or by a person without a prescription.

drug A chemical substance that alters the body physically or mentally for a non-nutritional purpose.

dynamic flexibility The ability to move quickly and fluidly through a joint's entire range of motion with little resistance.

dynamic stretching A type of slow movement stretching in which activities from a workout or sport are mimicked in a controlled manner, often to help "warm up" for a game or event.

dyslipidemia Disorder characterized by abnormal levels of blood lipids, such as high LDL cholesterol or low HDL cholesterol.

dysmenorrhea Pain during menstruation that is severe enough to limit normal activities or require medication.

dysthymic disorder (dysthymia) A milder, chronic type of depressive disorder that lasts two years or more.

E

eating disorders A group of mental disorders, including anorexia nervosa, bulimia nervosa, and binge eating disorder, that is characterized by physiological and psychological disturbances in appetite or food intake.

ecological footprint* The collective impact of an entity on its resources, ecosystems, and other key environmental features.

ecological model Any of a variety of behavior-change models that acknowledge the creation of a supportive environment as being equally important to achieving change as an individual's acquisition of health information and development of new skills.

ecosystem* A dynamic collection of organisms and their nonliving surroundings that function as a unit.

ectopic pregnancy A pregnancy that occurs when a fertilized egg implants within one of the fallopian tubes instead of the uterus; considered a medical emergency.

electrocardiogram (ECG) A test that measures the heart's electrical activity.

electroencephalograph (EEG)* Device that monitors the electrical activity of different regions of the cerebral cortex of the brain using electrodes placed on or in the scalp; a tracing of brain activity is called an *electroencephalogram*.

embryo The growing collection of cells that ultimately become a baby.

emergency contraception (EC; "morning after" pill) A pill containing levonorgestrel, a synthetic hormone that is used to prevent pregnancy after unprotected sex.

emotional health The "feeling" component of psychological health that influences your interpretation of and response to events.

emotional intelligence (EI) The capacity to perceive, express, and reason accurately with emotion and emotional information.

emphysema A chronic disease in which the air sacs in the lung become damaged, making breathing difficult.

empty calories Calories from solid fats, alcohol, and/or added sugars that provide few or no nutrients.

enabling factor A skill, social support, or resource that make it possible (or easier) to succeed in changing a targeted behavior.

endocrine disruptor* A substance that stops the production or blocks the use of hormones in the body and that can have harmful effects on health or development.

endometriosis A condition in which endometrial tissue grows in areas outside of the uterus.

endorphins Hormones that act as neurotransmitters and bind to opiate receptors, stimulating pleasure and relieving pain.

energy balance The state achieved when energy consumed from food is equal to energy expended, maintaining body weight.

environmental health* The discipline that addresses all the physical, chemical, and biological factors external to individual human beings, especially those that influence human health.

environmental mastery The ability to choose or create environments that suit you.

epididymis A coiled tube on top of each testicle where sperm are held until they mature.

erectile dysfunction (ED) The inability of a male to obtain or maintain an erection.

erection The process of the penis filling up with blood as a result of sexual stimulation.

essential fatty acids (EFAs) Polyunsaturated fatty acids that cannot be synthesized by the body but are essential to body functioning.

essential nutrients Nutrients you must obtain from food or supplements because your body either cannot produce them or cannot make them in sufficient quantities to maintain health.

estate A person's personal holdings, including money, property, and other possessions.

ethyl alcohol (ethanol) The intoxicating ingredient in beer, wine, and distilled liquor.

eustress Stress resulting from positive stressors.

evidence-based medicine Health-care policies and practices based on systematic, scientific study.

e-waste* Hazardous waste generated by the production or disposal of electronic or digital devices.

excitement The first phase of the sexual response cycle, marked by erection in men, and lubrication and clitoral swelling in women.

exercise A type of physical activity that is planned and structured.

F

failure rate The percentage of women who typically get pregnant after using a given contraceptive method for one year.

fallopian tubes A pair of tubes that connect the ovaries to the uterus.

family health history A detailed record of health issues in one's family that presents a picture of shared health risks.

fats (triglycerides) Lipids made up of three fatty acid chains attached to a molecule of glycerol; the most common types of food lipid.

fee-for-service plan A type of health insurance in which you choose your providers, and you and your insurer divide the costs of care.

fellatio Oral stimulation of the penis.

fertility awareness (rhythm or calendar method) The tracking of a woman's monthly menstrual cycle; may be used as a method of preventing pregnancy if the woman tracks carefully and has regular periods, although it is not fail-safe.

fertility rate* Within a given population, the average number of births per woman.

fetal alcohol syndrome A pattern of mental and physical birth defects found in some children of mothers who drank excessively during pregnancy.

fetus The name given to the developing embryo eight weeks after fertilization.

fiber A nondigestible complex carbohydrate that aids in digestion.

fight-or-flight response A series of physiological reactions to a stressor designed to enable the body to stand and fight or to flee.

FITT Exercise variables that can be modified in order to accomplish progressive overload: frequency, intensity, time, and type.

flexibility The ability of joints to move through their full ranges of motion.

flexible spending account (FSA) A consumer-controlled account, usually offered through employers, that uses pre-tax dollars to cover approved health-related purchases.

food allergy An adverse reaction of the body's immune system to a food or food component.

food intolerance An adverse food reaction that doesn't involve the immune system.

foodborne illness (food poisoning) Illness caused by pathogenic microorganisms consumed through food or beverages.

functional death The end of all vital physiological functions, including heartbeat, breathing, and blood flow.

fungi Multicellular or single-celled organisms that obtain their food from organic matter, in some cases human tissue.

G

gender roles Behaviors and tasks considered appropriate by society based on whether someone is a man or a woman.

general adaptation syndrome (GAS) An adaptive response consisting of three stages (alarm, resistance, exhaustion) through which the body strives to maintain or restore homeostasis.

generalized anxiety disorder (GAD) An anxiety disorder characterized by chronic worry and pessimism about everyday events that lasts at least six months and may be accompanied by physical symptoms.

genetic modification Altering a plant's or animal's genetic material in order to produce desirable traits such as resistance to pests, poor-soil tolerance, or lower fat.

genome sequencing The full decoding and readout of an entire genome.

genome The genetic material of any living organism.

genomics The study of genomes and their effects on health and development.

GHB (gamma-hydroxybutyric acid) A central nervous system depressant known as a "date rape drug" because of its use to impair potential victims of sexual assault.

glaucoma An age-related vision disorder arising from an increase in internal eye pressure that damages the optic nerve and reduces peripheral vision.

global warming* A sustained increase in the Earth's temperature due to an increase in the greenhouse effect resulting from pollution.

globalization* The interaction and integration of regional phenomena globally.

glycemic index Value indicating the potential of a food to raise blood glucose.

groundwater* The supply of fresh water beneath the Earth's surface, which is a major source of drinking water.

H

hallucinogens Drugs that alter perception and are capable of causing auditory and visual hallucinations.

hangover Alcohol withdrawal symptoms, including headache and nausea, caused by an earlier bout of heavy drinking.

hate crime A crime fueled by bias against another person's or group's race or ethnicity, religion, national origin, sexual orientation, or disability.

hazardous waste* Garbage or byproducts that can pose a hazard to human health or the environment when improperly managed.

hazing Initiation rituals to enter a fraternity or other group that can be humiliating, hazardous, or physically or emotionally abusive, regardless of the person's willingness to participate.

health belief model A model of behavior change emphasizing the influence of personal beliefs on the process of creating effective change.

health discount program A system of health discounts given to members of groups, such as employees of a particular company or students attending a particular college.

health disparities Gaps in the rate and burden of disease and the access to and quality of health care among various population groups.

health insurance A contract between an insurance company and a group or individual who pays a fee to have some or all health costs covered by the insurer.

health literacy The ability to evaluate and understand health information and to make informed choices for your health care.

health maintenance organization (HMO) A type of managed care in which most health care is funneled through and must be approved by the primary care doctor.

health savings account (HSA) A consumer-controlled account that comes attached to a high-deductible health insurance plan and covers the costs of the deductible and other health-related expense approved by the federal government.

health More than merely the absence of disease, a state of well-being that encompasses physical, social, psychological, and other dimensions and is a resource for everyday life.

healthful weight The weight at which health risks are lowest for an individual; usually a weight that will result in a BMI between 18.5 and 24.9.

health-related fitness The ability to perform activities of daily living with vigor.

Healthy Campus An offshoot of the Healthy People initiative, specifically geared toward college students.

Healthy People initiative A federal initiative to facilitate broad, positive health changes in large segments of the U.S. population every 10 years.

heat exhaustion A mild form of heat-related illness that usually occurs as the result of exercising in hot weather without adequate hydration.

heatstroke A life-threatening heat-related illness that occurs when your core temperature rises above 105 degrees Fahrenheit.

hemorrhagic stroke A stroke caused by a leaking or ruptured blood vessel.

hepatitis Inflammation of the liver that affects liver function.

herd immunity The condition where greater than 90% of a community is vaccinated against a disease, giving it little ability to spread through the community, providing some protection against the disease to members of the community who are not vaccinated.

heroin An illicit, highly addictive opioid.

heterosexual A person sexually attracted to someone of the opposite sex.

high-density lipoprotein (HDL) A cholesterol-containing compound that removes excess cholesterol from the bloodstream; often referred to as "good cholesterol."

homeostasis A physiologic ability to maintain the body's internal conditions within a normal, healthful range, usually achieved via hormonal and neurological mechanisms.

homonegativity Having a negative attitude toward homosexuality.

homophobia The irrational fear of, aversion to, or discrimination against homosexuals or homosexuality.

homosexual A person sexually attracted to someone of the same sex.

hooking up Casual, noncommittal, physical encounters that may range from kissing and "making out" to oral sex and intercourse.

hormone Chemical secreted by a gland and transported through the bloodstream to a distant target organ, the activity of which it then regulates.

hospice A home-care program or facility that focuses exclusively on the dying and their loved ones, with a goal of providing comfort rather than facilitating a cure.

host A person, plant, or animal in which or on which pathogens live and reproduce.

human sexual response cycle Distinct phases extending from the first moment of sexual desire until the calm after orgasm.

hunger The physiological sensation caused by the lack of food.

hyperglycemia A persistent state of elevated levels of blood glucose.

hypertension (high blood pressure) A persistent state of elevated blood pressure.

hypothermia A potentially fatal condition in which your core body temperature becomes too low.

I

illicit drugs Drugs regulated by the U.S. Drug Enforcement Agency as unlawful substances, including prescription medications used unlawfully.

illness A subjective state in which a person feels unwell. Disease may or may not be present.

immune system Your body's cellular and chemical defenses against pathogens.

immunization Creating immunity to a pathogen through vaccination or through the injection of antibodies.

implantation The lodging of a fertilized egg in the endometrium of the uterus.

individuality The principle that individuals will respond to fitness training in their own unique ways.

infant mortality rate A calculation of the ratio of babies who die before their first birthday to those who survive until their first birthday.

infection The invasion of body tissues by microorganisms that use the body's environment to multiply and cause disease.

infertility The inability to conceive after trying for at least a year.

inflammatory response A response to damaged body tissues designed to kill any pathogens in the damaged tissue, promote healing, and prevent the spread of infection to other parts of the body.

influenza A group of viruses that cause the flu, a contagious respiratory condition.

inhalants Chemical vapors that, when inhaled, produce mind-altering effects.

insomnia* Condition characterized by difficulty falling or staying asleep, a pattern of waking too early, or poor-quality sleep.

insulin A hormone necessary for glucose transport into cells.

intentional injury Physical harm that is purposefully inflicted through violence.

intervention A technique used by family and friends of an addict to encourage the addict to seek help for a drug problem.

intestate Dying without leaving a legal will.

intimacy A sense of closeness with another person formed by being emotionally open and caring.

intimate partner violence (IPV) An abusive situation in which one member of a couple or intimate relationship may physically, psychologically, or sexually abuse the other.

intrauterine device (IUD) A plastic, T-shaped device that is inserted in the uterus for long-term pregnancy prevention.

ischemic stroke A stroke caused by a blocked blood vessel.

isometric exercise Exercise where the muscle contracts but the body does not move.

isotonic exercise Exercise where the muscle contraction causes body movement.

J

jaundice A yellowing of the skin, mucous membranes, and sometimes the whites of the eyes often caused by liver malfunction.

jealousy The response to a threat to a relationship from an actual or imagined rival for a partner's attention.

L

labia Two pairs (majora and minora) of fleshy lips surrounding and protecting the clitoris and the vaginal and urethral openings.

labor The physical processes involved in giving birth.

leukemia Cancer of blood-forming tissue.

leukoplakia White spots on the mucous membranes in the mouth that may become cancerous.

life expectancy The average number of years a person may expect to live.

locus of control A person's belief about where the center of power lies in his or her life; it can be external or internal.

loneliness A feeling of isolation from others, often prompted by a real or perceived loss.

low birth weight The term given to birth weights less than 5 pounds, 8 ounces.

low-density lipoprotein (LDL) A cholesterol-containing compound that, as it degrades, releases its cholesterol load into the bloodstream; often referred to as "bad cholesterol."

LSD (lysergic acid diethylamide) A powerful hallucinogen manufactured from lysergic acid, a substance found in a fungus that grows on rye and other grains.

lymphoma Cancer of the lymphoid tissues.

M

mainstream smoke Smoke exhaled from the lungs of smokers.

major depressive disorder (unipolar depression) A type of depressive disorder characterized by experiencing five or more symptoms of depression, including either depressed mood or loss of interest or pleasure, for at least two weeks straight.

malaria A serious disease that causes fever and chills that appear in cycles. In some cases malaria can be life-threatening.

malignant melanoma An especially aggressive form of skin cancer.

malignant tumor A tumor that grows aggressively, invades surrounding tissue, and can spread to other parts of the body; all cancers are malignant.

managed-care plan A type of health insurance in which the insurer contracts with a defined group of health providers, which the consumer must use or face higher out-of-pocket costs.

marijuana The most commonly used illegal drug in the United States; derived from the plant *Cannabis sativa.*

mast cell A type of cell in the skin and mucous membranes that releases histamine and other chemicals into the bloodstream during an allergic reaction.

masturbation Manipulation of one's own genitals for sexual pleasure.

Medicaid A joint federal-state public insurance program that covers low-income individuals and families.

medical doctor (M.D.) A physician trained in conventional medicine, with many years of additional formal education and training and a professional license.

Medicare A federal public insurance program that covers people with long-term disabilities and anyone 65 or older.

menarche The first onset of menstruation.

menopause The permanent end of a woman's menstrual cycle and reproductive capacity.

menstrual cycle A monthly physiological cycle marked by *menstruation.*

menstrual phase Phase of the menstrual cycle characterized by menstrual flow, the release of follicle-stimulating hormone from the pituitary gland to the brain, and the release of estrogen into the bloodstream.

menstruation The cyclical discharge of blood and tissue from the vagina.

mental disorders Significant behavioral and psychological disorders that disrupt thoughts and feelings, impair ability to function, and increase risk of pain, disability, or even death.

mental health The "thinking" component of psychological health that allows you to perceive reality accurately and respond rationally and effectively.

metabolic syndrome A group of obesity-related factors that increase the risk of cardiovascular disease and diabetes, including large waistline, high triglycerides, low HDL cholesterol, high blood pressure, and high fasting blood glucose.

metabolism The sum of all chemical reactions occurring in body cells that break large molecules down into smaller molecules. Also, the breakdown of food and beverages in the body to transform them into energy.

metastasis The process by which a malignant tumor spreads to other body sites.

methamphetamine A highly addictive and dangerous stimulant that is chemically similar to amphetamine, but more potent and harmful.

methicillin-resistant *Staphylococcus aureus* (MRSA) A strain of staph that is resistant to the broad-spectrum antibiotics commonly used to treat staph infections.

methylenedioxymethamphetamine (MDMA) A synthetic drug, commonly called "ecstasy," that works as both a stimulant and a hallucinogen.

minerals Elements, with no energy value of their own, that regulate body processes and provide structure.

mini-med plan A type of managed-care plan, sold individually to younger people, which carries lower costs but does not cover many services.

miscarriage A pregnancy that suddenly terminates on its own before the 20th week.

modeling A behavior-change technique based on watching and learning from others.

mononucleosis A viral disease that causes fatigue, weakness, sore throat, fever, headaches, swollen lymph nodes and tonsils, and loss of appetite.

mons pubis The fatty, rounded areas of tissue in front of the pubic bone.

mood disorder Any chronic, pervasive emotional state that significantly alters the person's thoughts, behaviors, and normal functioning.

municipal solid waste (MSW)* Nonhazardous garbage or trash generated by industries, businesses, institutions, and homes.

murder The act of intentionally and unjustifiably killing another person.

muscular endurance The capacity of muscles to repeatedly exert force, or to maintain a force, over a period of time.

muscular strength The maximum force your muscles can apply in a single maximum effort of lifting, pushing, or pressing.

myeloma Cancer arising in plasma cells, a type of immune cell, and invading the bone marrow.

myocardial infarction (MI) (heart attack) A cardiac crisis in which a region of heart muscle is damaged or destroyed by reduced blood flow.

myocardium The heart's muscle tissue.

N

narcolepsy* A disorder in which the brain fails to regulate sleep–wake cycles normally.

near-death experience (NDE) A profound psychological event usually occurring in a person close to death and marked by a characteristic pattern of perceptions and common features such as movement through space and perception of light.

neurotoxin* A substance that interferes with or harms the functioning of the brain and nervous system.

neurotransmitters Chemicals that enable the transmission of messages from one neuron to another across synapses.

nicotine An alkaloid derived from the tobacco plant that is responsible for smoking's psychoactive and addictive effects.

nocturnal eating disorder* Condition characterized by significant food consumption at night, and typically accompanied by depression, insomnia, and a daytime eating disorder.

non-REM (NREM) sleep* Type of restful sleep during which the rapid eye movement characteristic of dreaming does not typically occur.

nonverbal communication Communication that is conveyed by body language.

nurse practitioner Registered nurses who have undergone additional training and can perform some of the care provided by a medical doctor.

nurse A licensed professional who provides a wide range of health-care services and supports the work of medical doctors.

nutrient-dense foods Any food in which the proportion of healthful nutrients is high relative to the number of calories.

nutrients Chemical substances in food that you need for energy, growth, and survival.

nutrition The scientific study of food and its physiological functions.

O

obese A weight disorder in which excess accumulations of nonessential body fat result in increased risk of health problems. A weight resulting in a BMI of 30 or higher.

obsessive-compulsive disorder (OCD) An anxiety disorder characterized by repeated and unwanted thoughts (obsessions) that lead to rituals (compulsions) in an attempt to control the anxiety.

oncogene A mutated gene that encourages the uncontrolled cell division that results in cancer.

opioids Drugs derived from opium or synthetic drugs that have similar sleep-inducing, pain-reducing effects.

opportunistic diseases Infections and other disorders that take advantage of a weakened immune system.

optimism The psychological tendency to have a positive interpretation of life's events.

optometrist (O.D.) A licensed professional who provides vision care.

oral sex Stimulation of the genitals by the tongue or mouth.

orgasm The peak, or climax, of sexual response, characterized by rhythmic muscle contractions of the genitals and surrounding areas, and ejaculation in men.

osteoporosis A disease characterized by low bone mass and deterioration of bone tissue, leading to fragile bones and an increased risk of fractures.

outercourse Sexual intimacy without penetration of the vagina or anus.

ovaries The two female reproductive organs where ova (eggs) reside.

overload Increasing the stress placed on your body through exercise, which results in an improved fitness level.

over-the-counter (OTC) medication A medication available for purchase without a prescription.

overweight The condition of having a body weight that exceeds what is generally considered healthful for a particular height. A weight resulting in a BMI of 25 to 29.9.

ovulate To release an egg from the ovary.

ozone depletion* Destruction of the stratospheric ozone layer, which shields the Earth from harmful levels of ultraviolet radiation, resulting from pollution.

P

palliative care Type of care that focuses on reducing pain and suffering and caring for the whole person, rather than prolonging life or curing disease.

pancreas An abdominal organ that produces insulin as well as certain compounds helpful in digestion.

pandemic A worldwide epidemic of a disease.

panic attacks Episodes of sudden terror that strike without warning.

panic disorder A mental disorder characterized both by recurring panic attacks and the fear of a panic attack occurring.

parasitic worms (helminths) Multicellular creatures that compete with a host body for nutrients.

parasomnia* Condition in which unusual events accompany sleep.

passive euthanasia Failure to begin or to maintain an intervention that is necessary to sustain a patient's life.

passive stretching Stretching performed with a partner who increases the intensity of the stretch by gently applying pressure to your body as it stretches.

pathogen An agent that causes disease.

PCP (phencyclidine) A dangerous synthetic hallucinogen that reduces and distorts sensory input and can unpredictably cause both euphoria and dysphoria.

penis The male sexual and reproductive organ.

percent Daily Value (% DV) Nutrient standards that estimate how much a serving of a given food contributes to the overall intake of nutrients listed on the food label.

personal safety The practice of making decisions and taking actions that reduce your risk of injury and death.

personalized medicine Health care based on the idea that because your individual DNA is unique, your health is as well, and your care and treatments should be tailored to you.

pesticides A chemical used to kill pests, including agricultural chemicals used to help protect crops from weeds, insects, fungus, slugs and snails, birds, and mammals.

pharmacogenomics The use of DNA information to choose medications and make prescribing decisions.

phobia An extreme, disabling, irrational fear of something that poses little or no actual danger.

physical activity Bodily movement that substantially increases energy expenditure.

physical fitness The ability to perform moderate to vigorous levels of activity and to respond to physical demands without excessive fatigue.

physician assistant (P.A.) A licensed health professional who practices under the supervision of a physician and provides a broad range of care.

phytochemicals Naturally occurring plant substances thought to have disease-preventing and health-promoting properties.

placenta The tissue that connects mother and baby.

plateau The second phase of the sexual response cycle, characterized by intense excitement, rapid heartbeat, genital sensitivity, the secretion of pre-ejaculatory fluid in men, and vaginal swelling in women.

podiatrist (D.P.M.) A licensed professional who specializes in the care of the feet.

point-of-service (POS) plan A type of managed care that lets HMO consumers see a broader list of providers for an additional fee.

pollution* Contamination of the natural environment as a result of human activities.

polyabuser A person who abuses more than one drug.

polypharmacy Simultaneous use of several prescription medications that can interact in dangerous ways.

positive psychotherapy A new field of psychology that focuses on increasing psychological strengths and improving happiness, rather than on psychological problems.

post-traumatic stress disorder (PTSD) An anxiety disorder characterized by recurrent fear, anger, and depression occurring after a traumatic event.

prebiotics Nondigestible food ingredients that benefit human health by stimulating the growth and/or activity of beneficial bacteria in the large intestine.

prediabetes A persistent state of blood glucose levels higher than normal, but not yet high enough to qualify as diabetes.

predisposing factor A physical, mental, emotional, or surrounding influence that affects the likelihood that a person will decide to change a current behavior.

preeclampsia A serious health condition characterized by high blood pressure in the pregnant woman.

pre-existing condition A health issue that existed prior to application to or enrollment in an insurance plan, which insurers sometimes use to restrict care or set the price paid for insurance.

preferred provider organization (PPO) A type of managed care in which the consumer is encouraged to stay within an approved network of providers but has more choice over who is seen when.

premature ejaculation (PE) A condition in which a male ejaculates earlier than he would like to.

premenstrual dysphoric disorder (PMDD) Severe and debilitating psychological symptoms experienced just prior to menstruation.

premenstrual syndrome (PMS) A collection of emotional and physical symptoms that occur just prior to menstruation.

premium The amount you pay an insurance company for an insurance policy, usually monthly.

prenatal care Nutritional counseling and regular medical screenings throughout pregnancy to aid the growth and development of the fetus.

presbycusis Age-related hearing loss, which usually develops gradually, often due to damage to or changes in the inner ear.

presbyopia Age-related decline in the ability to focus on objects up close, especially in low light.

probiotics Living, beneficial microbes that develop naturally in food and that help maintain digestive functions.

progressive overload Gradually overloading the body over time in order to avoid injury.

proliferative phase Phase of the menstrual cycle characterized by a thickening of the lining of the uterus and discharge of cervical mucus. This phase ends when luteinizing hormone triggers the release of a mature egg.

proof value A measurement of alcoholic strength, corresponding to twice the alcohol percentage (13% alcohol equals 26 proof).

prostate gland A walnut-sized gland that produces part of the semen.

protein A macronutrient that helps build many body chemicals and tissues, including muscle, bone, skin, and blood.

protozoa Single-celled parasites that rely on other living things for food and shelter.

psilocybin A hallucinogenic substance obtained from certain types of mushrooms that are indigenous to tropical regions of South America.

psychoactive drugs Drugs that affect the user's mood, perceptions, or other aspects of the mental state.

psychoactive Capable of altering feelings, mood, perceptions, or psychological functioning.

psychodynamic therapy A type of therapy that focuses on the unconscious sources for a patient's behavior and psychological state.

psychological health A broad dimension of health and wellness that encompasses both mental and emotional health.

psychoneuroimmunology The study of the interactions among psychological processes, the nervous system, hormones, and the immune system.

purging Behaviors, such as vomiting, laxative abuse, or overexercising, intended to reduce the calories absorbed by the body.

R

radiation* Energy that travels in the form of rays, waves, or particles.

rape Nonconsensual oral, anal, or vaginal penetration by body parts or objects, using force, threats of bodily harm, or taking advantage of circumstances that make a person incapable of consenting to sex.

rational suicide Action taken deliberately by a reasoned, terminally ill patient to hasten his or her own death.

recovery The period necessary for the body to recover from exercise demands and adapt to higher levels of fitness.

reinforcing factor An encouragement or a reward that promotes successful behavior change; negative reinforcers are barriers that oppose change.

relapse A return to the previous state or pattern of behavior.

religion A system of beliefs and practices related to the existence of a transcendent power.

REM behavior disorder (RBD)* Parasomnia characterized by failure of inhibition of muscle movement during REM sleep.

REM sleep* Type of wakeful sleep during which rapid eye movement and dreaming occur.

repetitions The number of times you perform an exercise repeatedly.

repetitive strain injury (RSI) An injury that damages joints, nerves, or connective tissue caused by repeated motions that put strain on one part of the body.

replacement-level fertility* The level of fertility at which a population exactly replaces itself from one generation to the next.

reservoir The natural environment for any particular pathogen, where it accumulates in large numbers.

resolution The stage of the response cycle in which the body returns to normal functioning.

restless legs syndrome (RLS)* Nervous system disorder characterized by a strong urge to move the legs, accompanied by creeping, burning, or other unpleasant sensations.

reversibility The principle that fitness levels decline when the demand placed on the body is decreased.

Rohypnol A powerful sedative known as a "date rape drug" because of its use to impair potential victims of sexual assault.

S

sarcoma Cancer of muscle or connective tissues.

satiety Physical fullness; the state in which there is no longer the desire to eat.

saturated fats Fats that typically are solid at room temperature; generally found in animal products, dairy products, and tropical oils.

schizophrenia A severe mental disorder characterized by delusions, hallucinations, and other aspects of psychosis.

scrotum The skin sac at the base of the penis that contains the testes.

secondhand smoke (environmental tobacco smoke) The smoke non-smokers are exposed to when someone has been smoking nearby; a combination of sidestream smoke and mainstream smoke.

secretory phase Phase of the menstrual cycle characterized by the degeneration of the follicle sac, rising levels of progesterone in the bloodstream, and further increase of the endometrial lining.

self-acceptance A sense of positive and realistic self-regard, resulting in elevated levels of self-confidence and self-respect.

self-actualization The pinnacle of Maslow's hierarchy of needs, which indicates truly fulfilling your potential.

self-care Actions you take to keep yourself healthy.

self-disclosure The sharing of honest feelings and personal information about yourself with another person.

self-efficacy The conviction that you can successfully execute the behavior required to make the change you desire.

self-medicating Using alcohol or drugs to cope with sadness, grief, pain, or mental health problems.

self-monitoring A behavior-change technique in which the individual observes and records aspects of his or her behavior-change process.

self-talk A person's internal dialogue.

semen The male ejaculate consisting of sperm and other fluids from the accessory glands.

sets Separate groups of repetitions.

sexting The use of cell phones or similar electronic devices to send sexually explicit text, photos, or videos.

sexual dysfunctions Problems occurring during any stage of the sexual response cycle.

sexual harassment Unwelcome language or contact of a sexual nature that explicitly or implicitly affects academic or employment situations, unreasonably interferes with work or school performance, or creates an intimidating, hostile, or offensive work or school environment.

sexual orientation Romantic and physical attraction toward others.

sexual violence Any form of nonconsensual sexual activity.

sexuality The biological, physical, emotional, and psychosocial aspects of sexual attraction and expression.

sexually transmitted infections (STIs) Infections transmitted mainly through sexual activity, such as vaginal, anal, or oral sex.

shaping A behavior-change technique based on breaking broad goals into more manageable steps.

shyness The feeling of apprehension or intimidation in social situations, especially in reaction to unfamiliar people or new environments.

sidestream smoke Smoke emanating from the burning end of a cigarette or pipe.

simple carbohydrates The most basic unit of carbohydrates, consisting of one or two sugar molecules.

skills-related fitness The capacity to perform specific physical skills related to a sport or other physically demanding activity.

sleep apnea* Disorder in which one or more pauses in breathing occur during sleep.

sleep bruxism* Clenching or grinding the teeth during sleep.

sleep debt* An accumulated amount of sleep loss that develops when the amount of sleep you routinely obtain is less than the amount you need.

sleep hygiene* The behaviors and environmental factors that together influence the quantity and quality of sleep.

sleep terror* Parasomnia characterized by the appearance of awakening in terror during a stage of NREM sleep.

sleep* A physiologically prompted, dynamic, and readily reversible state of reduced consciousness essential to human survival.

sleepwalking* Parasomnia in which a person walks or performs another complex activity while still asleep.

snoring* A ragged, hoarse sound that occurs during sleep when breathing is obstructed.

social anxiety disorder (social phobia) An anxiety disorder characterized by an intense fear of being judged by others and of being humiliated by your own actions, which may be accompanied by physical symptoms.

social physique anxiety Mental disorder characterized by extreme fear of having one's body judged by others.

social support A sufficient quantity of relationships that provide emotional concern, help with appraisal, information, and even goods and services.

specificity The principle that a fitness component is improved only by exercises that address that specific component.

spermicide A substance containing chemicals that kill or immobilize sperm.

spirituality That which is in total harmony with the perceptual and non-perceptual environment.

stalking A pattern of harassment and threats directed at a specific person that is intended to cause intimidation and fear, often through repeated, unwanted contact.

standard drink A drink containing about 14 grams pure alcohol (one 12-oz. can of beer, one 5-oz. glass of wine, or 1.5 oz. of 80-proof liquor).

static flexibility The ability to reach and hold a stretch at one endpoint of a joint's range of motion.

static stretching Gradually lengthening a muscle to an elongated position and sustaining that position.

status syndrome The disparity in health status and rates of premature mortality between the impoverished and the affluent within any given society.

statutory rape Any sexual activity with a person younger than the legally defined "age of consent," regardless of whether any coercion or force was involved.

stimulants A class of drugs that stimulate the central nervous system, causing acceleration of mental and physical processes in the body.

stress The collective psychobiological condition that occurs in reaction to a disruptive, unexpected, or exciting stimulus.

stressor Any physical or psychological condition, event, or factor that causes positive or negative stress.

stroke A medical emergency in which blood flow to or in the brain is impaired. Also called a *cerebrovascular accident* (*CVA*).

suction curettage A method of surgical abortion characterized by vacuum aspiration; typically used in the first 6 to 12 weeks of pregnancy.

sudden cardiac arrest A life-threatening cardiac crisis marked by loss of heartbeat and unconsciousness.

sudden infant death syndrome (SIDS) The sudden death of a seemingly healthy infant while sleeping.

Superfund* A federal program that funds and carries out emergency and long-term identification, analysis, removal, and cleanup of toxic sites.

sustainability* The ability to meet society's current needs without compromising future generations' abilities to meet their own needs; includes policies for ensuring that certain components of the environment are not depleted or destroyed.

T

tachycardia A fast arrhythmia.

tar A sticky, thick brown residue that forms when tobacco is burned and its chemical particles condense.

target heart rate range The heart rate range to aim for during exercise. A target heart rate range of 64–91% of your maximum heart rate is recommended.

terminal illness An irreversible condition that will result in death in the near future.

terrorism Premeditated, politically motivated violence against noncombatant individuals, usually as a means of influence.

testes (testicles) The two reproductive glands that manufacture sperm.

tolerance Reduced sensitivity to a drug so that increased amounts are needed to achieve the usual effect.

toxic shock syndrome A rare, serious illness caused by staph bacteria that begins with severe flu symptoms but can quickly progress to a medical emergency.

toxicity The dosage level at which a drug becomes poisonous to the body.

***trans* fat** A type of fat that is produced when liquid fat (oil) is turned into solid fat during food processing.

transgenderism The state in which someone's gender identity or gender expression is different from his or her assigned sex at birth.

transient ischemic attack (TIA) A temporary episode of strokelike symptoms, indicative of high stroke risk.

transition The final phase of the first stage of labor, characterized by the dilation of the cervix and strong, prolonged contractions.

transsexual A transgendered individual who lives as the gender opposite to his or her assigned sex.

transtheoretical model of behavior change A model of behavior change that focuses on decision-making steps and abilities. Also called the *stages of change* model.

traumatic brain injury (TBI) An injury that disrupts normal functioning of the brain, caused by a jolt or blow to the brain or a penetrating head wound.

tumor An abnormal growth of tissue with no physiological function.

type 1 diabetes A form of diabetes that usually begins early in life and arises when the pancreas produces insufficient insulin.

type 2 diabetes A form of diabetes that usually begins later in life and arises when cells resist the effects of insulin.

U

umbilical cord A vessel linking the bloodstream of the placenta to that of the baby and enabling the exchange of gases, nutrients, and wastes.

underweight A weight resulting in a BMI below 18.5.

unintentional injury (accidents) Bodily damage that is not deliberately caused.

unsaturated fats Fats that typically are liquid at room temperature; generally come from plant sources.

urethra A duct that travels from the bladder through the shaft of the penis, carrying fluids to the outside of the body.

uterus (womb) The pear-shaped organ where a growing fetus is nurtured.

V

vagina The tube that connects a woman's external sex organs with her uterus.

vaginal intercourse Intercourse characterized by the insertion of the penis into the vagina.

values Internal guidelines used to make decisions and evaluate the world around you.

vas deferens A tube ascending from the epididymis that transports sperm.

vector An animal or insect that transports pathogens from one point to another.

vegetarian A person who avoids some or all foods from animal sources: red meat, poultry, seafood, eggs, and dairy products.

veins Vessels that transport blood toward the heart, delivering oxygen-poor blood from the body periphery or oxygen-rich blood from the lungs.

ventricles The two lower chambers of the heart that pump blood to the body and lungs.

violence Use of physical force—threatened or actual—with the intent of causing harm.

violent crime One of four offenses involving force or the threat or force: murder and non-negligent manslaughter, forcible rape, robbery, and aggravated assault.

virus A microscopic organism that cannot multiply without invading body cells.

vitamins Compounds, with no energy value of their own, needed by the body in small amounts for normal growth and function.

vulva All of the female external organs collectively. Also called *genitals*.

W

water A liquid composed of hydrogen and oxygen that is necessary for life.

wellness An active process through which people become aware of, and make choices toward, a more successful existence.

whole grains Unrefined grains that contain bran, germ, and endosperm.

whole-genome scanning A form of genetic testing that looks for variants throughout a person's genome.

will A legally binding document stating what should be done with a person's property after death.

withdrawal (substance use) The process in which, and symptoms that develop when, a person stops using a drug.

withdrawal (sexuality) The withdrawal of the penis from the vagina before ejaculation.

Z

zygote A fertilized egg.

References

Chapter 1

i. Hoyert, D. L., & Xu, J. (2012, October 10). *National vital statistics reports 61* (6). Centers for Disease Control and Prevention. http://www.cdc.gov.
ii. Kvaavik, E., Batty, G., Ursin, G., Huxley, R., & Gale, C. (2010). Influence of individual and combined health behaviors on total and cause-specific mortality in men and women. *Archives of Internal Medicine, 170* (8), 711–718.
1. World Health Organization. (1948). Preamble to the Constitution of the World Health Organization as adopted by the International Health Conference, New York, 19–22 June, 1946; signed on 22 July 1946 by the representatives of 61 States (Official Records of the World Health Organization, no. 2, p. 100) and entered into force on 7 April 1948. http://www.who.int.
2. Dunn, H. L. (1959, June). High-level wellness for man and society. *American Journal of Public Health and the Nation's Health, 49* (6), 786–792. http://www.ncbi.nlm.nih.gov.
3. National Wellness Institute. (2013). *Defining wellness.* http://www.nationalwellness.org.
4. Hoyert, D. L., & Xu, J. (2012, October 10). *National vital statistics reports 61* (6). Centers for Disease Control and Prevention. http://www.cdc.gov.
5. Centers for Disease Control. (2000). *Leading causes of death, 1900–1998.* http://www.cdc.gov.
6. U.S. Centers for Disease Control. (2012, August 13). *Chronic diseases and health promotion.* http://www.cdc.gov.
7. U.S. Centers for Disease Control. (2012, August 7). *Facts about physical activity.* http://www.cdc.gov.
8. U.S. Centers for Disease Control. (2012, May). *Health, United States, 2011.* National Center for Health Statistics. DHHS Publication No. 2012-1232. http://www.cdc.gov.
9. U.S. Department of Health and Human Services. (2013). *About HHS.* http://www.hhs.gov.
10. U.S. Department of Health and Human Services. (2012, December 3). *What's new for 2020.* http://www.healthypeople.gov.
11. American College Health Association. (2013). *ACHA-NCHA II: Reference group executive summary, fall 2012.* http://www.acha-ncha.org.
12. Joint United Nations Program on HIV/AIDS. (2012). *UNAIDS report on the global AIDS epidemic 2012.* http://www.unaids.org.
13. U.S. Centers for Disease Control. (2010, July 19). *Antibiotic/Antimicrobial resistance.* http://www.cdc.gov.
14. Food and Agriculture Organization (FAO). (2012). *The state of food insecurity in the world, 2012.* FAO Media Centre. http://www.fao.org.
15. World Health Organization. (2011). *Nutrition: Controlling the global obesity epidemic.* http://www.who.int.
16. U.S. Department of Health and Human Services. (2012, September 20). *Determinants of health.* http://www.healthypeople.gov.
17. Centers for Disease Control and Prevention. (2011, January 14). CDC health disparities and inequalities report—United States, 2011. *Morbidity and Mortality Weekly Report, 60* (Supplement). http://www.cdc.gov.
18. Kvaavik, E., Batty, G., Ursin, G., Huxley, R., & Gale, C. (2010). Influence of individual and combined health behaviors on total and cause-specific mortality in men and women. *Archives of Internal Medicine, 170* (8), 711–718.
19. Marmot, M. G. (2006, March 15). Status syndrome: A challenge to medicine. *JAMA, 295* (11). http://www.psr.org.
20. U.S. Department of Health and Human Services. (2013, January 3). *The Affordable Care Act, section by section.* http://www.healthcare.gov.
21. National Network of Libraries of Medicine. (2012, November 20). *Health literacy.* http://nnlm.gov.
22. Green, L. W., & Mercer, S. L. (2002). Predisposing factors. *Gale Encyclopedia of Public Health.* Farmington Hills, MI: Gale Cengage Learning. http://www.healthline.com.
23. Green, L. W., & Mercer, S. L. (2002). Enabling factors. *Gale Encyclopedia of Public Health.* Farmington Hills, MI: Gale Cengage Learning. http://www.healthline.com.
24. Breslow, L., Ed. (2002). Health-related behavior. *Gale Encyclopedia of Public Health.* Farmington Hills, MI: Gale Cengage Learning.
25. Prochaska, J., & Velicer, W. (1997). The transtheoretical model of health behavior change. *American Journal of Health Promotion, 12* (1), 38–48.
26. Richard, L., Gauvin, L., & Raine, K. (2011). Ecological models revisited: Their uses and evolution in health promotion over two decades. *Annual Review of Public Health, 32,* 307–326. http://www.medsp.umontreal.ca.
27. Doran, G. T. (1981). There's a S.M.A.R.T. way to write management's goals and objectives. *Management Review, 70* (11) (AMA FORUM), 35–36.
28. National Institutes of Health. (2013, January 4). *Guide to behavior change.* http://www.nhlbi.nih.gov.
29. Bandura, A. (1977). Self-efficacy: Toward a unifying theory of behavior change. *Psychological Review 84* (2), 191–215. http://lnx.gaetanogioveni.it.
30. Rotter, J. B. (1954). *Social learning and clinical psychology.* Englewood Cliffs, NJ: Prentice Hall.
31. Marlatt, G. A., Larrimer, M. E., & Palmer, R. S. (2012, July 8). Relapse prevention: An overview of Marlatt's cognitive-behavioral model. Amazon Digital Services. Kindle edition.
32. American Cancer Society. (2011, November 30). Helping a smoker quit: Do's and don'ts. http://www.cancer.org.

Chapter 2

i. American College Health Association. (2013). *American College Health Association national college health assessment (ACHA-NCHA II): Reference group executive summary, fall 2012.* http://www.acha-ncha.org.
ii. National Institute of Mental Health. (n.d.). Panic disorder. Bipolar disorder. Obsessive-compulsive disorder. Retrieved from http://www.nimh.nih.gov.
iii. Hoyert, D. L., & Xu, J. (2012). Deaths: Preliminary data for 2011. *National Vital Statistics Reports, 61* (6), 52.
1. Ryff, C. D. (1989). Happiness is everything, or is it? Explorations on the meaning of psychological well-being. *Journal of Personality and Social Psychology, 57* (6), 1069–1081.
2. Stinson, D., Logel, C., Zanna, M., Holmes, J., Cameron, J., Wood, J., & Spenser, S. J. (2008). The cost of lower self-esteem: Testing a self- and social-bonds model of health. *Journal of Personality and Social Psychology, 94* (3), 412–428.
3. Payne, W. L. (1985). A study of emotion: Developing emotional intelligence. The Union Institute. *Dissertation Abstracts International, 47* (01A), 203.
4. Mayer, J. D., Salovey, P., Caruso, D. R., & Cherkasskiy, L. (2011). Emotional intelligence. In Sternberg, R. J., & Kaufman, S. B. (Eds.), *The Cambridge Handbook of Intelligence.* Cambridge University Press, 532, 545.
5. Day, A., Therrien, D., & Carroll, S. (2005). Predicting psychological health: Assessing the incremental validity of emotional intelligence beyond personality, type A behavior, and daily hassles. *European Journal of Personality, 19,* 519–536.
6. Seligman, M. (1998). *Learned optimism: Change your mind and change your life.* New York: Pocket Books, 5–6.
7. Burris, J. L., Brechting, E. H., Salsman, J., & Carlson, C. R. (2009). Factors associated with the psychological well-being and distress of university students. *Journal of American College Health, 57* (5), 536–543.
8. Segovia, F., Moore, J. L., Linnville, S. E., Hoyt, R. E., & Hain, R. E. (2012, June). Optimism predicts resilience in repatriated prisoners of war: A 37-year longitudinal study. *Journal of Traumatic Stress, 25* (3), 330–336.
9. Geers, A. L., Wellman, J. A., Fowler, S. L., Helfer, S. G., & France, C. R. (2010). Dispositional optimism predicts placebo analgesia. *Journal of Pain 11* (11), 1165–1171.
10. Rajandram, R. K., Ho, S. M., Samman, N., Chan, N., McGrath, C. & Zwahlen, R.A. (2011). Interaction of hope and optimism with anxiety and depression in a specific group of cancer survivors: A preliminary study. *BMC Research Notes 4,* 519. http://www.biomedcentral.com.
11. National Institutes of Health. (2011, September 26). Gene linked to optimism and self-esteem. *NIH Research Matters.* http://www.nih.gov.
12. Maslow, A. H. (1998). *Toward a psychology of being,* 3rd ed. New York: John Wiley & Sons.
13. Greene, L., & Burke, G. (2007, Fall). Beyond self-actualization. *Journal of the Health and Human Services Administration,* 116–128.
14. Cecero, J. J., Beitel, M., & Prout, T. (2008). Exploring the relationships among early maladaptive schemas, psychological mindedness and self-reported college adjustment. *Psychology and Psychotherapy: Theory, Research, and Practice 81,* 105–118.
15. Hefner, J., & Eisenberg, D. (2009, October). Social support and mental health among college students. *American Journal of Orthopsychiatry, 79* (4), 491–499.
16. Pew Forum on Religion and Public Life. (2012, October 9). "Nones" on the Rise: One-in-Five Adults Have No Religious Affiliation. http://www.pewforum.org.
17. Newport, F., Witters, D., & Agrawal, S. (2012, February 16). In U.S., very religious have higher well-being across all faiths. Gallup-Healthways Well-Being Index Jan 2, 2010–Dec 30, 2011. http://www.gallup.com.
18. Seaward, B. L. (2013). *Health of the human spirit: Spiritual dimensions for personal health,* 2nd ed. Burlington, MA: Jones & Bartlett Learning.
19. World Health Organization (WHO). (1992). *Health promotion and chronic illness: Discovering a new quality of health.* A. Kaplun, Ed. Geneva: WHO.
20. Post, S. G. (2011). It's good to be good: 2011 fifth annual scientific report on health, happiness, and helping others. *International Journal of Person Centered Medicine 1* (4), 814–829.
21. Johnstone, B., Yoon, D. P., Cohen, D., Schopp, L. H., McCormack, G., Campbell, J., & Smith, M. (2012, December). Relationships among spirituality, religious practices, personality factors, and health for five different faith traditions. *Journal of Religion and Health, 51* (4), 1017–1041.
22. National Cancer Institute. (2011). *Spirituality in cancer care.* http://www.cancer.gov.
23. Kohls, N., Sauer, S., Offenbacher, M., & Giordano, J. (2011, June 27).

Spirituality: An overlooked predictor of placebo effects? *Philosophical Transactions of the Royal Society B: Biological Sciences, 366* (1572), 1838–1848.

24. Weaver, A. J., & Koenig, H. G. (2006). Religion, spirituality, and their relevance to medicine: An update. *American Family Physician, 73,* 1336–1337.

25. Sieben, L. (2011, March 14). Nearly a third of college students have had mental health counseling, study finds. *The Chronicle of Higher Education.* http://chronicle.com.

26. Gonda, X., Fountoulakis, K. N., Rihmer, Z., Lazary, J., Laszik, A., & Akiskal, K. K. (2009, January). Towards a genetically validated new affective temperament scale: A delineation of the temperament phenotype of 5-HTTLPR using the TEMPS-A. *Journal of Affective Disorders, 112* (1–3), 19–29.

27. Lampert, R., Shusterman, V., Burg, M., McPherson, C., Batsford, W., Goldberg, A., & Soufer, R. (2009). Anger-induced T-wave alternans predicts future ventricular arrhythmias in patients with implantable cardioverter-defibrillators. *Journal of the American College of Cardiology, 53* (9), 774–778.

28. Chida, Y., & Steptoe, A. (2009, March 17). The association of anger and hostility with future coronary heart disease: A meta-analytic review of prospective evidence. *Journal of the American College of Cardiology, 53* (11), 947–949.

29. National Institute of Mental Health. (2013, January 22). The numbers count: Mental disorders in America. http://www.nimh.nih.gov.

30. National Institute of Mental Health. (2010, July 29). Annual total direct and indirect costs of serious mental illness (2002). http://www.nimh.nih.gov.

31. American College Health Association. (2013). *American College Health Association national college health assessment (ACHA-NCHA II): Reference group executive summary, fall 2012.* http://www.acha-ncha.org.

32. Blanco, C., Okuda, M., Wright, C., Hasin, D. S., Grant, B. F, Liu, S. M., & Olfson, M. (2008). Mental health of college students and their non-college-attending peers: Results from the National Epidemiologic Study on Alcohol and Related Conditions. *Archives of General Psychiatry, 65,* 1429–1437.

33. Kessler, R.C., Angermeyer, M., Anthony, J. C., De Graaf, R., Demyttenaere, K., Gasquet, I. . . . Ustun, T. B. (2007, October). Lifetime prevalence and age-of-onset distributions of mental disorders in the World Health Organization's World Mental Health Survey Initiative. *World Psychiatry, 6* (3), 168–176. http://www.ncbi.nlm.nih.gov.

34. Angell, M. (2011, June 23). The epidemic of mental illness: Why? *New York Review of Books,* 20–22.

35. Bear, M. F., Connors, B. W., & Paradiso, M. A. (2007). *Neuroscience: Exploring the brain,* 3rd ed. Baltimore: Lippincott Williams & Wilkins, 674–677.

36. American Psychiatric Association. (2000). *Diagnostic and statistical manual of mental disorders DSM-IV-TR* (4th ed.).

Arlington, VA: American Psychiatric Publishing.

37. Breene, G., Webb, B. T., Butler, A. W., van den Oord, E. J., Tozzi, F., Craddock, N. . . . McGuffin, P. (2011) A genome-wide significant linkage for severe depression on chromosome 3: The Depression Network Study. *American Journal of Psychiatry, 168* (8), 840–847.

38. Pergadia, M. L., Glowinski, A. L., Wray, N. R., Agrawal, A., Saccone, S. F., Loukola, A., . . . Madden, P. A. (2011). A 3p26-3p25 genetic linkage finding for DSM-IV major depression in heavy smoking families. *American Journal of Psychiatry, 168* (8), 848–852.

39. National Institute of Mental Health. (2011, July 27). *Depression.* http://www.nimh.nih.gov.

40. Centers for Disease Control and Prevention. (2008). Prevalence of self-reported postpartum depressive symptoms—17 states, 2004–2005. *Morbidity and Mortality Weekly Report, 57* (14), 361–366. http://www.cdc.gov.

41. National Center for Injury Prevention and Control. (2012). *Suicide: Facts at a glance.* http://www.cdc.gov.

42. Kline, N. (1964). The practical management of depression. *Journal of the American Medical Association, 190,* 122–130.

43. Posternak, M. A., & Miller, I. (2001). Untreated short-term course of major depression: A meta-analysis of outcomes from studies using wait-list control groups. *Journal of Affective Disorders, 66,* 139–146.

44. Mayo Clinic Staff. (2012, February 10). Depression (major depression): Treatments and drugs. Mayo Foundation for Medical Education and Research. http://www.mayoclinic.com.

45. Ioannidis, J. P. A. (2008). Effectiveness of antidepressants: An evidence myth constructed from a thousand randomized trials? *Philosophy, Ethics, and Humanities in Medicine, 3,* 14.

46. Kirsch, I. (2011). *The emperor's new drugs: Exploding the antidepressant myth.* New York: Basic Books.

47. National Institute of Mental Health. (2012, May 16). *Bipolar disorder.* http://www.nimh.nih.gov.

48. Spiegel, A. (2010, February 10). Children labeled bipolar may get a new diagnosis. National Public Radio. http://www.npr.org.

49. National Institute of Mental Health. (2009). *Panic disorder.* http://www.nimh.nih.gov.

50. National Institute of Mental Health. (2013, January 3). *Social phobia (social anxiety disorder).* http://www.nimh.nih.gov.

51. U.S. Department of Veterans Affairs, National Center for PTSD. (2012, May 29). *What is PTSD?* http://www.ptsd.va.gov.

52. Ratanasiripong, P., Sverduk, K., Prince, J., & Hayashino, D. (2012). Biofeedback and counseling for stress and anxiety among college students. *Journal of College Student Development, 53,* 742–749.

53. Cloos, J. M., & Ferreira, V. (2009, January). Current use of benzodiazepines in anxiety disorders. *Current Opinion in Psychiatry, 22* (1), 90–95.

54. Mayes, R., Bagwell, C., & Erkulwater, J. (2008). ADHD and the rise in stimulant use among children. *Harvard Review of Psychiatry, 16* (3), 151–166.

55. DuPaul, G. J., Weyandt, L. L., O'Dell, S., & Varejao, M. (2009, November). College students with ADHD: Current status and future directions. *Journal of Attention Disorders, 13* (3), 234–250.

56. WebMD. (2010, April 12). Stimulants for attention deficit hyperactivity disorder. http://www.webmd.com.

57. Substance Abuse and Mental Health Services Administration. (2009, May/June). Adderall and college students. *SAMHSA News, 17* (3). http://www.samhsa.gov.

58. Arria, A. M., & DuPont, R. L. (2010, October). Nonmedical prescription stimulant use among college students: Why we need to do something and what we need to do. *Journal of Addictive Diseases, 29* (4), 417–426.

59. National Institute of Mental Health. (2009). *Schizophrenia.* http://www.nimh.nih.gov.

60. Batey, H., May, J., & Andrade, J. (2010, February). Negative intrusive thoughts and dissociation as risk factors for self-harm. *Suicide and Life-Threatening Behavior, 40* (1), 35–49.

61. Swahn, M. H., Bina, A., Bossarte, R. M., Van Dulmen, M., Crosby, A., Jones, A. C., & Schinka, K. C. (2012, January). Self-harm and suicide attempts among high-risk, urban youth in the U.S.: Shared and unique risk and protective factors. *International Journal of Environmental Research and Public Health, 9* (1), 178–191.

62. Nixon, M. K., Cloutier, P., & Jansson, S. M. (2008, January 29). Non-suicidal self-harm in youth: A population-based survey. *Canadian Medical Association Journal, 178* (3), 306–312.

63. Kidger, J., Heron, J., Lewis, G., Evans, J. & Gunnell, D. (2012, June). Adolescent self-harm and suicidal thoughts in the ALSPAC cohort: A self-report survey in England. *BMC Psychiatry, 27* (12), 69.

64. Hoyert, D. L., & Xu, J. (2012). Deaths: Preliminary data for 2011. *National Vital Statistics Reports, 61* (6), 51.

65. National Institute of Mental Health. (2010, September 27). *Suicide in the U.S.: Statistics and prevention.* http://www.nimh.nih.gov.

66. Haas, A. P., Eliason, M., Mays, V. M., Mathy, R. M., Cochran, S. D., D'Augelli, A. R., . . . Clayton, P. J. (2010, December). Suicide and suicide risk in lesbian, gay, bisexual, and transgender populations: Review and recommendations. *Journal of Homosexuality, 58* (1), 10–51.

67. National Alliance on Mental Illness (2012). College students speak: Survey report on mental health. http://www.nami.org.

68. Hunt, J., & Eisenberg, D. (2010, January). Mental health problems and help-seeking behavior among college students. *Journal of Adolescent Health, 46* (1), 3–10. http://www.jahonline.org.

69. National Association of Cognitive-Behavioral Therapists. (2013). What is cognitive-behavioral therapy? http://www.nacbt.org.

70. Harvard Medical School. (2008, May). Positive psychology in practice. *Harvard Mental Health Letter.* http://www.health.harvard.edu.

71. Substance Abuse and Mental Health Services Administration. (2012, June 19). Acceptance and commitment therapy (ACT). *SAMHSA's National Registry of Evidence-Based Programs and Practices.* http://www.nrepp.samhsa.gov.

72. Lowry, F. (2011, February 2). FDA panel wants electroconvulsive therapy to retain high-risk class III status. *Medscape Medical News.* http://www.medscape.com.

73. Mayo Clinic. (2012). *Meditation: A simple, fast way to reduce stress.* http://www.mayoclinic.com.

Chapter 3

i. American College Health Association. (2013). *ACHA-NCHA II: Undergraduate students reference group executive summary, fall 2012.* http://www.acha-ncha.org.

ii. The American Psychological Association. (2013). *Stress in America: Missing the health care connection.* http://www.apa.org.

1. Selye, H. (1980). *Selye's guide to stress research* (vol. 1). New York: Van Nostrand Reinhold.

2. Selye, H. (1974). *Stress without distress.* New York: Lippincott.

3. Nixon, P. G. (1982). The human function curve—a paradigm for our times. *Activitas Nervosa Superior,* Suppl 3 (pt 1), 130–133.

4. McEwen, B. (September 0000). Stressed or stressed out: What is the difference? *Journal of Psychiatry and Neuroscience, 30* (5), 315–318.

5. Day, T. A. (2005, December). Defining stress as a prelude to mapping its neurocircuitry: No help from allostasis. *Progress in Neuro-Psychopharmacology and Biological Psychiatry, 29* (8), 1195–1200.

6. Juster, R., McEwen, B., & Lupien, S. (2009). Allostatic load biomarkers of chronic stress and impact on health and cognition. *Neuroscience and Biobehavioral Reviews, 35* (1), 2–16.

7. The American Psychological Association. (2013). *Stress in America: Missing the health care connection.* http://www.apa.org.

8. Marvar, P. J., & Harrison, D. G. (2012). Stress-dependent hypertension and the role of T lymphocytes. *Experimental Physiology, 97,* 1161–1167.

9. Von Kanel, R. (2012). Psychosocial stress and cardiovascular risk—current opinion. *Swiss Medical Weekly, 142* (1), 1–13.

10. Smith, T. G., Stoddard, C., & Barnes, M. G. (2009). Why the poor get fat: Weight gain and economic insecurity. *Forum for Health Economics & Policy, 12* (2), (Obesity), Article 5.

11. The American Psychological Association. (2012). *Stress in America: Our health at risk.* http://www.apa.org.

12. Vedhara, K., & Irwin, M. R. (2005). *Human psychoneuroimmunology.* Oxford University Press.

13. Segerstrom, S. (2010.) Resources, stress, and immunity: An ecological perspective on human psychoneuroimmunology. *Annals of Behavioral Medicine, 40* (1), 114–125.
14. Khanfer, R., Carroll, D., Lord, J. M., & Phillips, A. C. (2012). Reduced neutrophil superoxide production among healthy older adults in response to acute psychological stress. *International Journal of Psychophysiology, 86* (3), 238–244.
15. American College Health Association. (2013). *ACHA-NCHA II: Undergraduate students reference group executive summary, fall 2012.* http://www.acha-ncha.org.
16. American Academy of Sleep Medicine. (2008). *Insomnia.* http://www.aasmnet.org.
17. Randall, A. K., & Bodenmann, G. (2009). The role of stress in close relationships and marital satisfaction. *Clinical Psychology Review, 29,* 105–115.
18. Neff, L. A., & Karney, B. R. (2009). Stress and reactivity to daily relationship experiences: How stress hinders adaptive processes in marriage. *Journal of Personality and Social Psychology, 97* (3), 435–450.
19. Joiner, Jr., T. E., Wingate, L. R., Gencoz, T., & Gencoz, F. (2005). Stress generation in depression: Three studies on its resilience, possible mechanism, and symptom specificity. *Journal of Social and Clinical Psychology, 24* (2), 236–253.
20. Mayo Foundation. (2010). Panic attacks and panic disorder. http://www.mayoclinic.com.
21. Friedman, M. (1996). *Type A behavior: Its diagnosis and treatment.* New York: Plenum Press (pp. ix, 3, 4).
22. Friedman, M. (1996). *Type A behavior: Its diagnosis and treatment.* New York: Plenum Press (pp. ix, 3, 4).
23. Blatný M., & Adam, Z. (2008, June). Type C personality (cancer personality): Current view and implications for future research. *Vnitrní Lékarství, 54* (6), 638–645.
24. Polman, R., Borkoles, E., & Nicholls, A. R. (2010, September). Type D personality, stress, and symptoms of burnout: The influence of avoidance coping and social support. *British Journal of Health Psychology, 15* (3), 681–696.
25. Bissonette, M. (1998, August). Optimism, hardiness, and resiliency: A review of the literature. *The Child and Family Partnership Project.* http://www.reachinginreachingout.com.
26. Kobasa, S. (1982). The hardy personality: Toward a social psychology of stress and health. In G. S. Sanders & J. Suls (Eds.). *Social psychology of health and illness.* Hillsdale, NJ: Lawrence Erlbaum Associates (pp. 3–12).
27. Misra, R., McKean, M., West, S., & Russo, T. (2000). Academic stress of college students: Comparison of student and faculty perceptions. *College Student Journal, 34* (2), 236–246.
28. Murff, S. H. (2005, Sept./Oct.). The impact of stress on academic success in college students. *Association of Black Nursing Faculty Journal,* 102–104.

29. Wright, K. B., Craig, E. A., Cunningham, C. B., & Igiel, M. (2007). Emotional support and perceived stress among college students using facebook.com: An exploration of the relationship between source perceptions and emotional support. Paper presented at the annual meeting of the NCA, 93rd Annual Convention, TBA, Chicago, IL.
30. Braithwaite, S., Delevi, R. & Fincham, F. (2010). Romantic relationships and the physical and mental health of college students. *Personal Relationships, 17,* 1–12.
31. King, K. (2005). Why is discrimination stressful? The mediating role of cognitive appraisal. *Cultural Diversity and Ethnic Minority Psychology, 11* (3), 202–212.
32. Holmes, T. H., & Rahe, R. H. (1967). The social readjustment rating scale. *Journal of Psychosomatic Research, 11,* 213–218.
33. Rice, K. G., Leever, B. A., Christopher, J., & Porter, J. D. (2006). Perfectionism, stress, and social (dis)connection: A short-term study of hopelessness, depression, and academic adjustment among honors students. *Journal of Counseling Psychology, 33* (4), 524–534.
34. Lazarus, R. S., & Folkman, S. (1984). *Stress, appraisal, and coping.* New York: Springer.
35. American Council on Exercise. (2009). *Exercise can help control stress.* http://www.acefitness.org.
36. Vorvick, Linda. (2009). *Exercise and stress reduction.* National Institutes of Health. http://www.nlm.nih.gov.
37. Lande, R. G. (2009). *Caffeine-related psychiatric disorders.* eMedicine from WebMD. http://www.emedicine.medscape.com.
38. National Center for Complementary and Alternative Medicine. (2008). *Yoga.* http://www.nccam.nih.gov.
39. Zeitlin, D., Keller, S. E., Shiflett, S. C., Schleifer, S. J., & Bartlett, J. A. (2000). Immunological effects of massage therapy during academic stress. *Psychosomatic Medicine,* 83–84.
40. Wilkinson, L., Buboltz, Jr., W., & Seemann, E. (2001). Using breathing techniques to ease test anxiety. *Guidance and Counseling, 16* (3), 76–88.
41. Siedliecki, S. L., & Good, M. (2006, June). Effect of music on power, pain, depression, and disability. *Journal of Advanced Nursing, 54* (5), 553–562.
42. Staum, M. J., & Brotons, M. (2000, Spring). The effect of music amplitude on the relaxation response. *Journal of Music Therapy, 37* (1), 22–39.
43. Chafin, S., Roy, M., Gerin, W., & Christenfeld, N. (2004). Music can facilitate blood pressure recovery from stress. *British Journal of Health Psychology, 9,* 393–403.
44. Snow, D. L., Swan, S. C., Ragavan, C., Connell, C. M., & Klein, I. (2003). The relationship of work stressors, coping, and social support to psychological symptoms among female secretarial employees. *Work and Stress, 17* (3), 241–263.
45. Largo-Wright, E., Peterson, P. M., & Chen, W. W. (2005). Perceived problem

solving, stress, and health among college students. *American Journal of Health Behavior, 29* (4), 360–370.
46. Chu-Lien Chao, R. (2012). Managing perceived stress among college students: The roles of social support and dysfunctional coping. *Journal of College Counseling, 15* (1), 5–21.
47. Bender, E. (2010, August). Guide helps students, parents negotiate difficult passage. *Psychiatric News, 45* (16), 7. http://www.pn.psychiatryonline.org.

Chapter 4

i. Buzby, J. C., & Bentley, J. (2012, August 22). *Total caloric sweeteners.* Economic Research Service, USDA. http://www.ers.usda.gov.
ii. McDonald's USA. (2013, February 14). McDonald's USA nutrition facts for popular menu items. http://nutrition.mcdonalds.com.
iii. U.S. Food and Drug Administration. (2012). Food allergies: What you need to know. http://www.fda.gov.
1. Buzby, J. C., & Bentley, J. (2012, August 22). *Total caloric sweeteners.* Economic Research Service, USDA. http://www.ers.usda.gov.
2. Food and Nutrition Board, Institute of Medicine of the National Academies. (2005). *Dietary reference intakes for energy, carbohydrate, fiber, fat, fatty acids, cholesterol, protein, and amino acids.* Washington, D.C.: The National Academies Press. http://www.nap.edu.
3. O'Neil, C. E., Nicklas, T. A., Zanovec, M., & Cho, S. (2010, May). Whole grain consumption is associated with diet quality and nutrient intake in adults. *Journal of the Academy of Nutrition and Dietetics, 110,* 1461–1468.
4. Burris, J., Rietkerk, W., & Woolf, K. (2013, March). Acne: The role of medical nutrition therapy. *Journal of the Academy of Nutrition and Dietetics, 113* (3), DOI: 10.1016/j.jand.2012.11.016.
5. Linus Pauling Institute. (2010, April). *Glycemic index and glycemic load.* Oregon State University Micronutrient Information Center. http://lpi.oregonstate.edu.
6. American Heart Association. (2010). Fat. http://www.americanheart.org.
7. U.S. Department of Agriculture and Department of Health and Human Services. (2010). *Dietary guidelines for Americans, 2010,* 7th ed. Washington, DC: U.S. Government Printing Office.
8. U.S. Department of Agriculture. (2011, June 4). Protein foods. http://www.choosemyplate.gov.
9. Harvard School of Public Health. (2010). Fats and cholesterol: Out with the bad, in with the good. http://www.hsph.harvard.edu.
10. American College of Sports Medicine, American Dietetic Association, and Dietitians of Canada. (2009). Joint Position Statement. Nutrition and athletic performance. *Medicine and Science in Sports and Exercise, 41* (3), 709–731.
11. Manore, M. M., Meyer, N. L., & Thompson, J. T. (2009). *Sport nutrition for health and performance,* 2nd ed. Champaign, IL: Human Kinetics.

12. U.S. Department of Agriculture. (2011, June). With protein foods, variety is key. DG TipSheet No. 6. http://www.choosemyplate.gov.
13. Office of Dietary Supplements. (2011, June 24). Dietary supplement fact sheet: Vitamin D. http://ods.od.nih.gov.
14. Office of Dietary Supplements. (2012, December 14). Dietary supplement fact sheet: Folate. http://ods.od.nih.gov.
15. Thompson, J., & Manore, M. (2012). *Nutrition: An applied approach,* 3rd ed. San Francisco, CA: Pearson Education.
16. Gudeux, E. (2011, February 15). Coffee and kids. *Consumer Reports News.* http://news.consumerreports.org.
17. U.S. Food and Drug Administration. (2012, November 16). Energy "drinks" and supplements: Investigations of adverse event reports. http://www.fda.gov.
18. Institute of Medicine. (2004). *Dietary reference intakes for water, potassium, sodium, chloride, and sulfate.* Washington, DC: The National Academies Press.
19. Stasio, M., Curry, K., Sutton-Skinner, K., & Glassman, D. (2008). Over-the-counter medication and herbal or dietary supplement use in college: Dose frequency and relationship to self-reported distress. *Journal of the American College Health Association, 56* (5), 535–547.
20. Office of Dietary Supplements. (2013, January 7). Dietary supplement fact sheet: Multivitamin/mineral supplements. http://ods.od.nih.gov.
21. Thompson, J. L., Manore, M. M., & Vaughan, L. A. (2014). *The science of nutrition,* 3rd ed. San Francisco, CA: Pearson, 592–594.
22. Linus Pauling Institute. (2010). *Phytochemicals.* Micronutrient Information Center. http://lpi.oregonstate.edu.
23. American College Health Association. (2013). *National college health assessment (ACHA-NCHA II): Reference group executive summary, fall 2012.* http://www.acha-ncha.org.
24. U.S. Department of Agriculture, Agricultural Research Service. (2010, May). Oxygen radical absorbance capacity (ORAC) of selected foods, release 2. Nutrient Data Laboratory Home Page. http://www.ars.usda.gov.
25. National Institutes of Health. (2012, June 13). NIH Human Microbiome Project defines normal bacterial makeup of the body. *NIH News.* http://www.nih.gov.
26. Hemarajata, P., & Versalovic, J. (2013, January). Effects of probiotics on gut microbiota: Mechanisms of intestinal immunomodulation and neuromodulation. *Therapeutic Advances in Gastroenterology, 6* (1), 39–51. http://www.ncbi.nlm.nih.gov.
27. United States Food and Drug Administration. (2012, April 6). Regulatory information: Complementary and alternative medicine products and their regulation by the Food and Drug Administration. http://www.fda.gov.
28. U.S. Food and Drug Administration. (2012, February 15). How to understand

and use the Nutrition Facts label. http://www.fda.gov.

29. U.S. Food and Drug Administration. (2011, August 1). Food labeling guide. http://www.fda.gov.

30. U.S. Department of Agriculture. Food groups. http://www.choosemyplate.gov.

31. Rodriguez, N., DiMarco, N., & Langley, S. (2009). Position of the American Dietetic Association, Dietitians of Canada, and the American College of Sports Medicine: Nutrition and athletic performance. *Journal of the American Dietetic Association, 109* (31), 509–527.

32. Centers for Disease Control and Prevention (CDC). (2009, March 17). Investigation update: Outbreak of *Salmonella typhimurium* infections, 2008–2009. http://www.cdc.gov.

33. Hamburg, M. A. (2011, January 3). Food Safety Modernization Act: Putting the focus on prevention. http://www.whitehouse.gov.

34. Centers for Disease Control and Prevention. (2013, January 24). Tracking and reporting foodborne disease outbreaks. http://www.cdc.gov.

35. Hall, A. J. (2011, March 22). *Norovirus in the news.* FoodSafety.gov. http://www.foodsafety.gov.

36. U.S. Department of Agriculture, Food Safety and Inspection Service. (2011, May 25). Fact sheets: *Salmonella* questions and answers. http://www.fsis.usda.gov.

37. U.S. Department of Health and Human Services. (2011). Check your steps. http://www.foodsafety.gov.

38. *New York Times.* (2010, May 16). The squishy science of food allergies. http://www.nytimes.com.

39. U.S. Food and Drug Administration. (2012). Food allergies: What you need to know. http://www.fda.gov.

40. U.S. Environmental Protection Agency. (2012, May 9). Pesticides and food: Healthy, sensible food practices. http://www.epa.gov.

Chapter 5

i. Centers for Disease Control and Prevention. (2011). *Physical activity for everyone: Physical activity and health.* http://www.cdc.gov.

ii. Northwestern University. (2009, June 20). Aerobically unfit young adults on road to diabetes in middle age. *ScienceDaily.* http://www.sciencedaily.com.

iii. Liu-Ambrose, T., Nagamatsu, L. S., Graf, P., Beattie, B. L., Ashe, M. C., & Handy, T. C. (2010). Resistance training and executive functions: A 12-month randomized controlled trial. *Archives of Internal Medicine, 170* (2), 170–178.

1. Centers for Disease Control and Prevention. (2010). Exercise or physical activity. *FastStats.* http://www.cdc.gov.

2. William, P. T. (2008). Vigorous exercise, fitness and incident hypertension, high cholesterol, and diabetes. *Medicine & Science in Sports & Exercise, 40* (6), 998–1006.

3. Kaminsky, L. A., Arena, R., Beckie, T. M., Brubaker, P. H., Church, T. S., Forman, D. E., . . . Williams, M. A. (2013). The importance of cardiorespiratory fitness in the United States: The need for a national registry: A policy statement from the American Heart Association. *Circulation, 127,* 652–662.

4. Lang, T. F. (2011). The bone-muscle relationship in men and women. *Journal of Osteoporosis,* Article ID 702735, doi: 10.4061/2011/702735.

5. Ärnlöv, J., Ingelsson, E., Sundström, J., & Lind, L. (2010). Impact of body mass index and the metabolic syndrome on the risk of cardiovascular disease and death in middle-aged men. *Circulation, 121,* 230–236.

6. Knaepen, K., Goekint, M., Heym, E., & Meeusen. R. (2010). Neuroplasticity—Exercise-induced response of peripheral brain-derived neurotrophic factor: A systematic review of experimental studies in human subjects. *Sports Medicine, 40* (9), 765–780.

7. Williamson, J., & Pahor, M. (2010). Evidence regarding the benefits of physical exercise, *Archives of Internal Medicine, 170,* (2), 124–125.

8. Lee, D., Sui, X., Artero, G., Lee, I., Church, T. S., McAuley, P., . . . Blair, S. (2011). Long-term effects of changes in cardiorespiratory fitness and body mass index on all-cause and cardiovascular disease mortality in men. *Circulation, 124,* 2483–2490.

9. National Institutes of Health, National Institute of Diabetes and Digestive and Kidney Diseases. (2008, October). *Diabetes prevention program (DPP)* (NIH Publication No. 09-5099). Washington, DC: Government Printing Office.

10. Colberg, S., Sigal, R., Fernhall, B., Regensteiner, J., Blissmer, B., Rubin, R., . . . Braun, B. (2010). Exercise and type 2 diabetes: The American College of Sports Medicine and the American Diabetes Association joint position statement. *Diabetes Care, 33* (12), 147–167.

11. Remon, J., Bertoni, A., Connelly, S., Feeney, P., Glasser, S., Glick, . . . Montgomery, B. (2010). Effect of the Look AHEAD study intervention on medication use and related cost to treat cardiovascular disease risk factors in individuals with type 2 diabetes. *Diabetes Care, 33* (6), 1153–1158.

12. Friedenreich, C., Neilson, H., & Lynch, B. (2010). State of the epidemiological evidence on physical activity and cancer prevention. *European Journal of Cancer, 46* (14), 2593–2604.

13. Ibid.

14. Dallal, C., Sullivan-Halley, J., Ross, R., Wang, Y., Deapen, D., Horn-Ross, P., . . . Bernstein, L. (2007). Long-term recreational physical activity and risk of invasive and in situ breast cancer: The California teachers study. *Archives of Internal Medicine, 167* (4), 408–415.

15. Nieman, D. C. (2012). Clinical implications of exercise immunology. *Journal of Sport and Health Science, 1* (1), 12–17.

16. Medline Plus. (2008). *Exercise and immunity.* http://www.nlm.nih.gov.

17. Gunter, K. B., Almstedt, H. C., & Janz, K. F. (2012). Physical activity in childhood may be the key to optimizing lifespan skeletal health. *Exercise & Sport Science Reviews, 40* (1), 13–21.

18. Rozanski, A. (2012). Exercise as medical treatment for depression. *Journal of the American College of Cardiology, 60* (12), 1064–1066.

19. Sui, X., Laditka, J. N., Church, T. S., Hardind, J. W., Chase, N., Davis, K., & Blaira, S. N. (2009). Prospective study of cardiorespiratory fitness and depressive symptoms in women and men. *Journal of Psychiatric Research, 43* (5), 546–552.

20. Elliot, C., Kennedy, C., Morgan, G., Anderson, S., & Morris, D. (2012). Undergraduate physical activity and depressive symptoms: A national study. *American Journal of Health Behavior, 36* (2), 230–241.

21. Åberg, M. A. I., Pedersen, N. L., Torén, K., Svartengren, M., Bäckstrand, B., Johnsson, T., . . . Kuhn, H. G. (2009). Cardiovascular fitness is associated with cognition in young adulthood. *Proceedings of the National Academy of Sciences, 106,* 20906–20911.

22. Li, L., & Liu, L. (2012). Experimental studies of physical exercises to improve students' sleep quality and mental health. *Education and Educational Technology, 108,* 65–72.

23. Jespersen J. G., Nedergaard A., Andersen L. L., Schjerling P., & Andersen J. L. (2009). Myostatin expression during human muscle hypertrophy and subsequent atrophy: Increased myostatin with detraining. *Scandinavian Journal of Medicine & Science in Sports.* Published online November 9, 2009.

24. American College of Sports Medicine. (2010). *ACSM's guidelines for exercise testing and prescription* (8th ed.). Baltimore, MD: Wolters Kluwer/Lippincott Williams & Wilkins.

25. Centers for Disease Control and Prevention. (2009). *Physical activity for everyone: Target heart rate and estimated maximum heart rate.* http://www.cdc.gov.

26. Loprinzi, P., & Cardinal, B. (2013) Association between biologic outcomes and objectively measured physical activity accumulated in ≥10-minute bouts and <10-minute bouts. *American Journal of Health Promotion, 27* (3), 143–151.

27. Miyashita, M., Burns, S., & Stensel, D. (2008). Accumulating short bouts of brisk walking reduces postprandial plasma triacylgylcerol concentrations and resting blood pressure in healthy young men. *American Journal of Clinical Nutrition, 88* (5), 1225–1231.

28. Page, P. (2012). Current concepts in muscle stretching for exercise and rehabilitation. *International Journal of Sports Physical Therapy, 7* (1), 109–119.

29. Garber, C., Blissmer, B., Deschenes, M., Franklin, B., Lamonte, M., Lee, I., Nieman, D., & Swain, D. (2011). Quantity and quality of exercise for developing and maintaining cardiorespiratory, musculoskeletal, and neuromotor fitness in apparently healthy adults: Guidance for prescribing exercise. *Medicine & Science in Sports & Exercise, 43* (7), 1334–1359.

30. Centers for Disease Control and Prevention. (2008). *Physical activity guidelines for Americans.* http://www.health.gov.

31. McTiernan, A., Sorensen, B., Irwin, M., Morgan, A., Yasui, Y., Rudolph, R., . . . Potter, J. (2007). Exercise effect on weight and body fat in men and women. *Obesity, 15* (6), 1496–1512.

32. Patel, A., Bernstein, L., Deka, A., Feigelson, H., Campbell, P., Gapstur, S., Colditz, G., & Thun, M. (2010). Leisure time spent sitting in relation to total mortality in a prospective cohort of US adults. *American Journal of Epidemiology, 172,* 419–429.

33. Centers for Disease Control and Prevention. (2008). *Physical activity guidelines for Americans: Be active your way: A guide for adults* (ODPHP Publication No. U0037). http://www.health.gov.

34. Mayo Clinic. (2010). Eating and exercise: 5 tips to maximize your workouts. http://www.mayoclinic.com.

35. American Dietetic Association. (2009). Position of the American Dietetic Association, Dietitians of Canada, and the American College of Sports Medicine: Nutrition and athletic performance. *Journal of the American Dietetic Association, 109* (3), 509–527.

36. Manore, M. M., Meyer, N. L., & Thompson, J. L. (2009). *Sports nutrition for health and performance,* 2nd ed. Champaign, IL: Human Kinetics.

37. Hackney, K., Cook, S., Fairchild, T., & Ploutz-Snyder, L. (2012). Sketetal muscle volume following dehydration induced by exercise in heat. *Extreme Physiology & Medicine, 1* (3), 1–9.

38. Hampton, Tracy. (2006). Researchers address use of performance-enhancing drugs in nonelite athletes. *Journal of the American Medical Association, 295* (6), 607.

39. U.S. House of Representatives, U.S. Government Accountability Office, Committee on Oversight and Government Reform. (2007). *Federal efforts to prevent and reduce anabolic steroid abuse among teenagers.* Washington, DC: Government Printing Office.

40. MedlinePlus. (n.d.). *Creatine.* http://www.nlm.nih.gov.

41. Liu, H., Bravata, D., Olkin, I., Friedlander, A., Liu, V., Roberts, B., . . . Hoffman, A. (2008). Systematic review: The effects of growth hormone on athletic performance. *Annals of Internal Medicine, 148* (10), 747–758.

42. National Center for Complementary and Alternative Medicine. (2009). *Consumer advisory: Ephedra.* http://nccam.nih.gov.

43. Kumanyika, S., Wadden, T., Shults, J., Fassbender, J., Brown, S., Bowman, M., . . . Wu, X. (2009). Trial of family and friend support for weight loss in African American adults. *Archives of Internal Medicine, 169* (19), 1795–1804.

Chapter 6

i. Centers for Disease Control/National Center for Health Statistics. (2012). *FastStats: Obesity and overweight.* http://www.cdc.gov.

ii. Finkelstein, E., Trogdon, J., Cohen, J., & Dietz, W. (2009). Annual medical spending attributable to obesity: Payer- and service-specific estimates. *Health Affairs, 28* (5), 822–831.

iii. Murray, C., Vos, T., Lozano, R., Naghavi, M., Flaxman, A., Michaud, C., . . . Lopez, A. (2012.) Disability-adjusted life years (DALYs) for 291 diseases and injuries in 21 regions, 1990–2010: A systematic analysis for the Global Burden of Disease Study 2010. *The Lancet, 380* (5859), 2197–2227.

iv. American College Health Association. (2013). *American College Health Association national college health assessment II: Reference group data report, fall 2012.* http://www.acha-ncha.org.

1. Centers for Disease Control/National Center for Health Statistics. (2012). *FastStats: Obesity and overweight.* http://www.cdc.gov.

2. World Health Organization. (2009). *Obesity and overweight. Fact sheet number 311.* http://www.who.int.

3. Centers for Disease Control and Prevention. (2010). Health behaviors of adults: United States, 2005–2007. *Vital and Health Statistics, 10* (245). http://www.cdc.gov.

4. American College Health Association. (2013). *American College Health Association national college health assessment II: Reference group data report, fall 2012.* http://www.acha-ncha.org.

5. Benowitz-Fredericks, C., Garcia, K., Massey, M., Vasagar, B., & Borzekowski, D. (2012). Body image, eating disorders, and the relationship to adolescent media use. *Pediatric Clinics of North America, 59* (3), 693–704.

6. Keel, P., Baxter, M., Heatheron, T., & Joiner, T. (2007). A 20-year longitudinal study of body weight, dieting, and eating disorder symptoms. *Journal of Abnormal Psychology, 116* (2), 422–432.

7. Forrest, K., & Stuhldreher, W. (2007). Patterns and correlates of body image dissatisfaction and distortion among college students. *American Journal of Health Studies, 22* (1), 18–25.

8. Arciszewski, T., Berjot, S., & Finez, L. (2012). Threat of the thin-ideal body image and body malleability beliefs: Effects on body image self-discrepancies and behavioral intentions. *Body Image, 9* (3),334–341.

9. Halliwell, E., Easun, A., & Harcourt, D. (2011). Body dissatisfaction: Can a short media literacy message reduce negative media exposure effects amongst adolescent girls? *British Journal of Health Psychology, 16* (2), 396–403.

10. Freedman, D., Kettel Khan, L., Serdula, M., Dietz, W., Srinivasan, S., & Berenson, G. (2005). The relation of childhood BMI to adult adiposity: The Bogalusa heart study. *Pediatrics, 115* (1), 22–27.

11. Flegal, K., Kit, B., Orpana, H., & Graubard, B. (2013.) Association of all-cause mortality with overweight and obesity using standard body mass index categories: A systematic review and meta-analysis. *Journal of the American Medical Association, 309* (1), 71–82.

12. Ardern, C. I., Katzmarzyk, P. T., Janssen, I., & Ross, R. (2012). Discrimination of health risk by combined body mass index and waist circumference, *Obesity, 11* (1), 135–142.

13. Shape Up America! (2012.) Everything you want to know about body fat. http://www.shapeup.org/bfl/basics1.html.

14. Centers for Disease Control and Prevention (CDC). (2012). *Overweight and obesity: Adult obesity facts.* http://www.cdc.gov.

15. Finkelstein, E., Khavjou, O., Thompson, H., Trogdon, J., Pan, L., Sherry, B., & Dietz, W. (2012). Obesity and severe obesity forecasts through 2030. *American Journal of Preventive Medicine, 42* (6), 563–570.

16. Murray, C., Vos, T., Lozano, R., Naghavi, M., Flaxman, A., Michaud, C., . . . Lopez, A. (2012.) Disability-adjusted life years (DALYs) for 291 diseases and injuries in 21 regions, 1990–2010: A systematic analysis for the Global Burden of Disease Study 2010. *The Lancet, 380* (5859), 2197–2227.

17. Economos, C. D., Hildebrandt, M. L., & Hyatt, R. R. (2008). College freshman stress and weight change: Differences by gender. *American Journal of Health Behavior, 32* (1), 16–25.

18. Gropper, S., Simmons, K., Connell, L., & Ulrich, P. (2012.) Changes in body weight, composition, and shape: A 4-year study of college students. *Applied Physiology, Nutrition, and Metabolism, 37* (6), 1118–1123.

19. Wharton, C., Adams, T., & Hampl, J. (2008). Weight-loss practices and body weight perceptions among U.S. college students. *Journal of American College Health, 56* (5), 579–584.

20. Jung, M., Bray, S., & Ginis, K. (2008). Behavior change and the "freshman 15": Tracking physical activity and dietary patterns in 1st-year university women. *Journal of American College Health, (56)* 5, 523–530.

21. Kasparek, D., Corwin, S., Valois, R., Sargent, R., & Morris, R. (2008). Selected health behaviors that influence freshman weight change. *Journal of American College Health, 56* (4), 437–444.

22. Ogden, C. L., Carroll, M. D., Kit., B., & Flegal, K. (2012). Prevalence of overweight and obesity in the United States, 1999–2010. *Journal of the American Medical Association, 307* (5), 473–490.

23. National Heart, Lung, and Blood Institute. (2012). *What are the health risks of overweight and obesity?* http://www.nhlbi.nih.gov.

24. National Institute of Diabetes and Digestive and Kidney Diseases/National Institutes of Health. (2007). Do you know the health risks of being overweight? *NIH Publication No. 07–4098.* http://win.niddk.nih.gov.

25. Nguyen, N. T., Magno, C. P., Lane, K. T., Hinojosa, M. W., & Lane, J. S. (2008, December). Association of hypertension, diabetes, dyslipidemia, and metabolic syndrome with obesity: Findings from the National Health and Nutrition Examination Survey, 1999–2004. *Journal of the American College of Surgeons, 207* (6), 928–934.

26. U.S. Department of Health and Human Services, Office on Women's Health. (2010). *Polycystic ovary syndrome (PCOS) fact sheet.* http://www.womenshealth.gov.

27. Olshansky, S. J., Passaro, D. J., Hershow, R. C., Layden, J., Carnes, B. A., Brody, J., . . . Ludwig, D. S. (2005). A potential decline in life expectancy in the United States in the 21st century. *New England Journal of Medicine, 352*, 1103–1110.

28. Finkelstein, E., Trogdon, J., Cohen, J., & Dietz, W. (2009). Annual medical spending attributable to obesity: Payer- and service-specific estimates. *Health Affairs, 28* (5), 822–831.

29. Trogdon, J., Finkelstein, E., Feagan, C., . . . Cohen, J. (2011, June 16). State- and payer-specific estimates of annual medical expenditures attributable to obesity. *Obesity,* doi: 10.1038/oby.2011.

30. Dor, A., Ferguson, C., Langwith, C., & Tan, E. (2010). A heavy burden: The individual costs of being overweight and obese in the United States. The George Washington University School of Public Health and Health Services. http://www.gwumc.edu.

31. Duyff, R. L. (2012). *American Dietetic Association complete food and nutrition guide,* 4th, revised and updated edition. New York: John Wiley and Sons.

32. Levi, A., Chan, K., & Pence, D. (2006). Real men do not read food labels: The effects of masculinity and involvement on college students' food decisions. *Journal of American College Health, 55* (2), 91–98.

33. Power, M., & Schulkin, J. (2008). Sex differences in fat storage, fat metabolism, and the health risks from obesity: Possible evolutionary origins. *British Journal of Nutrition, 99* (5), 931–940.

34. Coutinho, T., Goel, K., Corrêa de Sá, D., Kragelund, C., Kanaya, A., Zeller, M., . . . Lopez-Jimenez, F. (2011). Central obesity and survival in subjects with coronary artery disease: A systematic review of the literature and collaborative analysis with individual subject data. *Journal of the American College of Cardiology, 57,* 1877–1886.

35. Mayo Clinic. (2011). *Belly fat in women: Taking—and keeping—it off.* http://www.mayoclinic.com.

36. Wang, K., Li, W., Zhang, C., Wang, Z., Glessner, J., Grant, S., . . . Price, R. (2012.) A genome-wide association study on obesity and obesity-related traits. *PLoS One, 6* (4), e18939.

37. Kaiser Family Foundation (2010). *Overweight and obesity rates for adults by race/ethnicity, 2010.* http://www.statehealthfacts.org.

38. Flegal, K. M., Carroll, M. D., Kit, B. K., & Ogden, C. L. (2012). Prevalance of obesity and trends in the distribution of body mass index among US adults, 1999–2010. *Journal of the American Medical Association, 307* (5), 491–497.

39. Beydoun, M., & Wang, Y. (2009). Gender-ethnic disparity in BMI and waist circumference distribution shifts in US adults. *Obesity, 17* (1), 169–176.

40. Duffey, K., & Popkin, B. (2011). Energy density, portion size, and eating occasions: Contributions to increased energy intake in the United States, 1977–2006. *PLoS Medicine, 8* (6), e1001050. doi: 10.1371/journal.pmed.1001050.

41. Wells, H., & Buzby. J. (2008.) Dietary assessment of major trends in U.S. food consumption, 1970–2005. *Economic Information Bulletin No. (EIB-33),* 1–27. http://www.ers.usda.gov.

42. Newman, C. (2004, August). Why are we so fat? *National Geographic, 206* (2), 46–61.

43. McDonald's. (2012.) McDonald's USA nutrition facts for popular menu items. (Electronic version.) http://nutrition.mcdonalds.com/getnutrition/nutritionfacts.pdf.

44. National Center for Health Statistics, Health Indicators Warehouse. (2010). Leisure-time physical activity—none (percent). http://www.healthindicators.gov.

45. Matthews, C. E., Chen, K. Y., Freedson, P. S., Buchowski, M. S., Bettina, M., Beech, B. M., Pate, R. R., & Troiano, R. P. (2008). Amount of time spent in sedentary behaviors in the United States, 2003–2004. *American Journal of Epidemiology, 167* (7), 875–881.

46. The Nielsen Company. The Cross Platform Report—Q4 2011. http://www.nielsen.com.

47. U.S. Census Bureau. (2011). Commuting characteristics by sex. American community survey, 2011. http://factfinder2.census.gov.

48. Christian, T. (2012.) Trade-offs between commuting time and health-related activities. *Journal of Urban Health, 89* (5), 746–757.

49. Moczulski, V., McMahan, S., Weiss, J., Beam, W., & Chandler, L. (2007). Commuting behaviors, obesity risk, and the built environment. *American Journal of Health Behaviors, 22* (1), 26–32.

50. O'Connor, D., Jones, F., Conner, M., & McMillan, B. (2008). Effects of daily hassles and eating styles on eating behavior. *Health Psychology, 27* (1), 20–31.

51. McDonald's. (2012). *McDonald's USA nutrition facts for popular menu items.* (Electronic version.) http://www.mcdonalds.com.

52. Food Research and Action Center. (2011). *Food insecurity and obesity: Understanding the connections.* http://frac.org.

53. Larson, N., & Story, M. (2011). Food insecurity and weight status among U.S. children and families: A review of the literature. *American Journal of Preventive Medicine, 40* (2), 166–173.

54. Gustat, J., Rice, J., Parker, K., Becker, A., & Farley, T. (2012.) Effect of changes to the neighborhood built environment on physical activity in a low-income African American neighborhood. *Preventing Chronic Disease, 9,* E57 (EPub).

55. Physicians Committee for Responsible Medicine. (2011). USDA's new MyPlate icon at odds with federal subsidies for meat, dairy. http://pcrm.org.

56. Dansinger, M., Gleason, J., Griffith, J., Selker, H., & Schaefer, E. (2005). Comparison of the Atkins, Ornish, Weight Watchers, and Zone diets for weight loss and heart disease risk reduction. *Journal of the American Medical Association, 293* (1), 43–53.
57. Mayo Clinic. (2011). *Trans fat is double trouble for your heart health.* http://www.mayoclinic.com.
58. Gardner, C., Kiazand, A., Alhassan, S., Kim, S., Stafford, R., Balise, R., Kraemer, H., & King, A. (2007). Comparison of the Atkins, Zone, Ornish, and LEARN diets for change in weight and related risk factors among overweight premenopausal women. *Journal of the American Medical Association, 297* (9), 969–977.
59. Paoli, A., Canato, M., Toniolo, L., Bargossi, A., Neri, M., Mediati, M., . . . Bianco, A. (2011). The ketogenic diet: An underappreciated therapeutic option? *La Clinica Terapeutica, 162* (5), 145–153.
60. Marketdata Enterprises, Inc. (2011). *U.S. weight loss market worth $60.9 billion.* (Electronic version.) http://www.prweb.com.
61. Harring, H., Montgomery, K., & Hardin, J. (2010). Perceptions of body weight, weight management, strategies, and depressive symptoms among U.S. college students. *Journal of American College Health, 59* (1), 43–50.
62. Hackett, A., & Krska, J. (2012). Is it time to regulate over-the-counter weight-loss formulations? *International Journal of Pharmacy Practice, 20* (3), 199–202.
63. U.S. Food and Drug Administration. (2011, December 6). *FDA, FTC act to remove "homeopathic" HCG weight loss products from the market.* FDA News Release. http://www.fda.gov.
64. U.S. Food and Drug Administration. (2009, May 1). FDA warns consumers to stop using Hydroxycut products. *FDA News.* http://www.fda.gov.
65. U.S. Food and Drug Administration. (2005). *FDA news release: FDA acts to seize ephedra-containing dietary supplements.* P05-94. http://www.fda.gov.
66. Hagobian, T., Yamashiro, M., Hinke-Lipsker, J., Streder, K., Evero, N., & Hackney, T. (2013). Effects of acute exercise on appetite hormones and ad libitum energy intake in men and women. *Applied Physiology, Nutrition, and Metabolism, 38* (999), 66–72.
67. National Institute of Diabetes and Digestive and Kidney Diseases. (First published 2008, updated 2013.) *Weight-control information network: Choosing a safe and successful weight-loss program.* http://win.niddk.nih.gov.
68. Weiss, F. (2004). Group psychotherapy with obese disordered-eating adults with body-image disturbances: An integrated model. *American Journal of Psychotherapy, 58* (3), 281–303.
69. U.S. Food and Drug Administration. (2010). *Questions and answers: Orlistat and severe liver injury.* http://www.fda.gov.
70. American Society for Metabolic and Bariatric Surgery. (2012). *Fact sheet:*

Metabolic and bariatric surgery. http://asmbs.org/asmbs-press-kit.
71. Ebell, M. (2008). Predicting mortality risk in patients undergoing bariatric surgery. *American Family Physician, 77* (2), 220–221.
72. Thomas, O. (2011, February 9). Apps to share your pride at the gym. *The New York Times.* http://www.nytimes.com.
73. Bair, C., Kelly, N., Serdar, K., & Mazzeo, S. (2012). Does the Internet function like magazines? An exploration of image-focused media, eating pathology, and body dissatisfaction. *Eating Behaviors, 13* (4), 398–401.
74. Mayo Clinic. (2010). *Body dysmorphic disorder.* http://www.mayoclinic.com.
75. Hart, E., Leary, M., & Rejeski, W. (1989). The measurement of social physique anxiety. *Journal of Sport Exercise Psychology, 11* (1), 94–104.
76. Hagger, M., & Stevenson, A. (2010). Social physique anxiety and physical self-esteem: Gender and age effects. *Psychology and Health, 25* (1), 89–110.
77. National Institute of Mental Health. (2011). *Eating disorders among children.* http://www.nimh.nih.gov.
78. National Institute of Mental Health. (Date of publication not reported.) *Eating disorders among adults—anorexia nervosa.* http://www.nimh.nih.gov.
79. Swanson, S., Crow, S., LeGrange, D., Swendsen, J., & Merikangas, K. (2011). Prevalence and correlates of eating disorders in adolescents: Results from the national comorbidity survey replication adolescent supplement. *Archives of General Psychiatry, 68* (7), 714–723.
80. Steinhausen, H. (2009). Outcomes of eating disorders. *Child and Adolescent Psychiatric Clinics of North America, 18,* 225–242.
81. Mayo Clinic. (2012). *Anorexia nervosa: Causes.* http://www.mayoclinic.com.
82. Gowers, S., Clark, A., Roberts, C., Byford, S., Barrett, B., Griffiths, A., . . . Roots, P. (2010.) A randomised controlled multicentre trial of treatments for adolescent anorexia nervosa including assessment of cost-effectiveness and patient acceptability—the TOuCAN trial. *Health Technologies Assessment, 14* (15), 1–98.
83. U.S. Department of Health and Human Services, National Guideline Clearinghouse. (2011). *Practice guideline for the treatment of patients with eating disorders.* http://guideline.gov.
84. Salahi, L. (2012, April 19). Internet crackdown on pro-anorexia sites. ABCNews.com. http://abcnews.go.com.
85. National Institute of Mental Health. (Date of publication not reported.) *Eating disorders among adults—bulimia nervosa.* http://www.nimh.nih.gov.
86. National Institute of Mental Health. (2011). *Eating disorders: What are the different types of eating disorders?* http://www.nimh.nih.gov.
87. U.S. Department of Health and Human Services, Office on Women's Health. (2009). *Bulimia nervosa fact sheet.* http://womenshealth.gov.
88. National Institute of Mental Health. (Date of publication not reported.) *Eating*

disorders among adults—binge eating disorder. http://www.nimh.nih.gov.
89. Eisenberg, D., Nicklett, E. J., Roeder, K., & Kirz, N. E. (2011). Eating disorder symptoms among college students Prevalence, persistence, correlates, and treatment-seeking. *Journal of American College Health, 59* (8), 700–707.
90. Rand, C., Macgregory, A., & Stunkard, A. (1997). The night eating syndrome in the general population and among postoperative obesity surgery patients. *International Journal of Eating Disorders, 22* (1), 65–69.
91. Nolan, L., & Geliebter, A. (2012). Night eating is associated with emotional and external eating in college students. *Eating Behaviors, 13,* 202–206.
92. American College of Sports Medicine. (2011). *The female athlete triad.* http://www.acsm.org.
93. Deimel, J., & Dunlap, B. (2012). The female athlete triad. *Clinical Journal of Sports Medicine, 2,* 247–254.

Chapter 7

i. Substance Abuse and Mental Health Services Administration. (2012). *Results from the 2011 National Survey on Drug Use and Health: Summary of National Findings* (NSDUH Series H-44, HHS Publication No. [SMA] 12-4713). Rockville, MD: Author. http://www.samhsa.gov
ii. Jones, C. M., Mack, K. A., & Paulozzi, L. J. (2013). Pharmaceutical overdose deaths, United States, 2010. *Journal of the American Medical Association, 309*(7), 657–659. doi: 10.1001/jama.2013.272
iii. American College Health Association. (2013). *American College Health Association national college health assessment (ACHA-NCHA II): Reference group executive summary, fall 2012.* http://www.acha-ncha.org
1. Jones, C. M., Mack, K. A., & Paulozzi, L. J. (2013). Pharmaceutical overdose deaths, United States, 2010. *Journal of the American Medical Association, 309*(7), 657–659. doi: 10.1001/jama.2013.272
2. Lawyer, S., Resnick, H., Bakanic, V., Burkett, T., & Kilpatrick, D. (2010, March–April). Forcible, drug-facilitated, and incapacitated rape and sexual assault among undergraduate women. *Journal of American College of Health, 58*(5), 453–460.
3. Substance Abuse and Mental Health Services Administration. (2012). *Results from the 2011 National Survey on Drug Use and Health: Summary of National Findings* (NSDUH Series H-44, HHS Publication No. [SMA] 12-4713). Rockville, MD: Author. http://www.samhsa.gov
4. National Council on Problem Gambling. (2013, March). *FAQs: Problem gamblers.* http://www.ncpgambling.org
5. American Society of Addiction Medicine. (2011, April 19). Definition of addiction. *ASAM Public Policy Statement.* http://www.asam.org

6. American Psychiatric Association. (2012). *DSM-5 development.* http://www.dsm5.org
7. National Center for Responsible Gaming. (2012). *Fact sheet: Gambling disorders among college students.* http://www.collegegambling.org
8. Society for the Advancement of Sexual Health. (2011). *Sexual addiction.* Retrieved from http://www.sash.net
9. Koran, L. M., Faber, R. J., Aboujaoude, E., Large, M. D., & Serpe, R. T. (2006). Estimated prevalence of compulsive buying behavior in the United States. *American Journal of Psychiatry, 163*(10), 1806–1812.
10. Weinstein, A., & Lejoyeux, M. (2010). Internet addiction or excessive Internet use. *American Journal of Drug and Alcohol Abuse, 36*(5), 277–283. doi: 10.3109/00952990.2010.491880
11. CTIA Media. (2011). *50 wireless quickfacts.* http://www.ctia.org
12. Lenhart, A. (2010, September 2). Adults, cell phones, and texting. *Pew Internet and American Life Project.* http://pewresearch.org
13. National Drug Intelligence Center. (2011, April). *The economic impact of illicit drug use on American society.* Washington DC: United States Department of Justice. http://www.justice.gov
14. American College Health Association. (2013). *American College Health Association national college health assessment (ACHA-NCHA II): Reference group executive summary, fall 2012.* http://www.acha-ncha.org
15. American Psychiatric Association. (1994). *Diagnostic and statistical manual of mental disorders* (4th ed.). Washington, DC: American Psychiatric Publishing.
16. United States Office of National Drug Control Policy. (2011). *Epidemic: Responding to America's prescription drug abuse crisis.* Washington, DC: Drug Enforcement Agency. http://www.whitehousedrugpolicy.org
17. Substance Abuse and Mental Health Services Administration, Center for Behavioral Health Statistics and Quality. (2010). *Drug abuse warning network, 2008: National estimates of drug-related emergency department visits.* http://www.oas.samhsa.gov
18. U.S. Food and Drug Administration and the Consumer Healthcare Products Association. (2010). *Over-the-counter medicines: What's right for you?* http://www.fda.gov
19. U.S. Food and Drug Administration. (2009, February 23). *A guide to safe use of pain medicine.* http://www.fda.gov
20. U.S. Food and Drug Administration. (2012, October 22). *Consumer updates: Using over-the-counter cough and cold products in children.* http://www.fda.gov
21. National Institute on Drug Abuse. (2012, December). *NIDA InfoFacts: Marijuana.* http://www.nida.nih.gov
22. Daling, J. R., Doody, D. R., Sun, X., Trabert, B. L., Weiss, N. S., Chen, C., . . . Schwartz, S. M. (2009, March 15). Association of marijuana use and the incidence of testicular germ cell tumors. *Cancer, 115*(6), 1215–1223.

23. Weng, X., Odouli, R., & Li, D. (2008). Maternal caffeine consumption during pregnancy and the risk of miscarriage: A prospective cohort study. *American Journal of Obstetrics & Gynecology, 198*(3), 279e1–279e8.

24. National Institute on Drug Abuse. (2010, March). *NIDA InfoFacts: Methamphetamine.* http://www.drugabuse.gov

25. National Institute on Drug Abuse. (2012, November). *DrugFacts: Synthetic cathinones ("bath salts").* http://www.drugabuse.gov

26. National Institute on Drug Abuse. (2012, December). *Club drugs.* http://www.drugabuse.gov

27. National Institute on Drug Abuse. (2012, December). *NIDA InfoFacts: MDMA (ecstasy).* http://www.drugabuse.gov

28. National Institute on Drug Abuse. (2012, December). *Inhalants.* http://www.drugabuse.gov

29. National Library of Medicine. (2013, February). Barbiturate intoxication and overdose. *MedlinePlus.* http://www.nlm.nih.gov

30. National Institute on Drug Abuse. (2010, March). *DrugFacts: Heroin.* http://www.drugabuse.gov

31. The Partnership at Drugfree.org. (2011). *Preventing teen abuse of prescription drugs.* http://www.drugfree.org

32. National Institute on Drug Abuse. (2010, August). *Drugs, brains, and behavior: The science of addiction* (NIH Pub. No. 10-5605). http://www.drugabuse.gov

33. Office of National Drug Control Policy. (2011). *National youth anti-drug media campaign.* http://www.mediacampaign.org

34. Occupational Safety and Health Administration. (2011). *Workplace substance abuse.* http://www.osha.gov

35. Executive Office of the President of the United States. (2010). *Executive summary: 2010 national drug control strategy.* http://www.whitehousedrugpolicy.gov

36. Narcotics Anonymous. (2010, May). *Information about NA.* http://www.na.org

37. Augsburg College. (2011). *StepUP program: Outcomes.* http://www.augsburg.edu

38. National Institute on Drug Abuse. (2009, September). *NIDA InfoFacts: Treatment approaches for drug addiction.* http://www.drugabuse.gov

39. Substance Abuse and Mental Health Services Administration, Center for Behavioral Statistics and Quality. (2012, July 12). *The DAWN report: Outcomes of drug-related emergency department visits associated with polydrug use.* Rockville, MD: Author. http://www.samhsa.gov

40. National Institutes of Health. (2012, March). *Diet and substance abuse recovery.* http://www.nlm.nih.gov

41. The Partnership at Drugfree.org. (2013). *6 Things you need to know about relapse.* http://www.drugfree.org

42. National Institute on Drug Abuse. (2012). *Principles of drug addiction treatment: A research-based guide* (3rd ed.) (NIH Publication No. 12–4180). http://www.drugabuse.gov

Chapter 8

i. National Institute on Alcohol Abuse and Alcoholism. (2010). *Rethinking drinking: Alcohol and your health.* http://rethinkingdrinking.niaaa.nih.gov

ii. American College Health Association. (2013). *American College Health Association National College Health Assessment (ACHA-NCHA II): UNDERGRADUATE STUDENTS— Reference Group Executive Summary, Fall 2012.* http://www.acha-ncha.org

iii. Centers for Disease Control and Prevention. (2012). *Fact Sheet—fast facts: Smoking and tobacco use.* http://www.cdc.gov

1. Substance Abuse and Mental Health Services Administration. (2012). *Results from the 2011 national survey on drug use and health: National findings.* http://www.samhsa.gov

2. National Institutes of Health. (2010). *Fact Sheet: Alcohol-related traffic deaths.* http://www.nih.gov

3. Carpenter, C., & Dobkin, C. (2011). The minimum legal drinking age and public health. *Journal of Economic Perspectives, 25*(2), 133–156.

4. McCartt, A. T., Hellinga, L. A., & Kirley, B. B. (2010). The effects of minimum legal drinking age 21 laws on alcohol-related driving in the United States. *Journal of Safety Research, 41*(2) 173–181.

5. Fell, J. C. (2008). The relationship of underage drinking laws to reductions in drinking drivers in fatal crashes in the United States. *Accident Analysis and Prevention, 40*(4), 1430–1440.

6. American College Health Association. (2013). *American College Health Association National College Health Assessment (ACHA-NCHA II): UNDERGRADUATE STUDENTS— Reference Group Executive Summary, Fall 2012.* http://www.acha-ncha.org

7. National Institute on Alcohol Abuse and Alcoholism. (2004, Winter). Binge drinking defined. *NIAAA Newsletter* (No. 3). http://pubs.niaaa.nih.gov

8. Silveri, M. M (2012). Adolescent brain development and underage drinking in the United States: Identifying risks of alcohol use in college populations. *Harvard Review of Psychiatry, 20*(4), 189–200.

9. National Institute on Alcohol Abuse and Alcoholism. (2010). *Rethinking drinking: Alcohol and your health.* http://rethinkingdrinking.niaaa.nih.gov

10. Hingson, R. W. (2010). Focus on: College drinking and related problems— magnitude and prevention of college drinking related problems. *Alcohol Research Health, 33*(1), 45–54.

11. National Institute on Alcohol Abuse and Alcoholism. (2010). Snapshot of annual high-risk college drinking consequences. http://www.collegedrinkingprevention.gov

12. Mikhailovich, K., George, A., Rickwood, D., & Parker, R. (2011). A duty of care: Non-drinkers and alcohol related harm among an Australian university sample. *Journal of Higher Education Policy and Management, 33*(6), 595–604.

13. Hingson, R. W., Zha, W., & Weitzman, E. R. (2009). Magnitude of and trends in alcohol-related mortality and morbidity among U.S. college students ages 18–24, 1998–2005. *Journal of Studies on Alcohol and Drugs* (Suppl. 16), 12–20.

14. Wechsler, H., & Nelson, T. F. (2008). What we have learned from the Harvard School of Public Health College alcohol study: Focusing attention on college student alcohol consumption and the environmental conditions that promote it. *Journal of Studies on Alcohol and Drugs, 69*(4), 481–490.

15. Courtney, K., & Polich, J. (2009). Binge drinking in young adults: Data, definitions, and determinants. *Psychological Bulletin, 135*(1), 142–156.

16. Turrisi, R., & Ray, A. E. (2010). Sustained parenting and college drinking in first-year students. *Developmental Psychobiology, 52*(3), 286–294.

17. Kerr, W. C., Greenfield, T. K., Tujague, J., & Brown, S. E. (2005). A drink is a drink? Variation in the amount of alcohol contained in beer, wine and spirits drinks in a U.S. methodological sample. *Alcoholism: Clinical and Experimental Research, 29*(11), 2015–2021.

18. Meier, P., & Seitz, H. K. (2008). Age, alcohol metabolism, and liver disease. *Current Opinion in Clinical Nutrition and Metabolic Care, 11*(1), 21–26.

19. Centers for Disease Control and Prevention. (2011.) *Injury prevention and control: Motor vehicle safety—effects of blood alcohol concentration.* http://www.cdc.gov

20. Lembke, A., Bradley, K. A., Henderson, P., Moos, R., & Harris, A. (2011). Alcohol screening scores and the risk of new-onset gastrointestinal illness or related hospitalization. *Journal of General Internal Medicine, 26*(7), 777–782.

21. Rohsenow, D. J., & Howland, J. (2010). The role of beverage congeners in hangover and other residual effects of alcohol intoxication: A review. *Current Drug Abuse Reviews, 3*(2), 76–79.

22. Penning, R., van Nuland, M., Fliervoet, L. A., Olivier, B., & Verster, J. C. (2010). The pathology of alcohol hangover. *Current Drug Abuse Reviews, 3*(2), 68075.

23. Nelson, D. E., Jaman, D. W., Rehm, J., Greenfield, T. K., Rey, G., Kerr, W. C., . . . Naimi, T. S. (2013). Alcohol-attributable cancer deaths and years of potential life lost in the United States. *American Journal of Public Health.* e-View Ahead of Print. doi: 10.2105/AJPH.2012.301199

24. Brooks, P. J., Enoch, M. A., Goldman, D., Li, T. K., & Yokoyama, A. (2009). The alcohol flushing response: An unrecognized risk factor for esophageal cancer from alcohol consumption. *PLoS Medicine, 6*(3), e1000050.

25. Yoon, Y., & Yi, H. (2012). *Liver cirrhosis mortality in the United States, 1970–2009.* National Institute on Alcohol Abuse and Alcoholism (Surveillance Report No. 93).

26. American Medical Association. (2010). *Harmful consequences of alcohol use on the brains of children, adolescents, and college students.* http://www.ama-assn.org

27. SAMHSA Fetal Alcohol Spectrum Disorders Center for Excellence. (2013). *The FASD Center.* http://fasdcenter.samhsa.gov

28. Substance Abuse and Mental Health Services Administration. (2012). *Results from the 2011 national survey on drug use and health: National findings.* http://www.samhsa.gov

29. National Highway Traffic Safety Administration. (2007, December). Fatalities related to alcohol-impaired driving during the Christmas and New Year's Day holiday periods. *Traffic Safety Facts* (DOT HS 810 870). http://www-nrd.nhtsa.dot.gov

30. National Highway Traffic Safety Administration. (2009). *Ignition interlocks: What you need to know.* www.nhtsa.gov

31. Wechsler, H., Lee, J. E., Kuo, M., Seibring, M., Nelson, T. F., & Lee, H. (2002). Trends in college binge drinking during a period of increased prevention efforts: Findings from 4 Harvard School of Public Health college alcohol study surveys: 1993–2001. *Journal of American College Health, 50*(5), 203–217.

32. Hingson, R., Heeren, T., Winter, M., & Wechsler, H. (2005). Magnitude of alcohol-related mortality and morbidity among U.S. college students ages 18–24: Changes from 1998 to 2001. *Annual Review of Public Health, 26,* 259–279.

33. Hufford, M. R. (2001). Alcohol and suicidal behavior. *Clinical Psychology Review, 21,* 797–811.

34. Grant, B., Dawson, D., Stinson, F., Chou, S., Dufour, M., & Pickering, R. (2004). The 12-month prevalence and trends in DSM–IV alcohol abuse and dependence in the United States, 1991–1992 and 2001–2002. *Drug and Alcohol Dependence, 74*(3), 223–234.

35. Moss, H. B., Chen, C. M., & Yi, H. Y. (2007). Subtypes of alcohol dependence in a nationally representative sample. *Drug and Alcohol Dependence, 91*(2–3), 149–158.

36. National Institute on Alcohol Abuse and Alcoholism. (2010, February). Alcoholism isn't what it used to be. *NIAAA Spectrum, 2*(1). http://www.spectrum.niaaa.nih.gov

37. Cronce, J. M. (2011). Individual-focused approaches to the prevention of college student drinking. *Alcohol Research and Health, 34*(2), 210–221.

38. National Institute on Alcohol Abuse and Alcoholism. (1989). Relapse and craving. *Alcohol Alert,* No. 6; PH 277. http://pubs.niaaa.nih.gov

39. National Institute on Alcohol Abuse and Alcoholism. (2010). *Rethinking drinking: Alcohol and your health: Tips to try.* http://rethinkingdrinking.niaaa.nih.gov

40. American Boating Association. (2010). *Alcohol & BWI: Why we must get BADD.* http://www.americanboating.org

41. University of Texas at Dallas. (2010). *How to help a friend.* http://www.utdallas.edu

42. Students Against Destructive Decisions. (2010). *SADD's mission.* http://www.sadd.org

43. Centers for Disease Control and Prevention. (2012). *Fact Sheet—fast facts: Smoking and tobacco use.* http://www.cdc.gov

44. National Center for Health Statistics. (2008). *Health, United States, 2008, with special feature on the health of young adults.* http://www.cdc.gov

45. Danaei, G., Ding, E., Mozaffarian, D., Taylor, B., Rehm, J., Murray, C., & Ezzati, M. (2009, April 28). The preventable causes of death in the United States: Comparative risk assessment of dietary, lifestyle, and metabolic risk factors. *PLoS Medicine, 6*(4), e1000058. doi: 10.1371/journal.pmed.1000058. Epub 2009 Apr 28.

46. Agrawal, A., & Lynskey, M. T. (2008). Are there genetic influences on addiction? Evidence from family, adoption and twin studies. *Addiction, 103*(5), 1069–1081.

47. Greenbaum, L., & Lerer, B. (2009). Differential contribution of genetic variation in multiple brain nicotinic cholinergic receptors to nicotine dependence: Recent progress and emerging open questions. *Molecular Psychiatry, 14,* 912–945.

48. Munafo, M. R., & Johnstone, E. C. (2008). Genes and cigarette smoking. *Addiction, 103*(6), 893–904.

49. Gilman, S., Rende, R., Boergers, J., Abrams, D., Buka, S., Clark, M., . . . Niaura, R. (2009.) Parental smoking and adolescent smoking initiation: An intergenerational perspective on tobacco control. *Pediatrics, 123*(2), 274–281.

50. Ling, P., Neilands, T., & Glantz S. (2009.) Young adult smoking behavior: A national survey. *American Journal of Preventive Medicine, 36*(5), 389–394.

51. Campaign for Tobacco-Free Kids. (2009). *The path to smoking addiction starts at very young ages.* http://www.tobaccofreekids.org

52. Song, A. V., Morrell, H. E. R., Cornell, J. L., Ramos, M. E., Biehl, M., Kropp, R. Y., & Halpern-Feisher, B. L. (2009, March). Perceptions of smoking-related risks and benefits as pre-dictors of adolescent smoking initiation. *American Journal of Public Health, 99*(3), 487–492.

53. Helweg-Larsen, M., & Nielsen, G. A. (2009, January). Smoking cross-culturally: Risk perceptions among young adults in Denmark and the United States. *Psychology and Health, 24*(1), 81–93.

54. Koval, J. J., Pederson, L. L., Zhang, X., Mowery, P., & McKenna, M. (2008, September). Can young adult smoking status be predicted from concern about body weight and self-reported BMI among adolescents? Results from a ten-year cohort study. *Nicotine and Tobacco Research, 10*(9), 1449–1455.

55. National Cancer Institute. (2008). The role of the media in promoting and reducing tobacco use. *NCI Tobacco Control Monograph Series.* http://cancercontrol.cancer.gov

56. U.S. Department of Health and Human Services. (2010). *How tobacco smoke causes disease: The biology and behavioral basis for smoking-attributable disease: A report of the Surgeon General.* Atlanta, GA: U.S. Department of Health and Human Services, Centers for Disease Control and Prevention, National Center for Chronic Disease Prevention and Health Promotion, Office on Smoking and Health. http://www.cdc.gov

57. Jha, P., Ramasundarahettige, C., Landsman, V., Rostron, B., Thun, M., Anderson, R. N., . . . Peto, R. (2013). 21st-Century hazards of smoking and benefits of cessation in the United States. *New England Journal of Medicine, 368,* 341–350.

58. American Cancer Society. (2009). *Cigarette smoking.* http://www.cancer.org

59. Kochanek, K., Xu, J., Murphy, S., Miniño, A, & Kung, H. (2011). Deaths: Final data for 2009. *National Vital Statistics Reports, 60*(3). http://www.cdc.gov

60. American Lung Association. (2012). *COPD.* Retrieved from http://www.lungusa.org/lung-disease/copd

61. Centers for Disease Control and Prevention. (2008, November 14). Smoking-attributable mortality, years of potential life lost, and productivity losses: United States, 2000–2004. *Morbidity and Mortality Weekly Report, 57*(45), 1226–1228. Retrieved from http://www.cdc.gov/mmwr/preview/mmwrhtml/mm5745a3.htm

62. Centers for Disease Control and Prevention. (2009). *Tobacco use and pregnancy.* http://www.cdc.gov

63. Salihu, H. M., Aliyu, M. H., Pierre-Louis, B. J., & Alexander, G. R. (2003). Levels of excess infant deaths attributable to maternal smoking during pregnancy in the United States. *Maternal and Child Health Journal, 7*(4), 219–227.

64. U.S. Department of Health and Human Services. (2006). *The health consequences of involuntary exposure to tobacco smoke: A report of the surgeon general.* http://www.surgeongeneral.gov

65. California Environmental Protection Agency. (2005). *Identification of environmental tobacco smoke as a toxic air contaminant: Executive Summary.*

66. American Cancer Society. (2009). *Cigar smoking.* http://www.cancer.org

67. National Cancer Institute. (2009). *Cigar smoking and cancer (Fact Sheet).* http://www.cancer.gov

68. Centers for Disease Control and Prevention. (2009). *Bidis and kreteks.* http://www.cdc.gov

69. Severson, H. H., Klein, K., & Lichtenstein, E. (2005). Smokeless tobacco use among professional baseball players: Survey results, 1998 to 2003. *Tobacco Control, 14,* 31–36.

70. Nemeth, J. M, Lui, S. T., Klein, E., Ferketich, A. K., Kwan, M. & Wewers, M. E. (2012). Factors influencing smokeless tobacco use in rural Ohio Appalachia. *Journal of Community Health, 37*(6), 1208–1217.

71. Centers for Disease Control and Prevention. (2012). Youth risk behavior surveillance—United States, 2011. *Morbidity and Mortality Weekly Report, 61*(4).

72. Centers for Disease Control and Prevention. (2010.) State-specific prevalence of cigarette smoking and smokeless tobacco use among adults—United States, 2009. *Morbidity and Mortality Weekly Report, 59*(43), 1400–1406.

73. Morrell, H., Cohen, L., Bacchi, D., & West, J. (2005). Predictors of smoking and smokeless tobacco use in college students: A preliminary study using web-based survey methodology. *Journal of American College Health, 54*(6), 108–115.

74. U.S. Food and Drug Administration. (2011). *Electronic cigarettes.* http://www.fda.gov

75. Centers for Disease Control and Prevention. (2012). Current cigarette smoking among adults: United States, 2011. *Morbidity and Mortality Weekly Report, 61*(44), 889–894.

76. Cosgrove, K. P. (2009). B2-nicotinic acetylcholine receptor availability during acute and prolonged abstinence from tobacco smoking. *Archives of General Psychiatry, 66*(6), 666–667.

77. National Cancer Institute. (2008, October). *Clearing the air: Quit smoking today* (NIH Publi-cation No. 08-1647). http://www.smokefree.gov

78. Harris, K. J., Stearns, J. N., Kovach, R. G., & Harrar, S. W. (2009, September/October). En-forcing an outdoor smoking ban on a college campus: Effects of a multicomponent approach. *Journal of American College Health, 58*(2), 121–126.

79. American College Health Association. (2011.) *ACHA guidelines—position statement on tobacco on college and university campuses.* http://www.acha.org

Chapter 9

i. Facebook Newsroom. (2013). *Key facts.* http://newsroom.fb.com

ii. Copen, C., Daniels, K., & Mosher, W. (2013.) First premarital cohabitation in the United States: 2006–2010 national survey of family growth. *National Health Statistics Reports, 64,* 1–16.

iii. Cohn, D., Passel, J., Wang, W., & Livingston, G. (2011). Barely half of U.S. adults are married—a record low. *Pew Research Social and Demographic Trends.* http://www.pewsocialtrends.org

1. Jourard, S. M. (1971). *The transparent self.* New York: D. Van Nostrand.

2. University of Pennsylvania Faculty/Staff Assistance Program. (n.d.). *Conflict resolution: How to fight fair so that everyone wins.* http://www.upenn.edu

3. Kimbrough, A. M., Guadgno, R. E., Muscanell, N. L., & Dill, J. (2012). Gender differences in mediated communication: Women connect more than do men. *Computers in Human Behavior, 29,* 896–900.

4. Tannen, D. (1991), *You just don't understand: Women and men in conversation.* New York: Ballantine Books.

5. Gray, J. (1992). *Men are from Mars, women are from Venus.* New York: HarperCollins.

6. Schuetz, A. (1998). Autobiographical narratives of good and bad deeds: Defensive and favorable self-description moderated by trait self-esteem. *Journal of Social and Clinical Psychology, 17,* 466–475.

7. Bellavia, G., & Murray, S. (2003). Did I do that? Self-esteem–related differences in reactions to romantic partners' moods. *Personal Relationships, 10*(1), 77–95.

8. Bowlby, J. (1982). *Attachment and loss: Vol. 1, attachment* (2nd ed.). New York: Basic Books.

9. Kilmann, P. R., Urbaniak, G. C., & Parnell, M. M. (2006). Effects of attachment-focused versus relationship skills-focused group interventions for college students with insecure attachment patterns. *Attachment & Human Development, 8*(1), 47–62.

10. Gurian, A. (n.d.). *Depression in adolescence: Does gender matter?* NYC Child Study Center. http://www.aboutourkids.org

11. Katz-Wise, S. L., Priess, H. A., & Hyde, J. S. (2010). Gender-role attitudes and behavior across the transition to parenthood. *Developmental Psychology, 46*(1), 18–28.

12. Ertel, K. A., Glymour, M., & Berkman, L.F. (2009). Social networks and health: A life course perspective integrating observational and experimental evidence. *Journal of Social and Personal Relationships, 26,* 73–92.

13. McPherson, M., Smith-Lovin, L., & Brashears, M. E. (2006). Social isolation in America: Changes in core discussion networks over two decades. *American Sociological Review, 71*(3), 353–375.

14. Swami, V., Chamorro-Premuzic, T., Sinniah, D., Maniam, T., Kannan, K., & Stanistreet, D. (2007). General health mediates the relationship between loneliness, life satisfaction and depression. *Social Psychiatry and Psychiatric Epidemiology, 42,* 161–166.

15. Hampton, K., Goulet, L., Her, E., & Rainie, B. (2009). Social isolation and new technology. *Pew Internet and American Life Project.* http://www.pewinternet.org

16. Hefner, J., & Eisenberg, D. (2009). Social support and mental health among college students. *American Journal of Orthopsychiatry, 79*(4), 491–499.

17. Ledbetter, A. M., Griffin, E. M., & Sparks, G. G. (2007). Forecasting "friends forever": A longitudinal investigation of sustained closeness between best friends. *Personal Relationships, 14*(2), 343–350.

18. Sternberg, R. J. (1986). A triangular theory of love. *Psychological Review, 93,* 119–135.

19. Association for Psychological Science. (2008, February 14). Beauty bias: Can people love the one they are compatible with?.*ScienceDaily.* http://www.sciencedaily.com

20. Swami, V., Furnham, A., Chamorro-Premuzic, T., Akbar, K., Gordon, N., Harris, T., Finch, J., & Tovee, M. J. (2010). More than just skin deep? Personality information influences men's ratings

of the attractiveness of women's body sizes. *The Journal of Social Psychology, 150*(6) 628–647.

21. Claxton, A., O'Rourke, N., Smith, J. Z., & Delongis, A. (2012). Personality traits and marital satisfaction within enduring relationships: An intra-couple discrepancy approach, *Journal of Social and Personal Relationships, 29*(3) 375–396.

22. Copen, C., Daniels, K., & Mosher, W. (2013). First premarital cohabitation in the United States: 2006–2010 national survey of family growth. *National Health Statistics Reports, 64*, 1–16.

23. Bradshaw, C., Kahn, A. S., & Saville, B. K. (2010). To hook up or date: Which gender benefits? *Sex Roles, 62*(9-10), 661–669.

24. Owen, J. J., Rhoades, G. K., Stanley, S. M., & Fincham, F. D. (2010). "Hooking up" among college students: Demographic and psychosocial correlates. *Achieves of Sexual Behavior, 39*, 653–663.

25. Owen, J. J., & Fincham, F. D. (2011). Young adults' emotional reactions after hooking up encounters. *Achieves of Sexual Behavior, 40*, 321–330.

26. Gates, G. (2011). *How many people are lesbian, gay, bisexual and transgender?* The Williams Institute, UCLA School of Law. http://williamsinstitute.law.ucla.edu

27. Gohn, L., & Albin, G. (2006). *Understanding college student subpopulations: A guide for student affairs professionals.* Washington, DC: National Association of Student Personnel Administrators.

28. Roisman, G. I., Clausell, E., Holland, A., Fortuna, K., & Elieff, C. (2008). Adult romantic relationships as contexts of human development: A multimethod comparison of same-sex couples with opposite-sex dating, engaged, and married dyads. *Developmental Psychology, 44*(1), 91–101.

29. Balsam, K. F., Beauchaine, T. P., Rothblum, E. D., & Solomon, S. E. (2008). Three-year follow-up of same-sex couples who had civil unions in Vermont, same-sex couples not in civil unions, and heterosexual married couples. *Developmental Psychology, 44*(1), 102–116.

30. Madureira, A. F. A. (2007). The psychological basis of homophobia: Cultural construction of a barrier. *Integrative Psychological & Behavioral Science, 41*, 225–247.

31. Cummings, E., El-Sheikh, M., Kouros, C. D., & Buckhalt, J. A. (2009). Children and violence: The role of children's regulation in the marital aggression-child adjustment link. *Clinical Child Family Psychological Review, 12*, 3–15.

32. Lyness, D. (2008). Am I in a healthy relationship? *TeensHealth from Nemours.* http://kidshealth.org

33. Barelds, D. P. H., & Dijkstra, P. (2006). Reactive, anxious and possessive forms of jealousy and their relation to relationship quality among heterosexuals and homosexuals. *Journal of Homosexuality, 51*(3), 183–198.

34. HealthyPlace.com. (2009, January 13). *How to deal with a jealous partner.* http://www.healthyplace.com

35. Lyness, D. (2010). Getting over a breakup. *TeensHealth from Nemours.* http://kidshealth.org

36. Harris Interactive. http://iac.mediaroom.com

37. Copen, C. E., Daniels, K., Vespa, J., & Mosher, W. D. (2012). First marriages in the United States: Data from the 2006–2010 national survey of family growth. *National Health Statistics Reports, 49*, 1–22.

38. Human Rights Campaign. (n.d.) *FAQs: Questions about same-sex marriage.* http://www.hrc.org

39. Hymowitz, K., Carroll, J., Wilcox, W., & Kaye, K. (2012.) *Knot yet: The benefits and costs of delayed marriage in America.* The National Marriage Project at the University of Virginia. http://nationalmarriageproject.org

40. Rhoades, G. K., Stanley, S. M., & Markman, H. J. (2009). The pre-engagement cohabitation effect: A replication and extension of previous findings. *Journal of Family Psychology, 23*(1), 107–111.

41. Goodwin, P. Y., Mosher, W. D., & Chandra, A. (2010). Marriage and cohabitation in the United States: A statistical portrait based on cycle 6 (2002) of the national survey of family growth. In *Vital and Health Statistics* (Series 23, No. 28). Atlanta, GA: National Center for Health Statistics, Centers for Disease Control and Prevention.

42. Karasu, S. R. (2007). The institution of marriage: Terminable or interminable? *American Journal of Psychotherapy, 61*(1), 1–16.

43. Wilcox, W. B., Doherty, W., Glenn N., & Waite, L. (2005). *Why marriage matters: Twenty-six conclusions from the social sciences* (2nd ed.). New York: Institute for American Values.

44. Koball, H. L., Moiduddin, E., Henderson, J., Goesling, B., & Besculides, M. (2010). What do we know about the link between marriage and health? *Journal of Family Issues, 31*(8), 1019–1040.

45. Popenoe, D., & Whitehead, B. D. (2007). *The state of our unions, 2007: The social health of marriage in America.* Piscataway, NJ: The National Marriage Project, Rutgers University.

46. Garrison, M. (2007). The decline of formal marriage: Inevitable or reversible? *Family Law Quarterly, 41*(3), 491–520.

47. Falke, S. I., & Larson, J. H. (2007). Premarital predictors of remarital quality: Implications for clinicians. *Contemporary Family Therapy, 29*, 9–23.

48. National Vital Statistics System, Centers for Disease Control and Prevention. (2013). *National marriage and divorce rate trends.* http://www.cdc.gov

49. Amato, P. R., & Hohmann-Marriott, B. (2007). A comparison of high- and low-distress marriages that end in divorce. *Journal of Marriage and Family, 69*, 621–638.

50. American Psychological Association. (2004). *Marital education programs help keep couples together.* http://www.apa.org

51. Kalmijn, M., & Monden, C. W. S. (2006). Are the negative effects of divorce on well-being dependent on marital quality? *Journal of Marriage and Family, 68*, 1197–1213.

52. Amato, P. A. (2010). Research on divorce: Continuing trends and new developments. *Journal of Marriage and Family, 72*, 650–666.

53. Riggio, H. R., & Fite, J. E. (2006). Attitudes toward divorce: Embeddedness and outcomes in personal relationships. *Journal of Applied Social Psychology, 36*(12), 2935–2962.

54. Copen, C., Daniels, K., & Mosher, W. (2013). First premarital cohabitation in the United States: 2006–2010 national survey of family growth. *National Health Statistics Reports, 64*, 1–16.

55. U.S. Census Bureau. (2008). *Marital status, 2006–2008 American community survey 3-year estimates* (S1201). http://factfinder.census.gov

56. Hymowitz, K., Carroll, J., Wilcox, W., & Kaye, K. (2012). *Knot yet: The benefits and costs of delayed marriage in America.* The National Marriage Project at the University of Virginia. http://nationalmarriageproject.org

57. DePaulo, B. (2008, February 8). *Single and happy.* National Sexuality Research Center. http://nsrc.sfsu.edu

58. National Center for Health Statistics, Centers for Disease Control and Prevention. (2009). Birth expectations. In *Key statistics from the national survey of family growth.* http://www.cdc.gov

59. Jiang, L., & O'Neill, B. C. (2007). Impacts of demographic trends on household size and structure. *Population and Development Review, 33*(3), 567–591.

60. U.S. Census Bureau. (2010). Table C3: Living arrangements of children under 18 years/1 and marital status of parents, by age, sex, race, and Hispanic origin/2 and selected characteristics of the child for all children: 2009. In *Current population survey, 2009, annual social and economic supplement.* http://www.census.gov

61. Holzworth, A. N., & Radunovich, H. L. (2007). *Questions to ask as you consider parenthood: A couples' guide* (Publication No. FCS2271). Department of Family, Youth, and Community Sciences, Florida Cooperative Extension Service, IFAS, University of Florida, Gainesville.

62. Ansari, A. S., Sharma, A., & Lohiya, N. K. (2007). Does paternal occupation and lifestyle affect embryo quality? *Journal of Endocrinology & Reproduction, 11*(1), 15–22.

63. Larson, J. (1992). Understanding stepfamilies. *American Demographics, 14*, 360.

64. Michaels, M. (2007, March). Remarital issues in couple therapy. *Journal of Couple & Relationship Therapy, 6*(1/2), 125–139.

65. National Stepfamily Resource Center. (2010). *Stepfamily fact sheet.* http://www.stepfamilies.info

66. Speer, R. B., & Trees, A. R. (2007). The push and pull of stepfamily life: The contribution of stepchildren's autonomy and connection-seeking behaviors to role development in stepfamilies. *Communication Studies, 58*(4), 377–394.

67. U.S. Census Bureau. (2010). Table C2: Living arrangements of children under 18 years/1 and marital status of parents, by age, sex, race, and Hispanic origin/2 and selected characteristics of the child for all children: 2009. In *Current population survey, 2009, annual social and economic supplement.* Washington, DC: DeNavas-Walt, C., Proctor, B. D., & Smith, J. C.

68. Kreider, R. M. (2008). *Living arrangements of children: 2004* (Publication No. P70-114). Washington, DC: U.S. Census Bureau.

69. Williams, K., Sassler, S., & Nicholson, L. M. (2008). For better or for worse? The consequences of marriage and cohabitation for single mothers. *Social Forces, 86*(4), 1481–1511.

70. Amato, P. R. (2005). The impact of family formation change on the cognitive, social, and emotional well-being of the next generation. *The Future of Children, 15*(2), 75–96.

71. Kalmijn, M., & Monden, C. W. S. (2006). Are the negative effects of divorce on well-being dependent on marital quality? *Journal of Marriage and Family, 68*, 1197–1213.

72. Jackson, M. (2007, November 4). Going solo. *The Boston Globe.* http://www.boston.com

73. Riciutti, H. N. (2004). Single parenthood, achievement, and problem behavior in white, black, and Hispanic children. *Journal of Educational Research, 97*(4), 196–207.

74. Day, R. D. (2010). Stephen Gavazzi: Strong families, successful students: Helping teenagers reach their full potential. *Journal of Youth Adolescence, 39*, 704–705.

75. DeFrain, J., & Asay, S. M. (2007). Strong families around the world: An introduction to the family strengths perspective. *Marriage & Family Review, 41*(1/2), 1–10.

76. King, M. L., Jr. (1964). Speech in St. Louis, Missouri, March 22, 1964. Reprinted by permission of Writer's House LLC on behalf of the Estate of Martin Luther King, Jr.

77. Granovetter, M. (1973, May). The strength of weak ties. *American Journal of Sociology, 78*(6), 1360–1380.

78. Wickramasinghe, S. (2011, February 4). Learning to live together. *NDSU Spectrum.* http://www.ndsuspectrum.com

79. Patchin, J. W., & Hinduja, S. (2012). School-based efforts to prevent cyberbullying. *The Prevention Researcher, 19*(1), 7–9.

Chapter 10

i. American College Health Association. (2013). *American College Health Association National College Health Assessment (ACHA-NCHA II) reference group executive summary, fall 2012.* http://www.acha-ncha.org

ii. National Campaign to Prevent Teen and Unplanned Pregnancy and CosmoGirl.com. (2009). *Sex and tech: Results from a survey of teens and young adults*. http://www.thenationalcampaign.org

iii. National Campaign to Prevent Teen and Unplanned Pregnancy. (2010). *National data*. http://www.thenationalcampaign.org

1. Centers for Disease Control and Prevention. (2002). Folate status in women of childbearing age, by race/ethnicity. *Morbidity and Mortality Weekly, 51*(36), 808–810.

2. American College Health Association. (2013). *American College Health Association National College Health Assessment (ACHA-NCHA II) reference group executive summary, Fall 2012*. http://www.acha-ncha.org

3. National Cancer Institute. (2008). *What you need to know about prostate cancer*. http://www.cancer.gov

4. National Women's Health Information Center. (2009). *Menstruation and the menstrual cycle*. http://www.womenshealth.gov

5. American Congress of Obstetricians and Gynecologists. (2008). *Premenstrual syndrome*. http://www.acog.org

6. Dennerstein, L., Lehert, P., & Heinemann, K. (2012). Epidemiology of premenstrual symptoms and disorders. *Menopause International, 18*, 48–51.

7. National Women's Health Information Center. (2010). *Premenstrual syndrome frequently asked questions*. http://www.womenshealth.gov

8. National Women's Health Information Center. (2008). *Menstruation, menopause, and mental health*. http://www.womenshealth.gov

9. Latthe, P. M., Champaneria, R., & Khan, K. S. (2011). Dysmenorrhoea. *Clinical Evidence (Online). 2011; 2011: 0813*. http://www.ncbi.nlm.nih.gov

10. French, L. (2005). Dysmenorrhea. *American Family Physician, 71*(2), 285–291.

11. American Congress of Obstetricians and Gynecologists. (2008). *Endometriosis*. http://www.acog.org

12. Masters, W. H., & Johnson, V. E. (1966). *Human sexual response*. New York: Bantam.

13. American Society for Reproductive Medicine. (2008). *Patient fact sheet: Sexual dysfunction and infertility*. http://www.asrm.org

14. MedlinePlus. (2010). *Female sexual dysfunction*. http://www.nlm.nih.gov

15. Mayo Foundation for Medical Education and Research. (2009). *Painful intercourse (dyspareunia)*. http://www.mayoclinic.com

16. Mayo Foundation for Medical Education and Research. (2009). *Low sex drive in women*. http://www.mayoclinic.com

17. Mayo Foundation for Medical Education and Research. (2009). *Anorgasmia*. http://www.mayoclinic.com

18. National Kidney and Urologic Diseases Information Clearinghouse. (2012). *Erectile dysfunction* (NIH Publication No. 09-3923). http://kidney.niddk.nih.gov

19. MedlinePlus. (2008). *Premature ejaculation*. http://www.nlm.nih.gov

20. Mayo Foundation for Medical Education and Research. (2009). *Premature ejaculation*. http://www.mayoclinic.com

21. Rosenbaum, J. E. (2009). Patient teenagers? A comparison of the sexual behavior of virginity pledgers and matched nonpledgers. *Pediatrics, 123*(1), 110–120.

22. Higgins, J. A., Trussell, J., Moore, N. B., & Davidson, J. K. (2010). Young adult sexual health: Current and prior sexual behaviours among non-Hispanic white U.S. college students. *Sexual Health, 7*(1), 35–43.

23. National Campaign to Prevent Teen and Unplanned Pregnancy and CosmoGirl.com. (2009). *Sex and tech: Results from a survey of teens and young adults*. http://www.thenationalcampaign.org

24. Lenhart, A. (2009). *Teens and sexting*. http://www.pewinternet.org

25. Newman, A. (2010. March 23). Senate passes Arizona sexting law. *Arizona Daily Wildcat*. http://wildcat.arizona.edu

26. Centers for Disease Control and Prevention. (2009). *Key statistics from the National Survey of Family Growth*. http://www.cdc.gov

27. American Pregnancy Association. (2010). *Statistics*. http://www.americanpregnancy.org

28. Pew Research Center. (2009). *Majority continues to support civil unions*. http://pewforum.org

29. Appleby, J. (2012, May 14). Many businesses offer health benefits to same-sex couples ahead of laws. *PBS Newshour*. http://www.pbs.org

30. Robinson, J. P., & Espelage, D. L. (2011). Inequities in educational and psychological outcomes between LGBTQ and straight students in middle and high school. *Educational Researcher, 40*, 315. doi: 10.3102/0013189X11422112

31. Federal Bureau of Investigation. (2012).*Hate crimes accounting: National report released*. http://www.fbi.gov

32. Ducker, D. J. (2012). Marking sexuality from 0–6: The Kinsey scale in online culture. *Sexuality & Culture, 16*, 241–262.

33. Diamond, L. M. (2008). Female bisexuality from adolescence to adulthood: Results from a 10-year longitudinal study. *Developmental Psychology, 44*(1), 5–14.

34. American Psychological Association. (2010). *Answers to your questions about transgendered individuals and gender identity*. http://www.apa.org

35. Bockting, W., Benner, A., & Coleman, E. (2009). Gay and bisexual identity development among female-to-male transsexuals in North America: Emergence of a transgender sexuality. *Archives of Sexual Behavior, 38*(5), 688–701.

36. McGuire, L. (2010). *New emergency contraceptive*. Mayo Foundation for Medical Education and Research. http://www.mayoclinic.com

37. Mayo Foundation for Medical Education and Research. (2010*).*

ParaGard (copper IUD). http://www.mayoclinic.com

38. Mayo Foundation for Medical Education and Research. (2010). *Mirena (hormonal IUD)*. http://www.mayoclinic.com

39. Mayo Foundation for Medical Education and Research. (2010). *Birth control pill FAQ: Benefits, risks and choices*. http://www.mayoclinic.com

40. Mayo Foundation for Medical Education and Research. (2009). *Vasectomy: Risks*. http://www.mayoclinic.com

41. National Campaign to Prevent Teen and Unplanned Pregnancy. (2010). *National data*. http://www.thenationalcampaign.org

42. National Campaign to Prevent Teen and Unplanned Pregnancy. (2008). *Policy brief: Thoughts for elected officials about teen and unplanned pregnancy*. http://www.thenationalcampaign.org

43. Jones, R. K., & Kooistra, K. (2011). Abortion incidence and access to services in the United States, 2008. *Perspectives on Sexual and Reproductive Health, 43*(1), 41–50. doi: 10.1363/4304111

44. World Health Organization. (2006). *Frequently asked clinical questions about medical abortion*. http://whqlibdoc.who.int

45. Raymond, E. G., & Grimes, D. A. (2012, February). The comparative safety of legal induced abortion and childbirth in the United States. *Obstetrics & Gynecology, 119*(2 Pt. 1), 215–219.

46. Pazol, K., Creanga, A., Zane, S., Burley, K., & Jamieson, D. (2012). Abortion surveillance—United States, 2009. *Morbidity and Mortality Weekly Report Surveillance Summaries, 61*(8), 1–12.

47. Coleman, P. (2011). Abortion and mental health: Quantitative synthesis and analysis of research published 1995–2009. *British Journal of Psychiatry, 199*(3), 180–186.

48. American Psychological Association, Task Force on Mental Health and Abortion. (2008). *Report of the APA Task Force on Mental Health and Abortion*. Washington, DC: Author. http://www.apa.org

49. American Congress of Obstetricians and Gynecologists. (2012). *Treating infertility*. http://www.acog.org

50. Cole, L. (2011). The utility of six over-the-counter (home) pregnancy tests. *Clinical Chemistry and Laboratory Medicine, 49*(8), 1317–1322.

51. U.S. Department of Health and Human Services, Health Resources and Services Administration, Maternal and Child Health Bureau. (2009). *A healthy start: Begin before baby's born*. http://mchb.hrsa.gov

52. Trabert, B., Holt, V. L., Onchee, Y., Van Den Eeden, S. K., & Scholes, D. (2011). Population-based ectopic pregnancy trends, 1993–2007. *American Journal of Preventive Medicine, 401*(5), 556–560.

53. Creanga, A., Shapiro-Mendoza, C., Bish, C., Zane, S., Berg, C., & Callaghan, W. (2011). Trends in ectopic pregnancy mortality in the United States 1980–2007. *Obstetrics and Gynecology, 117*, 837–843.

54. March of Dimes. (2009). *Miscarriage*. http://www.marchofdimes.com

55. American Congress of Obstetricians and Gynecologists. (2011). *High blood pressure during pregnancy*. http://www.acog.org

56. Young, B., Hacker, M. R., & Rana, S. (2012). Physicians' knowledge of future vascular disease in women with preeclampsia. *Informa Healthcare, 31*(1), 50–58.

57. National Vital Statistics System. (2013). *Birth data*. http://www.cdc.gov

58. World Bank. (2010). *Mortality rate, infant (per 1,000 live births)*. http://data.worldbank.org

59. Martin, J., Hamilton, B., Ventura, S., Osteman, M., Wilson, E., & Mathews, T. (2012). Births: Final data for 2010. *National Vital Statistics Reports, 61*(1), 1–71. http://www.cdc.gov

60. American Congress of Obstetricians and Gynecologists. (2011). *You and your baby: Prenatal care, labor and delivery, and postpartum care*. http://www.midtown-obgyn.com

61. MedlinePlus. (2009). *APGAR*. http://www.nlm.nih.gov

62. Martin, J. A., Hamilton, B. E., Sutton, P. D., Ventura, S. J., Menacker, F., Kirmeyer, S., & Mathews, T. J. (2009). Births: Final data for 2006. *National Vital Statistics Reports, 57*(7), 1–104. http://www.cdc.gov

63. Centers for Disease Control and Prevention. (2012). *National survey of family growth*. http://www.cdc.gov

64. MedlinePlus. (2009). *Infertility*. http://www.nlm.nih.gov

65. U.S. Department of Health and Human Services, Administration for Children & Families. (2009). *Trends in foster care and adoption—FY 2002–FY 2008*. http://www.acf.hhs.gov

66. Feminist Majority Foundation. (2010). *Birth control access campaign*. http://www.feministcampus.org.

Chapter 11

i. Centers for Disease Control and Prevention. (2011). *Seasonal flu: Questions and answers*. http://www.cdc.gov

ii. Centers for Disease Control and Prevention. (2013). *CDC fact sheet: Incidence, prevalence, and cost of sexually transmitted infections in the United States*. http://www.cdc.gov

iii. Centers for Disease Control and Prevention. (2008). *It helps to know* [Audio podcast]. http://www.cdc.gov

1. Centers for Disease Control and Prevention, National Center for Zoonotic, Vector-Borne, and Enteric Diseases. (2009). *Did you know . . .* http://www.cdc.gov

2. Busscher, H. J., & van der Mei, H. C. (2012). How do bacteria know they are on a surface and regulate their response to an adhering state? *PLoS Pathogens, 8*(1), e1002440. doi:10.1371/journal.ppat.1002440

3. American College Health Association. (2013). *American College Health Association National College Health*

Assessment (ACHA-NCHA II) reference group executive summary, Fall 2012. Linthicum, MD: American College Health Association. http://www.acha-ncha.org

4. American Academy of Allergy, Asthma & Immunology. (n.d.). *Tips to remember: Allergic reactions.* Retrieved from http://www.aaaai.org/patients/publicedmat/tips/whatisallergicreaction.stm

5. American Academy of Allergy, Asthma & Immunology. (2013). *Asthma statistics.* http://www.aaaai.org

6. Directors of Health Promotion and Education. *Addressing infectious disease threats.* http://www.dhpe.org

7. Baccam, P., Beauchemin, C., Macken, C., Hayden, F., & Perelson, A. (2006). Kinetics of influenza A virus infection in humans. *Journal of Virology, 80*(15), 7590–7599.

8. Centers for Disease Control and Prevention. (2011). *Seasonal Flu: Questions and answers.* http://www.cdc.gov

9. Centers for Disease Control and Prevention. (2009). *Hepatitis C FAQs for the public.* http://www.cdc.gov

10. National Institutes of Health, National Institute of Allergy and Infectious Diseases. (2009). *Understanding microbes in sickness and in health* (NIH Publication No. 06-4914). http://www.niaid.nih.gov

11. World Health Organization. (2010). *Meningococcal meningitis* (Fact sheet No. 141). http://www.who.int

12. Centers for Disease Control and Prevention. *Toxic shock syndrome.* http://www.cdc.gov

13. Centers for Disease Control and Prevention, National Center for Health Statistics. (2013). *Leading causes of death.* http://www.cdc.gov

14. World Health Organization. (2009). *Pneumonia* (Fact sheet No. 331). http://www.who.int

15. Centers for Disease Control and Prevention. (2009). *The difference between latent TB infection and active TB disease.* http://www.cdc.gov

16. Centers for Disease Control and Prevention. (2012). *Tuberculosis: Trends in tuberculosis, 2011.* http://www.cdc.gov

17. National Institutes of Health. *TB still declining in U.S., but at slower rate.* http://www.nlm.nih.gov

18. World Health Organization. (2010). *Malaria* (Fact sheet No. 94). http://www.who.int

19. World Health Organization. (2007). *Sexually transmitted infections* (Fact sheet No. 110). http://www.who.int

20. World Health Organization. (2007). *Global strategy for the prevention and control of sexually transmitted infections: 2006–2015. Breaking the chain of transmission.* Geneva, Switzerland: WHO Press.

21. Centers for Disease Control and Prevention. (2013). *CDC fact sheet—incidence, prevalence, and cost of sexually transmitted infections in the United States.* http://www.cdc.gov

22. Forhan, S. E., Gottlieb, S. L., Sternberg, M. R., Fujie, X., Datta, S. D., McQuillan, G. M., . . . Markowitz, L. E. (2009). Prevalence of sexually transmitted infections among female adolescents aged 14 to 19 in the United States. *Pediatrics, 124*(6), 1505–1512. doi: 10.1542/peds.2009-0674

23. *Global report: UNAIDS report on the global AIDS epidemic by the Joint United Nations Programme on HIV/AIDS (UNAIDS) and World Health Organization (WHO).* (2012). http://www.unaids.org

24. World Health Organization. (n.d.). *Mother-to-child transmission of HIV.* http://www.who.int

25. Word Health Organization. (2009). *Rapid advice: Use of antiretroviral drugs for treating pregnant women and preventing HIV infection in infants.* Geneva, Switzerland: WHO Press.

26. World Health Organization. (2009). *Love in the era of HAART. HIV/AIDS Prevention and Care Newsletter, 2*(1), 1. http://www.who.int

27. Centers for Disease Control and Prevention. (2009). *Hepatitis B FAQs for the public.* http://www.cdc.gov

28. Centers for Disease Control and Prevention. (2010). *CDC study finds U.S. herpes rates remain high* [Press release]. http://www.cdc.gov

29. American Social Health Association. (n.d.). *Treatment for oral herpes.* http://www.ashastd.org

30. Centers for Disease Control and Prevention. (2011). *HPV and men: Fact sheet.* http://www.cdc.gov

31. Centers for Disease Control and Prevention. (2013). *Genital HPV infection: Fact sheet.* http://www.cdc.gov

32. American Cancer Society. (2009). *Overview: Cervical cancer. How many women get cancer of the cervix?* http://www.cancer.org

33. U.S. Food and Drug Administration. (2009, October 16). *FDA approves new indication for Gardasil to prevent genital warts in men and boys* [News release]. http://www.fda.gov

34. American Social Health Association. (n.d.). *Chlamydia: Questions & answers.* http://www.ashastd.org

35. Centers for Disease Control and Prevention. (2010). What are the symptoms of chlamydia? *CDC fact sheet: Chlamydia.* http://www.cdc.gov

36. U.S. Preventive Services Task Force. (2007). Screening for chlamydial infection: U.S. Preventive Services Task Force recommendation statement. *Annals of Internal Medicine, 147*(2), 128–134.

37. Mayo Clinic. (2009). *Gonorrhea.* http://www.mayoclinic.com

38. Centers for Disease Control and Prevention. (2010). *CDC fact sheet: Pelvic inflammatory disease.* Retrieved from http://www.cdc.gov/std/PID/STDFact-PID.htm

39. Centers for Disease Control and Prevention, National Center for HIV, STD, and TB Prevention (NCHSTP), Division of STD/HIV Prevention. (2011).*Selected STDs by age, race/ethnicity, and gender, 1996–2009.* CDC WONDER On-line Database. http://wonder.cdc.gov

40. Ginocchio, C. C., Chapin, K., Smith, J. S., Aslanzadeh, J., Snook, J., Hill, C. S., & Gaydos, C. A. (2011, July). Prevalence of *Trichomonas vaginalis* and coinfection with *Chlamydia trachomatis* and *Neisseria gonor rhoea* in the USA as determined by the aptima *Trichomonas vaginalis* nucleic acid amplification assay. *Sexually Transmitted Infections, 87*(1), A72–A73.

41. Centers for Disease Control and Prevention. (2011, November 11). *CDC fact sheet: Trichomoniasis.* http://www.cdc.gov

42. Tuller, D. (2009, January 19). After hook ups, e cards that warn, 'get checked.' *The New York Times.* http://www.nytimes.com

Chapter 12

i. Centers for Disease Control and Prevention. (2011). *National diabetes fact sheet: National estimates and general information on diabetes and prediabetes in the United States, 2011.* Atlanta, GA: U.S. Department of Health and Human Services, Centers for Disease Control and Prevention. http://www.cdc.gov

ii. Hoyert, D. L., & Xu, J. (2012, October 10). Deaths: Preliminary data for 2011. *National Vital Statistics Reports, 61*(6). Centers for Disease Control and Prevention.

iii. American Cancer Society. (2013). *Cancer facts and figures 2013.* Atlanta, GA: American Cancer Society. http://www.cancer.org

1. Centers for Disease Control and Prevention. (2011). *National diabetes fact sheet, 2011.* http://www.cdc.gov

2. Centers for Disease Control and Prevention. (2013, March). *Heart disease facts.* http://www.cdc.gov

3. Centers for Disease Control and Prevention. (2013, March). *Stroke facts.* http://www.cdc.gov

4. American Cancer Society. (2013). *Cancer facts and figures 2013.* Atlanta GA: American Cancer Society. http://www.cancer.org

5. Centers for Disease Control and Prevention. (2012, August). *Chronic diseases and health promotion.* http://www.cdc.gov

6. Hoyert, D. L., & Xu, J. (2012, October 10). Deaths: Preliminary data for 2011. *National Vital Statistics Reports, 61*(6). Centers for Disease Control and Prevention.

7. Centers for Disease Control and Prevention. (2011, April). *Rising health care costs are unsustainable.* http://www.cdc.gov

8. U.S. Department of Heath and Human Services. (2013, April). *Smoking and your health.* http://betobaccofree.hhs.gov

9. Centers for Disease Control and Prevention. (2012, August). *Adult obesity facts.* http://www.cdc.gov

10. Centers for Disease Control and Prevention. (2013, March). *Diabetes data and trends.* http://www.cdc.gov

11. National Diabetes Information Clearinghouse. (2011). *National diabetes statistics, 2011.* http://diabetes.niddk.nih.gov

12. Gebel, E. (2010, May). The other diabetes: LADA, or type 1.5. *Diabetes Forecast.* American Diabetes Association. http://forecast.diabetes.org

13. Mayo Foundation. (2013, January). *A1C test.* http://www.mayoclinic.com

14. Luo, M., Guan, X., Luczak, E.D., Lang, D., Kutschke, W., Gao, Z., . . . Anderson, M. E. (2013). Diabetes increases mortality after myocardial infarction by oxidizing CaMKII. *Journal of Clinical Investigation, 123*(3),1262–1274.

15. The Emerging Risk Factors Collaboration. (2011, March 3). Diabetes mellitus, fasting glucose, and risk of cause-specific death. *New England Journal of Medicine, 364*, 829–841. http://www.nejm.org

16. Gebel, E. (2011, September). Obesity and type 2 diabetes. American Diabetes Association: *Diabetes Forecast.* http://forecast.diabetes.org

17. Basu, S., Yoffe, P., Hills, N., & Lustig, R. H. (2013). The relationship of sugar to population-level diabetes prevalence: An econometric analysis of repeated cross-sectional data. *PLoS ONE, 8*(2), e57873. doi:10.1371/journal.pone.0057873

18. Manenschijn, L., Schaap, L., van Schoor, N.M., van der Pas, S., Peeters, G.M.E.E., et al. (2013). High long-term cortisol levels, measured in scalp hair, are associated with a history of cardiovascular disease. *The Journal of Clinical Endocrinology & Metabolism.* April 17, 2013 jc.2012-3663.

19. American College Health Association. (2013). *National College Health Assessment II: Reference Group Executive Summary Fall 2012.* Hanover, MD: American College Health Association. http://www.acha-ncha.org

20. Smith, M. L., Dickerson, J. B., Sosa, E. T., McKyer, L. J., & Ory, M. G. (2012). College students' perceived disease risk versus actual prevalence rates. *American Journal of Health Behavior, 36*(1), 96–106.

21. National Heart, Lung, and Blood Institute. (2013). *Disease statistics.* http://www.nhlbi.nih.gov

22. Mayo Foundation. (2011, March 22). *High blood pressure.* http://www.mayoclinic.com

23. National Heart, Lung, and Blood Institute. (n.d.). *Your guide to lowering high blood pressure: Prevention.* http://www.nhlbi.nih.gov

24. Go, A. S., Mozaffarian, D., Roger, V. L., Benjamin, E. J., Berry, J. D., Borden, W. B., . . . Turner, M. B.; on behalf of the American Heart Association Statistics Committee and Stroke Statistics Subcommittee. (2013). Heart disease and stroke statistics—2013 update: A report from the American Heart Association. *Circulation, 127*, e6–e245. http://circ.ahajournals.org

25. American Heart Association. (2012, October 25). *Arrhythmia: Understand your risk for arrhythmia.* http://www.heart.org

26. MedlinePlus. (2013, March 22). *Heart attack.* http://www.nlm.nih.gov

27. Levy, D., Larson, M., Vasan, R., Kannel, W., & Ho, K. (1996). The progression from hypertension to congestive heart failure. *Journal of the American Medical Association, 275* (20), 1557–1562.

28. Medline Plus. (2012, June 23). *Heart failure.* http://www.nlm.nih.gov

29. Centers for Disease Control and Prevention. (2013, January). *Faststats: Cerebrovascular disease or stroke.* http://www.cdc.gov

30. Mayo Foundation. (2012, July 03). *Stroke.* http://www.mayoclinic.com

31. American Heart Association. (2013, February 4). *Understand your risk for congenital heart defects.* http://www.heart.org

32. National Institute on Drug Abuse. (2012, December). *Medical consequences of drug abuse.* http://www.drugabuse.gov

33. American Heart Association. (2013, January). *Understand your risk of heart attack.* http://www.heart.org

34. Gangwisch, J. E., Malaspina, D., Babiss, L. A., Opler, M. G., Posner, K., Shen, S., . . . Ginsberg, H. N. (2010). Short sleep duration as a risk factor for hypercholesterolemia: Analyses of the national longitudinal study of adolescent health. *Sleep, 33*(7), 956–961.

35. Vgontzas, A. N., Duanping, L., Bixler, E. O., Chrousos, G. P., & Vela-Bueno, A. (2009). Insomnia with objective short sleep duration is associated with a high risk for hypertension. *Sleep, 32*(4), 491–497.

36. International Chair on Cardiometabolic Risk. (2011). *Global cardiometabolic risk: Historical perspective.* http://www.myhealthywaist.org

37. Agency for Healthcare Research and Quality National Guideline Clearinghouse. (2012, April 13). *Cardiometabolic risk management in primary care.* http://www.guideline.gov

38. Klien, S., Allision, D. B., Heymsfield, S. B., Kelley, D. F., Leibel, R. L., Nonas, C., & Kahn, R. (2007). Waist circumference and cardiometabolic risk: A consensus statement from Shaping America's Health: Association for Weight Management and Obesity Prevention; NAASO, The Obesity Society; the American Society of Nutrition; and the American Diabetes Association. *American Journal of Clinical Nutrition, 85,* 1197–1202.

39. Morrell, J. S., Lofgren, I. E., Burke, J. D., & Reilly, R. A. (2012). Metabolic syndrome, obesity, and related risk factors among college men and women. *Journal of American College Health, 60*(1), 82–89.

40. Dalleck, L. C., & Kjelland, E. M. (2012). The prevalence of metabolic syndrome and metabolic syndrome risk factors in college-aged students. *American Journal of Health Promotion, 270*(1), 37–42.

41. American Cancer Society. (2013). *Cancer facts and figures 2013.* Atlanta, GA: American Cancer Society.

42. American Cancer Society. (2012, June 13). *Known and probable human carcinogens.* http://www.cancer.org

43. National Cancer Institute. (2009). *National Cancer Institute fact sheet: BRCA1 and BRCA2: Cancer risk and genetic testing.* http://www.cancer.gov

44. American Cancer Society. (2012, August 13). *Signs and symptoms of cancer.* http://www.cancer.org

45. FDA. (May 6, 2013). FDA issues proposal to increase consumer awareness of tanning bed risks. FDA News Release. http://www.fda.gov

46. U.S. Environmental Protection Agency. (2013, January 10). *A citizen's guide to radon.* http://www.epa.gov

47. American Cancer Society. (2013, February 6). *American Cancer Society recommendations for early breast cancer detection in women without breast symptoms.* http://www.cancer.org

48. American Cancer Society. (2013). *Treatment types.* http://www.cancer.org

49. Shi, L., Morrison, A., Wiecha, J., Horton, M., & Hayman, L. L. (2011). Healthy lifestyle factors associated with reduced cardiometabolic risk. *British Journal of Nutrition, 105*(5), 747–754.

50. Ford, E. S., Zhao, G., Tsai, J., & Li, C. (2011). Low-risk lifestyle behaviors and all-cause mortality: Findings from the National Health and Nutrition Examination Survey III Mortality Study. *American Journal of Public Health, 101*(10), 1922–1929.

51. U.S. Centers for Disease Control and Prevention. (2012, January 10). *Health effects of cigarette smoking.* http://www.cdc.gov

52. Rohrmann, S., Overvad, K., Bueno-de-Mesquita, H. B., Jakobsen, M. U., Egeberg, R., Tiønneland, A., . . . Linseisen, J. (2013). Meat consumption and mortality—results from the European prospective investigation into cancer and nutrition. *British Medical Journal, 11,* 63–75.

53. Fung, T., McCullough, M., van Dam, R., & Hu, F. (2007). A prospective study of overall diet quality and risk of type 2 diabetes in women. *Diabetes Care, 30,* 1753–1757.

54. Pan, A., Sun, Q., Bernstein, A. M., Schulze, M. B., Manson, J. E., Stampfer, M. J., Willett, W. C., & Hu, F. B. (2012). Red meat consumption and mortality: Results from 2 prospective cohort studies. *Archives of Internal Medicine, 172,* 555–563.

55. Estruch, R., Ros, E., Salas-Salvado, J., Covas, M.-I., Corella, D., Arós, F., . . . Martínez-González, M. A. (2013). Primary prevention of cardiovascular disease with a Mediterranean diet. *New England Journal of Medicine, 368,* 1279–1290.

56. Goodpaster, B. H., Delany, J. P., Otto, A. D., Kuller, L., Vockley, J., South-Paul, J. E., . . . Jakicic, J. M. (2010). Effects of diet and physical activity interventions on weight loss and cardiometabolic risk factors in severely obese adults. *Journal of the American Medical Association, 304*(16), 1795–1802.

57. Guinhouya, B. C., Samouda, H., Zitouni, D., Vilhelm, C., & Hubert, H. (2011). Evidence of the influence of physical activity on the metabolic syndrome and/or on insulin resistance in pediatric populations: A systematic review. *International Journal of Pediatric Obesity,* published online. doi: 10.3109/17477166.2011.605896

58. Kushi, L. H., Doyle, C., McCullough, M., Rock, C. L., Demark-Wahnefried, W., Bandera, E. V., . . . Gansler, T. (2012). American Cancer Society guidelines on nutrition and physical activity for cancer prevention. *CA: Cancer Journal for Clinicians, 62,* 30–67.

59. Winzer, B. M., Whiteman, D. C., Reeves, M. M., & Paratz, J. (2011). Physical activity and cancer prevention: A systematic review. *Cancer Causes Control, 22,* 811–826.

60. Jorgensen, R., & Maisto, S. (2008). Alcohol consumption and prehypertension: An investigation of university youth. *Behavioral Medicine, 34,* 21–26.

61. Fan, A. Z., Russell, M., Stranges, S., Dorn, J., & Trevisan, M. (2008, January). Association of lifetime alcohol drinking trajectories with cardiometabolic risk. *Journal of Clinical Endocrinology and Metabolism, 93*(1), 154–161.

62. Nelson, D. E., Jarman, D. W., Rehm, J., Greenfield, T. K., Rey, G., Kerr, W. C., . . . Naimi, T. S. (2013, April). Alcohol-attributable cancer deaths and years of potential life lost in the United States. *American Journal of Public Health, 103*(4), 641–648.

63. Latinio-Martel, P., Arwidson, P., Ancellin, R., Druesne-Pecollo, N., Hercberg, S., Le Quellec-Nathan, M., Le-Luong, T., & Maraninchi, D. (2011). Alcohol consumption and cancer risk: Revisiting guidelines for sensible drinking. *Canadian Medical Association, 183*(16), 1861–1865.

64. Lockhart, P. B., Bolger, A. F., Papapanou, P. N., Osinbowale, O., Trevisan, M., Levison, M. E., . . . Baddour, L. M. (2012). Periodontal disease and atherosclerotic vascular disease: Does the evidence support an independent association? American Heart Association Scientific Statement. *Circulation, 125,* 2520–2544.

65. Chida, Y., & Steptoe, A. (2009, March 17). The association of anger and hostility with future coronary heart disease: A meta-analytic review of prospective evidence. *Journal of the American College of Cardiology, 53*(11), 947–949.

66. National Cancer Institute. (2012, December). *Psychological stress and cancer.* http://www.cancer.gov

67. Rubin, R. R. (2011). *Tips for really helping a person who has diabetes.* American Diabetes Association. http://www.diabetes.org

68. American Cancer Society. (2013, January 25). *Listen with your heart: Talking with the person who has cancer.* http://www.cancer.org

69. National Collegiate Cancer Foundation. (2009). *History.* http://www.collegiatecancer.org

Chapter 13

i. Pew Internet & American Life Project. (2009). *Generational differences in online activities.* http://www.pewinternet.org

ii. Centers for Disease Control and Prevention. (2013). *FastStats—therapeutic drug use.* http://www.cdc.gov

iii. LaCaille, R. A., & Kuvaas, N. J. (2011). Coping styles and self-regulation predict complementary and alternative medicine and herbal supplement use among college students. *Psychology, Health & Medicine, 16*(3), 323–332.

1. Kwan, M., Arbour-Nicitopoulos, K., Lowe, D., Taman, S., & Faulkner, G. (2010). Student reception, sources, and believability of health-related information. *Journal of American College Health, 58*(6), 555–562.

2. University of California, San Francisco. (2012). *Evaluating health information.* http://www.ucsfhealth.org

3. Slone Epidemiology Center at Boston University. (2006). *Patterns of medication use in the United States: A report from the Slone survey.* http://www.bu.edu

4. American College of Preventive Medicine. (2011). *Over-the-counter medications: Use in general and special populations, therapeutic errors, misuse, storage and disposal.* www.acpm.org

5. U.S. Food and Drug Administration, Center for Drug Evaluation and Research. (2009). *Regulation of nonprescription products.* http://www.fda.gov

6. Stasio, M., Curry, K., Sutton-Skinner, K., & Glassman, D. (2008). Over-the-counter medication and herbal or dietary supplement use in college: Dose frequency and relationship to self-reported distress. *Journal of the American College Health Association, 56*(5), 535–547.

7. Kittinger, P., & Herrick, D. (2005). Patient power: Over-the-counter drugs. *National Center for Policy Analysis, Brief Analysis, 524.* http://www.ncpa.org

8. American Academy of Family Physicians. (2010). *When should I go to the emergency department?* http://www.acep.org

9. Porter, R. S. (Ed.). (2007). *The Merck manual of medical information—home edition.* Whitehouse Station, NJ: Merck & Co., Inc. http://www.merck.com

10. American Academy of Family Physicians. (2009). *Tips for talking to your doctor;* and *Medical errors: Tips to help prevent them.* http://familydoctor.org

11. American College Health Association. (2013). *American College Health Association national college health assessment II: Reference group executive summary fall 2012.* http://www.acha-ncha.org

12. Centers for Disease Control and Prevention. (2011). *Vital signs—prescription painkiller overdoses in the US.* http://www.cdc.gov

13. Centers for Disease Control and Prevention. (2012). *Injury prevention and control. Saving lives and protecting people: Preventing prescription painkiller overdoses.* http://www.cdc.gov

14. Jones, C. M., Mack, K. A., & Paulozzi, L. J. (2013). Pharmaceutical overdose deaths, United States, 2010. *Journal of the American Medical Association, 309,* 657–659.

15. Centers for Disease Control and Prevention. (2013). *Vital signs. Prescription painkiller overdoses: A growing epidemic, especially among women.* http://www.cdc.gov

16. National Center for Complementary and Alternative Medicine. (2007). *CAM basics: What is CAM?* http://nccam.nih.gov

17. National Center for Complementary and Alternative Medicine. (2009). *CAM basics: Are you considering*

complementary and alternative medicine? http://nccam.nih.gov

18. National Center for Complementary and Alternative Medicine. (2009). *CAM basics: Selecting a complementary and alternative medicine practitioner.* http://nccam.nih.gov

19. World Health Organization. (2008). *World health statistics: Global health indicators.* http://www.who.int

20. California Healthcare Foundation. (2012). *Healthcare costs 101.* http://www.chcf.org

21. Kaiser Family Foundation. (2011). *Employer health benefits 2011 annual survey.* http://kff.org

22. U.S. Government Accountability Office. (2008). *Health insurance: Most college students are covered through employer-sponsored plans, and some colleges and states are taking steps to increase coverage* (Report GAO-08-389). http://www.gao.gov

23. Jost, T. (2008). Access to health care: Is self-help the answer? *Journal of Legal Medicine, 29,* 23–40.

24. U.S. Department of Health and Human Services. (2011). *New rule ensures students get health insurance protections of the Affordable Care Act.* http://www.hhs.gov

Chapter 14

i. Hoyert, D. L., & Xu, J. Q. (2012, October 11). Deaths: Preliminary data for 2011. *National Vital Statistics Reports, 61*(6). Hyattsville, MD: National Center for Health Statistics. http://www.cdc.gov

ii. National Highway Traffic Safety Administration. (2012, June). *Blueprint for ending distracted driving* (DOT HS 811 629). Retrieved from http://www.distraction.gov/download/campaign-materials/8747-811629-060712-v5-Opt1-Web-tag.pdf

iii. Centers for Disease Control and Prevention. (2011). *National intimate partner and sexual violence survey: Highlights of 2010 findings.* http://www.cdc.gov

1. Hoyert, D. L. & Xu, J. Q. (2012, October 11). Deaths: Preliminary data for 2011. *National Vital Statistics Reports, 61*(6). Hyattsville, MD: National Center for Health Statistics. http://www.cdc.gov

2. Centers for Disease Control and Prevention. (2012, January 17). *Injuries and violence are leading causes of death: Key data and statistics.* http://www.cdc.gov

3. Centers for Disease Control and Prevention. (2012). *2010 Emergency department summary tables. National hospital ambulatory medical care survey.* http://www.cdc.gov

4. National Safety Council. (2013). *Injury facts 2011 edition.* http://www.nsc.org

5. Centers for Disease Control and Prevention. (2012). CDC WISQARS (Web-based Injury Statistics Query and Reporting System). Atlanta, GA: U.S. Department of Health and Human Services, CDC. http://www.cdc.gov

6. National Institute on Alcohol Abuse and Alcoholism. (2010). *Rethinking*

drinking: Alcohol and your health. http://rethinkingdrinking.niaaa.nih.gov

7. National Highway Traffic Safety Administration. (2012, September). *Distracted driving 2011. Key facts and statistics.* http://www.distraction.gov

8. National Highway Traffic Safety Administration. (2013, April). *The impact of hand-held and hands-free cell phone use on driving performance and safety-critical event risk* (DOT HS 811 757). http://www.distraction.gov

9. AAA Foundation for Traffic Safety. (2013, June). *Measuring cognitive distraction in the automobile.* https://www.aaafoundation.org

10. Governors Highway Safety Association. (2013, May). *Distracted driving laws.* http://www.ghsa.org

11. Harrison, M. A. (2011). College students' prevalence and perceptions of text messaging while driving. *Accident Analysis & Prevention, 43*(4), 1516–1520.

12. Atchley, P., Atwood, S., & Boulton, A. (2011). The choice to text and drive in younger drivers: Behavior may shape attitude. *Accident Analysis & Prevention, 43*(1), 134–142.

13. National Transportation Safety Board. (2013, May 14). *Reaching zero: Actions to eliminate alcohol-impaired driving.* http://www.ntsb.gov

14. Governors Highway Safety Association. (2013, May). *Drug impaired driving laws.* http://www.ghsa.org

15. American Automobile Association Foundation for Traffic Safety. (2012, March). *Two out of five drivers admit to falling asleep at the wheel, finds AAA Foundation study.* http://www.aaafoundation.org

16. National Conference of State Legislatures. (2013, February). *Summaries of current drowsy driving laws.* http://www.ncsl.org

17. American College Health Association. (2013). *American College Health Association—National College Health Assessment (ACHA-NCHA II) reference group executive summary, fall 2012.* http://www.acha-ncha.org

18. National Highway Traffic Safety Administration. (2010). *The top 5 things you should know about buckling up* (DOT HS 811 257). http://trafficsafetymarketing.gov

19. California Department of Motor Vehicles. (2010). Seat belts: Mistaken beliefs about seat belts. In *California Driver Handbook* (p. 19). http://www.dmv.ca.gov

20. National Highway Traffic Safety Administration. (2013). *Aggressive driving.* http://www.nhtsa.gov

21. Faul, M., Xu, L., Wald, M. M., & Coronado, V. G. (2010). *Traumatic brain injury in the United States: Emergency department visits, hospitalizations, and deaths.* Atlanta, GA: Centers for Disease Control and Prevention, National Center for Injury Prevention and Control. http://www.cdc.gov

22. National Highway Traffic Safety Administration. (2012, August). *Pedestrians. Traffic safety facts: 2010 data* (DOT HS 811 625). http://www.nhtsa.gov

23. National Highway Traffic Safety Administration. (2013, May). *Motorcycles. Traffic safety facts: 2011 data* (DOT HS 811 765). http://www.nhtsa.gov

24. National Highway Traffic Safety Administration. (2013, April). *Bicyclists and other cyclists. Traffic safety facts: 2011 data* (DOT HS 811 743). http://www.nhtsa.gov

25. Governors Highway Safety Association. (2013, June). *Helmet laws.* http://www.ghsa.org

26. Centers for Disease Control and Prevention. (2012, June 29). *Poisoning in the United States: Fact sheet.* http://www.cdc.gov

27. Centers for Disease Control and Prevention. (2013, March 29). QuickStats: Number of deaths from poisoning, drug poisoning, and drug poisoning involving opioid analgesics, 1999–2010. *Morbidity and Mortality Weekly Report, 62*(12), 234. http://www.cdc.gov

28. Solomon, D. H., Rassen, J. A., Glynn, R. J., Garneau, K., Levin, R., Lee, J., & Schneeweiss, S. (2010, December). The comparative safety of opioids for nonmalignant pain in older adults. *Archives of Internal Medicine, 170*(22), 1979–1986.

29. National Institutes of Health. (2011, July 16). Choking: Adult or child over 1 year. *MedlinePlus.* http://www.nlm.nih.gov

30. American Academy of Pediatrics. (2010, March 1). Prevention of choking among children. *PEDIATRICS, 125*(3), 601–607.

31. Centers for Disease Control and Prevention. (2012, November 29). *Unintentional drowning: Fact sheet.* http://www.cdc.gov

32. Sleet, D. A., Ballesteros, M. F., & Borse, N. N. (2010). A review of unintentional injuries in adolescents. *Annual Reviews, 31,* 195–212.

33. Centers for Disease Control and Prevention. (2011, October). *Fire deaths and injuries: Fact sheet.* http://www.cdc.gov

34. U.S. Fire Administration. (2013, January 29). *Campus fire safety: Tips for students and parents.* http://www.fema.gov

35. Bureau of Labor Statistics. (2013, June 3). *Injuries, illnesses, and fatalities—2011 data.* http://www.bls.gov

36. Berolo, S., Wells, R. P., & Amick, B. C. (2011). Musculoskeletal symptoms among mobile hand-held device users and their relationship to device use: A preliminary study in a Canadian university population. *Applied Ergonomics, 42*(2), 371–378.

37. Centers for Disease Control and Prevention. (2013, March 14). *Youth violence: National statistics.* http://www.cdc.gov

38. Federal Bureau of Investigation, Criminal Justice Information Services Division. (2012, October 29). *Crime in the United States: 2011: Violent crime.* http://www.fbi.gov

39. U.S. Department of Justice, Bureau of Justice Statistics. (2012, April 17). *National crime victimization survey.* http://www.bjs.gov

40. National Institute on Alcohol Abuse and Alcoholism. (2012, April). *College drinking.* http://niaaa.nih.gov

41. Krug, E. G., Dahlberg, L. L., Mercy, J. A., Zwi, A. B., & Lozano, R. (Eds.). (2010, June). *World report on violence and health.* Geneva: World Health Organization. http://who.int

42. Bureau of Justice Statistics & National Center for Education Statistics. (2012). *Indicators of school crime and safety: 2012.* http://www.bjs.gov

43. Allan, E. J., & Madden, M. (2011). The nature and extent of college student hazing. *International Journal of Adolescent Medicine and Health, 24*(1), 83–90.

44. Newer, H. (2012). *The hazing reader.* Bloomington: Indiana University Press.

45. Federal Bureau of Investigation, Criminal Justice Information Services Division. (2012, December 10). *Hate crime statistics, 2011.* http://www.fbi.gov

46. National Counterterrorism Center. (2012). *2011 report on terrorism.* http://www.cfr.org

47. Centers for Disease Control and Prevention. (2013, May 10). *National intimate partner and sexual violence survey: Highlights of 2010 findings.* http://www.cdc.gov

48. Centers for Disease Control and Prevention. (2012). *Understanding intimate partner violence: Fact sheet 2012.* http://www.cdc.gov

49. McDermott, R. C., & Lopez, F. G. (2013). College men's intimate partner violence attitudes: Contributions of adult attachment and gender role stress. *Journal of Counseling Psychology, 60*(1), 127–136.

50. National Network to End Domestic Violence. (2013). *National summary: Domestic violence counts 2012: A 24-hour census of domestic violence shelters and services.* http://www.nnedv.org

51. Nabors, E., Dietz, T., & Jasinski, J. (2006). Domestic violence beliefs and perceptions among college students. *Violence and Victims, 21*(6), 779–795.

52. McNamara, C. L., & Marsil, D. F. (2012). The prevalence of stalking among college students: The disparity between researcher-and self-identified victimization. *Journal of American College Health, 60*(2), 168–174.

53. Reyns, B. W., Henson, B., & Fishers, B. S. (2012). Stalking in the twilight zone: Extent of cyberstalking victimization and offending among college students. *Deviant Behavior, 33*(1), 1–25.

54. Kraft, E. M., & Wang, I. (2010). An exploratory study of the cyberbullying and cyberstalking experiences and factors related to victimization of students at a public liberal arts college. *International Journal of Technoethics, 1*(4), 74–91.

55. Centers for Disease Control and Prevention. (2010, September). *Intimate partner violence: Risk and protective factors.* http://www.cdc.gov

56. Franklin, C. A., Bouffard, L. A., & Pratt, T. C. (2012). Sexual assault on the college campus: Fraternity affiliation, male peer support, and low self-control. *Criminal Justice and Behavior, 39*(11), 1457–1480.

57. Krebs, C., Lindquist, C., Warner, T., Fisher, B., & Martin, S. (2009). College women's experiences with physically forced, alcohol- or other drug-enabled, and drug-facilitated sexual assault before and since entering college. *Journal of American College Health, 57*(6), 639–647.
58. Core Institute. (2013, April 24). *Core alcohol and drug survey: 2011 data.* http://core.siu.edu/pdfs/report0911.pdf
59. O'Byrne, R., Hansen, S., & Rapley, M. (2007). If a girl doesn't say 'no' . . .: Young men, rape, and claims of 'insufficient knowledge.' *Journal of Community and Applied Social Psychology, 18,* 168–193.
60. U.S. Equal Employment Opportunity Commission. (2013). *Sexual harassment charges: FY 2011.* http://www.eeoc.gov
61. U.S. Equal Employment Opportunity Commission. (n.d.). *Sexual harassment.* http://www.eeoc.gov
62. Hill, C., & Silva, E. (2005). *Drawing the line: Sexual harassment on campus.* American Association of University Women Educational Foundation. http://www.aauw.org
63. U.S. Department of Justice. (2000). *The sexual victimization of college women.* https://www.ncjrs.gov
64. Center for Public Integrity. (2010, February 24). *Sexual assault on campus: A frustrating search for justice: Key findings.* http://www.publicintegrity.org
65. Department of Health and Human Services. (2011, May 18). *Violence against women: How to help a friend who is being abused.* http://womenshealth.gov

Chapter 15

i. Administration on Aging. (2013, April 17). *A profile of older Americans: 2012.* http://www.aoa.gov
ii. Rocheleau, M. (2010, July 26). Seniors get their tech on. *Christian Science Monitor, 102*(35), 29.
1. Administration on Aging. (2013, April 17). *A profile of older Americans: 2012.* http://www.aoa.gov
2. Centers for Disease Control and Prevention. (2012, January 26). *Health-related quality of life: National trend – Percentage with fair or poor self-rated health: Age group.* http://apps.nccd.cdc.gov
3. Hoyert, D. L., & Xu, J. (2012, October 10). Abstract: Deaths: Preliminary data for 2011. *National Vital Statistics Reports, 61*(6). National Center for Health Statistics. http://www.cdc.gov
4. Kulkarni, S. C., Levin-Rector, A., Ezzati, M., & Murray, C. J. L. (2011). Falling behind: Life expectancy in US counties from 2000 to 2007 in an international context. *Population Health Metrics, 9,* 16. http://www.pophealthmetrics.com
5. Olshansky, S. J., Antonucci, T., Berkman, L., Binstock, R. H., Boersch-Supan, A., Cacioppo, J. T. . . . Rowe, J. (2012, August). Differences in life expectancy due to race and educational differences are widening, and many may not catch up. *Health Affairs, 3*(8), 1803–1813.

6. Murray, C. J. L., Kulkarni, S. C., Michaud, C., Tomijima, N., Bulzacchelli, M. T., Iandiorio, T. J., & Ezzati, M. (2006, September). Eight Americas: Investigating mortality disparities across races, counties, and race-counties in the United States. *PLoS Medicine.* http://www.plosmedicine.org
7. Central Intelligence Agency. (2012). Country comparison: Life expectancy at birth. In *The World Factbook.* https://www.cia.gov
8. Central Intelligence Agency. (2012). Field listing: Life expectancy at birth. In *The World Factbook.* https://www.cia.gov
9. Centers for Disease Control and Prevention. (2012, November 9). Current cigarette smoking among adults: United States, 2011. *Morbidity and Mortality Weekly Report, 61*(44),889-894. http://www.cdc.gov
10. Pinkhasov, R. M., Wong, J., Kashanian, J., Lee, M, Samadi, D. B., Pinkasov, M. M., & Shabigh, R. (2010). Are men shortchanged on health? Perspective on health care utilization and health risk behavior in men and women in the United States. *Internal Journal of Clinical Practice, 64*(4), 475-487.
11. American Academy of Ophthalmology. (2011, April). *Eye health statistics at a glance.* http://www.aao.org
12. Glaucoma Research Foundation. (2012, May 24). *Glaucoma facts and stats.* http://www.glaucoma.org
13. National Eye Institute. (2013, May). *Age-related eye disease study 2.* http://www.nei.nih.gov
14. Centers for Disease Control and Prevention. (2011). *Arthritis: Data and statistics.* http://www.cdc.gov
15. National Osteoporosis Foundation. (2011). *About osteoporosis: Bone health basics.* http://www.nof.org
16. National Institutes of Health, Osteoporosis and Related Bone Diseases National Resource Center. (2011). *What is osteoporosis? Fast facts.* http://www.niams.nih.gov
17. The North American Menopause Society. (2012). Position statement: The 2012 hormone therapy position statement of the North American Menopause Society. *Menopause: The Journal of the North American Menopause Society, 19*(3), 257–271. doi: 10.1097/gme.0b013e31824b970a
18. U.S. Food and Drug Administration. (2011). *FDA drug safety communication: Ongoing safety review of oral osteoporosis drugs (bisphosphonates) and potential increased risk of esophageal cancer.* http://www.fda.gov
19. Mayo Foundation. (2011, July 23). *Male menopause: Myth or reality?* http://www.mayoclinic.com
20. O'Connor, A. (2013, June 3). Men's use of testosterone on the rise. *The New York Times.* http://www.nytimes.com
21. Basaria, S., Coviello, A. D., Travison, T. G., Storer, T. W., Farwell, W. R., Jette, A. M., . . . Bhasin, S. (2010). Adverse events associated with testosterone administration. *New England Journal of Medicine, 363*(2), 109–122.
22. Minichiello, V., Rahman, S., & Hawes, G. (2012). STI epidemiology in the global

older population: Emerging challenges. *Perspectives in Public Health, 132*(4),178-181.
23. Tomasi, D., & Volko, N. D. (2012). Aging and functional brain networks. *Molecular Psychiatry, 17,* 549–558.
24. National Institute on Aging. (2011, November 14). *Looking for the causes of AD.* http://www.nia.nih.gov
25. Alzheimer's Association. (2012). *2012 Alzheimer's disease facts and figures.* http://www.alz.org
26. Aarts, S. (2012). *Multimorbidity in general practice: Adverse health effects and innovative research strategies.* Maastricht, The Netherlands: Maastricht University Press, pp. 31–48.
27. Kimchi, E., Desai, A. K., & Grossber, G. T. (2012). New Alzheimer's disease guidelines: Implications for clinicians. *Current Psychiatry, 11*(3), 15–22.
28. Centers for Disease Control and Prevention. (2013, March 21). *Healthy places terminology.* http://www.cdc.gov
29. Social Security Administration. (2011). *Facts and figures about Social Security, 2011.* http://www.socialsecurity.gov
30. Browning, E. S. (2011, February 19). Retiring boomers find 401(k) plans fall short. *The Wall Street Journal.* http://online.wsj.com
31. National Institute of Mental Health. (2013). *Suicide in the U.S.: Statistics and Prevention.* http://www.nimh.nih.gov
32. Substance Abuse and Mental Health Services Administration. (2011, September 1). *Illicit drug use among older adults* (NSDUH_013). National Survey on Drug Use and Health. http://samhsa.gov
33. National Institutes of Health. (2010, August). Alcohol and aging. *NIH Senior Health.* http://nihseniorhealth.gov
34. American Society of Consultant Pharmacists. (2011). *Senior ASCP fact sheet.* https://www.ascp.com
35. Barondess, J. (2008). Toward healthy aging: The preservation of health. *Journal of the American Geriatrics Society, 56*(1), 145–148.
36. Kempermann, G., Fabel, K., Ehninger, D., Babu, H., Leal-Galicia, P., Garthe, A., & Wolf, S. A. (2010). Why and how physical activity promotes experience-induced brain plasticity. *Frontiers in Neuroscience, 4,* 189. doi: 10.3389/fnins.2010.00189
37. Swain, R. A., Berggren, K. L., Kerr, A. L., Patel, A., Peplinski, C., & Sikorski, A. M. (2012). On aerobic exercise and behavioral and neural plasticity. *Brain Science, 2,* 709–744.
38. Centers for Disease Control and Prevention. (2011, December 1). *Physical activity for everyone: How much physical activity do older adults need?* http://www.cdc.gov
39. Tufts University. (2011, November 1). Tufts University nutrition scientists unveil MyPlate for older adults. *Tufts Now.* http://now.tufts.edu
40. American Lung Association. (2010, February). *Smoking and older adults.* http://www.lung.org
41. Ja, P., Ramasundarahettige, C., Landsman, V., Rostron, B., Thun, M., Anderson, R. N., . . . Peto, R. (2013). 21st-Century hazards of smoking and

benefits of cessation in the United States. *The New England Journal of Medicine, 368*(4), 341–350.
42. Dregan, A., Stewart, R., & Gulliford, M. C. (2012). Cardiovascular risk factors and cognitive decline in adults age 50 and older: A population-based cohort study. *Age and Ageing, 0,*1–8. http://ageing.oxfordjournals.org
43. Friedrich, M. J. (2013, February 20). Tobacco smoke and dementia. *Journal of the American Medical Association, 309*(7), 649. doi:10.1001/jama.2013.503
44. Schoenfeld, T. J., Rada, P., Pieruzzini, P. R., Hsueh, B., & Gould, E. (2013). Physical exercise prevents stress-induced activation of granule neurons and enhances local inhibitory mechanisms in the dentate gyrus. *Journal of Neuroscience, 33*(18), 7770–7777.
45. Speece, M. W. (1995). Children's concepts of death. *Living and Dying: Family Decisions: Michigan Family Review, 15*(1), 1. http://quod.lib.umich.edu/m/mfr
46. Howarth, G. (2011). Dying as a social relationship. In D. Oliviere, B. Monroe, & S. Payne (Eds.), *Death, dying, and social differences* (pp. 9–10). London: Oxford University Press.
47. Monroe, B., Oliviere, D., & Payne, S. (2011). Introduction: Social differences: The challenge for palliative care. In D. Oliviere, B. Monroe, & S. Payne (Eds.), *Death, dying, and social differences* (p. 4). London: Oxford University Press.
48. International Association for Near-Death Studies. (2011, April 26). *Impact of the near-death experience on grief and loss.* http://iands.org
49. U.S. Department of Health and Human Services. (2012). *Organ procurement and transplantation network: Transplant history.* http://optn.transplant.hrsa.gov
50. U.S. Department of Health and Human Services. (2012). *Organ procurement and transplantation network: Data.* http://optn.transplant.hrsa.gov
51. Greenhough, J. (2011, March 31). 57% of adults don't have a will—Are you one of them? Estate planning survey results announced. *Rocket Lawyer Insider.* http://insider.rocketlawyer.com
52. American Academy of Hospice and Palliative Medicine. (n.d.). *What is palliative care?* http://www.palliativedoctors.org
53. Hall, M. J., Levant, S., & DeFrances, C. J. (2013). Trends in inpatient hospital deaths: National hospital discharge survey, 2000–2010 (NCSH Data Brief 118). Hyattsville, MD: National Center for Health Statistics.
54. National Hospice and Palliative Care Organization. (2012). *NHPCO facts and figures: Hospice care in America.* http://www.nhpco.org
55. Hospice Foundation of America. (2010). *Choosing hospice.* http://www.hospicefoundation.org
56. Tarzian, A. J., & ASBH Core Competencies Update Task Force. (2013). Health care ethics consultation: An update on core competencies and emerging standards from the American

society of bioethics and humanities' core competencies update task force. *The American Journal of Bioethics, 13*(2), 3–13.

57. Stöppler, M. C. (2012). Autopsy (post-mortem examination, obduction). *MedicineNet.com.* http://www.medicinenet.com

58. Funeral Consumers Alliance. (2011, March 2). *Earth burial, tradition in simplicity.* http://www.funerals.org

59. Maciejewski, P., Zhang, B., Block, S., & Prigerson, H. (2007). An empirical examination of the stage theory of grief. *Journal of the American Medical Association, 297*(7), 716–723.

60. Corr, C. A., Nabe, C. M., & Corr, D. M. (2009). *Death & dying, life & living* (6th ed., pp. 340–343). Belmont, CA: Wadsworth.

61. Buckley, T., Sunari, D., Marshall, A., Bartrop, R., McKinley, S., & Tofler, G. (2012). Physiological correlates of bereavement and the impact of bereavement interventions. *Dialogues of Clinical Neuroscience, 14*(2), 129–139.

62. Vaillant, G. E. (2002). *Aging well: Surprising guideposts to a happier life from the landmark Harvard study of adult development.* Boston: Little, Brown.

63. Kübler-Ross, E. (1997). *On death and dying* (reprint edition). New York: Collier Books.

64. Byock, I. (2004). *The four things that matter most.* New York: Free Press.

65. U.S. Census Bureau. (2011, June 27). *Facts for features: Back to school.* http://www.census.gov

66. Kvaavik, E., Batty, G. D., Ursin, G., Huxley, R., & Gale, C. R. (2010). Influence of individual and combined health behaviors on total and cause-specific mortality in men and women: The United Kingdom health and lifestyle survey. *Archives of Internal Medicine, 170*(8), 711–718.

Chapter 16

i. National Sleep Foundation. (2011, March 7). 2011 *Sleep in America poll: Communications technology in the bedroom.* http://www.sleepfoundation.org

1. Lund, H. G., Reider, B. D., Whiting, A. B., & Prichard, J. R. (2009). Sleep patterns and predictors of disturbed sleep in a large population of college students. *Journal of Adolescent Health, 46*(2), 124–132.

2. Silverthorn, D. (2010). *Human physiology: An integrated approach* (5th ed.). San Francisco: Benjamin Cummings.

3. Bear, M. F., Connors, B. W., & Paradiso, M. A. (2007). *Neuroscience: Exploring the brain* (3rd ed.). Baltimore: Lippincott Williams & Wilkins, p. 596.

4. American Academy of Sleep Medicine. (2008, December 31). *Seven signs you need sleep.* http://yoursleep.aasmnet.org

5. Harvard Health Publications. (2009, November). *Napping may not be such a no-no.* http://www.health.harvard.edu

6. Bonnet, M. H., & Arand, D. L. (2010). How much sleep do adults need? *White paper, National Sleep Foundation.* http://www.sleepfoundation.org

7. Jones, M. (2011, April 15). How little sleep can you get away with? *The New York Times.* http://www.nytimes.com

8. Kamdar, B., Kaplan, K., Kezirian, E., & Dement, W. (2004). The impact of extended sleep on daytime alertness, vigilance, and mood. *Sleep Medicine, 5,* 441–448.

9. National Sleep Foundation. (2009, March 2). 2009 *Sleep in America poll: Health and safety.* http://www.sleepfoundation.org

10. National Sleep Foundation. (2011, March 7). 2011 *Sleep in America poll: Communications technology in the bedroom.* http://www.sleepfoundation.org

11. American College Health Association. (2013). *American College Health Association National College Health Assessment (ACHA-NCHA II) reference group executive summary, Fall 2012.* http://www.acha-ncha.org

12. Mann, D. (2011). Can better sleep mean catching fewer colds? *WebMD.* http://www.webmd.com

13. Ackermann, K., Revell, V. L, Lao, O., Rombout, E., Skene, D., & Kayser M. (2012.) Diurnal rhythms in blood cell populations and the effect of acute sleep deprivation in healthy young men. *Sleep, 35*(7), 933–940.

14. Centers for Disease Control. (2011, January 27). *Sleep and sleep disorders.* http://www.cdc.gov

15. Luyster, F., Strollo Jr., P., Zee, P., & Walsh, J. (2012.) Sleep: A health imperative. *SLEEP, (35)*6, 727–734.

16. Regestein, Q., Natarajan, V., Pavlova, M., Kawasaki, S., Gleason, R., & Koff, E. (2010). Sleep debt and depression in female college students. *Psychiatry Research, 176*(1), 34–39.

17. Brooks, P. R., Girgenti, A. A., & Mills, M. J. (2009). Sleep patterns and symptoms of depression in college students. *College Student Journal, 43*(2), 464–472.

18. Ahrberg, K., Dresler, M., Niedermaier, S., Steiger, A., & Genzel, L. (2012). The interaction between sleep quality and academic performance. *Journal of Psychiatric Research, 46*(12), 1618–1622.

19. Patel, S. R., & Hu, F. B. (2008). Short sleep duration and weight gain: A systematic review. *Obesity, 16*(3), 643–653.

20. Mitchell, J., Rodriguez, D., Schmitz, K., & Audrain-McGovern, J. (2013.) Sleep duration and adolescent obesity. *Pediatrics, 131,* e1428.

21. Greer, S., Goldstein, A., & Walker, M. (2013.) The impact of sleep deprivation on food desire in the human brain. *Nature Communications, 4.* doi:10.1038/ncomms3259

22. Vail-Smith, K., Felts, W., & Becker, C. (2009). Relationship between sleep quality and health risk behaviors in undergraduate college students. *College Student Journal, 43*(3), 924–930.

23. Gilbert, S. P., & Weaver, C. C. (2010). Sleep quality and academic performance in university students: A wake-up call for college psychologists. *Journal of College Student Psychotherapy, 24*(4), 295–306.

24. Curcio, G., Ferrara, M., & De Dennaro, L. (2006). Sleep loss, learning capacity and academic performance. *Sleep Medicine, 10*(5), 323–337.

25. Gomes, A., Tavares, J., & Azevedo, M. (2011.) Sleep and academic performance in undergraduates: A multi-measure, multi-predictor approach. *Chronobiology International, 28*(9), 786–801.

26. Gaultney, J. F. (2010, September–October). The prevalence of sleep disorders in college students: Impact on academic performance. *Journal of Am Coll Health, 59*(2), 91–97.

27. Thacher, P. V. (2008). University students and the "all nighter": Correlates and patterns of students' engagement in a single night of total sleep deprivation. *Behavioral Sleep Medicine, 6*(1), 16–31.

28. Becker, C. M., Adams, T., Orr, C., & Quilter, L. (2008). Correlates of quality sleep and academic performance. *Health Educator, 40*(2), 82–89.

29. American Academy of Sleep Medicine. (2011, January 7). Sleep: Nature's study aid. *Sleep Education.* Retrieved from http://yoursleep.aasmnet.org/Article.aspx?id=2030

30. Rasch, B., & Born, J. (2013.) About sleep's role in memory. *Physiology Reviews, 93,* 681–766.

31. Greer, M. (2004, July). Strengthen your brain by resting it. American Psychological Association. *Monitor, 35*(7), 60.

32. Carpenter, S. (2001, October). Research confirms the virtues of "sleeping on it." American Psychological Association. *Monitor, 32*(9), 49.

33. National Sleep Foundation. (2011, July 27). *Drowsy driving prevention week highlights prevalent and preventable accidents.* http://drowsydriving.org

34. Uehli, K., Mehta, A. J., Miedinger, D., Hug, K., Schindler, C., Holsboer-Trachsler, E., . . . Künzli, N. (2013, May 20). Sleep problems and work injuries: A systematic review and meta-analysis. *Sleep Medicine Reviews,* pii: S1087-0792(13)00008-7. doi: 10.1016/j.smrv.2013.01.004. ePub ahead of print.

35. Guindalin, C., & Tufik, S. (2012). Genetic aspects of sleep in humans. *Sleep Science, 5*(4), 125–130.

36. Tomfohr, L., Pung, M. A., Edwards, K., & Dimsdale, J. E. (2012). Racial differences in sleep architecture: The role of ethnic discrimination. *Biological Psychology, 89*(1), 34–38.

37. Thompson, J., & Manore, M. (2012). *Nutrition: An applied approach* (3rd ed., p. 85). San Francisco: Benjamin Cummings.

38. Fujiwara, Y., Arkawa, T., & Fass, R. (2012). Gastroesophageal reflux and sleep disturbances. *Journal of Gastroenterology, 47,* 760–769.

39. Edwards, S. J., Montgomery, I. M., Colquhoun, E. Q., Jordan, J. E., & Clark, M. G. (1992, September). Spicy meals disturb sleep: An effect of thermoregulation? *International Journal of Psychophysiology, 13*(2), 97–100.

40. U.S. Fire Administration. (2010, September 23). *Smoking and fire safety.* http://www.usfa.dhs.gov

41. Ruxton, C. H. S. (2008). The impact of caffeine on mood, cognitive function, performance and hydration: A review of benefits and risks. British Nutrition Foundation. *Nutrition Bulletin, 33,* 15–25.

42. WedMD Medical Reference. (2011, February 27). *Caffeine myths and facts.* http://www.webmd.com

43. Substance Abuse and Mental Health Services Administration, Office of Applied Studies. (2010, September). *Results from the 2009 national survey on drug use and health: Volume I: Summary of national findings.* http://oas.samhsa.gov

44. Clegg-Kraynok, M. M., McBean, A. L., & Montgomery-Downs, H. E. (2011). Sleep quality and characteristics of college students who use prescription psychostimulants nonmedically. *Sleep Medicine, 12,* 598–602.

45. Roehrs, T., & Roth, T. (2008, July). *Sleep, sleepiness, and alcohol use.* National Institute on Alcohol Abuse and Alcoholism. http://pubs.niaaa.nih.gov

46. Myllymaki, T., Kyrolainen, H., Savolainen, K., Hokka, L., Jakonen, R., Juuti, T., . . . Rusko, H. (2011, March). Effects of vigorous late-night exercise on sleep quality and cardiac autonomic activity. *Journal of Sleep Research, 20*(1 pt. 2), 146–153.

47. American Academy of Sleep Medicine. (2010). *Sleep disorders.* http://yoursleep.aasmnet.org

48. National Institutes of Health. (2009, March). *Insomnia.* http://www.nhlbi.nih.gov

49. Mayo Foundation. (2010, May 25). *Snoring.* http://www.mayoclinic.com

50. National Institutes of Health. (2009, March). *Sleep apnea.* http://www.nhlbi.nih.gov

51. Young, T., Finn, L., Peppard, P., Szklo-Coxe, M., Austin, D., Nieto, F. J., Stubbs, R., & Hla, K. M. (2008). Sleep disordered breathing and mortality: Eighteen-year follow-up of the Wisconsin sleep cohort. *SLEEP, 31*(8), 1071–1078.

52. National Sleep Foundation. (2011). *Narcolepsy and sleep.* http://www.sleepfoundation.org

53. Townsend, D. R. (2005, October 21). *Nightmares.* American Academy of Sleep Medicine. http://yoursleep.aasmnet.org

54. National Library of Medicine. (2009, June 20). *Sleepwalking.* MedlinePlus. http://www.nlm.nih.gov

55. Mayo Foundation. (2011, May 19). *Sleep bruxism.* http://www.mayoclinic.com

56. Winkelman, J. W. (2006). Sleep-related eating disorder and night-eating syndrome: Sleep disorders, eating disorders, or both? *SLEEP, 29*(7), 876–877.

57. Postuma, R. B., Montplaisir, J. Y., Pelletier, A., Dauvilliers, Y., Oertel, W., Iranzo, A., . . . Wolfson, C. (2012). Environmental risk factors for REM sleep behaviour disorder: A multicenter case-control study. *Neurology, 79*(5), 428–434.

58. National Institutes of Health. (2010, November). *Restless legs syndrome.* http://www.nhlbi.nih.gov

59. Austin, E. (2008). Addressing sleep deprivation in college students. *American Journal for Nurse Practitioners, 12*(6), 34.

60. Brown, F. C., Buboltz, W. C., & Soper, B. (2006). Development and evaluation of the sleep treatment and education program for students (STEPS). *Journal of American College Health, 54*(4), 231–237.

61. Kloss, J. D., Nash, C. O., Horsey, S., & Taylor, D. J. (2011). The delivery of behavioural sleep medicine to college students. *Journal of Adolescent Health, 48*(6), 553–561.

62. National Sleep Foundation. (2011). *Sleep aids and insomnia.* http://www.sleepfoundation.org

63. American Academy of Sleep Medicine. (2011). *Sleep hygiene: The healthy habits of good sleep.* http://yoursleep.aasmnet.org

64. WebMD. (2005, June 1). *Addictive sleep medications remain popular.* http://www.webmd.com

65. Sleep complaints: Whenever possible, avoid the use of sleeping pills. (2008, October). *Prescrire International, 17*(97), 206–212.

66. Kloss, J. D., Nash, C. O., Horse, S. E., & Taylor, D. J. (2011). The delivery of behavioral sleep medicine to college students. *Journal of Adolescent Health, 48*(6), 553–561.

67. Carney, C. E., & Waters, W. F. (2006). Effects of a structured problem-solving procedure on pre-sleep cognitive arousal in college students with insomnia. *Behavioral Sleep Medicine, 4*(1), 13–28.

68. National Center for Complementary and Alternative Medicine. (2010, December). *Sleep disorders and CAM: What the science says.* http://nccam.nih.gov

69. Kozasa, E. H., Hachul, H., Monson, C., Pinto, L., Jr., Garcia, M. C., de Araujo Moraes Mello, L. E., & Tufik, S. (2010, December). Mind–body interventions for the treatment of insomnia: A review. *Revista Brasileira de Psiquiatria, 32*(4), 437–443.

70. Caldwell, K., Harrison, M., Adams, M., & Triplett, N. (2009). Effect of Pilates and taiji quan training on self-efficacy, sleep quality, mood, and physical performance of college students. *Journal of Bodywork and Movement Therapies, 13*(2), 155–163.

71. Harmon, K. (2011, March 8). Short on sleep, the brain optimistically favors long odds. *Scientific American.*

72. National Sleep Foundation. (2011). *Sleep hygiene.* http://www.sleepfoundation.org

73. Lack, L. C., Gradisar, M., Van Someren, E. J., Wright, H. R., & Lushington, K. (2008, August). The relationship between insomnia and body temperatures. *Sleep Medicine Reviews, 12*(4), 307–317.

Chapter 17

i. U.S. Census Bureau. (2013, May 3). *U.S. and world population clock.* http://www.census.gov.

ii. Marcott, S. A., Shakun, J. D., Clark, P. U., & Mix, A. C. (2013, March 8). A reconstruction of regional and global temperature for the past 11,300 years. *Science, 399*(6124), 1198–1201.

iii. Environmental Protection Agency. (2012, November 15). *Municipal solid waste.* http://www.epa.gov

1. World Health Organization. (2013). *Environmental health.* http://www.who.int

2. World Health Organization. (2010). *10 facts on preventing disease through healthy environments.* http://www.who.int

3. Environmental Protection Agency. (2013, April 10). *About EPA: EPA's mission.* http://www2.epa.gov

4. Wong, E. (2013, April 1). Air pollution linked to 1.2 million premature deaths in China. *The New York Times.* http://www.nytimes.com

5. National Research Council. (2009). *Global sources of local pollution: An assessment of long-range transport of key air pollutants to and from the United States.* Washington, DC: The National Academies Press. http://www.nap.edu

6. Lewis, J. (1985, November). The birth of EPA. *EPA Journal.* http://www.epa.gov

7. Kjellstrom, T., & McMichael, A. J. (2013, April 3). Climate change threats to population and well-being: The imperative of protective solutions that will last. *Global Health Action, 6,* 1–9.

8. Medez-Lazaro, P. (2012). Potential impacts of climate change and variability on public health. *Geology & Geosciences, 1,* 2. http://dx.doi.org/10.4172/jgg.1000e104

9. World Health Organization. (2012). Climate change. *Health and Environment Linkages Initiative.* http://www.who.int

10. World Health Organization. (2013). *Global health observatory: Life expectancy.* http://www.who.int

11. Pimentel, D. (2011). World overpopulation. *Environmental Development and Sustainability.* doi: 10.1007/s10668-011-9336-2. http://www.springerlink.com

12. Worldwatch Institute. (2011). *Worldwatch Institute's state of the world 2011.* http://www.worldwatch.org

13. International Energy Agency. (2012). *World energy outlook 2012: Executive summary.* http://www.iea.org

14. U.S. Energy Information Administration. (2013). *International energy statistics: Total primary energy consumption.* http://www.eia.gov

15. International Energy Agency. (2012). CO_2 *emissions from fuel combustion: Highlights.* http://www.iea.org

16. World Bank. (2012, March 9). *Data: Fertility rate.* http://data.worldbank.org

17. U.S. Census Bureau. (2013, May 3). *U.S. and world population clock.* http://www.census.gov

18. United Nations Population Division. (2013). *World population prospects: The 2012 revision population database.* http://esa.un.org

19. Population Reference Bureau. (2010). *Human population.* http://www.prb.org

20. Eberstadt, N., & Shah, A. (2011, December 7). Fertility decline in the Muslim world: A veritable sea-change, still curiously unnoticed. *The American Enterprise Institute Working Paper Series on Development Policy.* http://www.aei.org

21. Peters, G. L. (2012). Depopulation in some rich nations: Good news for planet earth? *Yearbook of the Association of Pacific Coast Geographers, 74,* 122–140.

22. The National Academies. (2013). Our energy sources: Fossil fuels. *What you need to know about energy.* http://needtoknow.nas.edu

23. Environmental Protection Agency. (2012, November 7). *Pollutants and sources.* http://www.epa.gov

24. Environmental Protection Agency. (2013, April 22). *Overview of greenhouse gases: Carbon dioxide emissions.* http://www.epa.gov

25. Gillis, J. (2013, May 10). Heat-trapping gas passes milestone, raising fears. *The New York Times.* http://www.nytimes.com

26. Environmental Protection Agency. (2011, July 21). *Bad nearby.* http://www.epa.gov

27. American Lung Association. (2013). *State of the air 2013.* http://www.stateoftheair.org

28. Global Warming Policy Foundation. (2011, November 19). IPCC introduces new "climate change" definition. *GWPF Science News.* http://thegwpf.org

29. Marcott, S. A., Shakun, J. D., Clark, P. U., & Mix, A. C. (2013, March 8). A reconstruction of regional and global temperature for the past 11,300 years. *Science, 399*(6124), 1198–1201.

30. Environmental Protection Agency. (2013, April 22). *Climate change indicators in the United States.* http://www.epa.gov

31. Nature Conservancy. (2011, January 31). *Brazil: Atlantic forest.* http://www.nature.org

32. Pelletier, N., & Tyedmers, P. (2010). Forecasting potential global environmental costs of livestock production 2000–2050. *Proceedings of the National Academy of Sciences, 107*(43), 18371–18374.

33. United Nations Environment Programme: Ozone Secretariat. (2010). *The 2010 assessment of the scientific assessment panel.* http://ozone.unep.org

34. Environmental Protection Agency. (2011, January 13). *Health and environmental effects of ozone layer depletion.* http://www.epa.gov

35. Environmental Protection Agency. (2010, August 19). *Myth: Ozone depletion occurs only in Antarctica.* http://www.epa.gov

36. Environmental Protection Agency. (2012, December 4). *Acid rain.* http://www.epa.gov

37. Environmental Protection Agency. (2012, March). *Light-duty automotive technology, carbon dioxide emissions, and fuel economy trends, 1975 through 2011.* http://www.epa.gov

38. United Nations Framework Convention on Climate Change. (2012). *The international response to climate change.* http://unfccc.int

39. Global Carbon Project. (2011). *Carbon budget: Highlights: Emissions from fossil fuel and cement.* http://www.globalcarbonproject.org

40. United Nations. (2012). *Water scarcity.* http://www.un.org

41. World Health Organization. (2013, January 26). *Water quality and health strategy: 2013-2020.* http://who.int

42. Environmental Protection Agency. (2013, January 31). *Polychlorinated biphenyls (PCBs).* http://www.epa.gov

43. Food and Drug Administration. (2012, February). *Questions and answers about dioxins and food safety.* http://www.fda.gov

44. Environmental Protection Agency. (2012, May 9). *Assessing health risks from pesticides.* http://www.epa.gov

45. Environmental Protection Agency. (2013, January 17). *Public drinking water systems programs.* http://water.epa.gov

46. Latif, R. (2013, April 25). *U.S. bottled water sales totalled 11.8 billion in 2012.* http://www.bevnet.com

47. Kaye, D. (2010). Bottled water found contaminated with high levels of bacteria. *Clinical Infectious Diseases, 51*(4), pi–ii.

48. NOAA Marine Debris Program. (2011, July). *Marine debris: What we know about the "garbage patches."* http://marinedebris.noaa.gov

49. Environmental Protection Agency. (2012, November 15). *Municipal solid waste.* http://www.epa.gov

50. Foderaro, L. (2009, April 28). Without cafeteria trays, colleges find savings. *The New York Times.* http://www.nytimes.com

51. San Francisco Department of the Environment. (2003). *Resolution setting zero waste date.* http://www.sfenvironment.org

52. City and County of San Francisco, Office of the Mayor. (2012, October 5). *Mayor Lee announces San Francisco reaches 80 percent landfill waste diversion, leads all cities in North America* (News release). http://sfmayor.org

53. Acaroglu, L. (2013, May 4). Where do old cellphones go to die? *The New York Times.* http://www.nytimes.com

54. Environmental Protection Agency. (2012). *Superfund national accomplishments summary fiscal year 2012.* http://epa.gov

55. Environmental Protection Agency. (2012, February 23). *Household hazardous waste management: A manual for one-day community collection programs.* http://www.epa.gov

56. Food and Drug Administration. (2012, March 30). *FDA continues to study BPA.* http://www.fda.gov

57. Environmental Protection Agency. (2012, March 14). *Phthalates: Action plan.* http://www.epa.gov

58. Luz, C. (2012, June). Our food: Packaging and public health. *Environmental Health Perspectives, 120*(6), A232–A237.

59. Environmental Protection Agency. (2013, April 16). *Asbestos: Protect your family.* http://www2.epa.gov

60. National Cancer Institute. (2011, December 6). *Radon and cancer.* http://www.cancer.gov

61. Environmental Protection Agency. (2013, March 14). *An introduction to*

indoor air quality (IAQ): carbon monoxide (CO). http://www.epa.gov

62. Environmental Protection Agency. (2012, July 9). *An introduction to indoor air quality (IAQ): Volatile organic compounds (VOCs).* http://www.epa.gov

63. Environmental Protection Agency. (2011, March 10). *Report on the environment: Indoor air.* http:// cfpub.epa.gov

64. Matsui, E.C. (2009, September). Role of mouse allergens in allergic disease. *Current Allergy and Asthma Reports, 9*(5), 370–375.

65. Centers for Disease Control and Prevention. (2010). *Fourth national report on human exposure to environmental chemicals.* http://www.cdc.gov

66. Harrison, R. V. (2012). The prevention of noise-induced hearing loss in children. *International Journal of Pediatrics, 2012*(2012). Article ID 473541, 13 pages. doi:10.1155/2012/473541. http://www .hindawi.com

67. American Speech-Language-Hearing Association. (2012). *The prevalence and incidence of hearing loss in adults.* http://www.asha.org

68. National Cancer Institute. (2010, June 1). Tanning bed study shows strongest evidence yet of increased melanoma risk. *NCI Cancer Bulletin, 7*(11), 2. http://www.cancer.gov

69. Orr, D. W. (2007). Optimism and hope in a hotter time. *Conservation Biology, 21*(6), 1392–1395.

70. Association for the Advancement of Sustainability in Higher Education. (2012). *Resources for campus sustainability: Resources for students.* http://www .aashe.org

Index

Note: Page references in *italics* refer to figures and tables. An asterisk (*) following a page number indicates a page found in electronic Chapters 16 or 17.

A

Abdominal aortic aneurysm, tobacco use and, 192
Abortion, 244–246, *246*
Absorption, alcohol, 178
Abstinence, 255, 271
Academic performance
    impediments to, 54
    sleep and, 394*
Academic pressure, 56
Academy of Nutrition and Dietetics, 97, 150
Acamprosate, 185
Acceptable Macronutrient Distribution Range (AMDR), 85, *85*
Acceptance and commitment therapy (ACT), 40
Accessory glands, 225–227
Accidents, *5,* 343–347
Acetaminophen, 158
Acid rain, 417*
Acquired immunity, 262
Action, behavior change, 13
Active euthanasia, 379
Active immunity, 262
Active Minds, 46
Active stretching, 110
Activity, physical
    aging and, 372–373
    benefits of, 12–103
    cardiorespiratory fitness, 101–104
    diabetes, risk of, 100
    Dietary Guidelines for Americans, 88, 97
    fitness, components of, 100–102
    fitness training principles, 103–104
    flexibility, 101, 110–111
    frequency recommendations, 111, 114
    muscular strength and endurance, 101, 107
    safety issues, 115–120
    weight management, 102, 103
Acupuncture, *331*
Acyclovir, 274
Adaptation, 50
Adderall, 37, 158, 159, 173, 396*
Addiction
    behavioral, 154
    coping with, 167
    defined, 153
    to technology, 154, *155*
    warning signs of, 154
Addictive behaviors. *See* Alcohol use and abuse; Drug use and abuse
Additive interactions, drugs, 157
Adele, 151, *151*
Adequate Intake (AI), 85
Administration on Aging, 386
Adoption, 253
Adult neurogenesis, 372
Adult-onset diabetes, 287
Advance directives, 377
Advertising, smoking and, 189, 190
Advocacy, 17
Affordable Care Act, 10, 332, *332,* 333, 334, 335
African-Americans
    aging population, 365
    alcohol use and abuse, 176

cancer, 288, 303
cardiovascular disease, 288
diabetes, 288
health disparities, 6
HIV/AIDS and, 272
hypertension, 9
life expectancy, 366
mental health, 32
overweight and obesity, 134
poverty, 288
sexually transmitted infections, 276
sleep, 395*
tobacco use, 191
Age
    alcohol use and abuse, 176, 185
    basal metabolic rate, 134
    cardiovascular disease, 299
    drug use, 155
    health and, 8
    infertility, 253
    sexually transmitted infections, 276
    stress and, 60
    tobacco use, 189, 191
    unintentional injuries, 343
    violent crime, 351
    weight gain and, 134
Ageism, 369
Agency for Healthcare Research and Quality (AHRQ), 302, 340
Age-related macular degeneration (AMD), 367
Aggravated assault, 351, 352–353
Aggressive driving, 345
Aging
    in Blue Zones, 373
    body composition changes, 367
    campus advocacy, 383
    chronic disease, 368–370
    cognition and memory, 370
    current trends, 366
    end-of-life issues, 376–380
    gender and longevity, 366–367
    grief, 381–382, *383*
    hearing loss, 367
    life expectancy, 366
    nutrition needs, 373–374
    personal choices, 380–381
    psychosocial changes, 370–372
    sexuality, 369
    statistics on, 364
    successful, tips for, 372–375
    trends in health and health care, 366
    in United States, *365,* 365–366
    vision loss, 367
    weight management, 374
Aging in place, 371
Agoraphobia, 35
AIDS, 8, *8,* 232, 258, 272
Airborne pathogens, 259
Air pollution, 305, 410*, 413–419*, *415*
Air Quality Index (AQI), 414*, *414*
Alanon-Alateen, 200
Alarm phase, stress response, *50,* 50–51
Alaska Natives, sexually transmitted infections, 276
Alcohol dehydrogenase (ADH), 178
Alcohol dependence, 184
Alcoholic cirrhosis, 182
Alcoholic hepatitis, 182
Alcoholics Anonymous, 186, 200

Alcohol intoxication, 180
Alcohol poisoning, 181, 184
Alcohol use and abuse, 64, *64*
    age and, 179, 185
    alcohol, metabolism of, *178,* 178–179
    alcoholism, 184–185
    behavioral effects, 183–184
    benefits of alcohol, 182, 314
    binge drinking on campus, 175–177
    blood alcohol concentration, 179, *179*
    burn injuries, 349
    campus advocacy, 187
    campus use statistics, 177
    chronic disease, 286, 313
    defined, 184
    driving and, 183–184, 344–345
    effects on body, *180,* 180–183
    friends, 187
    gender and, 179, 185
    hypertension, 294
    injuries and, 343
    intoxication, 180
    makeup of alcohol, 177–178
    media and, 190
    older adults, 372
    peer pressure, 177, 188
    personal choices, 187
    pregnancy, 183
    serving sizes, 178, *178*
    sexual violence, 184, 358–359
    sleep and, 396*, 403*
    statistics, 174, 175
    treatment options, 185–186
    violent crime, 352
Alcohol use disorders identification test (AUDIT), 186
Allergens, 264
Allergic asthma, 264
Allergies, 70, 91–92, *92,* 263–264
Allopathic medicine, 327
Allostatic overload, 52
Alpha waves, sleep and, 390*, 391*
Alternative medicine, 329–330
Altruism, 28, *28*
Alzheimer's Association, 386
Alzheimer's disease (AD), 370, *370*
Ambien, 400*, 407*
Amenorrhea, 229
American Academy of Pediatrics (AAP), 221
American Academy of Sleep Medicine, 400*
American Academy of Sleep Medicine's Consumer Information Site, 406*
American Association for Marriage and Family Therapy, 220
American Association of Poison Control Centers, 362
American Association of Retired Persons (AARP), 386
American Association of University Women, 360
American Cancer Society, 17, 191, 315, 318
American College Health Association, 7, 157, 197
American College of Sports Medicine (ACSM), 105, 111, 115, *115,* 123, 150
American Congress of Obstetricians and Gynecologists (ACOG), 225
American Council on Exercise, 123
American Diabetes Association, 315, 318
American Heart Association, 100, 295, 298, 301, 315, 318
American Institute for Cancer Research, 313
American Lung Association, 193, 414*
    Freedom from Smoking Online, 200

American Medical Association, 183, 387
American Psychiatric Association (APA), 30, 34, 35, 37, 154, 157, 233, 246
American Psychiatric Foundation, 65
American Psychological Association, 46, 60, 68, 220, 236, 246
   Active Minds, 46
   Psychologist Locator, 46
American Social Health Association, 282
American Society of Addiction Medicine, 153
Amino acids, 77
Amniotic fluid, 248
Amphetamines, 161–162, *162, 165*
Anabolic steroids, 118–119
Anaerobic exercise, 106–107
Anal intercourse, 232, 272, 273, 274. *See also* Sexually transmitted infection
Anaphylactic shock, 92, 264
Anaphylaxis, 264
Andropause, 369
Androstenedione, 120
Aneurysm, 298
Anger, *29,* 29–30
Angina, 293
Angina pectoris, 295
Animals, infections from, 259, 269
Anorexia nervosa, 125, 145, *145*
Antagonistic interactions, drugs, 157
Antibiotic resistance, 266
Antibodies, 261
Anticonvulsant medications, 34
Antidepressant medications, 33–34, 37, 369
Antigens, 261
Antioxidants, 83–84, *84*
Antiretroviral drugs, 273
Anxiety and Depression Association of America, 46
Anxiety disorders, 23, 34–37, 54–55
Apgar score, 251
Aphasia, 299
Appetite, 136–137
Arable land, 412*
Armstrong, Lance, 124, *124*
Arrhythmia, 295
Arsenic, 419*
Arteries, 292, *292, 293. See also* Cardiovascular disease
Arthritis, 368
Artificially acquired immunity, 262
Artificial sweeteners, 140
Asbestos, 427*, *428**
Asbestosis, 427*
Asian Americans
   aging population, 365
   alcohol use and abuse, 176
   cancer, 288
   cardiovascular disease, 288
   diabetes, 288
   health disparities, 6
   life expectancy, 366
   overweight and obesity, 134
   poverty, 288
   sleep, 395*
   tobacco use, 191
Assault, 352–353
Assertiveness, 25
Assortative mating, 210
Asthma, 192, 264
Atherosclerosis, 131, 132, *293,* 293–294
Athletes. *See also* Exercise
   ergogenic aids, 82
   gay, 256
   nutrition needs, 90, 116
   performance-enhancing drugs, 118–120, 124
Athletic shoes, 118, *118*
Atkins, Robert, 138

Atkins diet, 137, *138*
Atria, 292, *292*
Attachment theory, 206
Attention deficit hyperactivity disorder (ADHD), 37, 158, 159, 173
Attention disorders, 37
Attraction, 210
Autism, 263
Automated external defibrillator (AED), 296, 298
Autonomy, 25, *25*
Autopsy, 379
Aversion therapy, 40
Avian influenza, 259, 269
Ayurveda, *331*

B

Baby Boomers, 60
BACCHUS Network, 187
Back extension, *109*
Back injuries, 350–351
Backpacks, 351, *352*
Bacteria, 266
   foodborne illness, 90
   infections from, 260
Bacterial infection
   chlamydia, 252
   gonorrhea, 231
   immunizations, 262–263
   Lyme disease, 267, *267*
   meningitis, 266–267, 326
   overview of, 266
   pelvic inflammatory disease, 252, 277
   pneumonia, 267–268
   Staphylococcus, 267
   Streptococcus, 267
   syphilis, 277–278, *273*
   tuberculosis, 258, 268, 272
Ballistic stretching, 110
Balloon angioplasty, 296
Bandura, Albert, 16
Barbiturates, 164, *166*
Bariatric surgery, 142, 290
Basal metabolic rate (BMR), 134
Bath salts, 162
B cells, 261, 272
Behavioral addictions, 154
Behavioral therapy, 39–40
Behavior change
   barriers to, *16*
   factors related to, 12–13
   models of, 13–14
Behavior-change contract, 17
Beliefnet, 46
Benign tumors, 304
Benzene, tobacco, 192
Benzodiazepines, 37, 164
Beta-carotene, 83
Beverages
   caffeine content of, *161*
   pollutants in, 426–427*
Beyoncé, 22, *22*
Bianchi, Suzanne, 217
Biceps curl, *108*
Bicycle accidents, 347
Bicycling, 105, *105,* 121
Biden, Joe, 214
Bidis, *194,* 194–195
Binge drinking, 175–177. *See also* Alcohol use and abuse
Binge eating disorder, 146
Biofeedback, 36
Biofuels, 418*
Biologic therapy, 311

Biology, health and, 8–10
Biomagnification, 426*, *426**
Biomonitoring, 428*
Bipolar disorder, 23, 34
Birth control, 237–244, *238–239, 241, 242, 243,* 244
Birth control pills, 236, *238,* 242–243, *243*
Bisexuality, 211, 232, 235–236
Bisphenol A, 427*
Bisphosphonates, 369
Blackberry thumb, 350
Blastocyst, 248
Blood alcohol concentration (BAC), 175, 179, *179,* 180, 183, 344
Blood glucose, 301. *See also* Diabetes
Blood glucose monitors, 323
Blood lipids, 131, 300–301, *301*
Blood pressure, 293, *294,* 300
Blood pressure kits, 323
Blue Zones, aging in, 373
Boating accidents, 348
Body, The: The Complete HIV/AIDS Resource, 282
Body burden, 428*
Body composition, 129
Body dysmorphic disorder, 144
Body image, *144*
   defined, 126
   disorders, 144
   factors related to, 127
   positive, developing, 147
   support and, 147
Body language, 204, *204*
Body mass index (BMI), 127, *129,* 130, 290
Body measurements, 127–128
Body weight
   healthful, defining, 127–130
   statistics, 125
   websites, 150
   weight trends, 130–131
Bone-building medications, 369
Bones
   activity, benefits of, 102–103
   muscular strength, 101
   osteoporosis, 80
   vitamin D and, 78, 80
Borrelia burgdorferi, 267
Boston Marathon bombing, 355
Botanicals, 82, 330, *331*
Bottled water, 80, 421*, 422*
Botulism, 90
Bovine growth hormone (rBGH), 93
Bovine spongiform encephalitis, 90
BPA, 427*
Bradycardia, 295
Brain
   cancer in, *306*
   cell phone and, 432*
   drugs and effects on, 156
Brain death, 376
Brain fitness, 375
Brain stem, sleep and, 389*, 390*
Braxton Hicks contractions, 248
BRCA1 gene, 9, 310, 337
BRCA2 gene, 9, 310, 337
Breast cancer, 9, 102, 182, 304, 319, 337. *See also* Cancer
Breast self-exam (BSE), 312
Bronchitis, tobacco use and, 192
Bronchoconstriction, 264
Bruxism, 399*
Bryant, Kobe, 256
Budget Worksheet for College Students, 68
Built environment, 10, 136
Bulimia nervosa, 125, 145–146
Bupropion, 196

Burial, 379
Burn injuries, 349
Burnout, 52
Byock, Ira, 382

C

Caffeine, 61, 80, 160–161, *161,* 396*, 402*
Calcium, 79, 80
Calendar method, 237, *238*
Calories. *See also* Energy
　dietary guidelines, 88
　empty, 89
　energy and, 71–72
　healthful weight gain diet, 143, *143*
　reducing, 140
　weight gain, causes of, 135
　weight-loss diets, 137
Campus Men of Strength Clubs, 360
Campus Pride, 218
Campylobacter, 90
Cancer
　activity, benefits of, 102
　aging and, 368, 374
　alcohol use, 182
　breast cancer, 310, 337
　cervical cancer, 275, 306, 311, 326
　colorectal cancer, 308
　defined, 303
　detecting, 306
　excess body weight and, 132
　lung cancer, 307–308, 427*
　oral cancer, 309
　ovarian cancer, 310–311
　overview of, 303
　pancreatic cancer, 308–309
　progression of, *304*
　prostate cancer, 309
　risk factors for, 286, 304–306
　skin cancer, 307, *307,* 417*
　statistics on, 284, *303*
　testicular cancer, 309
　tobacco use and, 192
　treating, 311
　types of, 306–307
　uterine cancer, 311
　websites, 318
Candida albicans, 225, 270
Cannabis, *165*
Cannon, Walter B., 49, 51
Capillaries, 292, 293
Carbohydrates, 72–74, *74*
　complex, 73, 74
　defined, 72
　fiber, 73
　glycemic index, 74
　low-carbohydrate diets, 138–139
　recommended intake, 74
　simple, 73
　whole grains, 73–74, *74*
Carbon dioxide, 413*, *417*,* 419*
Carbon emissions, 411*
Carbon footprint, 417*
Carbon monoxide (CO), 189, 192, 413*, 427*, *428**
Carcinogens, 189, 303, *304,* 305
Carcinomas, 306
Cardiac rehabilitation, 296
Cardiometabolic risk (CMR), 132, 301–303, *302, 313*
Cardiorespiratory fitness, 100–101, 104, 105
Cardiovascular disease (CVD). *See also* Cardiovascular
　　　system
　aging and, 368, 374
　alcohol use, 182
　forms of, 293, *293,* 294–299
　overview of, 291

physical inactivity and, 100
risk factors for, 286, 299–301
saturated fats and, 75
statistics, 284, *295*
tobacco use and, 192
Cardiovascular system, *292. See also*
　　　Cardiovascular disease
　chronic stress, 52
　normal function, 292–293
　target heart rate, 105, 106
　tobacco use and, 192
Caring Connections Advance Directive Forms, 386
Carotenoids, 83
Carpal tunnel syndrome (CTS), 350
Carrier, infection transmission, 258
Carrying capacity, 412*
Carson, Rachel, 410*
Cataracts, 367, *368*
Cathinone, 162
Caucasians
　alcohol use, 175, 176
　cancer, 288
　cardiovascular disease, 288
　diabetes, 288
　health disparities, 6
　life expectancy, 365, 366
　mental health, 32
　overweight and obesity, 134
　poverty, 288
　sleep, 395*
　suicide, 38
　tobacco use, 191
CD4 T cells, 272
Celebrity endorsements, 98
Cell phones, 57, 344, *344,* 423*, 424*, 432*
Cellular death, 376
Center for Public Integrity, 359
Center for Science in the Public Interest, 97
Center for Young Women's Health, 282
Centers for Disease Control and Prevention (CDC), 5, 9, 21,
　　　126, 197, 200, 232, 259, 262, 282, 318, 394*, 435*
　Overweight and Obesity website, 150
Central Intelligence Agency (CIA), 355
Central nervous system cancers, 306
Cerebrum, sleep and, 390*, *390**
Cervarix, 275, 311
Cervical cancer, 225, 275, 306, 311, 326
Cervical cap, *238,* 242
Cervical mucus, 228
Cesarean section (C-section), 252
Chain of infection, 258, *259*
Chancre, syphilis, 277, *277*
Chantix, 196
Checkups, medical, 324
Chemical imbalance theory, of mental disorders, 30
Chemotherapy, 311
Chewing tobacco, 195, *195*
Chickenpox, *262*
Childbearing age, 224
Childbirth, 250–252
Children, 194, 216–217
　body image, 126
　choking incidents, 348
　grief in, 380
Chilean miners, rescue of, 69
China, "one child policy," 413*
Chinese medicine, traditional, 330
Chiropractic medicine, 330, *331*
Chlamydia, 252, 275, 277, 278
Chlamydia trachomatis, 275
Chloride, 79
Chlorofluorocarbons (CFCs), 417*
Choking, 343, 347–348, *349*
Cholera, 8
Cholesterol, 75, 293

healthy diet, 137–138
home tests, 323
ChooseMyPlate.gov, 87, *87*
Choose This, Not That
　conflict resolution, 206
　exercise *vs.* alcohol, 64, *64*
　fitness level, 119
　healthful *vs.* high-fat lunch, 82, *82*
　healthy food choices, 142
　safe driving, 346
Chromium, 79
Chromosomes, 337
Chronic disease, 5. *See also* Cancer; Cardiovascular
　　　disease; Diabetes
　aging and, 366, 368–370, 374
　campus advocacy, 315
　diversity and disparities in, 288
　overview of, 285–288
　personal choices, 312–314
　risk factors for, 286, *286*
　sleep difficulties and, 394*
　supporting friends with, 314
　websites, 318
Chronic obstructive pulmonary disease (COPD), 192
Chronic severe subtype, alcoholism, 185
Chronic stress syndrome, 52–55, *53*
Cialis, 230
Cigars/cigarettes
　aging and, 374, 380
　chemical contents, 189
　forms of, *194,* 194–195
　"light" cigarettes, 194
　warning labels, 201
Cilia, 260
Circadian rhythm, 390*
Circumcision, 225, *225,* 226
Cirrhosis, liver, 182
Civil Rights Act of 1964, 357
Clean Air Act of 1963, 418*
Cleaning products, environmentally friendly, 423*
Climate change, 410*, 411*, 414–417*
Clinical death, 376
Clinton, Hillary, 214
Clitoris, 223, *224*
Clooney, George, 283, *283*
Clostridium botulinum, 90
Clothing, physical activity, 115–116
Clove cigarettes, 194, *194*
Club drugs, 163–164, *166*
COBRA, 335
Cocaine, 161, *161, 165. See also* Drug use
　　　and abuse
Codeine, 158
Coffee, 181
Cognition, aging and, 370, 375
Cognitive-behavioral therapy (CBT), 36, 37, 39, 400*
Cognitive distortion, 39
Cohabitation, 210, 213
Coitus, 232
Colds, 264
Cold virus, *259*
College Diabetes Network, 315
CollegeTown, 253
Collins, Jason, 256, *256*
Colorectal cancer, 102, 304, 308, 323
Columbine High School, Colorado, shooting at, 353
Commitment, 208, *208*
Communication skills
　relationships and, 203–205, *204*
　sex, communication about, 244
　social media, 209
Companionate love, 208, *208*
Complementary and alternative medicine (CAM),
　　　400*, 401*
　defined, 329

evaluating therapies, 330, 332
types of, *331*
Complete proteins, 77
Complex carbohydrates, 73, 74
Compliance, blood pressure and, 294
Comprehensive Environmental Response and Liability Act, 424*
Compulsive spending, 154
Conception, 236–237
Concerta, 37
Condoms, 232, 236, *238,* 240–241, *241,* 243, 253, 274, 279
Conflict avoidance, 205
Conflict escalation, 205
Conflict Management Information Source, 220
Conflict resolution, 205, 206
Congenital heart disease, 299
Congestive heart failure, 294, 298
Consumer Corner
    athletic shoes, 118, *118*
    beverages, 81
    bicycle helmets, 348
    bottled water, 422*
    choosing a therapist, 40
    "light" cigarettes, 194
    organic, local, all natural, and fair trade choices, 93
    over-the-counter medications, 324
    sleep aids, 401*
Consumer health
    being smart patient, 328–329
    campus advocacy, 338
    checkups and preventive care, 324
    emergency situations, 326
    genomics, 336–338
    herbal and dietary supplements, 330
    home health tests, 323–324, *324*
    information sources, evaluating, 322–323
    paying for care, 332–336
    personal choices, 338
    physicians, when to seek help, 324–326
    providers, choosing, 328
    providers, complementary and alternative medicine, 329–330, *331, 332*
    providers, conventional, 327–328
    screenings, recommended, *325*
    self-care, defined, 321
    statistics, 320
    vaccinations, 326, *326*
    websites, 322, 340
    wellness habits, 321–322
Consummate love, 208, *208*
Contaminated objects, infections from, 259
Contemplation, behavior change, 13
Continuation rate, birth control, 243
Contraception, 237–244, *238–239, 241, 242, 243, 253,* 413*
Contraceptive sponge, *238,* 241, *242*
Conventional health care, finding, 327–328
Conventional medicine, 327
Cool-down, physical activity, 115
Co-pays, medical services, 332–333
Copper, 79
Core muscle strength, building, 107, *107*
Coronary angiography, 296
Coronary arteries
    atherosclerosis, 293
    coronary heart disease, 295–296
    normal function, 292–293
Coronary artery bypass grafting (CABG), 296
Coronary heart disease (CHD), 52, 295
    angina, 295
    arrhythmia and sudden cardiac arrest, 295
    clinical management of, 295–296, 298
    excess body weight and, 132

myocardial infarction, 295
    tobacco use and, 192
Coronaviruses, 264
Corpus luteum, 228
Cortisol, 51
Cotinine, 193, 428*
Counselors, 39
Counter-conditioning, 17
Cowper's glands, *225, 227*
CPAP machine, sleep apnea, 397*, *398*
CPR, 297, 298
Cramps, 118
Craving, drug addiction, 153, 154, 157
C-reactive protein (CRP), 301
Creatine, 119
Credit card debt, 56, 57, 65
Cremation, 379
Crystal meth, 162
Cue control, 17
Cues to action, behavior change, 13
Cunnilingus, 231
Curl-up, *109*
Cyber-bullying, 209
Cyberstalking, 356–357
Cycle of violence, 356
Cytokines, 260
Cytotoxic T cells, 261, 262

D

Daily hassles, 56
Dairy foods, 89, 98
Danger zone, food-borne illness, 91
DASH diet, 294
Date (acquaintance) rape, 358
Date rape drugs, 163–164, *164,* 358, 359
Dating, 210–211
Davis, Kelly, 407*
Day of the Dead, Mexico, 376, *377*
DDT, 410*
Death
    definitions of, 376
    developing concepts of, 376–377
    end-of-life issues, 377–379
    grief, 379–380
    leading causes of, 1, *4, 7*
    psychology of the dying, 381
Debt, 65
Decibels, noise pollution, 429–430*, *430*
Deductibles, health care, 333
Deep breathing, 63
Defense of Marriage Act (DOMA), 214
Deforestation, 416*
Dehydration, 116, 180
Delta sleep, 391*
Delusions, 37
Dementia, 370, 372
Dental hygiene, 321, *322*
Dentists, 327
Department of Homeland Security, 355
Dependence, drugs, 157
Depressants, 164–165, *166*
Depression, 23, 54, 394*, 396*
Depressive disorders, 31, 33–34
Destructive thoughts, 41
Determinants of health, 8–10
    biology and genetics, 8–9
    individual behaviors, 9
    physical determinants, 10
    social determinants, 9–10
Diabetes, 52
    aging and, 368
    chronic disease, overview, 285–286
    chronic stress and, 290
    clinical management of, 290–291

detecting, 289
    diabetes mellitus, 286
    excess body weight and, 131, 289, *289*
    exercise and, 290
    long-term effects of, 289
    managing, 324
    physical inactivity and, 100
    statistics, 284
    trans fats and, 76
    types of, 286–288
    websites, 318
Diagnostic and Statistical Manual of Mental Disorders (DSM), 30
Diaphragm, *238, 242, 242*
Diastolic pressure, 294
Diencephalon, sleep and, 389*, *390*
Diet. *See also* Nutrients; Weight management
    chronic disease and, 312
    complex carbohydrates, 74
    defined, 71
    diabetes, 290
    drug addiction, 169
    guidelines, 88
    for healthful weight gain, *143*
    healthy food choices, 142, 342
    heart health, 301
    low-calorie, 137
    low-sodium, 294
    popular, *138*
    premenstrual syndrome, 228
    stress and, 61
    vegetarian, 91
    weight-loss, 137, *137*
Dietary Guidelines for Americans, 88, 97, 294
Dietary Reference Intakes (DRIs), 85, *85*
Dietary supplements, 81–82, 83, 330
Diethylpropion, 141
Dieting, on campus, 132
Diet pills, 139–141
Digestive system
    digestive process, *72*
    stress response, 52
Dilation and evacuation (D&E), 245–246
Dioxins, 420*, 427*
Diphtheria, *262*
Disease
    definition of, 2
    health *vs.,* 2–3
Disordered eating, 146
Disorder of sexual development, 236
Disorganized thinking, 37
Distress, 49
Distribution half-life, drugs, 157
Disulfiram, 185
Diversity & Health
    aging in the Blue Zones, 373
    alcohol use, 176
    chronic disease, 288
    drug use, 155
    health disparities, 6
    heart disease, 300
    injuries and violence, 353
    men, women, and building muscle, 101
    mental health, 32
    overweight, obesity, ancestry, and the "thrifty gene," 135
    safe exercise for special populations, 120
    same-sex marriage, 214
    sexually transmitted infection, 276
    sleep, 395*
    stress, 60
    tobacco use, 191
    vegetarian diets, 91
    working for environmental justice, 425*, *425*
Divorce, 214–215

DNA (deoxyribonucleic acid), 236, 303, 336
Dodson, John, 52
Domestic partnerships, 215
Domestic violence, 355
Do Not Resuscitate (DNR) order, 377
Dopamine, 30, 156, 158, 161, 191
Dreaming sleep, 390*, 391*, *391*
Driving
    alcohol use and, 183–184
    drowsy, 394*
    texting and, 344, *344*
Drought, 415*
Drowning, 343, 348–349
Drowsiness, 390*, *391*
Drug Enforcement Agency (DEA), 156
Drugs
    defined, 155
    misuse, defined, 156
    tainted, 160
Drugs of Abuse Information, 172
Drug testing, 165, 167
Drug use and abuse
    amphetamines, 161–162
    body response to, 156–157
    caffeine, 160–161, *161*
    campus advocacy, 169
    cardiovascular disease, 301
    club drugs, 163–164
    cocaine, 161, *161*
    commonly abused drugs, 157–158, 160–165,
        165–166, 167
    common methods of drug administration, *157*
    "date rape drugs," 163–164, *164*
    defined, 156
    depressants, 164
    hallucinogens, 162–163
    heroin, 165
    inhalants, 164
    injuries and, 343
    LSD, 162
    marijuana, 158, 160, *160*
    MDMA (ecstasy), 163
    methamphetamine, 162, *162*
    older adults, 372
    overview of addiction, 153–154
    patterns of, 155–156
    PCP, 163, *163*
    personal choices, 168–169
    prescription and over-the-counter medications,
        157–158, *158*
    prevention and treatment, 167–168
    statistics on, 152, 153
    stimulants, 160–162, 396*
    "study drugs," 159
    violent crime, 352
    websites, 172
DWI, 183–184
Dynamic flexibility, 110
Dynamic muscular endurance, 101
Dynamic stretching, 110
Dyslipidemia, 300
Dysmenorrhea, 229
Dysphoria, 228
Dysthymic disorder, 31

E

Ears
    aging, hearing loss, 367
    noise pollution, 429–430*
Eartheasy Non-Toxic Home Cleaning, 435*
Eating disorders, 125, 144–146, *145*
    amenorrhea and, 229
    anorexia nervosa, 145, *145*

bulimia nervosa, 145–146
    getting help for, 147
Eat Right for Your Type diet, *138*
ECG (EKG), 295
Echocardiogram, 296
Ecological footprint, 412*
Ecological models, behavior change, 13–14, *14*
Economics, aging and, 371
Ecosystem, 409*
Ecstasy, club drugs, 163, *166*
Ectopic pregnancy, 250, 277
Education level
    alcohol use and abuse, 176
    tobacco use, 191
Edwards, John, 159
EEG, 295–296
Effacement, 251
Ejaculation, premature, 230–231
Ejaculatory duct, 225, *225*
Electrocardiogram, 295
Electroconvulsive therapy (ECT), 40–41
Electroencephalograph (EEG), 389*
Electrolytes, 116
Electronic cigarettes, 195
Embryo, development of, 248, *249*
Emergency contraception (EC), *238, 239,* 242, 243
Emergency response, cardiac events, 297
Emotional abuse, 356
Emotional health. *See also* Psychological health
    chronic disease and, 313
    defined, 24
    heart health, 301
    premenstrual dysphoric disorder, 228–229
    premenstrual syndrome, 228
    schizophrenia, 37
    stress and, 63–64
Emotional intelligence (EI), 25
Emphysema, tobacco use and, 192
Employment, aging and, 371
Empty calories, 89
Empty love, 208, *208*
Empty nest syndrome, 371
Enabling factors, behavior, 12
Endocrine disruptors, 427*
End-of-life issues, 377–379
Endometrial cancer, 311
Endometriosis, 229, 252
Endometrium, 224
Endorphins, 168
Energy, calories and, 71–72
Energy balance, 133, *133*
Energy consumption, reducing, 417–418*
Energy drinks, 80
Energy therapies, 330, *331*
Environment, defining, 410*
Environmental health, *3, 4*
    air pollution, 413–419*, *415*
    campus advocacy, 432–433*
    evolution of, 410–411*
    as global issue, 410*
    land pollution, 422–424*
    noise pollution, 429–430*
    overview, 409–410*
    personal choices, 432*
    pollution at home, 426–429*, *428*
    population growth, *411*, 411–413*, *413*
    radiation, 431*, *431*
    statistics about, 408*
    sustainability, 411*
    water pollution, 419–422*, *421*
    websites, 435*
Environmental justice, 425*, *425*
Environmental mastery, 25, *25*
Environmental Protection Agency (EPA), 92, 308, 410*, 435*

Environmental stressors, 57
Environmental tobacco smoke, 193
Environmental Working Group, 435*
Enzyme immunoassay (EIA), 273
Ephedra, 120
Epididymis, 225, *225*
Epstein-Barr virus, 265
Erectile dysfunction (ED), 230
Erection, 225
Ergogenic aids, 82
Ergot, 162
Escherichia coli (E. coli), 90
Essential fatty acids (EFAs), 75
Essential nutrients, 71
Estate, 378
Estimated Average Requirement (EAR), 85
Estimated Energy Requirement (EER), 85
Estrogen, 242, 300, 368
Ethanol, 177. *See also* Alcohol use and abuse
Ethics, genomics and, 338
Ethnicity
    alcohol use and abuse, 176
    chronic disease, 288
    health, 9
    health disparities, 6
    life expectancy, 366
    mental health, 32
    sleep, 395*
    suicide, 38
    tobacco use, 191
    weight gain, 134
Ethyl alcohol, 177. *See also* Alcohol use and abuse
Eustress, 49
Euthanasia, active and passive, 379
Evaluating Health Information on the Internet, 340
Evidence-based medicine, 323, 327
e-waste, 423*, *423*
Excitement phase, human sexual response
        cycle, 229
Exercise, 41, 64, *64,* 88
    ACSM guidelines, *115*
    aerobic, 105–106
    aging and, 372–373, *374*
    anaerobic, 106–107
    benefits of, 102–103
    body composition and, 101–102
    campus advocacy, 121
    cancer, reducing risk of, *305*
    cardiorespiratory fitness and, 100–101, 104, 105
    chronic disease, preventing, 313
    defined, 100
    diabetes, management of, 290–291
    diabetes, risk of, 290
    fitness training principles and, *103,* 103–104, *104*
    flexibility, 101, 110–111
    frequency recommendations, 111, 114
    heart health, 301
    intensity levels, *105*
    isometric and isotonic, 107
    menopause and, 369
    muscular strength and endurance, 101,
        106–107, 110
    nutrition and, 90
    personal choices, 120–121
    pregnancy, 248
    safety issues, 115–120
    for special populations, 120
    stress and, 61, 62, *62*
    websites, 123
    weight gain, causes of, 135
    weight loss and, 141
Exhaustion stage, stress response, *50, 52*
Exposure therapy, 40
External locus of control, 16

Eye contact, 204
Eyes
    aging and, 367
    cataracts, 367
    diabetes, 289

F

Facebook, 47, 202, 209
Failure rate, birth control, 243
Fair trade, 93
Fallopian tubes, 224, *224*, 252
Falls, 343
Family health history, 9, 337
Family life
    aging and, 370–371
    choosing children, 216
    happy families, characteristics, 217
    single parenthood, 217
    stepfamilies, 216–217
Fantasy, sexual, 231
Fasting blood glucose test (FBG), 289
Fatigue, 344–345
Fats, dietary, 74–77
    as food lipids, 75
    "good," 138
    healthful, *76,* 140
    recommended intake of, 76–77
    saturated, 75
    trans fats, 76, 137–138
    unsaturated, 75
Fat soluble, 426*
Fat-soluble vitamins, 77, *78–79*
"Fat Studies," 144
Fatty acids, 75
Fatty liver, 132, 182
Fatuous love, 208, *208*
Federal Bureau of Investigation (FBI), 351, 355
Federal Comstock Act, 246
Federal Trade Commission (FTC), 139
Federal Uniform Drinking Age Act (FUDAA), 175
Fee, Richard, 173, *173*
Fee-for-service plans, 333
Fellatio, 231
Female athlete triad, 147
Female sexual anatomy, 223–224, *224*
Female-to-male (FTM) transsexuals, 236
Fermentation, 177
Fertility, 132, 216, 237, *238, 240*
Fertility drugs, 252
Fertility rate, 412*, 413*
Fertilization, 237, *237,* 248
Fetal alcohol syndrome, 183
Fetal development, 248, *249*
Fetus, 248
Fiber, dietary, 73, 83, 314
Fibrillation, 295
Fight-or-flight response, *50,* 50–51, 55
Financial stressors, 56
Fire injuries, *349,* 349–350
FitDay, 150
Fitness apps, 117
FITT principle, 103–104, *104*
Flat affect, 37
Flavonoids, 83
Flexibility, 101, 110–111
Flexible spending accounts (FSAs), 333, 335
Flexitarians, 91
Fluid balance, 374
Fluorescent light bulbs, *418**
Fluoride, 79
Flu shots, 326
Folic acid, 78
Follicle-stimulating hormone (FSH), 227–228

Food
    allergies, 91–92, *92*
    caffeine content of, *161*
    groups, 89
    intolerances, 92
    labels, 85–87, *86,* 88
    pollutants in, 426–427*
    residues, 92
    supply, safety of, 90
Food and Drug Administration (FDA), 5, 34, 80, 83, 87, 90, 97, 120, 139, 140, 141, 142, 158, 195, 201, 243, 245, 255, 323, 427*
Foodborne illness, 90–91
Foodsafety.gov, 97
Food Safety Modernization Act, 90
Forcible rape, 358
Foreplay, 231
Foreskin, 225, *225,* 226
Formaldehyde, *428**
Fossil fuels, 413*, *417**
Fractures, osteoporosis and, 368
Freebase cocaine, 161
Free radicals, 83
Frequency, FITT principle, 103, *104*
Freud, Sigmund, 24, 27, 40
Friedman, Meyer, 55
Friendships, 42, 65, 144, 207–208, 314–315, 360. *See also* Relationships
Fructose, 73
Fruits, 84, *84,* 87, *87*
Fun, 42
Functional death, 376
Functional foods, 83
Functional subtype, alcoholism, 185
Funerals, 379
Fungal infections, 270
Fungi, 270
Fusion inhibitors, 273

G

GABA, 375
Galactose, 73
Gallbladder disease, 132
Gambling, pathological, 154
Games, high-tech, 375
Gamete intrafallopian transfer (GIFT), 252
Garbage, 422–423*
Gardasil, 275, 311
Gastric banding, 142
Gastric bypass, 142
Gastroesophageal reflux disease (GERD), 396*
Gastrointestinal system, alcohol, effects of, 180
Gay people, 6, 38, 211
Gender
    alcohol use and abuse, 176, 179, 185
    attention deficit hyperactivity disorder, 37
    body image, 126–127
    building muscle, 101
    cardiovascular disease, 299–300
    communication and, 205
    death and dying, 376
    depressive disorders, 31, 33, *33*
    drug use, 155
    generalized anxiety disorder, 35
    health, 8
    heart attacks, 296
    longevity, 366–367
    mental health, 31, 33
    roles, relationships and, 207
    sexually transmitted infections, rates of, 276
    sleep, 395*
    stress and, 52, 56, 60
    tobacco use, 191

    violent crime, 351
    weight gain, 134
Gender identity, 236
General adaptation syndrome (GAS), 50, *50*
Generalized anxiety disorder (GAD), 34–35
Genes
    cancer and, 303
    defined, 336
Genetically modified foods, 92
Genetic counselor, 337
Genetic factors
    Alzheimer's disease, 370
    bipolar disorder, 34
    cancer, 304
    cardiovascular disease, 300
    depressive disorders, 31
    diabetes, risk of, 290
    genomics, 336
    health and, 8–9
    schizophrenia, 37
    sleep patterns, 395–396*
    weight gain, 134
Genetic Information Nondiscrimination Act (GINA), 338
Genital warts, 326
Genome, 336
Genome sequencing, 337
Genomics, 336, 337, 338
Gen Xers, 60
Geography
    alcohol use and abuse, 176
    drug use, 155
    stress, 60
    tobacco use, 191
Germ theory of disease, 410*
Gestational diabetes, 287–288
GHB (gamma-hydroxybutyric acid), 163, *166,* 184
Glaucoma, 367, *368*
Globalization, 411*, 412*
Global warming, 414–415*
"Globesity," 8
Glucose, 50, 73, 74
Glucose monitoring, 290
Gluteal stretch, *113*
Glycated hemoglobin test (A1C test), 289
Glycemic index, 74
Glycogen, 73
Go Ask Alice, 21, 220, 255
Gonorrhea, 231, 252, 277, 278
Google, 12
Google Plus, 209
Grades, 65
Grains, 87, *87*
"Granny pods," 371
Granovetter, Mark, 218
Great American Condom Campaign (GACC), 253
Green burials, 379
Greenhouse effect, *416**
Greenhouse gases, 413*, *417**, 419*
Greenpeace, 432*, 436*
Grief, 380, 382
Ground-level ozone, 414*
Groundwater, 419*
Growth hormone, 391*
Gum disease, diabetes and, 289
Gummas, 278
Guns, 352

H

Habits, 1, 321–322, *322. See also* Self-Assessment
Hallucinations, 37
Hallucinogens, 162–163, *166*
Hamstrings stretch, *113*
Hand washing, 90, 260

Hangover, 180, 181
Hannah, Daryl, 436*
Hardiness, 56
Hate crimes, 355
Hazardous waste, 423–424*
Hazing, 355, 363
HDL, 131, 137
Health
    across America, 4–6
    aging and trends in, 366
    on America's campuses, 6–7
    definitions of, 2–3
    determinants of, 8–10
    disease *vs.*, 2–3
    global, 7–8
    keys to, *5*
    wellness and, dimensions of, 3–4
    wellness *vs.*, 3
Health belief model, 13
Health care
    paying for, 332–336
    trends in, 366
Health-care directive, 377
Health-care proxy, 377
Health discount program, 332
Health disparities, 6
Health exchanges, state, 333
Healthful weight, 127
Health history, 9
Health information
    accurate, 322–323
    in media, evaluating, 11
Health insurance, 10, 288, 328, 332–333
Health Insurance Marketplace, 335, 336
Health literacy, 10, 12
Health maintenance organizations (HMOs), 333
Health on the Net Foundation, 11
Health-related fitness, 100. *See also*
        Physical fitness
Health savings accounts (HSAs), 333, 335
Health services, access to, 10
Healthy Campus Initiative, 7
Healthy People 1990, 5–6
Healthy People 2020, 5–6
Healthy People Initiative, 5–6
Hearing loss, 367, 429*, 430*
Heart, 292, *292*
    activity, benefits of, 102
    cardiorespiratory fitness, 100–101, 104
    normal cardiovascular function, 292–293
    target heart rate, 105, 106
Heart attack, 289, 291, 295, 297
Heart disease, 52, 294, 337
    excess body weight and, 131
    omega-3 and omega-6 fatty acids, 75
    sleep difficulties and, 394*
    tobacco use and, 192
    trans fats and, 76
Heart valve disorders, 299
Heat exhaustion, 117
Heatstroke, 117–118
Heavy episodic drinking, 175
Heavy metals, 429*
Helicobacter pylori, 53
Helmets, 347, 348
Helminths, 271
Helper T cells, 261, 272
Hemophilia, 337
Hemorrhagic stroke, 298, *298*
Hepatitis, 182, 266
Hepatitis A, 90, 262, *262,* 266
Hepatitis B, 231, *262,* 273, 306
Hepatitis C, 266
Herbal supplements, 59, 330

Herbicides, 420*, *428*,* 429*
Herbs, 82
Herd immunity, 263
Heroin, 158, 165, *165, 166. See also* Drug use
        and abuse
Herpes, genital, 273–274, *275*
Hertz, Rosanna, 217
Heterosexuality, 211, 232–233
H5N1 virus, 269
Hierarchy of needs (Maslow), *26,* 26–27
High-density lipoprotein (HDL), 300
High-fructose corn syrup (HFCS), 73, 80
Highly active antiretroviral therapy (HAART), 273
High-tech games, 375
Hip flexor stretch, *113*
Hippocratic Oath, 387
Hip stretch, *113*
Hispanics
    aging population, 365
    alcohol use and abuse, 176
    cancer, 288
    cardiovascular disease, 288
    diabetes, 288
    health disparities, 6
    mental health, 32
    overweight and obesity, 134
    poverty, 288
    sexually transmitted infections, 276
    tobacco use, 191
Histamine, 264
HIV (human immunodeficiency virus), 8, *8,* 232, 306
    incidence of, 272, *272*
    preventing, 273
    statistics, 257
    testing and treatment, 272–273, 323
    transmission of, 272–273, *273*
Holmes, Thomas, 57
Home, pollution in, 426–429*, *428**
Home care, end of life, 378
Home health tests, 323–324, *324*
Homeopathy, *331*
Homeostasis, 49–50
Homicides, 355
Homocysteine, 301
Homonegativity, 211, 235
Homophobia, 235, 253
Homo sapiens, 412*
Homosexuality, 211, 232, 233, 235
HONcode certification, 322
H1N1 flu pandemic, 265, 269
Hooking up, 210
Hormones
    birth control pills, 242–243
    childbirth, 251
    depressive disorders, 33
    menstrual cycle, *227,* 227–228
    pregnancy, 247
    stress response, 51
    weight gain, 134
Hormone therapy (HT), 369
Hospice, 378
Hospitals, 328, 378
Host, infection transmission, 258
Hot flashes, 369
Household hazardous waste, 424*
Howarth, Glennys, 376
H7N9 virus, 269
Human chorionic gonadotropin (hCG), 228, 247
Human genome, 336
Human Genome Project, 341
Human growth hormone (HGH), 119
Human papillomavirus (HPV), *262,* 274–275, 306,
        311, 326
Human Rights Campaign, 220

Human sexual response cycle, 229
Humor, 63–64
Hunger, 8, 136, 396*
Hybrid electric vehicles (HEVs), 420*
Hydration, 116. *See also* Fluid balance
Hydrocodone, 158
Hydrogenation, oils, 76
Hydroxycut diet supplements, 139
Hygiene hypothesis, 264
Hyperglycemia, 287, 289
Hypersexual disorder, 154
Hypertension, 79, 132, 250, 291, 294–295
Hypertrophic cardiomyopathy (HCM), 299
Hypoglycemia, 181
Hypothalamus, 51, 389*, 390*, *390**
Hypothermia, 117, 181
Hysterectomy, *239,* 243

I

Illicit drugs, 155–156
Illness, defined, 2
Illness-wellness continuum, *3*
Immune disorders, 263–264
Immune response, *261*
Immune system
    activity, benefits of, 102
    chronic stress and, 54
    response, overview, 260–262
Immunizations, 262–263
Immunoglobulins, 264
Immunotherapy, 311
Implantable cardioverter defibrillator (ICD), 298
Implantation, 237, *237*
Implants, contraceptive, *239*
Incomplete proteins, 77
Individuality, fitness training, 104, 193
Infant mortality, 250
Infatuation, 208, *208*
Infections, defined, 258
Infectious agents, cancer and, 306
Infectious disease. *See also* Sexually
        transmitted infection
    bacterial infections, 266–268
    emerging, 269
    fungal infections, 270
    immunizations, 262–264
    parasitic worm infections, 270
    protection against, 260–264, 270
    protozoan infections, 270
    spread of, 258–260
    viral infections, 264–266
Infertility, 225, 252–253
Inflammation, atherosclerosis and, 293, 301
Inflammatory markers, 301
Inflammatory response, 260
Influenza, 257, 258, *262,* 264–265, *265*
Ingestion, drugs, *157,* 162, *165*
Inhalation, drugs, *157,* 162, 164, *165, 166*
Injection, drugs, *157,* 162, 165, *165*
Injections, contraceptive, *239*
Injury
    activity, benefits of, 103
    bicycling, 347
    campus advocacy, 360
    care for, 118
    choking and suffocation, 347
    drowning and other water injuries, 348–349
    fire injuries, *349,* 349–350
    intentional, 343, 351–352
    motor vehicle accidents, 343–346
    personal choices, 359–360
    poisoning, 347
    sleep problems, 394*

statistics on, 342, 343
stretching and, 116
traumatic brain injury, 346, 347
unintentional, overview of, 343
violence, 351–352, 353
websites, 362
work safety, 350–351
Injury Prevention Web, 362
Inner-thigh butterfly stretch, 113
Insecticides, 410*, 429*
Insects, infections from, 259
Insomnia, 397*, 397*
Insulin, 286, 287
Insulin-dependent diabetes, 287
Insulin resistance, 287, 301
Insulin therapy, 291
Intellectual health, 3, 3
Intensity, FITT principle, 103, 104
Intentional injury, 343
Intercourse, 230, 232. See also Sexual health; Sexually
    transmitted infection
Intergovernmental Panel on Climate Change
    (IPCC), 410*
Intermediate familial subtype, alcoholism, 185
Internal locus of control, 16
Internal stressors, 59
International Association for Near-Death Studies, 377
Internet
    addiction to, 154
    information on, 11, 12, 322–323
Intersex, 211
Intervention, drug treatment, 169
Intestate, 378
Intimacy, 25, 25, 208, 208
Intimate partner violence (IPV), 355–356
Intracytoplasmic sperm injection (ICSI), 252
Intrauterine device (IUD), 238, 242
Intrauterine insemination, 252
Intrinsic asthma, 264
In vitro fertilization (IVF), 252
Iodine, 79
Ionizing radiation, 431*, 431*
Iron, 79
Ischemic stroke, 298, 298
Isometric exercise, 107
Isotonic exercise, 107

J

Jaundice, 266
Jealousy, 212–213
Jeanne Clery Act, 355
Jed Foundation, 46, 65
Jenny Craig, 138
Jet lag, 390*, 401*
Jobs
    injuries, 350–351
    stress and, 56
Jogging, 105
Johnson, Virginia E., 229
Jolie, Angelina, 311
Jourard, Sidney M., 203
Journaling, stress and, 61

K

Kaposi's sarcoma, 272
Karate, 105
Keystone XL pipeline, 436*
Kickboxing, 105
Kidneys, diabetes and, 289
King, Martin Luther, Jr., 217
Kinsey, Alfred, 232
Kinsey Scale, 232, 235

Kobasa, Suzanne, 56
Kreteks, 194
Kübler-Ross, Elisabeth, 381
Kyoto Protocol, 419*

L

Labels
    food, 85–87
    OTC medications, 324
Labia majora, 223, 224
Labia minora, 223, 224
Labor, childbirth, 250–252, 251
Lactobacillus acidophilus, 266
Lacto-ovo-vegetarians, 91
Lactose, 73
Lagerfeld, Karl, 151
Land pollution, 422–424*
LAP-BAND, 143
Latent autoimmune diabetes of adults (LADA), 288
Latinos
    alcohol use, 176
    cardiovascular disease, 288
    diabetes, 288
    health disparities, 6
    mental health, 32
    overweight and obesity, 134
    sexually transmitted infections, 276
    tobacco use, 191
Laughter, 63–64
Lawless, Lucy, 436*
Lead, 428*, 428*
Learning, sleep and, 394*
Ledger, Heath, 158
Left ventricular hypertrophy, 301
Leg abduction, 108
Legumes, 84, 87
Leisure, stress and, 61
Lesbians, 6, 38, 211
Let's Move campaign, 22
Leukemias, 307
Leukoplakia, 195
Levitra, 230
LGBT population
    mental health, 32
    suicide, 38
Life expectancy, 1, 4, 366
    economics and, 371
    obesity, 132–133
Lifestyle
    Alzheimer's disease and, 370
    cancer and, 304–306
    coronary heart disease and, 296
    effect on health, 2, 9
    stress and, 61
Lifting, proper vs. improper, 350
Liking, 208, 208
Lipids, 75
Listening, 204–205
Lithium, 34
Liver
    alcohol, effects of, 180, 182
    hepatitis, 182, 266
Living wills, 377
Local food, 93
Locus of control, 16
Loneliness, 29, 207
Longevity, 373, 392*
Love, 203, 371, 379. See also Relationships
    Sternberg's triangular theory of, 208–209, 209
Low birth weight, 250
Low-carbohydrate diets, 138–139
Low-density lipoproteins (LDLs), 131, 137, 300
Lowe, Sean, 233, 233

Low-fat diets, 137–138
LSD (lysergic acid diethylamide), 162, 166
Lung cancer, 192, 304, 307–308, 312, 427*
Lunge, 108
Lungs, 292, 292
    activity, benefits of, 102
    cardiorespiratory fitness, 100–101
Luteinizing hormone (LH), 228
Lyme disease, 267, 267
Lymphocytes, 261
Lymphomas, 306, 307

M

Macronutrients, 71
Macrophages, 260
Macula, 367
Mad cow disease, 90
Magnesium, 79
Maintenance, behavior change, 13
Major depressive disorder, 31
Major life events, stress and, 57
Malaria, 258, 270, 283, 411*
Male sexual anatomy, 225, 225–227
Male-to-female (MTF) transsexuals, 236
Malignant melanoma, 307, 307
Malignant tumors, 304. See also Cancer
Maltose, 73
Managed-care plans, 333
Manganese, 79
Mania, 34
Manic-depressive disorder, 34
Manipulative therapies, 330, 331
Marijuana, 158, 160, 160, 165, 301, 372. See also Drug
    use and abuse
Marriage, 54, 202
Maslow, Abraham, hierarchy of needs, 26, 26–27
Massage, 63, 330
Mast cells, 264
Masters, William H., 229
Masturbation, 231
Mature adults, 60. See also Aging
Maximum heart rate, 106
Mayo Clinic, 21, 282
McCarthy, Jenny, 263, 263
McCartney, Paul, 381
MDMA (Ecstasy), 163, 166
Measles, 262
Meat, 77
Meat consumption, 416*
Media
    alcohol and tobacco use and, 190
    smoking and, 189, 190
    violence in, 352
Media and aging, high-tech games, 375
Media and body image, beauty in age of Photoshop,
    128, 128
Media and fitness, fitness apps, 117
Media and health, evaluating health information, 11
Media and sexuality, pornography, 234
Media and violence, studies on, 354
Media Literacy Project, 21
Medicaid, 12, 333, 335
Medical abortion, 245
Medical devices, 323
Medical doctors (M.D.s), 327
Medical Library Association's Top 100 List: Health
    Websites You Can Trust, 340
Medical marijuana, 160
Medicare, 12, 333, 335, 366
Medications
    bone-building, 369
    diabetes, 291
    driving and, 344

heart, 296
hypertension, 294
menopause, 369
over-the-counter medications, 323, 324
pain, 378
proper handling of, 329
sleep, 400*, 401*
stimulants, 396*
testosterone therapy, 369
Meditation, 42
Medline Plus, 21, 282, 318
Melanoma, 417*, 431*
Melatonin, 390*, 401*
Memorial Day, 376
Memorial services, 379
Memory, aging and, 370
Memory B cells, 262
Memory T cells, 262
Men
    alcohol use and abuse, 176, 179, 185
    body image, 126–127
    building muscle, 101
    caloric needs of, 72
    communication, 205
    contraception, 237–244, 238–239, 240, 241, 242, 243
    depression, 33, 33
    fiber intake, 73
    heart attack, 296
    heart disease, 300
    infertility, 252
    life expectancy, 366
    obesity, 133
    prostate cancer, 309
    sexual anatomy, 225, 225–227
    sexual dysfunctions, 230
    sexually transmitted infections, rates of, 276
    sleep, 395*
    steroid use, 119
    stress, 56
    testicular cancer, 309, 310
    tobacco use, 191
    unintentional injuries, 343
    violent crime, 351
    weight gain, 134
Menarche, 227
Men Can Stop Rape, 360
Meningitis, 326
Meningococcal disease, 262
Menopause, 227, 300, 304, 369
Menstrual cycle, 224, 225, 227, 227
Menstrual phase, 227, 227–228
Menstruation, 227
Mental disorders
    attention disorders, 37
    bipolar disorder, 23, 34
    depressive disorders, 33–34
    mood disorders, 31
    obsessive-compulsive disorder (OCD), 35–36
    overview, 30–31
    post-traumatic stress disorder, 34
    schizophrenia, 37
Mental health. See also Psychological health
    chronic stress and, 54–55
    defined, 24
    statistics on, 23, 30
Mental Health America, 46
Men who have sex with men, sexually transmitted infections, 276
Mercury, 428*, 429*
Metabolic syndrome, 132, 302
Metabolism, 72
    activity, benefits of, 103
    alcohol, 178, 178–179

Metastasis, 304. See also Cancer
Methamphetamine, 162, 162, 165
Methane, 416*
Methicillin-resistant Staphylococcus aureus (MRSA), 267, 268, 268
Methylphenidate, 37
Micronutrients, 71
Microorganisms, 258
Midwife, 250
Mifepristone, 245
Milk and milk substitutes, 80, 80, 98
Millennials, 60
Minamata, Japan, contaminated seafood, 409*
Mind-body medicine, 330, 331
Minerals, 78, 78, 79, 79
Mini-med plans, 333, 335
Mini-pill, 239
Mirena IUD, 242
Mirren, Helen, 372
Miscarriage, 250
Modeling, 16
Models, behavior change, 13–14
Modified push-ups, 109
Mold, 428*
Money, financial stress, 48
Mononucleosis, 265–266
Monosaturated fats, 75
Mons pubis, 223, 224
Mood changes, aging and, 372
Mood disorders, 31, 33–34
Morning after pill, 238, 242
Morphine, 158
Mortality, 4
Mothers Against Drunk Driving (MADD), 183
Mother-to-child transmission (MTCT), HIV, 273
Motorcycle accidents, 347
Motorcycle Safety Foundation, 362
Motor vehicle accidents (MVA), 343–347, 395, 407*
Movement disorders, 37
"Move Your Body" video (Beyoncé), 22, 22
Mucosal absorption, drugs, 157
Multivitamin/mineral supplements (MVMs), 81
Mumps, 262
Municipal solid waste (MSW), 422–423*
Murder, 351, 352, 353
Murray, Christopher J. L., 366
Muscular endurance, 101, 107
Muscular strength, 101, 107
Music, 63
Mutations, cancer, 303, 304
Mycobacterium tuberculosis, 268
Myelomas, 306, 307
My Family Health Portrait, 318
MyFitnessPal, 144
Myocardial infarction (MI), 295
Myocardium, 292, 292. See also Cardiovascular disease
My Physical Activity & Exercise Pyramid, 114
MyPlate for Older Adults, 374
MyPlate website, 97
MySpace, 209
Myth or Fact?
    cell phone and your brain, 432*
    circumcision, need for, 226
    coffee and hangover, 181
    hybrid electric vehicles, 420*
    stress and ulcers, 53
    stretching and injury, 116
    vaccines and autism, 263

N

NA. See Narcotics Anonymous
Naltrexone, 185
Naps, 392*, 403*

Narcolepsy, 398*
Narcotics, 158. See also Drug use and abuse
Narcotics Anonymous, 167, 172
Nash, Steve, 98
National Aging in Place Council, 371
National Alliance on Mental Illness (NAMI), 42
National Association to Advance Fat Acceptance (NAAFA), 144
National Cancer Institute (NCI), 190, 194, 197, 200, 313, 318, 427*, 431*
National Center for Complementary and Alternative Medicine (NCCAM), 330
National Center for Environmental Health (NCEH), 435*
National Center for Injury Prevention & Control, 362
National Center on Addiction and Substance Abuse at Columbia University, 172
National Coalition on Health Care, 332
National Collegiate Cancer Foundation (NCCF), 315
National Domestic Violence Hotline, 357, 362
National Drug Control Strategy, 167
National Educational Association of Disabled Students (NEADS), 218
National Eye Institute, 367
National Institute on Alcohol Abuse and Alcoholism, 175, 186
National Institute of Mental Health, 46, 150
National Institute on Aging, 372, 373
National Institutes of Health (NIH), 5, 15
National Institutes of Health Senior Health, 386
National Marriage Project, 220
National Safety Council (NSC), 343, 344, 362
National Sleep Foundation, 395*, 406*
National Student Campaign Against Hunger and Homelessness, 95
National Suicide Prevention Lifeline, 46, 47
National Survey on Drug Use and Health, 158
National Teen Dating Abuse Helpline, 220
National Transportation Safety Board, 344
National Wellness Institute, 3
Native Americans
    alcohol use and abuse, 176
    cardiovascular disease, 288
    diabetes, 288
    health disparities, 6
    mental health, 32
    overweight and obesity, 134
    sexually transmitted infections, 276
    suicide, 38
    tobacco use, 191
Natural foods, 93
Natural killer (NK) cells, 260, 262
Naturally acquired immunity, 262
Natural products, 330, 331
Natural Resources Defense Council, 432*, 435*
Naturopathy, 331
Near-death experiences (NDEs), 376–377
Neck stretches, 112
Negative population growth, 413*
Neisseria gonorrhoeae, 277
Neisseria meningitidis, 266
Nervous system, 183
Neural tube development, 78
Neurotoxins, 427*, 429*
Neurotransmitters, 30, 50
Neutrophils, 260
Newtown, Connecticut, school violence in, 353
Nicotine, 189, 191, 192, 193, 195, 301
Nicotine replacement therapies, 196
Night blindness, 8
Night-eating syndrome, 146
Nitrogen oxides, 414*
Nitroglycerin, 296

Nixon, Peter, 52
Nocturnal eating disorder, 399*, *399*
Noise pollution, 429–430*
Non-ionizing radiation, 431*, *431*
Nonlove, 208, *208*
Nonoxynol-9, 241
Nonprofit clinics, 327
Non-REM (NREM) sleep, 391*
Nonspecific immune response, 260, *261*
Non-suicidal self-injury (NSSI), 38
Nonverbal communication, 204
Noradrenaline, 50
Norovirus, 90
No Woman Left Behind, 362
Nurse practitioners, 327
Nurses, 327
Nursing homes, 371
Nutrient-dense foods, 89
Nutrients
    antioxidants, 83–84
    carbohydrates, 72–74, *74*
    defined, 71
    fats, dietary, 74–77
    fiber, 73
    minerals, 78–80
    phytochemicals, 83
    prebiotics and probiotics, 84
    proteins, 77
    vitamins, 77–78
    water, 80–81
Nutrition
    aging and, 373–374
    campus advocacy, 95
    ChooseMyPlate.gov, 87, *87*
    chronic disease and, 286, 312
    defined, 71
    Dietary Reference Intakes (DRIs), 85, *85*
    food labels, reading, 85–87, *86*
    healthy food choices, 314
    personal choices, 93, 95
    physical activity, 116
    pregnancy, 248
    shopping smart, 95
    statistics on, 70
    stress and, 61
    variation for different groups, 90
    websites, 97
Nutrition Facts panel, 85, *86*
Nuts, food allergies, 92, *92*

O
Obama, Barack, 214
Obama, Michelle, 22
Obesity, 8
    aging and, 374
    on campus, 131, 132
    cardiometabolic risk, 301–302, *302*
    cardiovascular disease, 301
    chronic disease and, 312
    clinical options for, 141–143
    financial burden of, 133
    healthful weight, defining, 127
    health risks with, 131–132, *133*
    physical activity, 100, 114
    sleep difficulties and, 394*
    statistics on, 125, 130
    stress and, 53
    "thrifty gene" and, 135
    type 2 diabetes and, 287
    weight gain, causes of, 133–136
Obsessive-compulsive disorder (OCD), 23, 35–36
Occupational health, 3, 4
Occupational Safety and Health Administration, 167
Oils, 89

Older adults. *See* Aging
Olive oil, *76*
Omega-3 fatty acids, 75, 76, 314
Omega-6 fatty acids, 75, 76
Oncogenes, 304
On Death and Dying (Kübler-Ross), 381
Online dating, 210–211
Online information, evaluating, 322
Opioids, 157–158, *158, 166*
Opportunistic diseases, 272
Optimism, 25–26, 56
Optometrists, 327
Oral cancer, 309, *309*
Oral hygiene, 321, *322*
Oral sex, 210, 231, 233, 272, 274, 309. *See also*
        Sexually transmitted infection
Organ donation, 377
Organic foods, 93
Organosulfur compounds, 83
Orgasm, 229, 230
Oristat, 141
Ornish diet, 137
Orr, David, 432*
Osteoarthritis, 132, 368
Osteoporosis, 80, 102–103, 192, *368,* 368–369
Ounce-equivalent, *89*
Outercourse, 231
Ovarian cancer, 9, 102, 304, 310–311
Ovaries, 224, *224,* 236
Overdose, drug, 158, 167
Overeaters Anonymous, 144
Overload, fitness training, 193
Over-the-counter (OTC) medications, 157, 158, 323,
        324, 401*
Overweight
    on campus, 131, 132
    chronic disease and, 312
    diabetes, risk of, 289
    financial burden of, 133
    healthful weight, defining, 127
    physical activity, 114
    statistics on, 125
    "thrifty gene" and, 135
    weight gain, causes of, 133–136
Ovulation, 228, 237, *237,* 252
Oxidation reactions, 83
Oxycodone, 158
OxyContin, 158
Oxytocin, 251
Ozone (O₃), 414*, 417*

P
Pain medications, end of life, 378
Palliative care, 378
Pancreas, 286, *287*
Pancreatic cancer, 308–309
Pandemics, 265, 269
Panic attacks, 35, 54, 55
Panic disorder, 23, 35
Pap smear, 225, 311
ParaGard IUD, 242
Parasitic worm infections, 271
Parasomnias, 399–400*
Particulates, 414*
Passion, 208, *208*
Passive euthanasia, 379
Passive immunity, 262
Passive smokers, 193
Passive stretching, 110
Pathogens, 90, 258, 259, 262, *265*
PCBs, 429*
PCP (phencyclidine), 160, 163, *166*
Pedestrian safety, 347
Peer mentoring associations, 169

Peer pressure, 17, 188
Pelvic inflammatory disease (PID), 252, 277
Penicillin, 270
Penis, 225, *225*
Perceived benefit, behavior change, 13
Perceived severity, behavior change, 13
Perceived threat, behavior change, 13
Percent daily value (%DV), 85–86
Percocet, 158
Percodan, 158
Performance-enhancing drugs, 82, 118–120, 124
Perimenopause, 369
Persistent vegetative state, 379
Personal choices, 15–17
Personal growth, 25, *25*
Personality types, stress and, 55–56
Personalized medicine, 336
Personal safety
    assault, 352–355
    defined, 343
    domestic and intimate partner violence, 355
    hate crimes, 355
    murder, 351, 352, 353
    school and campus violence, 353, 355
    sexual violence, 357–359
    websites, 362
    work safety, 350–351
Personal values, 28
Pertussis, *262*
Pesco-vegetarians, 91
Pesticides, 92, 420*, *428*
Petroleum products, in water, 419*
Pets, infection from, 259
Pharmacogenomics, 337–338
Pharmacologic therapy, 40
Phendimetrazine, 141
Phentermine, 141
Phobias, 35
Phospholipids, 75
Phosphorus, 79
Photosynthesis, 416*
Phthalates, 427*, 429*
Physical abuse, 213, 356
Physical activity
    ACSM guidelines, *115*
    aerobic exercise, 105–106
    aging and, 372–373, 374
    benefits of, 102–103
    body composition, 101–102
    campus advocacy, 121
    cardiorespiratory fitness, 100–101, 104, 105
    chronic disease, 286, 313
    defined, 100
    diabetes, risk of, 100
    fitness, components of, 100–102
    fitness training principles, *103,* 103–104, *104*
    flexibility, 101, 110–111
    frequency recommendations, 111, 114
    heart health, 301
    intensity levels, *105*
    muscular strength and endurance, 101, 106–107, 110
    personal choices, 120–121
    safety issues, 115–120
    statistics on, 99
    websites, 123
    weight loss and, 141
Physical Activity Guidelines for Americans, 111
Physical dependence, drugs, 157
Physical fitness, defined, 100. *See also*
        Physical activity
Physical health, 3, *3*
Physical inactivity
    cancer and, 102
    diabetes, risk of, 290
    weight gain, causes of, 135

Physician-aid-in-dying (PAD), 378–379, 387
Physician assistants, 327
Physician-assisted suicide, 378–379
Physicians, 327
Phytochemicals, 83
Phytoplankton, 417*
Pilates, 101, 111
Pineal gland, sleep and, 389*, 390*, 390*
Pink Ribbons, Inc. (film), 319
Pinworms, 271
Pituitary gland, 51
Placebo, 26
Placenta, 248, 251, 251
Plan B, 242
Plank, 109
Planned Parenthood, 255, 282
Plaque, 293, 295
Plasmodium, 270
Plateau, human sexual response cycle, 229–230
Plaza, Aubrey, 299
PMAs. See Peer mentoring associations
Pneumococcal polysaccharide (PPV), 262
Pneumonia, 267–268
Podiatrists, 327
Point-of-service plans (POSs), 333
Poisoning, unintentional, 343, 347
Policy-making, 12
Polio, 262, 262
Pollution. See also Environmental health
    air, 305, 410*, 413–419*, 415*
    defined, 409*
    at home, 426–429*, 428*
    land, 422–424*
    noise, 429–430*
    oil spills, 410*
    water, 419–422*, 421*
Polyabusers, 167–168
Polychlorinated biphenyls (PCBs), 420*
Polypharmacy, 372
Polyunsaturated fats, 75
Polyvinyl chloride (PVC), 427*
Pons, REM sleep and, 389*, 391*
Population growth, 411*, 411–413*, 413*
Pornography, 234
Portion control, 140
Positive psychotherapy, 40
Postabortion traumatic stress syndrome, 246
Postmenopause, 369
Postpartum depression, 33
Post-traumatic stress disorder (PTSD), 36, 54, 55
Potassium, 79
Poverty, 288, 352
Practical Strategies
    affordable health care, 336
    antidepressant medications, 34
    building optimism, 26
    communicating effectively about sex and birth
        control, 244
    complex carbohydrates, 74
    cutting calories, not nutrition, 140
    eating right on the run, 95
    financial stress, 57
    grief, 382
    healthful fats, 76
    healthy food choices, 314
    infectious diseases, 270
    quitting smoking, 198
    reducing energy consumption, 418*
    reducing pollution at home, 429*
    reducing risk of STIs, 274
    repetitive strain injuries, 351
    risky alcohol-related behavior, 184
    safe weight lifting, 110
    spotting destructive thoughts, 41

    stress overload, 55
    strong relationships, 212
    warning signs of addiction, 154
Prebiotics, 84
Precontemplation, behavior change, 13
Prediabetes, 289
Predisposing factors, behavior, 12
Preeclampsia, 250
Pre-existing condition, 332
Preferred provider organizations (PPOs), 333
Pregnancy, 228
    alcohol and, 183
    complications, 250
    early signs of, 247
    ectopic, 277
    excess body weight and, 132
    gestational diabetes, 287–288
    home tests, 247, 323
    overview of, 246–250, 247, 249
    prenatal care, 247, 248
    sleep and, 395–396*
    smoking and, 192–193, 248
    trimesters, 246, 248
    unintended, 236, 244
    weight gain and, 134
Premature ejaculation (PE), 230–231
Premenstrual dysphoric disorder (PMDD), 228–229
Premenstrual syndrome (PMS), 228
Premium, health insurance, 332
Prenatal care, 247, 248
Preparation, behavior change, 13
Presbycusis, 367
Presbyopia, 367
Prescription medications
    abuse of, 372
    antidepressants, 369
    driving and, 344
    obesity and overweight, 141–142
    proper handling of, 329
    sleep medications, 400–401*
    stimulants, 396*
Prescription stimulants (PS), 158, 159
President's Challenge Program, 123
Prevention, practicing, 321–322
Primary care facilities, 327
Prions, 90
Probiotics, 84, 330
Problem solving, 63
Prochaska, James O., 13
Professional trainers, 115
Progestin, 242
Progressive muscle relaxation (PMR), 62
Progressive overload, fitness training, 103, 103
Proliferative phase, menstrual cycle, 227, 227, 228
Proof value, 177
Prostaglandins, 229
Prostate cancer, 304, 309
Prostate gland, 225, 226
Prostatitis, 227
Protease inhibitors, 273
Protein, dietary, 77, 87, 87, 116, 139
Protozoa, 270
Protozoan infections, 260, 270
Psilocybin (magic mushrooms), 163, 163
Psychiatrists, 39
Psychoactive drugs, 30, 31, 155
Psychodynamic therapy, 40
Psychological dependence, drugs, 157
Psychological health, 3, 4
    activity, benefits of, 103
    aging and, 370–372
    anger, 29, 29–30
    anxiety disorders, 34–37
    attention disorders, 37

    bipolar disorder, 34
    campus advocacy, 42
    components of, 24
    defined, 24
    depressive disorders, 31, 33–34
    emotional intelligence, 25
    facets of, 24–25
    factors related to, 26–29
    family history, 27
    helping friends, 42
    loneliness, 29
    mental disorders, overview, 30–31
    optimism, 25–26
    overview, 24–25
    professional help, 39–41
    reaching out, 41
    schizophrenia, 37
    self-care, 41
    self-esteem, 42, 42
    shyness, 29
    social support, 27
    spirituality, 27–29
    statistics on, 23, 30, 30
    suicide and self-injury, 38
    websites, 46
Psychologists, 39
Psychoneuroimmunology, 54
Psychosis, 37
Psychotherapy, 33, 141
Pthirus pubis, 278, 278
Pubic lice, 278, 278
Public health, 4, 327, 410*
Public health insurance programs, 333
Purging, 146
Purpose in life, 25, 25, 29
Push-ups, modified, 109

Q

Quadriceps stretch, 113
Queer or questioning, 211
Quinto, Zachary, 235

R

Race
    alcohol use and abuse, 176
    chronic disease, 288
    drug use, 155
    health, 9
    health disparities, 6
    life expectancy, 366
    mental health, 32
    sexually transmitted infections, rates of, 276
    suicide, 38
    tobacco use, 191
    weight gain, 134
Racism, 253
Radiation absorbed doses (rads), 431*, 431*
Radiation exposure, 305, 431*, 431*
Radiation therapy, 311
Radon, 308, 427*, 428*
Rahe, Richard, 57
Rape, 184, 351, 358–359
Rape, Abuse, & Incest National Network (RAINN), 362
Rapid eye movement (REM) sleep, 390*, 391*, 391*, 394*
Rational suicide, 378–379
Ray, Rachel, 76
Real Food Challenge, 144
Recommended Dietary Allowance (RDA), 85
Recovery, exercise, 107
Recycling, 422–423*
Refractory period, sexual response cycle, 230

Regulatory T cells, 262
Reinforcing factors, behavior, 12–13
Relapse, 17
    alcohol abuse, 186
    drug abuse, 169
    tobacco use, 196
Relationships, 56
    attraction, causes of, 210
    campus advocacy, 218
    chronic stress and, 54
    cohabitation, 210, 213, *213*
    communication in, 203–205
    conflict resolution, 205
    dating, 210–211
    developing, 205
    domestic partnerships, 215
    dysfunctional, 211–213
    early, 206–207
    ending, 213
    friendships, maintaining, 207–208
    gender roles, 207
    healthy, 211
    marriage, 213–214
    personal choices, 217–218
    same-sex marriage, 221
    same-sex relationships, 211
    single, remaining, 215–216
    statistics on, 202, 215
    Triangular Theory of Love, 208, *208*
    violence within, 355–357
    websites, 220
Relaxation techniques, 40
Reliability, of research studies, 323
Religion, *27,* 27–28
REM behavior disorder (RBD), 399*
Repetitions, 107
Repetitive strain injuries (RSIs), 350, 351
Replacement-level fertility, 412*
Research studies, understanding, 323
Reservoir, infection transmission, 258
Residence changes, aging and, 371
Resiliency, 56
Resistance stage, stress response, *50,* 51–52
Resistance training, 101, 107
Resolution phase, human sexual response cycle, 230
Respiratory disease, tobacco use and, 192
Resting metabolic rate (RMR), 134
Restless legs syndrome (RLS), 399–400*
Retail clinics, 327, *328*
Rethinking Drinking: Alcohol and Your
        Drinking, 200
Reticular activating system (RAS), 389*
Retirement, 371
Reuse, 422*
Reverse curl, *109*
Reverse transcriptase inhibitors, 273
Reversibility, fitness training, 104
Rewards, 16–17
Rheumatic heart disease, 299
Rhinoviruses, 264
Rhythm method, 237, *238*
Riciutti, Henry, 217
Ritalin, 37, 158, 159, 396*
Robbery, 351
Roe v. Wade, 246
Rohypnol, 164, *166,* 184
Romantic love, 208, *208*
Rosenman, Ray, 55
Rotter, Julian B., 16
RU-486, 242, 245
Rubella, 262
Ruffalo, Mark, 436*
Ryff, Carol D., 25
Ryff Scales of Psychological Well-Being, 24–25, *25*

S

SafeRides program, 345
Safety
    assault, 352–355
    domestic and intimate partner violence, 355
    hate crimes, 355
    murder, 351, 352, 353
    physical activity, 115–120
    school and campus violence, 353, 355
    sexual violence, 357–359
    work safety, 350–351
Safe Zone, campus, 253
Salmonella, 90
Salmonellosis, 90
Saltow, Donna, 65
Saltow, Jed, 65
Saltow, Phil, 65
Same-sex marriage, 214, 221
Sarcomas, 306
Satiety, 137
Saturated fats, 75, *75*
SAVE (Suicide Awareness Voices of Education), 47
Scabies, 278
Schedule II drugs, 162
Schizophrenia, 37
School and campus violence, 353, 355
ScienceDaily: Mind & Brain, 46
Science of Addiction, The, 172
Scientific method, 323, 327
Scrotum, 225, *225*
Seat belts, 345
Seaward, Brian Luke, 28
Secondhand smoke, 193–194, 308
Secretory phase, menstrual cycle, 227, *227,* 228
Sedentary lifestyle, 111, 136
Selenium, 79
Self-acceptance, 25, *25*
Self-actualization, 27
Self-Assessment
    aggressive driving, 345
    alcohol use disorders identification test, 186
    anxiety assessment, 36
    cancer risk, 305
    death, 377
    eating disorders, 146
    eating well, 94
    health of current lifestyle, 18
    healthy relationships, 211
    heart attack risk, 302
    loud music, 431*
    maximum heart rate and target heart rate range, 106
    negative event scale for university students, 58
    preventive health care, 338
    readiness for sex, 235
    seeking drug treatment, 168
    sexually transmitted infections, 271
    sleep, 403*
    type 2 diabetes, 290
    weight-related health risks, 130
Self-care, 41, 321
    options, 323–324
    wellness habits, 321–322, *322*
Self-disclosure, 203
Self-efficacy, 16
Self-esteem, 25, 41, 42, 63, 205
Self-exams
    breast, 312
    testicular, 310
Self-injury, 38
Self-medicating, alcohol, 185
Self-monitoring, 17
Self-perception, relationships and, 205–206
Self-talk, 17

Seligman, Martin, 25
Selye, Hans, 50, 51
Semen, 226
Seminal fluid, 226
Semivegetarians, 91
Separation and divorce, 214–215
September 11, 2001, terrorist attacks, 355
Serious mental illness (SMI), 30
Serotonin, 30
Serving sizes, estimating, 86, *86*
Sets, 107
Sex assignment, 236
Sexism, 253
Sexting, 231, *232*
Sexual desire, low level of, 230
Sexual harassment, 357–358
Sexual health. *See also* Sexually transmitted infection
    abortion, 244–246
    abstinence and celibacy, 231, 233
    aging and, 369
    alcohol use and abuse, 176, 184
    campus advocacy, 253
    common problems in females, 225
    communicating about sex, 232
    conception and contraception, 236–244, *237, 238–
        239, 241, 242, 243*
    health problems in males, 227
    hooking up, 210
    infertility, 252–253
    intimacy without intercourse, 237, *238*
    menstrual cycle, *227,* 227–229
    non-intercourse sexual activity, 231
    personal choices, 253
    pregnancy and childbirth, 246–252, *247, 249, 251*
    readiness for sex, 235
    sexual anatomy, 223–227
    sexual dysfunctions, 230–231
    sexual intercourse, 232
    sexual orientation and identity, 232–233, 235–236
    sexual response cycle, 229
    statistics on behavior, 222, 240
    understanding sexuality, 223
Sexually transmitted infection, 225, 232. *See also*
        Infectious disease
    aging and, 369
    asking potential partner about, 245
    campus advocacy, 279
    chlamydia, 252, 275, 277
    condoms and, 241, 243, 271–272
    diaphragm and cervical cap, 242
    genital herpes, 273–274
    gonorrhea, 252, 277
    hepatitis B, 273
    HIV/AIDS, 272–273
    human papillomavirus, 274–275
    incidence of, 271
    infertility, 252
    intrauterine device, 242
    oral sex, 210, 231
    pelvic inflammatory disease, 277
    personal choices, 279
    pubic lice and scabies, 278, *278*
    risk factors for, 271–272
    statistics, 257
    syphilis, *277,* 277–278
    trichomoniasis, 278–279
Sexual orientation, 32, 232–233, 235–236, 253, 276
Sexual violence, 357–359
Shaping, 15
Shopping, compulsive, 154
Shoulder stretch, *112*
Shyness, 29
Sidestream smoke, 193
Silent Spring (Carson), 410*

Simple carbohydrates, 73
Single-gene testing, 337
Single parenthood, 217
Skills-related fitness, 100
Skin, 260
Skin cancer, 304, 307, *307,* 417*
Sleep, 313
    academic performance, 394*
    activity, benefits of, 103
    alcohol, effects of, 180, 403*
    alcohol and, 396*
    in America, 393*, *393*
    campus advocacy, 403*
    cardiovascular disease, 301
    chronic stress and, 54
    complementary and alternative medicine, 400–401*
    cycles of, 391*
    defined, 389*
    disorders, 397–400*
    health effects, 393–394*
    individual behaviors and, 396*
    personal choices, 401*, 403*
    regions and rhythms of, 338–390*, *390*
    short and long, research on, 392–393*
    sleep debt, 392*
    stages of, 390–391*, *391*
    statistics on, 388*
    stress and, 61, *61,* 395*, 397*
    websites, 406*
Sleep apnea, 395*, 397, *398**
    defined, 397*
    diagnosis of, 397*
    excess body weight and, 132
    treatment of, 397–398*
    types of, 397*
Sleep bruxism, 399*
Sleep deprivation, 14
Sleep disorders, 406*
Sleep hygiene, 401*
Sleep studies, 400*, *400**
Sleep terrors, 399*
Sleep Treatment and Education Program for Students
        (STEPS), 400*
Sleepwalking, 399*
Slim-Fast diet, *138*
Slow-wave sleep, 391*
SMART goal, 15
Smart Grid, 418*
Smog, 414*
Smoke detectors, 349
Smokeless ("spit") tobacco, *194,* 195
Smoking, tobacco
    age and, 189
    benefits of quitting, *196*
    birth control pills and, 244
    on campus, 187, 189
    campus advocacy, 197
    cancer and, 192, 308
    cardiometabolic risk and, *313*
    cardiovascular disease and, 301
    cessation programs, 195–196, 198
    chemical contents, 189
    chronic disease and, 286, 312
    fire-related deaths, 349
    health effects, 191–192, *193*
    hypertension, 294
    media and, 190
    menopause and, 369
    personal choices, 197
    pregnancy and, 192–193, 248
    sleep and, 396*
    statistics on, 174, 187
    stress and, 189
    treatment options, 196
Snoring, 397*

Snuff, 195
Social anxiety disorder, 35, *35*
Social health, *3,* 4
Social media, 209
Social physique anxiety, 144
Social Readjustment Rating Scale (SRRS), 57
Social Security, 371
Social stressors, 56
Social support, *16, 27, 41,* 186
Social withdrawal, 37
Socioeconomic status
    cardiovascular disease, 301
    life expectancy, 371
Sodium, 79, 294, 314
South Beach Diet, *139*
Spears, Britney, 128, *128*
Special Feature
    Affordable Care Act, 334–335
    campus safety, 360
    CVD emergency, 297
    dietary guidelines, 88
    peer pressure: alcohol use and abuse, 188
    sleep, 402*
    social media, communication, and cyber-bullies, 209
Specialists centers, 328
Specific immune response, *261,* 261–262
Specificity, fitness training, 104, 193
Speeding, 345
Sperm, 225, 236, 252
Spermicides, *238,* 241–242
Sphygmomanometer, 294
Spicy foods, sleep and, 396*
Spiritual health, *3,* 4. *See also* Psychological health
Spirituality, 28–29
Spiritual well-being, Seaward's pillars of, 28, *28*
Sponge, contraceptive, *238, 242*
Spontaneous abortion, 250
Sports beverages, 80
Spotlight
    alcohol, health benefits of, 182
    breast awareness and self-exam, 312
    celibacy, 233
    core strengthening, 107
    exercise, 374
    feeding your bones, 80
    hand washing and hand sanitizers, 260
    MRSA, 268*
    naps, 392*
    stress, research on, 51
    testicular self-exam, 310
    vaccinations, 326, *326*
Squat, *108*
Stalking, 356–357
Standard drink, 178, *178*
Stanford University, Center for Sleep and Dreams
        Sleep Guide, 406*
Staphylococcus aureus, 267
Starches, 73
Static flexibility, 110
Static muscular endurance, 101
Static stretching, 110
Status syndrome, 9–10
Statutory rape, 358
Stepfamilies, 216–217
Sterilization, 243
Sternberg, Robert, 208
Steroids, anabolic, 82, 118–119
Stimulants, 158, 159
    amphetamines, 161–162, *162*
    caffeine, 160–161, *161*
    cocaine, 161, *161*
    commonly abused drugs, *165*
    defined, 160
Stomach cancer, 304
Stratosphere, 413*

Strength training, 101, 107
Streptococcus, 267
Streptococcus pneumoniae, 266, 267
Stress
    academic pressure, 56
    activity, benefits of, 103
    aging and, 375
    body's response to, 49–52
    campus advocacy, 65
    cardiovascular disease, 301
    cardiovascular system and, 52
    changing thinking, 63–64
    chronic, health effects of, 52
    common causes of, 56–57, 59
    daily hassles, 56
    defined, 49
    diabetes, risk of, 290
    digestive system and, 52
    environmental, 57
    exercise, 62, *62*
    financial, 56, 57
    general adaptation syndrome, 50, *50*
    grief and, 380
    health professionals, 59
    immune system and, 54
    internal, 59
    job-related, 56
    lifestyle and, 59, 61
    major life events, 57
    managing, 59, 61–65
    mental health and, 54–55
    overload, signs of, 55
    personality types and, 55–56
    post-traumatic stress disorder, 36, 54, 55
    relationships and, 54
    research on, 51
    self-assessment, 58
    sleep and, 54, 61, *61,* 395*, 397*
    smoking and, 189
    social, 56
    statistics on, 48
    tension relievers, 62–63
    test-taking skills, 61–62
    thought process and, 63–64
    ulcers and, 53
    violent crime and, 352
    websites, 68
    weight and, 53
Stressors, 49, 56
Stress test, 296
Stretching, 110, *112–113,* 116
Stroke, 52, 76, 132, 192, 289, 291, 294, 297, 298–299
Student health centers, 327
Student loans, 56
Students, health insurance and, 335–336
Students Active for Ending Rape (SAFER), 360
Students Against Destructive Decisions (SADD), 187
Students Against Violence Everywhere (SAVE), 360
Students Health Organizing Coalition (SHOC), 338
Student Stats
    alcohol use on campus, 177
    CAM use among college students, 330
    causes of death among people aged 15-24, 344
    common health problems, 7
    drug use among young adults, 156
    herb and supplement use, 81
    impediments to academic performance, 54
    overweight, obesity, and dieting on campus, 132
    psychological health on campus, 30, *30*
    sex and the college student, 240
    sexually transmitted infection in people aged 15-24, 278
    sleepless on campus, 393*
    smoking on campus, 189
    students and relationships, 215
    thinking green, 411*